Applications in
MEDICAL
NUTRITION
THERAPY

SECOND EDITION

SECOND EDITION

Applications in
MEDICAL
NUTRITION
THERAPY

Frances J. Zeman, Ph.D., R.D.
University of California at Davis

Denise M. Ney, Ph.D., R.D.
University of Wisconsin—Madison

Merrill
an imprint of Prentice Hall
Upper Saddle River, New Jersey   Columbus, Ohio

Every effort has been made to ensure that drug-dosage schedules and indications are correct at time of publication. Since ongoing medical research can change standards of usage, and also because of human and typographical error, it is recommended that readers check the PDR or package insert before prescription or administration of the drugs mentioned in this book.

Library of Congress Cataloging–in–Publication Data

Zeman, Frances J.
    Applications in medical nutrition therapy / Frances J. Zeman,
Denise M. Ney.—2nd ed.
        p. cm.
    Rev. ed. of: Applications of clinical nutrition. ©1988.
    Includes bibliographical references and index.
    ISBN 0-13-375015-9
    1. Diet therapy. 2. Food—Analysis—Tables. 3. Diet therapy—Examinations, questions, etc.
I. Ney, Denise M., 1953
II . Zeman, Frances J. Applications of clinical nutrition.
III. Title.
[DNLM: 1. Diet Therapy. 2. Nutrition.   WB 400 Z526a 1995]
RM216.Z46   1996
615.8 ' 54—dc20
DNLM/DLC
for Library of Congress
                                         95-34138
                                           CIP

Editor: *Kevin M. Davis*
Production Services: *Aksen Associates*
Text Designer: *Susan Brown Schmidler*
Cover Designer: *Tammy Johnson*
Production Manager: *Pamela D. Bennett*
Illustrations: *Pasini Graphics*

This book was set in Times Roman by Aksen Associates
and was printed and bound by The Banta Company.
The cover was printed by Phoenix Color Corp.

Printed in the United States of America

10 9 8 7 6

ISBN: 0-13-375015-9

PRENTICE-HALL INTERNATIONAL (UK) LIMITED, *LONDON*
PRENTICE-HALL OF AUSTRALIA PTY. LIMITED, *SYDNEY*
PRENTICE-HALL CANADA INC., *TORONTO*
PRENTICE-HALL HISPANOAMERICANA, S.A., *MEXICO*
PRENTICE-HALL OF INDIA PRIVATE LIMITED, *NEW DELHI*
PRENTICE-HALL OF JAPAN, INC., *TOKYO*
PEARSON EDUCATION ASIA PTE. LTD., *SINGAPORE*
EDITORA PRENTICE-HALL DO BRASIL, LTDA., *RIO DE JANEIRO*

Contents

Preface

This volume is designed to help teach the procedures of nutritional care. It is intended to serve as an adjunct to a standard text in diet therapy, not as the sole text. Therefore, the chapters containing the relevant background material in several texts are listed at the end of the Introduction.

Since this volume has potential use for students in dietetics, public health nutrition, nursing, medicine, and the allied health professions, we have chosen to use the generic term "nutritional care specialist" in referring to individuals participating in nutritional care. We have organized this volume to provide for maximum flexibility in its use, not only for various groups but also for courses of variable length. Part I is basic to those that follow. For the remaining chapters, the sequence in which they are studied can be rearranged in order to coordinate study with the chosen text.

For each chapter, exercises entitled "To Test Your Understanding" give the reader an opportunity for review and practice. "Case Studies," included at intervals, provide the student an opportunity for review and integration of material from an entire chapter or several chapters. Alternatively, these questions can be used by the instructor for evaluation of progress. Some questions require modification of diets; for this purpose, it is assumed that the reader will have a diet manual for information on details of individual diets. In Appendix M, one copy of forms are provided. These may be photocopied when the same form is needed for several purposes. Current menus may be obtained from cooperating institutions when menus are modified in the exercises included here.

We have also included at the end of most chapters a section entitled "Topics for Further Discussion". This section suggests additional topics for inclusion in the course that are not included in the text due to space limitations. Also at the end of each chapter, sources of information are given in the "References" and "Additional Sources of Information" sections.

We would appreciate suggestions and comments from readers and course instructors using this book.

Acknowledgments

We gratefully acknowledge the careful review of selected case studies for medical accuracy by Theodore G. Ganiats, M.D., School of Medicine, University of California, San Diego.

We wish also to express our appreciation to the following for giving us the benefit of their advice:

Barbara Bayard, Ph.D., R.D., University of Wisconsin-Stout, Menomonie, WI

Barbara Dale, R.D., Veterans Administration Hospital, Madison, WI

Sally Gleason, M.S., R.D., University of Wisconsin, Madison, WI

Mary H. Hager, Ph.D., R.D., College of Saint Elizabeth, Morristown, NJ

Lynette Karls, M.S., R.D., University of Wisconsin, Madison, WI

Julie Kong, R.D., University of Illinois, Chicago, IL;

Kristine G. Koski, Ph.D., R.D., McGill University, Montreal, Quebec, Canada

Rosa Mak, M.S., R.D., C.N.S.D., University Hospital, University of Wisconsin, Madison, WI

Cathy C. Monsma, M.S., R.D., University Hospital, University of Wisconsin, Madison, WI

Bruce Rengers, Ph.D., R.D., University of Northern Colorado, Greeley, CO

Leslie F. Tinker, Ph.D., R.D., University of Washington, Seattle, WA

Sandy Van Calcar, M.S., R.D., Waisman Center, Madison, WI

Introduction for the Reader

The purpose of this manual is to give you an understanding of the objectives and procedures of nutritional care. It will introduce the skills required of the professional nutritional care specialist and provide you with an opportunity to integrate knowledge of nutritional care with related aspects of clinical care.

When you have completed the assignments in this manual, you will have an understanding of the importance and effect of medical nutritional therapy, which is defined as the assessment of patient nutritional status followed by therapy, ranging from diet modification to administration of specialized nutritional therapies such as intravenous or tube feedings. Some of the skills expected of an entry-level professional in nutritional care, as well as the medical vocabulary and the means to communicate in the medical record, should become familiar. You also should be able to evaluate laboratory data and other patient information, understand the purpose of the main aspects of treatment of the conditions discussed, assess the nutritional status of a patient and the nutritional adequacy of the diets in terms of specific medical conditions, plan the most frequently used diet modifications, recognize the interrelationships between diet and other forms of treatment, and integrate sociological factors into the nutritional care plan. We provide an introduction to some techniques of patient interviewing and patient education. We assume that these skills will be sharpened by further practice and clinical experience.

Within each chapter, exercises labeled "To Test Your Understanding" provide an opportunity to test mastery of the immediately preceding subject matter and to integrate material from previous assignments and from an accompanying text.

The "Case Studies" were designed to develop an appreciation of the contribution of nutrition to the overall care of the patient. They provide a vehicle by which to learn to relate diagnostic procedures, medications, and other forms of treatment to nutritional care. Suggested additional questions and reading resources appear at the end of each chapter.

We assume that you will use this volume in coordination with a textbook that provides background reading on the subject of the assignment. The chapters in several texts providing relevant background for each chapter in this book are indicated at the end of this section. You will sometimes find it necessary to seek additional information from standard reference materials; this structure has been planned in order to introduce you to useful references and encourage you to develop skills in their use. As you prepare for a professional career in nutrition, you should assemble a professional library. For the work required in this book, you should refer to a typical diet manual; a manual from any number of institutions or regional associations is suitable, and we provide below a list of some that are generally available.

Some questions require you to seek information elsewhere. These sources may vary from pharmacology textbooks in the medical library to the local supermarket. It will be helpful to have a medical dictionary. Suggested choices follow. Food values tables are also necessary; we list some available sources of these tables. In the process of using these resources and completing the work in this volume, you will develop the ability to seek information independently.

SUGGESTED REFERENCES

Textbooks in Diet Therapy

Zeman, F.J. *Clinical Nutrition and Diet Therapy*, 2d ed., Englewood Cliffs: Merrill/Prentice Hall, 1991.

Mahan, L.K., and M. Arlin. *Krause's Food, Nutrition and Diet Therapy*, 8th ed. Parts 2, 3, and 4. Philadelphia: Saunders, 1992.

Cataldo, C.B., S. R. Rolfes, and E.N. Whitney. *Understanding Normal and Clinical Nutrition*, 3d ed. St. Paul, MN: West, 1991.

Diet Manuals

American Dietetic Association. *Handbook of Clinical Dietetics* 2d ed., New Haven, CT: Yale University Press, 1992.

Chicago Dietetic Association and South Suburban Dietetic Association. *Manual of Clinical Dietetics*. 6th ed., Chicago: American Dietetic Association, 1988.

Pemberton, C.M., et al. *Mayo Clinical Diet Manual*, 6th ed. Toronto: B.C. Decker, 1988.

University of California Center for Health Sciences. *Manual of Clinical Dietetics*. Los Angeles: University of California, 1986.

Medical Dictionaries

Dorland's Illustrated Medical Dictionary, 27th ed. Philadelphia: Saunders, 1988.

Stedman's Medical Dictionary, 25th ed. Baltimore: Williams and Wilkens, 1990.

Mosby's Medical, Nursing and Allied Health Dictionary, 4th ed. St. Louis: Mosby-Year Book, Inc., 1994.

Tables of Food Values

Consumer and Food Economics Institute. *Composition of Foods*. Agricultural Handbooks No. 8–1 to 8–16. Washington, D.C.: U.S. Dept. of Agriculture, 1976–1987.

Leveille, G.A., M.E. Zabik, and K.V. Morgan. *Nutrients in Foods*. Cambridge, MA: The Nutritional Guild, 1983.

Pennington, V.A.T. and H.N. Church. *Bowes and Church's Food Values of Portions Commonly Used*, 16th ed. St. Louis: Lippincott, 1994.

Science and Education Administration. *Nutritive Value of Foods*. Home and Garden Bulletin No. 72. Washington, DC: U.S. Department of Agriculture, 1986.

Pharmacology References

American Medical Association, Department of Drugs, *Drug Evaluations*, 6th ed. Chicago: American Medical Association, 1988.

Compendium of Pharmaceuticals and Specialties, 20th ed., (C.M.E. Krogh ed.), Ottawa: Canadian Pharmaceutical Association, 1985.

Drug Facts and Comparisons (J.R. Boyd, ed.) St. Louis: Lippincott, 1985.

Handbook of Nonprescription Drugs, 7th ed. Washington, DC: American Pharmaceutical Association, 1982.

Physician's Desk Reference, 49th ed. Oradell, NJ: Medical Economics, 1995.

Zimmerman, D.R. *Zimmerman's Complete Guide to Non-prescription Drugs*, 2d ed. Detroit, MI: Gale Research, Inc., 1993.

Sources of Laboratory Values and Interpretation

Bakerman, S. *ABC's of Interpretive Laboratory Data*, 2d ed. Greenville, NC: Interpretive Laboratory Data, 1984.

Bennington, J.L. *Saunders Dictionary and Encyclopedia of Laboratory Medicine and Technology*. Philadelphia: Saunders, 1984.

Clinical Guide to Laboratory Tests, 2d ed. (N.W. Tietz, ed.) Philadelphia: Saunders, 1990.

Fischbach, F. *A Manual of Laboratory and Diagnostic Tests*, 4th ed. Philadelphia: J.B. Lippincott, 1992.

Jacobs, D.S., B.L. Kastin, W.R. Demott and W.L. Wolfson. *Laboratory Test Handbook*, 2d ed. Baltimore:Williams and Wilkins, 1990.

The Laboratory in Clinical Medicine, 2d ed. (J.A. Halsted and C.H. Halsted.eds.) Philadelphia: Saunders, 1981.

Ravel, R. Clinical Laboratory Medicine. *Clinical Application of Laboratory Data*, 5th ed. Chicago: Year Book Medical, 1989.

Tilkian, S.M. and M.H. Conover. *Clinical Implications of Laboratory Tests*, 3d ed. St. Louis: Mosby, 1983.

Widmann, F.K. *Clinical Interpretations of Laboratory Tests*, 10th ed. Philadelphia: Davis, 1989.

REFERENCES TO BACKGROUND TEXTS

Zeman & Ney, *Applications in Medical Nutrition Therapy,* 2d ed. Prentice Hall, 1996	Zeman, *Clinical Nutrition and Dietetics*, 2d ed. Macmillan, 1992	Krause & Mahan, *Food, Nutrition Diet Therapy*, 8th ed. Saunders, 1992	Cataldo, Rolfes & Whitney, *Understanding Clinical Nutrition*. West, 1991
Chapter	Chapter	Chapter	Chapter
4	2	8	
5	3, 18, 4	17, 32	1, 2
6	3	16	2
8	9		
9	10, 11, 12, 13		
12	5		
13	5	30	4
14	6	30	5
15	7	38	20
16	8	26	4, 7
17	8	27	8
18	8	27	31
19	11	31	10
20	10	20, 21, 33	11
21	9	35	12
22	14, 15, 16	29	6, 13
23	17	41, 34, 36	9

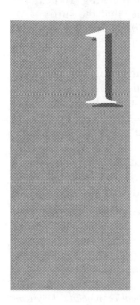

1 Medical Terminology

The acquisition of vocabulary is an important part of learning a new subject. In clinical nutrition, the nutritional care specialist must acquire an extensive medical vocabulary to function effectively. This can seem to be an overwhelming task at first.

This chapter will introduce you to medical terminology and provide some tools to promote easier and faster learning, but learning new vocabulary will continue throughout the use of this manual.

Most medical terms are derived from Greek or Latin; fewer terms are derived from modern languages. As medicine advances, new words must be coined and may be derived from any of these sources. Some terms are composed of elements combined from more than one language.

It is possible to simplify learning, promote understanding of reading material, and increase the ability to communicate by learning to analyze the component parts of words—the root words, prefixes, and suffixes. For example, *tonsillitis* refers to inflammation (*-itis*) of the tonsils. In other cases, the result of such analysis cannot be taken literally but can be used to suggest the meaning. For example, an analysis of the word *anemia* suggests that *an-* (without) *-emia* (blood) means *without blood*. Absence of blood, of course, is incompatible with life, and the term *anemia* is actually used to indicate a deficiency of red blood cells or hemoglobin.

ROOT WORDS

The root word of a medical term indicates the organ or body part that is modified by the prefixes and suffixes. A vowel—a, i, or o—may be inserted in combined forms

for easier pronunciation. Some of the root words of particular use to nutritional care specialists include the following:

cardi-	heart	hepat-	liver
enter-	intestine	nephr-	kidney
gastr-	stomach	osteo-	bone

SUFFIXES AND COMPOUNDING WORDS

Suffixes may be prepositions or adverbs added to root words to modify their meaning. Alternatively, adjectives or nouns are used as suffixes to form compound words. Many suffixes indicate a diagnosis, procedure, or symptom. The following are some diagnostic suffixes, with examples of their use:

Suffix	Definition	Examples
-ectasis	dilation of	bronchiectasis
-iasis	presence of	lithiasis
-itis	inflammation of	appendicitis
-megaly	enlargement of	cardiomegaly
-oma	tumor of	hepatoma
-osis	condition	nephrosis
-pathy	disease	cardiopathy

The following are commonly used suffixes indicating procedures:

-ectomy	removal of	appendectomy
-scopy	examination of	gastroscopy
-stomy	opening	ileostomy
-tomy	incision	lithotomy

Symptoms may be indicated by suffixes such as the following:

-algia	pain	myalgia
-genic	originate	cardiogenic
-lysis	breaking down	lipolysis
-oid	resembling	carcinoid
-osis	increase	leukocytosis
-penia	decrease	leukopenia
-spasm	involuntary contraction	cardiospasm

Some suffixes mean "pertaining to." These include -al, -ic, -eal, -ary, or -ous. Examples are these:

renal	pertaining to the kidneys
gastric	pertaining to the stomach
peritoneal	pertaining to the peritoneum
pulmonary	pertaining to the lungs
serous	pertaining to the serum

Practitioners may be indicated by -er or -ist, for example, pathologist, one who studies (-ology) disease (path-).

PREFIXES

A prefix may precede a root word to modify its meaning. Some prefixes that are frequently used by nutrition care specialists include the following:

Prefix	Definition	Example
dys-	difficult, painful	dyspnea
endo-	within	endocardium
hemi-, semi-	half	hemiplegic
hyper-	above, excessive	hyperglycemia
hypo-	beneath, below, deficient	hypodermic
para-	beside, around, near, abnormal	parathyroid
peri-	around	perinatal

Some terms have more than one meaning. You can see in the foregoing lists, for example, that the suffix *-osis* can refer to a *condition* or to an *increase*. Also, you can see that both *-osis* and *hyper-* indicate a higher level or amount.

It is also necessary for the nutritional care specialist to be familiar with the abbreviations used in patients' medical records. Many commonly used abbreviations are listed and defined in Appendix D. They will be used in the case studies contained in the succeeding chapters. Most of the assignments associated with the case studies require that a chart note be written. You should use appropriate abbreviations in writing these notes to become familiar with the medical terminology and the accepted means of communicating in the medical record.

REFERENCES

1. **Brooks, M.L.** *Exploring Medical Language*, 3d ed. St. Louis: Mosby–Year Book, 1994.
2. **Gylys, B.A.,** and **M.E. Wedding.** *Medical Terminology. A Systems Approach*, 2d ed. Philadelphia: Davis, 1988
3. **Leonard, P.C.** *Building a Medical Vocabulary*, 3d. ed. Philadelphia: Saunders, 1993
4. **Smith, G.L., P.E. Davis,** and **J.T. Jennerll.** *Medical Terminology, A Programmed Text*, 6th ed. Albany, NY: Delman Publishers, 1991.

ADDITIONAL SOURCES OF INFORMATION

Chabner, D.E. *The Language of Medicine*, 4th ed. Philadelphia: Saunders, 1991.
Dunmore, C.W., and **R.M. Fleischer.** Medical Terminology. *Exercises in Etymology*, 2d ed. Philadelphia: Davis, 1985.
Frenay, Sr., A.C., and **R.M. Mahoney, Sr.** *Understanding Medical Terminology*, 8th ed. St. Louis: Catholic Hospital Association, 1989.

TO TEST YOUR UNDERSTANDING

1. Using the examples in this chapter, define the following terms. The hyphens indicate the separate portions of the words.
   a. Gastr-itis
   b. Hepat-oma
   c. Nephr-ectomy
   d. Osteo-genic
   e. Cardio-megaly

2. Using the examples of root words, suffixes, and prefixes in the chapter, compose terms with the following meanings:
   a. Inflammation of the intestine
   b. Enlargement of the liver
   c. Examination of the interior of the stomach
   d. Inflammation of the interior lining of the heart
   e. Incision into or opening into the stomach
   f. Removal of the spleen

3. A more extensive listing of terms is contained in Appendix D. Using this list, define the following terms:
   a. Hyperglycemia
   b. Arteriosclerosis
   c. Cholelithiasis
   d. Stomatitis
   e. Nephrolithotomy
   f. Erythropoiesis
   g. Lymphocytosis
   h. Leukocytopenia
   i. Ileostomy
   j. Dysphagia
   k. Hematemesis
   l. Tachycardia

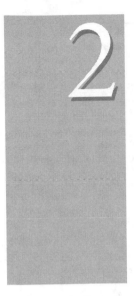

The Medical Record

The patient's *medical record,* or *chart,* is an ongoing collection of information that documents a patient's medical care. It is considered a legal document and therefore must be accurate. It includes a complete assessment of a patient's medical condition, including the history, results of the physical examination, summary of the patient's condition at the time of discharge, and results of all diagnostic and laboratory tests. A *patient care plan* followed by *progress notes* monitoring the status of the care plan are also part of the record.

The purpose of the medical record is threefold, to:

1. Document medical care
2. Facilitate communication between members of the health care team
3. Serve as a basis for the evaluation of health care delivery, including hospital accreditation and quality of care monitoring programs.

The professional personnel who provide patient care constitute the *health care team,* which consists, at least, of a physician, a nurse, a nutrition care specialist, and a pharmacist. Depending on the patient's needs, others who may be included are physical therapists, occupational therapists, and social workers. As the member of the health care team most knowledgeable in the field of nutrition, it is essential that you be skilled in documenting relevant nutrition information in the medical record. Such information is useful in coordinating nutrition care with the care provided by other members of the team.

In this chapter you will learn the appropriate *content* of a medical record entry and the correct *format* in which to record the information. We will focus on the *Problem-Oriented Medical Record (POMR).* In the completion of case studies in subsequent chapters, you will be asked to use the skills developed in this chapter to summarize your findings and suggestions for medical nutrition therapy in a chart note.

FINANCIAL IMPLICATIONS OF DOCUMENTATION

Documentation of nutritional care serves two important functions that have financial implications. First, documentation is essential for quality of care monitoring, which is required by the Joint Commission on Accreditation of Healthcare Organizations (JCAHO) (1,2). Second, documentation in the medical record and on client billing forms is the basis for assessing the economic costs and benefits of nutrition services (3). Explicit documentation of *patient* or *client outcomes* is needed to assess the benefits of nutrition services, for example, documenting that a client participating in a weight reduction program has lost 20 pounds and has also experienced a decrease in blood pressure. Documentation for quality-of-care monitoring programs requires more of a *process-oriented* approach rather than focusing on patient outcomes. For example, documentation of nutrition care activities such as the results of completed nutrition assessment, evaluation of the appropriateness of the dietary prescription, development and implementation of a nutrition care plan, or the status of patient education efforts.

The escalating cost of health care in America has renewed interest in the economic costs and benefits associated with nutrition services. Several current issues have resulted in cost reduction measures for health care. In 1983, legislation was approved to establish a Medicare

Prospective Payment System that reimburses hospitals for inpatient services as categorized by *diagnosis-related groups* (DRGs). The DRG scheme is intended to control federal spending for health care and requires that hospital departments define their costs according to the diagnoses of the patients served. Another change involves the federal government shifting a greater share of the responsibility for health and medical care to state governments (3), many of which have inadequate revenues to assume the additional expenses. Health care professionals are being asked to justify the benefits of the services that they provide, and documentation is the key to generating data for this purpose. In the words of one chief clinical dietitian, "If a dietitian doesn't chart recommendations for nutrition care and the progress of the nutrition care plan, it's as if the patient was never seen." Clinical dietitians commonly spend 1 to 2 hours of the work day charting in the medical record.

Accreditation by the JCAHO provides official recognition that a health care organization conforms to an acceptable standard of patient care. It is extremely important that a health care organization maintain JCAHO accreditation, because reimbursement for patient care by federal and state agencies, as well as by private insurance companies, usually requires that the institution be accredited. JCAHO has ongoing programs and standards for monitoring the quality of health care. An understanding of current JCAHO definitions of quality and the processes for quality measurement and monitoring are needed to prepare for accreditation (1,2). Definitions of terms used for monitoring the quality of patient care are provided in Table 2-1.

TYPES OF MEDICAL RECORDS

There are two major styles for organization of the medical record: *source oriented* and *problem oriented*. In the *Source-Oriented Medical Record*, the chart is organized according to the category of personnel writing in the record. These charts tend to have numerous sections and may, for example, contain three sets of progress notes—one for physicians, one for nurses, and one for allied health personnel.

The Problem-Oriented Medical Record (POMR) is in widespread use, although many institutions have chosen to combine elements of the source-and problem-oriented approaches. The POMR organizes the chart around a patient's problems. A major advantage of the problem-oriented approach is greater use of allied health professionals, including nutritional care specialists, in the health care team, which is headed by the primary care physician. A second advantage of the POMR arises from the fact that the documentation of problem-oriented thought processes is an educational tool for other health professionals and tends to enhance communication among members of the health care team.

TABLE 2-1   Definitions of Terms for Monitoring the Quality of Patient Care

Quality assurance, a preplanned and systematic process that monitors and evaluates the quality and appropriateness of patient care actually provided

Quality control, activities, methods, or procedures that ensure that the results of a program meet preestablished accepted standards; a part of quality assurance

Quality assurance program, program(s) organized and administered to certify continuously quality and cost-effective care through implementation of ongoing problem identification, analysis, and solution systems

Quality improvement, value or belief system about the capability of the organization to improve the care or service it provides; a process, not a plan or program, that considers the human element; the level of quality is not predetermined as with quality assurance

Clinical indicator, quantitative measure that can be used as a guide to monitor and evaluate the quality of patient care; not a direct measure of quality but rather a "flag" that identifies or directs attention to specific performance issues

Thresholds, points at which intensive evaluation of care is triggered

Adapted from: *Nutrition in Clinical Practice*, 1991; 6:131-41; *Accreditation Manual for Hospitals*, Chicago: JCAHO, 1991, p. 218; and *Manual for Food and Nutrition Services*, Rockville, MD: Aspen Publishers, Inc., 1989, p. 212.

COMPONENTS OF THE POMR

The POMR has four components: the database, a problem list, the initial care plan, and progress notes (4).

THE DATABASE

The database, which is established at the time care is initiated, is the foundation for the diagnosis and care plan. It includes the history and the results of a physical examination (H&P). The H&P is usually dictated by the admitting physician, and a typed copy is placed in the chart. The history includes the following:

The chief complaint (CC), or the *patient's* perception of his purpose in seeking medical care
    The history of the present illness (HPI)
    The previous medical history (PMH)
    The patient profile (PP), which describes the patient's social and family history
    The review of systems (ROS), which consists of a series of focused screening questions organized by organ system

The results of laboratory tests and diagnostic procedures and the nutrition history and initial nutritional assessment are also part of the database. Information included in the database is found in various parts of the chart.

THE PROBLEM LIST

The problem list is kept at the front of a patient's chart and acts as a table of contents. The master problem list is usually established by the physician, although in many institutions other professionals may add to the problem list. A problem can be defined as anything that requires diagnostic procedures or management. Problems are dated and numbered consecutively, and are dated again when resolved. Problems may be stated in a variety of ways. Here are some examples:

Classification of Problem	Medical Problem	Nutritional Problem
Diagnosis	Hypertension	Anorexis nervosa
Physiological finding	Heart Failure	Malnutrition
Symptom	Chest Pain	Weight loss
Abnormal lab finding	Elevated fasting blood sugar	Elevated serum cholesterol
Behavior	Refuses medication	Poor compliance with prescribed diet

INITIAL CARE PLAN

For each problem identified, an initial care plan is developed. The plan may include obtaining more information for diagnosis and management, specific intervention measures, and patient education. Physicians, nurses, physical therapists, and nutritional care specialists may each have a care plan to deal with a specific problem with which they are concerned.

In planning for nutritional care, the nutritional care specialist must establish goals and objectives. The objectives should be *patient centered* and should specify *measurable*, verifiable steps toward achieving the overall goal. Specific activities or interventions must be planned to help the patient achieve the objectives identified. Space limitations in the chart do not usually allow for a detailed discussion of goals and objectives. Instead, patient-centered activities or interventions that are planned or completed are usually charted in the progress notes. In nutrition care, the general types of activity or intervention include the following:

1. Prescription of a diet or special supplement
2. Recommendation for the route—either parenteral or enteral—and frequency of nutrient delivery
3. Recommendation for more comprehensive nutrition assessment, including additional laboratory work and measures of food intake
4. Nutrition education
5. Referrals for public aid, nutrition follow-up or other social services

Here are examples of two different types of care plans for two common nutritional problems:

Example 1: Patient refuses to eat hospital food.
Goals:
1. Patient's nutrition intake is adequate.

Objectives:
1. Patient will select proper foods from the regular hospital menu, adjusted according to preferences.
2. Patient will demonstrate adequate nutrient intake.

Activities or interventions:
1. Complete a baseline nutrition assessment, including diet history and food preferences.
2. Estimate caloric needs.
3. Modify menus according to patient preferences.
4. Monitor patient-selected menus.
5. Quantify food intake via calorie count or other means.

Example 2: Patient lacks knowledge of low-fat diet for management of cholecystitis.
(Note: The physician would include cholecystitis in the problem list, and the item described would be charted under this problem number by the nutrition care specialist.)
Goals:
1. Patient is able to apply the principles of the low-fat diet.

Objectives:
1. Patient will verbalize the rationale for a low-fat diet in the management of cholecystitis.
2. Patient will apply the principles of a low-fat diet by selecting proper foods from the hospital menu.
3. Patient will complete a correct sample low-fat menu to be used at home.

Activities or interventions:
1. Instruct patient and significant others in the rationale for the diet and the fat content of the various food groups.
2. Develop a meal plan in accordance with the quantity of fat prescribed.

PROGRESS NOTES

Progress notes are contributed by the various members of the health care team to document the status of the care plan in relation to the initial problem. Notes are of three types: (1) narrative, which are always dated, timed, and headed by the number and name of the problem with which they are associated; (2) flow sheets, or records of data that are obtained periodically; and (3) the discharge summary, which summarizes the level of resolution of the various problems at the time the patient is discharged.

A standardized format for narrative progress notes is described by the acronym **SOAP*** and contains the following elements:

Subjective: information that is pertinent to a listed problem and that is obtained from the patient or patient's family or significant others. Information may be recorded as a direct quote—"I can't drink that canned milkshake"—or it may be paraphrased—"Patient refuses supplemental feedings." The key characteristic of the subjective data is that it expresses the *patient's perception* of a problem.

Objective: factual information relevant to the problem that can be *confirmed by others*, including laboratory and physical findings and observations by health professionals. Factual nutrition information often found in this section of a progress note includes prescribed diet (Diet Rx), height (ht), weight (wt), ideal body weight (IBW), pertinent laboratory values, results of measured food intake, calculation of nutrient needs, and observed difficulties with eating. As a minimum, initial chart notes should state Diet Rx, ht, wt, and IBW under **O**.

Assessment: the health care team member's evaluation or interpretation of subjective and objective data. In this section the nutrition care specialist's judgment about a particular problem, based on patient-provided and factual information, is presented. Examples include the following:

"Patient does not accept value of diet in relation to medical care."

"Present intake is inadequate for nutritional needs."

"Pt demonstrates little knowledge of Na content of foods."

Plan: The specific course of action to be taken, based on **S**, **O**, and **A**, to resolve the patients problem. The plan may include all or part of the following components:

Dx (diagnosis)—further workup needed, such as a nutrition history, calorie count, lactose tolerance test, or serum albumin or lipid measurement.

Rx (therapy)—suggested diet or diet changed (diet order would have to be written by the physician), supplemental feedings, request for an eating aid.

Pt Ed (patient education)—plans for future individual or group instruction, and notation of teaching just completed, including major instructional materials provided and plans for follow-up.

An example of the components of a progress note is given here:

8-6-95, 1000 hr.
Problem 2: Anorexia
- **S**: Pt says doesn't eat because "has no appetite," no C/O food.
- **O**: Diet Rx-Reg; ht- 5 ft, 3 in, wt- 90#, 8# wt loss since admission; present intake is 600–800 kcal/day.
- **A**: Pt is 25# below IBW of 115 #, with continued wt loss; inadequate nutritional intake while hospitalized secondary to general disinterest in food.

- **P**: Pt Ed-Daily visits to patient, with emphasis on importance of nutritional intake and positive feedback.
- Rx1. Recommend daily multivitamin and mineral supplement.
- 2. Offer 4 oz of Ensure Plus t.i.d. between meals.
- Dx—Recommend examination of factors responsible for patient's anorexia (depression, meds, treatments).

Jane Doe, R.D.

CONTENT OF A NUTRITIONAL CARE PROGRESS NOTE

There is an essential core of nutrition information that belongs in every chart, regardless of format, in which a nutrition care specialist makes entries (5). Throughout this section, the content of a chart note will be linked with the POMR system of SOAP progress notes.

SUBJECTIVE AND OBJECTIVE INFORMATION

Significant History
Any historical data that relate to a patient's nutritional status should appear in a chart note labeled with the number of the problem to which it relates. Historical data may include medical, psychological, social, economic, and environmental factors, such as diet history information (see evaluation of prior or current dietary intake section), a statement reflecting a patient's previous experience with a particular diet regimen, an account of a previous nutritional problem, or details of a patient's lifestyle.

Many nutritional care specialists make the mistake of failing to restate pertinent data or of restating data that have no bearing on the problem. A good deal of judgment and knowledge is required to glean the *significant* information from patients and from their medical records.

Patient Comments About Prescribed Diet
Noting patient's own observations and opinions about their nutritional problems and dietary management provides valuable information in analyzing and diagnosing problems. It also enhances communication between the patient and the health care team by enabling team members to relate to the patient's problems as the patient perceives them.

Contraindicated Foods
Foods that interact with a patient's prescribed medications or precipitate allergic reactions should be prominently indicated in the chart.

Anthropometric Data
The initial chart notes should state Diet Rx. Measurements of height, weight, skinfold thicknesses, and calculation of ideal body weight (see Chapter 5) should also be recorded under **O**.

Accidents or Unusual Occurrences

An *unusual occurrence* can be defined as any incident, such as an error in patient care, from which medicolegal action may stem. Whenever an unusual incident occurs, the following should be noted: time of the occurrence, time the physician was notified, name of the physician contacted, and confirmation of the filing of an incident report.

For example:

> O: Pt served brk at 8:15 AM before 9:30 scheduled surgery by food service error. Dr. Smith notified 8:30 AM and incident report filed.

Impaired Ability to Feed Self and Eat

Any physical disabilities that limit a patient's ability to feed himself, masticate, or swallow should be noted in the chart, along with any adaptive equipment used or recommended. Disabilities may include new, poorly fitting, or absent dentures, amputation, use of a prosthesis, paralysis, or perceptual dysfunction.

For example

> O: Pt requires plate-guard and swivel utensils developed by OT for impaired shoulder motion.

ASSESSMENT OF SUBJECTIVE AND OBJECTIVE INFORMATION

Evaluation of Pertinent Prior Intake

This usually includes a summary of *pertinent* aspects of the diet history, including eating habits and lifestyle influences, and an evaluation of the adequacy of the prior intake and its relationship to the current problem.

For example

> S: Pt states lives alone and was too sick to go shopping last week so "just didn't eat very much." Summary of 24-hr recall: 800-1,000 kcal/day and less than 20 g pro/day.
> O: Diet Rx-Reg; Ht-6 ft, Wt-140#, IBW 175#-185#, estimated calorie needs -2,500 kcal/day
> A: Poorly nourished male 35-45# below IBW; intake PTA inadequate in most nutrients.

Note that the 24-hour recall results are part of **S** because they were calculated from what the patient *said* he ate. The *calculation* of nutritional needs is based on fact and thus is part of **O**, and the *evaluation* of the prior intake is part of **A**. (See Chapter 6 for other techniques, such as food records or food frequency lists, that can be used to evaluate prior intake.)

Evaluation of Current Dietary Intake and Diet Prescription

Current intake usually refers to food consumed within the preceding 72 hours. For a hospitalized patient, then, current intake would be based on the diet received in the hospital. The appropriateness of the dietary prescription should also be evaluated and noted in the medical record. For hospitalized patients, the calorie count allows for a more objective and quantitative estimate of nutrient intake than is provided by food recall methods. An example of quantification and evaluation of the diet of a hospitalized patient follows:

> S: "I'm just not hungry."
> O: Diet Rx-Reg, ht-5 ft, 6 in, wt-100#, IBW -120#-130#. 2# wt loss since admission 10 days ago. Calorie count: average of 3 days-40 g pro, 1,200 kcal/day. Estimated calorie needs : 1,500—1,800 kcal/day.
> A: Underweight female undergoing CA therapy consuming inadequate calories secondary to anorexia.

Evaluation of Current Nutritional Status

This involves the evaluation of prior and current diet, and of the anthropometric, laboratory, and physical findings summarized in S and O and interpreted under A.

For example:

> A: Wt loss of 10% in past month, low serum albumin, and inadequate calorie and protein intake indicate nutritional depletion.

The dietitian should interpret laboratory values or diagnostic findings (see Chapter 4) only in terms of their relationship to diet and nutritional problems. Laboratory and physical assessment findings should be used to support the diagnosis of a nutrition problem or to monitor an identified nutritional problem.

For example:

> O: serum albumin = 2.5 mg/dL
> A: Visceral protein depletion indicated by low serum albumin level

Evaluation of Patient's Ability to Accept and Understand Diet Instruction

This part of the note documents the nutrition care specialist's assessment of a patient's attitude about and understanding of the prescribed diet. It is important to describe how the patient's attitude was assessed and how understanding of the diet was demonstrated.

For example:

> A: Pt demonstrates adequate knowledge of 2-g-Na diet based on completion of three sample menus for home use and ability to verbalize high-Na "foods to avoid."

ASSESSMENT OR PLAN

Recommendation for Consultation or Evaluation by Others

Institutional policies differ concerning referral or to

consultation by nonphysician health professionals. The rationale for a referral or consultation would be stated under **A** and the recommendation under **P**lan Rx.

For example:

A: Pt unable to purchase special dietary items necessary for 500-mg-Na diet due to financial constraints.

P: Rx—Contact social worker to explore possible financial resources with patient.

Implementing, Monitoring, and Revising the Nutritional Care Plan to Achieve Patient Outcomes

The establishment of a nutritional care plan, including goals and patient-centered objectives, is essential to the treatment of a nutritional problem. However, time and space limitations in the medical record usually do not allow for a detailed discussion of goals and objectives. Instead, the patient-centered activities or interventions that are *planned* or *completed* are usually stated, and the goals and objectives are implied. The advantages of stating patient-centered activities are twofold: (1) other health professionals, including other nutritional care specialists, know what has been done and can provide follow-up, and (2) activities are more measurable than goals and can thus be used for audit purposes.

The following is an example of a series of chart notes which state the plans for nutritional care and the progress of the care plan:

9-2-95, 1000 hr.
Problem 1: Excess Body Weight

S: "I want to lose weight while I'm in traction."

O: Diet Rx-House: ht-5 ft, 2 in, wt-160# (bed scale), IBW range-110#-120#. Estimated maintenance calorie needs, 2,000, kcal/day. Nursing intake records reflect 50% meal consumption. S/P pin placement for compound fracture; 3-6 weeks hospitalization required for traction and antibiotic Rx.

A: Obese, immobilized 20 y.o. female w/o major food preferences. Motivated to lose wt but needs education regarding weight reduction diet allowing for 1#/week wt loss during recovery from skeletal fracture.

P: Rx—Contact MD to suggest change to 1,500 kcal wt reduction diet and weekly weight checks. Dx—Obtain diet history.

Jane Doe R.D.

9-22-95, 1400 hr.
Problem1: Excess Body Weight

S: Diet history reflects usual intake of 3,000 kcal/day with high intake of sweetened beverages. No C/O 1,500 kcal diet.

O: Diet Rx—1,500 kcal; weigh weekly on bed scale.

A: Prescribed diet is acceptable to pt; will begin pt ed re principles of wt reduction diet.

P: Pt Ed—1. Reviewed concept of exchange lists with elimination of sweetened foods.

2. Gave pt exchange booklet with 1,500-kcal

meal plan to study.

3. Asked pt to categorize a list of foods according to exchange list and to state appropriate portion size.

4. F/U next week.

Rx—1. Maintain flow sheet of pt's weekly weights to be kept in chart.

Jane Doe R.D.

9-28-95, 0930 hr.
Problem 1: Excess Body Weight

S: "I finished categorizing that list of foods."

O: Diet Rx-1,500 kcal; wt-157#

A: Pt correctly used exchange lists to classify foods according to calorie content.

P: Pt Ed—1. Explained 1,500-kcal meal plan in relation to hospital menu.

2. Asked pt to complete sample menus for use at home using 1,500-kcal meal plan.

3. F/U next week.

Jane Doe R.D.

10-4-95, 0915 hr.
Problem 1: Excess Body Weight

S: "I feel like I lost some weight, and the doctor says my fracture is healing OK."

O: Diet Rx-1,500 kcal; wt-155#. 5# wt loss since 9-2-95.

A: Adequate understanding of diet demonstrated by completion of selective menus and sample menus for home. Pt verbalizes value of diet. No further instruction needed.

P: Pt Ed—1. Pt given R.D. name and phone number to contact with future questions.

Jane Doe R.D.

Disposition Indicated

Nutrition progress notes should come to some logical conclusion. Discharge, referral, or follow-up should be specifically indicated under **P** at the end of a progress note.

Change in Standard Procedure

Variations from standard dietary policy should be documented in the medical record to alert other health professionals that the change has been planned and is not an oversight or error. Examples of such variations or changes in food service procedure include a renal patient's being allowed to have a salt packet on his tray, a patient on a clear liquid diet being allowed to have sherbet, or a patient's being permitted to go to the hospital cafeteria to supplement her dietary intake.

Table 2.2 summarizes the content of a progress note and provides guidelines for placement in the SOAP format. Placement of data in the SOAP format varies somewhat, but the general format, previously outlined in the section on Components of the POMR-Progress Notes, should help to clarify the placement of data.

TABLE 2-2 Content of a Progress Note According to Placement in the SOAP Format

Component	Placement
Significant history	S or O
Patient comments about prescribed diet	S
Contraindicated foods	S or O
Anthropometric data	O
Accidents or unusual occurrences	O
Impaired motor ability to feed self and eat	O
Evaluation of pertinent prior intake	S, O, and A*
Evaluation of current dietary intake	S, O, and A*
Evaluation of currrent nutritional status	A
Evaluation of client's ability to accept and understand diet instruction	A
Recommendation for consultation or evaluation by other professionals	A and P
Implementation, monitoring, and revision of the nutrition care plan	P
Disposition indicated	P
Change in standard procedure	A and P†

* Summary of diet history information should be included under **S**, calculations of nutritional needs and results of measured food intake under **O**, and the evaluation of data under **A**.
† Rationale should be included under **A**, and recommendations under **P-Rx**.

OTHER FORMATS FOR PROGRESS NOTES

No one format is the correct format for meeting the required legal standard of care for patient documentation. The key feature is that the format must promote effective communication among the members of the health care team about the patient's health and the status of the care plan (6). Several formats other than the SOAP format have been suggested for documentation of patient care as outlined below.

A non-SOAP format suggested for the documentation of nutrition care is described by the acronym **PIE**. PIE charting states the **p**roblem, identifies the nutrition **i**nterventions, and then describes the **e**valuation of the patient's responses to the interventions. A sample of the PIE charting format is shown here:

P: Inadequate energy intake with associated wt. loss due to poor appetite.
I: Examine factors responsible for patient's lack of appetite-depression, meds or treatments. Offer 4 oz. Ensure Plus t.i.d. between meals. Recommend daily multivitamin and mineral supplement.
E: Monitor food intake and review selective menu with patient daily.

Many practitioners feel that the PIE format is more succinct than the SOAP format and that it facilitates follow-up charting and the evaluation of nutrition outcomes.

Nutritional diagnostic charting is another format for recording progress notes. This method uses the SOAP format as a basis and expands the assessment portion to include a nutritional diagnostic statement. The diagnostic statement is a written expression using components described by the acronym **PES** - **p**roblem, **e**tiology and **s**igns and symptoms (7). A nutritional diagnostic statement might read, "caloric deficit related to poor tolerance of bolus enteral feedings and shown by intake meeting 60 to 75 % of estimated energy needs and continued wt loss"

A charting format described by the acronym **SCIP** has also been suggested. SCIP states the **s**pecific **c**riteria, **i**ssues, and **p**lan. In follow-up notes using the SCIP format, only the issue and plan sections are required.

WRITING STYLE IN PROGRESS NOTES

Dark ink, usually black, should be used for progress notes. Pencil or other colors of ink should not be used. Handwriting should be legible and dark enough to photocopy or put on microfilm. The date, time of entry, and associated problem should precede every note in the chart. All components of the SOAP format need not be used in each entry unless charting is infrequent. The dietitian's signature and credentials should be affixed to the bottom of the chart note.

The objective style, rather than personal pronouns such as *I*, *my*, or *me*, should be used in the medical record. For example, "Pt's need for protein is increased" is preferable to "I recommend an increase in protein intake." Phrases commonly used in charting are listed in Table 2.3. Accurate spelling and correct medical abbreviations should be used. Medical records departments usually maintain a list of acceptable medical abbreviations. For our purposes, the abbreviations listed in Appendix D, will be used.

In general, the traditional rules of grammar are not strictly applied in medical charting. For instance, complete sentences need not be used consistently as long as complete thoughts are expressed. However, subjects and verbs must agree, and verb tenses must be correct. For example, "pt *eats* adequate amounts" is acceptable. "Pt *eat* adequate amounts" is not.

A chart note must be accurate, clear, and concise. The entry should be as brief as it can be without omission of essential elements. Medical personnel do not have time to read rambling chart notes, and you want your notes to be read. In addition, most dietitians record between six and ten short notes a day, so there just isn't time to record information that is not pertinent to the assessment of nutritional problems. For example, listing certain lab values as objective data, but failing to use these data in the assessment, would be adding nonessential data.

FUTURE TRENDS

In the future, documentation of patient care will most likely be automated by computer systems and utilize computer-generated spread sheets, graphs and patient-specific care plans or care maps. Multidisciplinary

TABLE 2-3 Phrases Commonly Used in Charting

Admits to eating poorly
Admitted for evaluation of
Appetite good, wt. stable
Appetite was good
As described previously on (in)
Associated with
Because of the history of
Characterized by
Consistent with
Continuous with
Demonstrated that
Despite these findings
Disregard
Impression at time
Improved with
In consultation with_____, we suggest the following
Inform
Initially seen at
Instruct
Is not remarkable
It is felt that pt. is a candidate for
Markedly increased
Need
Nutritional workup included
Observed
Old records confirm
On this basis
On this regimen she continued to
Oral intake was
Pt. continues to have
Pt. exhibits difficulty chewing
Pt. has no past history
Pt. was initially started on
Pt. was noted to be
Pertinent dietary findings
Previously in good health
Recommend
Request
Revealed evidence of
Reviewed previous
Should be followed very carefully
Suggest
To be followed by
Was not felt to be significant

methods of documentation will be introduced to reduce duplication of documentation among the various members of the health care team. For example, members of the health care team may all record on the same patient care plan which has been individualized for the patient and is accessed from a computer database. Some practitioners predict that progress notes will simply document "exceptions" in the responses and progress of the patient from their original individualized care plan. This approach is described by the term *exception documentation* (7). A bedside "paperless" charting system with a computer screen at each patient's bedside is being evaluated at some hospitals. In a bedside charting system the members of the health care team simply enter the patient's identification code and are provided access to the total patient care record. Discipline-specific menus such as a nutrition-related menu would be available to standardize information provided in the initial progress notes. In summary, future patient care documentation systems will be automated by computer technology and will utilize a multidisciplinary format which minimizes duplication.

TOPICS FOR FURTHER DISCUSSION

1. Review the literature for studies that demonstrate a positive relationship between nutritional services and reduced total health care costs. How strong are the data, and how could the methodology be improved?
2. Review the most recent "Guidelines for Dietetic Services" published by the Joint Commission on Accreditation of Healthcare Organizations. What kind of nutritional care documentation is required to meet the standards of care specified in these guidelines?
3. Discuss the types of activities required in effective quality-assurance or quality-improvement programs for nutritional care.
4. Review the International Classification of Disease, ninth revision, Clinical Modification Codes (ICD-9-CM), to become familiar with codes for nutrition problems such as marasmus or kwashiorkor.

REFERENCES

1. JOINT Commission on Accreditation of Healthcare Organizations. *Accreditation Manual for Hospitals.* Chicago: JCAHO, 1995.
2. **Clark, K., A.M. Hunter**. Quality assessment and improvement. In *Nutrition Support Dietetics*, 2d ed. Rockville, MD: Aspen, 1993.
3. **Disbrow, D.D.** The costs and benefits of nutrition services: A literature review. *J. Amer. Dietet. Assoc.*, (supplement) 89:(1989)S6–S9.
4. **Weed, L.L.** *Medical Records, Medical Education, and Patient Care: The Problem-Oriented Medical Record as a Basic Tool.* Cleveland: Case-Western Reserve University Press, 1969.
5. **Zimmerman, T.P., S.L. Sayers, M. Price, A. Laduca, J.D. Engel, M.E. Risley, and G. Giannini.** *Medical Dietetics: Medical Recording Skills Manual.* Revised by S. Sayers. Chicago: Center for Educational Development, University of Illinois, 1978.
6. **Scott, R.W.** *Legal Aspects of Documenting Patient Care.* Gaithersburg, MD: Aspen Publishers, 1994

7. **Dougherty, O.** Nutrition intervention documentation. Hospital Food & Nutrition Focus 11: (1994)1–7

ADDITIONAL SOURCES OF INFORMATION

The American Dietetic Association. *Costs and Benefits of Nutritional Care: Phase 1.* Chicago: ADA, 1979.

The American Dietetic Association *Nutrition Services Payment System: Guidelines for Implementation.* Chicago: ADA, 1985.

Blackburn, S.A., and S.P. Himburg. Nutrition care activities and drugs. *J. Am. Dietet. Assoc.* 87:(1987)1535.

Dowling, R., and A. Smith. *Benefits of Nutrition Services: A Costing and Marketing Approach;* Report of the Seventh Ross Roundtable of Medical Issues. Columbus, OH: Ross Laboratories, 1987.

Schiller, M.R., K. Miller-Kovach, and M.A. Miller. *Total Quality Management for Hospital Nutrition Services.* Gaithersburg, MD: Aspen Publishers, 1994.

Splett, P.L. Effectiveness and cost effectiveness of nutrition care: a critical analysis with recommendations: *J Amer Dietet. Assoc.* 91 (supplement): (1991)S-3–S-53.

Srp, F., E.A. Ayello, E. Andujar, and N.N. Konstantinides. Quality of Care Concepts and Nutrition Support. *Nutrition in Clinical Practice*, 6:(1991)131.

TO TEST YOUR UNDERSTANDING

1. For each of the following problems, state a goal, a patient-centered measurable objective, and a specific activity or intervention to help reach the goal.
  a. Problem 1: Poorly fitting dentures
  b. Problem 2: Excessive weight gain during pregnancy

2. List four items that must be included in initial chart notes under **O**.

3. A problem and background information are provided for this exercise. For each component listed, extract any appropriate information and fill in the chart. If a factor is not applicable or if the information is not available, state N/A (not applicable). This exercise is designed to help you practice selecting key information to include in the SOAP note; it is not critical that you correctly categorize the selected information.

Problem 1: Obesity

Mr. Toone is referred by his physicians to the Nutrition Outpatient Clinic for counseling on a weight-reduction diet. While talking to Mr. Toone, you obtain a quick diet history that you feel is reasonably accurate. You calculate that the diet contains 2,800 kcal per day. Mr. Toone tells you that he is 52 years old, dislikes sweets and fats, is fairly inactive, and eats two large meals a day. You measure Mr. Toone and find that he is 5 feet, 7 inches tall and weighs 195 pounds. You recommend that Mr. Toone eat three meals a day and bring a 3-day dietary record back to the clinic next week for your evaluation.

Significant history

Patient comments about prescribed diet

Contraindicated foods

Anthropometric data

Accidents or unusual occurrences

Impaired motor ability to feed self and eat

Evaluation of pertinent prior intake

Evaluation of current nutritional status

Evaluation of client's ability to accept and understand diet instruction

Recommendation for consultation or evaluation by other professionals

Implementation, monitoring, and revision of the nutritional care plan

Disposition indicated

Change in usual procedure

4. Now write a SOAP progress note for Problem 1 (above in Question 3) based on the information in question 3. Be sure to use correct and complete format.

5. Write a SOAP progress note for Problem 2 given below.

Problem 2: Tantrums

While working as a consultant at a small nursing home, you are referred by the nursing department to a resident, Ms. Smith, who has started throwing her tray on the floor whenever it is served. You talk with Ms. Smith and she tells you that the hospital food is terrible and that her favorite foods are buttermilk, cheese, and ham. Upon checking the patient's chart, you find that a mild sodium-restricted diet (3 g Na) had been ordered for her at about the time her disruptive behavior began. Some quick calculations indicate that Ms. Smith could have a 6 ounce glass of buttermilk with each meal if she eats salt-free vegetables and meat. You decide to try this and see if it will improve Ms. Smith's appetite. You will return during the evening meal tomorrow to assess whether the patient is accepting her diet.

3 Interviewing the Patient

Betsy B. Holli, Ed.D., R.D.

Interviewing is a communication skill used frequently by health professionals. In conversations with patients and clients, it is often necessary to obtain selected information in the course of professional practice. An interview may be defined as a conversation between two parties in which one questions the other in seeking information to evaluate as a basis for treatment. Knowledge of the principles of interviewing and practice in the process enhance the ability of the nutrition care specialist to work effectively with others.

PURPOSE OF INTERVIEWS

Having the specific purpose of the interview clearly in mind has several advantages. Because the nutritional care specialist asks a number of questions in the interview process, it is important for both the interviewer and the client or patient to understand the purpose of the interview. Frequently the purpose of nutrition interviews is to obtain information about the individual's current eating habits or behaviors as baseline information and as a basis for suggesting changes, as a part of nutritional assessment, or as a basis for nutrition care plans, nutrition counseling, and education. Having been told that the nutrition care specialist needs some basic information on eating habits in order to help effectively, the individual is more comfortable and also likely to respond more fully. Chapter 6 discusses the types of information needed to evaluate an individual's dietary intake using a variety of techniques. In addition, the questions asked in the interview should be related to the purpose in order to use time most efficiently. Questions unrelated to the purpose may be a waste of everyone's time.

KNOWLEDGE, BEHAVIORS, FEELINGS

A client's current daily food intake is the result of long-standing eating habits or behaviors. During the interview, questions can differentiate between eating behaviors, knowledge, and feelings. For example: "Do you know why it is important to eat dietary fiber? is a knowledge question, while "What foods do you eat to include fiber in your diet?" is an eating behavior question. "Are you aware of the effect of sodium in your body?" is a knowledge question, but "What foods do you eat that are high in salt or sodium content?" is an eating behavior question. Since time is limited, you need to focus most on eating behaviors.

When clients are not adhering to their dietary regimens or when people are just starting new dietary changes, questions dealing with feelings may provide important insights. You may ask, for example: "How do you feel about making these dietary changes?" The client may reply: "I feel that it will be difficult for me to have to eat different foods from the rest of my family." Or you may inquire: "You seem to be having problems following your diet. How do you feel about trying to eat fruit for dessert instead of cake and cookies?" A reply of "I'm willing to give it a try" is one client response, while "I love to bake, and cookies are one of my favorite foods" gives you different information. Clients' reactions, as expressed by feelings, provide additional understanding necessary for the counseling process.

CONFIDENTIALITY/PRIVACY

Information obtained in interviews must be treated confidentially. Clients with eating disorders, obesity, and other medical problems may be reluctant to disclose their problems fully and honestly. They may be embarrassed by what they have been eating and wonder why the questions are important. Besides clarifying the purpose of the interview, the nutrition care specialist may need to reassure the client that the information obtained will be treated confidentially.

Better results are also obtained in a private setting where others cannot overhear the individual's story. Whenever possible, a private office or room where there are no interruptions and phone calls are held creates a better atmosphere where clients feel more free to talk. While this is not always possible in a hospital setting, one can still rearrange a chair to create the most privacy and the opportunity of listening with undivided attention.

OPENING THE INTERVIEW

There are three basic parts to an interview: (1) the opening, (2) the body of the interview, and (3) the closing (1). While the opening and closing take less time than the body of the interview, none-the-less they both serve important functions and should not be overlooked.

In the opening, several things need to be established. Introducing oneself by name and occupation and meeting the hospitalized patient are usually first. The patient needs to know who you are and what your credentials are. For example: "Good morning. I'm Susan Smith, your registered dietitian. Please call me Susan."

Some adults may not like to be called by their first names. They may consider it another reduction in their control of the circumstances or a lack of respect for their age or status in life. It is well to clarify how the person prefers to be addressed so that rapport is not damaged unnecessarily.

The opening provides an opportunity to establish a degree of rapport and a supportive, nonjudgmental environment that must be maintained during all phases of the interview. Both the client and the counselor need to feel at ease. Rapport suggests a harmonious, supportive relationship. Individuals are reluctant to speak frankly with people whom they do not know or trust. Thus a few minutes need to be spent in getting acquainted and developing a friendly climate. "Small talk" about the weather, local or national events, sports teams, holidays, or a bit of information noticed in reading the medical record can break the ice. Afterwards, the purpose of the interview should be clarified and discussed.

BODY OF THE INTERVIEW

During the main part of the interview, the nutrition care specialist uses questions to obtain information about the individual's dietary habits or behaviors. Several kinds of questions may be used, and these questions may be organized into a specific sequence.

Types of Questions

The types of questions used in interviews may be classified as: (1) primary or secondary, (2) open or closed, and (3) neutral or leading. Some questions are rephrased as directives. There are advantages and disadvantages to each type of question (1).

Primary Questions

Primary questions are used to introduce new topics. The following are examples:

"Now that we have discussed your meals, can you tell me about any snacks that you eat between meals?"

"Besides eating at home, where else do you eat and what do you eat there?"

Secondary Questions

Secondary questions are also called follow-up questions. Their purpose is to clarify what has been said or to elicit further information. The following are examples:

"When you have chocolate-chip cookies for a snack, how many do you eat?"

"When you eat in restaurants, how are your meats and potatoes prepared?"

Open Questions

Open questions are those that are phrased broadly. Examples are:

"Can you tell me about what you usually eat at meals?"

"Can you tell me about how your weekend meals differ from what you eat during the week?"

Open questions have the advantage of being less threatening to people. Individuals are given more control and broad leeway to express themselves. The limitations are, however, that open questions may consume more time, and the patient may stray far from the facts needed.

Closed Questions

Closed questions, on the other hand, give the interviewer more control and help obtain specific information. The following are examples:

"What do you put in your coffee?"
"What kinds of breakfast cereal do you eat?"

They have the disadvantage of obtaining a brief answer that then requires the interviewer to ask another question. Too many closed questions in sequence may seem like an interrogation.

Neutral and Leading Questions

Neutral questions are preferred to leading questions because one receives more accurate answers. Leading questions reveal the interviewer's personal biases and suggest the answer expected. The expected answer is the one the patient or client is most likely to give you. Examples of leading questions are:

"You eat three meals a day, don't you?" "Yes."
"You know that pregnant women should drink milk, don't you?" "Yes, of course."

Directives

Directives can break the feeling of interrogation which may arise from the overuse of questions. Of course, they should not sound too direct. Directives can suggest more subtly what you would like to know about. The following are examples:

"Tell me about your lunches at work."
"Now that we have discussed your meals during the week, I'd like to hear about your meals on weekends."

PREPLANNING

Good interviewers plan their questions in advance. Preplanning is especially important for the less-experienced interviewer. Each question should be related in some way to the purpose of the interview. With the questions well in mind, you can concentrate on the interaction, listen carefully to the client or patient, and remember what was said rather than worrying about the next question you have to ask or interrupting the relationship with constant note taking.

The sequence in which the questions are asked should be preplanned as well. Not that it is necessary to follow the outline strictly. Certainly, an individual's response may suggest a different direction for a follow-up question. Experience will show which questions are most productive and should be retained in one's repertoire, and which may be eliminated.

WORDING QUESTIONS

Now look back at the examples of questions and directives and notice that many questions are phrased with "what," "where," "how," and "tell me about." Questions starting with "do you" are avoided because they result in a one-word answer, such as "yes" or "no," which is not productive. The following are examples:

"Do you like milk?" "Yes."
"Do you cook the meals at home?" "Yes."
"Do you fry your foods?" "Seldom."

These questions need rephrasing. See if you can change them to broader questions.

A second type of question usually avoided begins with "why." These questions may indicate disapproval or appear to force people into a defensive posture of justifying their actions (2). Examples are:

"Why don't you drink milk?"
"Why do you eat so many salty foods?"
"Why haven't you lost any weight since I last saw you?"

Nothing is likely to be gained with a "why" question, and rapport may be lost.

RESPONSES

As the interview progresses, and rapport is maintained through a supportive environment, the nutrition care specialist may consider responses other than another question. Three possible responses to a client's statements are: (1) probing, (2) an understanding response, and (3) confrontation (1).

Probing

The probing response is an attempt to gain further information or clarification. Several approaches may be useful. One of these is paraphrasing. The interviewer may summarize and rephrase what has been said, and then pause for confirmation and further clarification. For example:

"You indicate that you cook mostly Italian foods for your family's evening meals and that your family prefers home-cooked foods. And when you eat in restaurants, do you usually go to your favorite Italian restaurants?"

A summary sentence stated as a question may encourage elaboration, such as the following:

"You say you only have cereal for breakfast?"

Echoing the person's previous statement should not be overdone, however, or it can have a parrotlike effect.

Although an inexperienced interviewer may not be comfortable with using silence, a 30 to 60 second silence with eyes temporarily averted may help patients gather their thoughts before elaborating further. It is better not to push ahead with a subsequent question too fast, or parts of the story may be missed. Other nonverbal probes include nodding the head as a reply, a quizzical look, and leaning forward slightly.

Examples of other probes are:

"Tell me more about…"
"I don't think I fully understand…"
"Go on."
"That's interesting."
"I see."
"Uh huh."
"Good for you."
"And what else…"

Understanding Response

An understanding response may enhance the supportive environment and rapport. Patients have more rapport with those who try to understand them. They feel more accepted even though they may not be following a dietary regimen perfectly. In this response, the interviewer supposes what the client is either thinking or feeling and tentatively expresses this in words. For example:

"You seem to be feeling that your dietary regimen is difficult to follow."

"You seem to be worried about how you can cook for your family and still follow your diabetic diet."

"You are concerned that you won't be able to find low-sodium foods at your favorite restaurant."

The patient will then feel safe in discussing this response and exploring problems and solutions. It is possible, of course, that you have misunderstood the person's thoughts or feelings. However, there is no need to worry. The client perceives you as an understanding person and will correct any misunderstanding.

Confrontation

Confrontation is an authority-laden response that should not be used unless you know the person well and have established good rapport. This response calls to the person's attention, in a dramatic fashion, some behavior, habit, or discrepancy the client uses to hide from understanding of self or from constructive behavior change. It is self-defeating, and the individual may not be facing or recognizing it (3). The nutrition care specialist could say to an obese client, for example:

"You really don't seem to take your diet seriously. You keep eating bags of potato chips."

A challenge to action is implied. The goal is to explore areas that the client has been reluctant to explore. Unless done carefully by an experienced interviewer, however, confrontation may inhibit the rapport and relationship between the client and the dietitian, which hinders more than helps.

Other Responses

Other responses are not recommended because they are ineffective. A reassuring response inhibits problem solving with the patient, as for example: "Don't worry. You will find your sodium-restricted diet easier to follow as the weeks go on." Evaluative responses indicate that the counselor approves or disapproves, are judgmental, and lead to giving advice rather than solving problems, such as: "I think that you would find it easier to follow your diabetic diet if you would plan a week's menus in advance." And a hostile response, said in frustration or anger, may lead to humiliation of the patient, such as: "How many times have I told you to be more careful of what you order in restaurants."

CLOSING THE INTERVIEW

The final part of the interview is the closing. Several important tasks are accomplished in the closing. A few words of appreciation for the patient's time and cooperation are appropriate. You may want to review the initial purpose and discuss the next steps, i.e., what you plan to do with the information obtained. An inquiry concerning whether the patient has any questions or additional thoughts may bring out overlooked information or a new perspective, which is helpful. Be sure to allow adequate time for this. It is not an afterthought. And plans for future appointments should be completed. For example:

"Well, Mrs. Jones, I think I have a good picture of what you eat currently. I appreciate your cooperation. Do you have any questions or any other thoughts that you would like to add?" (Allow time for the response.) "I'll stop by your hospital room tomorrow, and we can begin to discuss your diabetic diet and how to manage it at home."

Because it is a skill, interviewing improves with repeated practice. Observing a skilled interviewer can be very helpful as can having a skilled interviewer observe you and make suggestions. Inexperienced interviewers may benefit from tape recording or video taping their interviews, with permission of the client, for later analysis of the kinds of responses and questions used and the effectiveness of the process.

REFERENCES

1. **Holli, B.B.,and R.M. Calabrese.** *Communication and Education Skills: The Dietitian's Guide*, 2d ed. Philadelphia: Lea & Febiger, 1991.

2. **Bernstein, L., and R.S. Bernstein.** *Interviewing: A Guide for Health Professionals*, 4th ed. Norwalk, CT: Appleton-Century-Crofts, 1985.

3. **Engen, H.B., L. Iasiello-Vailas, and K. L. Smith.** Confrontation: a new dimension in nutrition counseling. *J. Amer. Dietet. Assoc.* 83:(1983)34–38.

 ## TO TEST YOUR UNDERSTANDING

1. a. Fill in the blanks: The three parts of an interview are the ———, ———, and ———.

b. List the types of information that should be included in each of the three parts of the interview.

2. Classify the following questions as to type, such as open, closed, neutral, or leading. Rephrase those that are closed or leading questions.

a. Can you tell me about your previous experiences with dieting?

b. You follow your diabetic diet, don't you?

c. How many cups of coffee do you drink at breakfast?

d. Don't you know how important it is to drink milk during pregnancy?

e. Now that we have discussed your meals, what about snacks between meals?

3. Provide a probing response to the following client statements:

a. I have dieted twice before, but I have always regained the weight I lost.

b. I've been on a diabetic diet for 2 years already.

c. The doctor thinks that I should cut down on my salt intake.

4. Provide an understanding response to the following client statements:

a. I'm too old to change the way I eat. What does it matter anyway?

b. I don't have time to prepare meals from scratch. When I get home from work, my children are hungry.

c. I eat so many meals in restaurants that I don't know how I can manage this diet.

5. Reword the following questions:

a. Why don't you drink milk?

b. Why do you eat so many salty foods?

c. Why haven't you lost any weight since I last saw you?

6. Identify the following responses as reassuring, evaluative, or confrontational. Rewrite each.

a. You don't seem to be making any effort to lower the amount of fat and cholesterol in your diet.

b. Don't worry if you have not been following your diet perfectly. It gets easier with time.

c. Skipping breakfast is a big mistake. You would feel much better if you ate something in the morning.

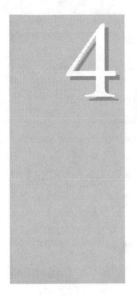

4 Water, Electrolytes, and Acid-Base Balance

Disorders of fluid, electrolyte, and acid-base balances occur in association with many pathological conditions. Therefore, their general principles will be discussed in this chapter, and applications will be noted in later chapters concerning specific organ systems.

FLUIDS

Water participates in regulation of body temperature and is a major component of cells, blood, lymph, mucus, and digestive juices. The water in the body also serves as a carrier of nutrients and waste materials and as a medium for chemical reactions. It is thus important that appropriate amounts of fluids be present in each compartment.

BODY WATER CONTENT AND DISTRIBUTION

Approximately 60-percent of the body weight of an average adult male is water. Water content varies, however, with age, sex, and body fat content. The adult female body, for example, is about 50-percent water. There is a direct relationship between lean body mass (LBM) and total body water (TBW):

$$LBM = \frac{TBW}{0.732} \qquad (4\text{-}1)$$

Children's bodies have higher proportions of body fluid, a newborn's body at term is composed of 75- to 80-percent water, an amount that decreases progressively with age.

Of the 60-percent total fluid in an adult male, about two-thirds, or 40-percent, of body weight is within the cells (*intracellular fluid,* or *ICF*). In dehydration, fluid shifts out of the cells, and total ICF is decreased. The remaining one-third of total fluid, or 20 percent of body weight, is the *extracellular fluid (ECF)*. It is divided between the 3 to 5 percent within the blood vessels (*intravascular*) and the 12 to 15 percent in intercellular space (*interstitial fluid* or *ISF*). Lymph is included in the ISF and comprises 3 to 5 percent of body weight. In some conditions, the ISF increases, resulting in edema. A small quantity, 1 to 5 percent, is categorized as *transcellular*, which includes water in cerebrospinal and intraocular fluids and water in the glands, excretory portion of the kidney, secretions of the gastrointestinal tract, bone, and "potential spaces."

Potential spaces, also called *third spaces*, are important in that they can expand to hold large quantities of fluid that accumulate in some disease states. These spaces include the pericardial and peritoneal cavities, joint space and bursae, and the thoracic cavity. In the burned patient, for example, a fluid shift to "third space" can result in shock and circulatory collapse as blood volume decreases.

Potential spaces communicate easily with the intercellular space. The intravascular and interstitial fluids mix freely through the highly porous capillary walls, but the intracellular fluid is separated from extracellular fluid by semipermeable membranes, that is, cell membranes. Table 4-1 summarizes values for these fluid compartments.

FLUID REQUIREMENTS

Estimates of water requirements for normal persons have been based on calorie intake, body surface area, or body weight. Methods of estimation are shown in Table 4-2.

TABLE 4-1 Water Compartments in the Adult Male Human Body

Water Compartment	% Total Body Weight	Volume in 70-kg Man, L
Extracellular fluid	20–23	14.0
Intravascular	3–5	3.0
Intercellular (Interstitial)	12–15	10.0
Transcellular	1–5	1.0
Intracellular fluid	35–40	28.0
Total	~55–60	42.0

TABLE 4-2 Methods of Estimation of Daily Fluid Requirements

Basis of Estimation	Calculation
Body Weight	
Adults	
Young Active. 15–30 years	40 mL/kg
Average. 25–55 years	35 mL/kg
Older. 55–65 years	30 mL/kg
Elderly >65 years	25 mL/kg
Children	
1–10 kg	100 mL/kg
11–20 kg	an additional 50 mL/each kg >10
21 kg or more	an additional 20 mL/each kg >20 at age 50 or less or an additional 15 mL/kg.>20 at age >50
Energy intake	1 mL/kcal for adults 1.5 mL/kcal for infants
Nitrogen plus energy intake	100 mL/g nitrogen intake PLUS 1 mL/kcal[*]
Body surface area	1,500 mL/M^{2}[†][‡]

[*] Especially useful with high protein feedings.
[†] Body surface area may be calculated from the following formula:
$$S = W^{0.425} \times H^{0.725} \times 71.84$$ or
$$\log X = (\log W \times 0.425) + (\log H \times 0.725) + 1.8564$$
where $X = cm^2$ body surface area, $W = kg$ body weight, and $H = cm$ height.
[‡] Body surface often used for "average" adult is 1.73M^2.

These methods vary in their results, but the differences are within the range of the compensatory ability of the normal kidney. The estimates are not applicable to patients with diarrhea, renal disease, fever, or catabolic diseases. These will be discussed in later chapters.

FLUID INTAKE

Fluid is supplied to the body via three routes (Table 4-3):

1. by ingestion of liquids.
2. from preformed fluid in solid foods such as meats, fruits, and vegetables.
3. from the production of water from the metabolism of proteins, fats, and carbohydrates.

In metabolism to carbon dioxide and water, 100 g of fat produce 107 g of water; 100 g of carbohydrate yield 55 g of water; and 100 g of protein produce 41 g of water. In some pathological conditions, human muscle is catabolized and contributes to water. This is not calculated into the fluid balance since the exact amount of muscle catabolized is not accurately measurable in clinical situations.

FLUID TRANSFER

There are two processes, diffusion and osmosis, by which transfer of water and some solutes from one fluid compartment to another can occur without expenditure of energy. Filtration and active transport also transfer water across membranes but require energy expenditure.

Diffusion
Diffusion refers to the movement of a substance from an area of high concentration to an area of low concentration. If a membrane is permeable to a substance, diffusion can take place across the membrane.

Osmosis
Some membranes in the body are semipermeable, that is, water and some solutes, *but not all*, will pass through freely. *Osmosis* is the movement of *solvent* molecules across a semipermeable membrane. The solvent (water) moves from the area of low concentration of solute to an area of high concentration of solutes *that cannot cross the membrane*. The movement of the water equalizes the concentration of the solute on the two sides of the membrane.

The force that pulls the water through the semipermeable membrane toward the concentrated solution is called *osmotic pressure*. It is directly proportional to the *number* of particles in the solution and inversely proportional to their molecular weights. In biological materials, the osmotic pressure of a solution is measured

TABLE 4-3 Representative Fluid Balance

Water Intake	(mL)	Water Loss	(mL)
Sensible		Sensible	
Oral fluids	1,600	Urine	1,600
Solid foods	800	Intestinal	300
Insensible		Insensible	
Metabolic water	300	Lungs and skin	800
Total	2,700	Total	2,700

in *milliosmols* (*mOsm*). One millimole (mmol) of a substance that does not dissociate in solution, such as glucose, exerts an osmotic pressure of 1 mOsm. One mmol of a substance that dissociates into two particles, such as sodium chloride, has an osmotic pressure of 2 mOsm. In substances producing three ions, 1 mmol = 3 mOsm.

Although the S.I. units, recently adopted in medical practice (see Appendix E), would measure osmolarity in mmol/kg, it is suggested that the previous units of Osm/kg continue to be used "so that clinical understanding is not lessened" (1). Therefore, in this book we will continue to use the milliosmol as the unit.

In clinical practice, the most commonly used term is *osmolality*, defined as the number of osmotic particles per *kilogram* of solvent, which, in biological systems, is water. Osmolarity, less commonly used, is measured per *liter* of solution (solute plus solvent). In tissue fluids that are very dilute, the difference between osmolality and osmolarity is small and can be ignored. In feeding solutions, which contain large amounts of solute, the values are significantly different, with osmolarity as low as 80 percent of osmolality. *Osmolality* is the preferred term for liquid formulas.

When sufficient water has moved across the semipermeable membrane so that the concentration of particles is equal on both sides of the membrane, the solutions are called *isotonic*. For clinical purposes, an example of an isotonic solution is 5 percent glucose. Another example of an isotonic solution is 0.85 percent sodium chloride (NaCl), also known as *normal saline*. A *hypotonic* saline solution has less NaCl than does an isotonic solution, while a *hypertonic* saline solution has a higher NaCl concentration. It is important to remember that, in clinical usage, a 5-percent solution consists of 5 g of material in 100 mL of solution.

FLUID EXCRETION

Routes of fluid excretion, summarized in Table 4-3, are urine, feces, respiratory water loss (via the lungs), and perspiration (via the skin). Urinary fluid excretion may be divided into two parts. *Obligatory* excretion represents the minimum necessary to remove the waste materials to be excreted in the urine. The amount of obligatory excretion is dependent on the concentrating ability of the kidney. *Facultative* excretion depends on the tubular resorption rate and fluctuating body needs.

The materials that normally must be excreted in largest amount by the kidney are products of protein metabolism, mainly *urea*. In addition, sodium, potassium, and chloride must be excreted. These materials, which together constitute the *renal solute load (RSL)*, determine the volume of fluid needed for excretion. Carbohydrate and fat normally do not contribute to the RSL because they are metabolized to carbon dioxide and water and do not appear in the urine.

The kidneys of a normal adult are able to concentrate urine to 1,200 to 1,400 mOsm/L. The immature kidneys of infants or diseased kidneys with low concentrating ability are not able to do so. They require more fluid for an equivalent amount of load. Diets producing a large solute load—high-protein or high-salt diets, for example—result in higher fluid requirement.

To calculate the RSL, the following values are useful. Each gram of protein (or amino acids) yields an RSL of 5.7 mOsm in adults. On the other hand, in young children, the yield from each gram of protein is less and varies with the rate of growth (2). Anabolic patients would also excrete less urea. Conversely, the catabolic patient would have an increased RSL as a result of catabolism of body protein. The catabolized protein is assumed to be excreted as urea. In all patients, in addition to the osmolality of the nitrogen compounds, each millequivalent of electrolyte yields 1 mOsm.

The total renal solute load of an adult may be estimated from a simplified equation:

$$mOsm = (g\ protein \times 5.7) + mEq\ (Na + K + Cl)$$
$$\textbf{(4-2)}$$

Total RSL is calculated as milliosmole per day, and all values used in the formula refer to the amount per day.

Kidneys work most efficiently when urine output in milliliters is 1.5 to 2 × RSL, justifying additional water intake. This does not apply if mild dehydration is desired, as in the case of head injury. In the unfed patient, the dietary RSL is zero, but we do not expect urine output to cease since catabolism continues. Obligatory urine output for these patients is estimated to be 700 mL per day, or 30 mL per hour.

Filtration

In filtration, water and dissolved substances are transferred from a region of high pressure to a region of low pressure. For example, in the capillary bed, hydrostatic pressure resulting from the beating of the heart causes the transfer by filtration of water and electrolytes to the interstitial fluid, which has low pressure.

Active Transport

The expenditure of energy is also necessary to move materials against a chemical or electrical gradient. For example, active transport expends energy (ATP) to move sodium from the ICF to the ECF, and potassium in the opposite direction. In general, a gain or loss of sodium in a compartment is accompanied by a gain or loss of water.

HYDRATION STATUS

The normal osmolality of plasma is usually given as 280 to 295 mOsm/kg for adults and 270 to 285 mOsm/kg for children. However, a range of 280 to 320 mOsm/kg in adults is generally considered acceptable and not of clinical concern.

Serum osmolality can be calculated from values found in a patient's chart. Osmotic pressure is dependent on the numbers, *not* weight, of particles in a given unit of water.

Large numbers of small molecules, such as glucose and electrolytes, exert the greatest osmotic pressure, while small numbers of large molecules, such as proteins, exert little osmotic pressure in most body fluids. The electrolyte sodium is the source of 90 to 95 percent of the osmotic pressure of the *extracellular* fluid. This is reflected in the calculation of serum osmolality using the equation:

$$\text{Serum osmolality} = (2 \times \text{serum Na})$$
$$+ \frac{\text{BUN}}{2.8} + \frac{\text{Plasma Glucose}}{18} \tag{4-3}$$

where serum osmolality is in mOsm/kg, serum Na is in mEq/L, and plasma glucose and BUN (as a measure of urea) are in mg/dL.

The Na^+ concentration is multiplied by 2, because each Na^+ cation is accompanied by an unmeasured anion. The constant 2.8 is derived from the two nitrogen molecules (mol wt = 14) in urea. Thus, each 28 mg per dL will raise serum osmolality by 10 mOsm/L. The constant 18 is derived from the molecular weight (180) of glucose. The remainder of the osmotic pressure is provided by potassium (K), calcium (Ca), and magnesium (Mg) cations, again with matching anions to maintain electrical neutrality in body fluids. These are commonly chloride (Cl^-) or bicarbonate HCO_3^-).

Intracellular osmotic pressure is provided mainly by potassium as the cation, with small contributions by magnesium and sodium. The major anion is phosphate. We assume that the total intracellular osmotic pressure is equal to that in the extracellular fluid, even though it is not measured.

HORMONAL CONTROL OF FLUID BALANCE

There are two hormones that function in fluid and electrolyte balance by regulation of the osmolality of the extracellular fluid (ECF).

Antidiuretic Hormone
Secretion of antidiuretic hormone (ADH or vasopressin) by the posterior pituitary gland tends to result in the retention of fluid. Increased ADH secretion is caused by

1. Reduced volume of the ECF (hypovolemia)
2. Increased osmolality of the ECF (hyperosmolality)
3. Increased serum sodium (hypernatremia)

ADH secretion may be increased by abnormal conditions such as acute or chronic lung disease, oat cell carcinoma of the lung, meningitis, encephalitis or heat trauma affecting the central nervous system, and myxedema (advanced adult thyroxin deficiency). It also occurs as the result of the action of some drugs, e.g., morphine (analgesic), chlorpropamide (hypoglycemic agent), cyclophosphamide, and vincristine (antineoplastics).

The ADH decreases the permeability of the renal tubules to water, so water is reabsorbed. As a consequence, urine volume is decreased and urine osmolality is increased. The dilutional effect of the reabsorbed fluid in the body fluids results in both lowered sodium concentration and osmolality.

Diminished ADH secretion, on the other hand, occurs because of

1. Increased IVF or ECF volume (hypervolemia)
2. Decreased osmolality of the ECF and hyponatremia

Reduced ADH action results in increased volume of urine with low osmolality. The loss of fluid and reduced diutional effect thus counteract the hypervolemia and hypo-osmolality.

Deficient ADH secretion occurs in diabetes insipidus (ADH deficiency in pituitary or hypothalamic lesion), head injury, renal tubular hormone resistance, or use of drugs such as alcohol, narcotic antagonists, and lithium carbonate (psychotropic drug) (3).

Aldosterone
Aldosterone, secreted from the adrenal cortex, affects fluid balance by controlling sodium absorption from the kidney tubules. It increases sodium and chloride reabsorption as well as excretion of potassium and hydrogen from the tubules.

Aldosterone secretion is increased in sodium deprivation, increased potassium, trauma, burns, surgery, decreased cardiac output, and hypovolemia. An adrenal tumor can result in *primary hyperaldosteronism,* while congestive heart failure, cirrhosis of the liver, and nephrotic syndrome may be accompanied by secondary hyperaldosteronism. The sodium excess of high aldosterone levels, accompanied by water reabsorption, presents as thirst, increased ICF and ECF, hypertonicity, and hypernatremia.

When aldosterone secretion is decreased, a primary sodium deficit results with decreased ECF, increased ECF, and hyponatremia. This condition can result from salt loading, potassium deficit, and hypervolemia (3).

FLUID IMBALANCES

Disturbances in body fluids are the result of abnormal differences between gains and losses of water and electrolytes and of shifts between compartments. Often, fluid imbalances are accompanied by changes in electrolytes. These will be discussed later in this chapter.

Extracellular Fluid Volume Deficit
This deficit, also known as *hypovolemia* (low plasma volume), or *dehydration*, may be caused by a sudden decrease in fluid intake, by acute loss of secretions or increased volume of excretions from the body, or a combination of both. It occurs, for example, in severe or prolonged vomiting, diarrhea, fistula draining, intestinal obstruction, polyuria, third space

losses, and any condition accompanied by elevated body temperature. Normally, about 8 liters of water are secreted and absorbed from the gastrointestinal tract daily. In disease states with vomiting and diarrhea, the loss may be as much as 30 liters, producing severe dehydration.

The dehydrated patient has weight loss (2 percent, mild; 5 percent, moderate; 8 percent, severe), dry skin and mucous membranes, rapid pulse, decreased venous pressure, subnormal body temperature, low blood pressure, and altered sensorium. Decreased perfusion of the kidney results in lower urine output. As fluid content of the plasma decreases, other substances in the blood become more concentrated (*hemoconcentration*), and plasma protein, hemoglobin and red cell levels rise.

The objective of treatment is to restore fluid volume while maintaining normal electrolyte composition. In particular, normal perfusion in the kidney must be restored and maintained. Restoration of fluid volume greater than mild thirst is usually done with intravenous fluid and electrolytes, e.g., lactated Ringer's solution. See Chapter 22 for further discussion.

Patients who are at risk of dehydration, must be monitored carefully:

1. Daily body weight can indicate large fluid losses or gains. For example, a weight loss of 2 kilograms in 48 hours indicates a corresponding loss of 2 liters of fluid.
2. Measure all gastrointestinal losses, urinary output, fluid absorbed into dressings.
3. Record incidents of diaphoresis (excessive perspiration).
4. Review laboratory values for serum sodium, potassium, chloride, BUN, creatinine, and glucose.

Most of these data are provided by the nursing staff and by laboratory results that can be found in the patient's medical record.

Extracellular Fluid Volume Excess

Fluid excess is also referred to as *overhydration* or *hypervolemia* (abnormal increase in plasma volume). It is most commonly caused by the inability of the kidneys to excrete excess water and electrolytes. It may also result from administration of excess normal saline to the patient or to chronic renal disease, congestive heart failure, or the portal hypertension seen in liver failure.

The objective of therapy of fluid excess is to remove the excess water without changing normal electrolyte concentrations. The patient is often restricted in fluid intake, and many are given diuretic medications to increase urine output.

Many of the monitoring procedures for patients with fluid excess are similar to those used with the dehydrated patients. Body weight, records of fluid intake and output, and laboratory values are useful. The amount of edema can be estimated by feeling with light pressure of the fingers (*palpation*) and, in the case of ascites, measuring abdominal circumference.

Shifts from Plasma to Interstitial Fluid

Capillary membranes consist of a single layer of endothelial cells with cement-filled spaces between them. The capillaries behave as though they had "pores" through which water and electrolytes can pass. Transfer of fluid and small molecules from the vascular to interstitial space occurs by (1) diffusion and (2) filtration. The rate of filtration is proportional to the filtration pressure, that is, hydrostatic pressure in the capillary minus hydrostatic pressure in the ISF. On the other hand, the capillaries are not permeable to plasma proteins and other compounds except those of very small size (e.g., urea). Small amounts of proteins cross the capillary wall, apparently via pinocytosis and exocytosis.

The filtration pressure is opposed by the osmotic effect of the protein in the capillary. This osmotic effect is known as *oncotic pressure*. At the arteriolar end of the capillary, hydrostatic pressure exceeds oncotic pressure, and fluid moves out of the capillary. At the venous end, hydrostatic pressure has dropped below oncotic pressure, and fluid moves back into the capillary. There is normally a slight balance in favor of fluid movement *out* of the capillary. The resulting accumulated excess is moved via the lymphatic system to the thoracic duct and then to the blood.

An abnormal increase in fluid shift to the ISF results in a condition(s) known as:

> **edema**, abnormal accumulation of intercellular fluid,
> **anasarca**, generalized massive edema or, sometimes,
> **ascites**, an abnormal accumulation of edema fluid in the peritoneal cavity.

These abnormalities occur in a number of conditions which have one or more of the following in common:

> Increased hydrostatic pressure, general or localized
> Decreased oncotic pressure
> Increased capillary permeability

Specific conditions in which these occur will be discussed in later chapters.

As fluid shifts out of the vascular system and into the interstitial space, the clinical manifestations are hypovolemia, pallor, weakness, tachycardia, and oliguria, all indicating a drop in blood volume and blood pressure. Also, as the fluid component of the blood decreases, the hemoglobin, hematocrit and red cell counts increase as the blood becomes less dilute.

In conditions in which this fluid shift occurs, the vascular volume must be restored and maintained while the underlying disorder is treated. Progress in restoring the intravascular fluid deficit may be evaluated by monitoring body weight, blood pressure, central venous pressure, heart rate, and urine output, which would rise. Heart rate and hemoglobin and hematocrit levels would decrease as the fluid deficit is corrected.

Shifts from Interstitial Fluid to Plasma

In recovery from the condition described in the section above, fluid is returned to the vascular system. Administration of large amounts of plasma protein may also cause a fluid shift to the blood stream.

Clinical evidence includes hypervolemia, venous engorgement, bounding pulse, cardiac dilation, and moist lung rales, an abnormal sound indicating fluid in the air passages. Hematocrit, hemoglobin, and red cell counts decrease as the returning fluid dilutes their concentration. Progress is frequently monitored by measuring body weight.

ELECTROLYTE BALANCE

The term *electrolytes* refers to substances that develop an electric charge when dissolved in water. The principle positively charged electrolytes are sodium, potassium, calcium, and magnesium. Principal negative ions are chloride, bicarbonate, and phosphate.

Intracellular fluid contains principally potassium and phosphate, while extracellular fluid contains mostly sodium and chloride. Plasma also contains protein, which maintains the oncotic pressure.

INDIVIDUAL ELECTROLYTES

A derangement in one electrolyte or in water usually results in a change in one or more of the others. However, for greater ease of understanding, each is described individually. Tables 4-4 to 4-9 are text tables summarizing functions, causes, and clinical manifestations of deficiencies and excesses. These may be consulted when reading later chapters.

The sum of the cations in serum or plasma is normally 155 mEq/L, and the sum of the anions also equals 155 mEq/L. These totals can be greater when water loss occurs, or smaller when electrolytes are low. Regardless of these conditions, electrical equivalence is maintained.

Electrolyte disturbances will also be discussed in later chapters in relation to specific diseases.

RELATIONSHIPS BETWEEN WATER, ELECTROLYTES, AND ENERGY

The complex interrelationships among water, electrolyte and energy balances, and distribution are disturbed in many pathological conditions. These include malnutrition, burns, cancer, trauma, hypertension, and some diseases of the kidneys, liver, heart, and gastrointestinal tract. Some of the relationships among sodium, potassium fluid, and energy will be described more specifically in ensuing chapters.

Sodium and Fluid

The size of the ECF space is largely controlled by sodium balance. As a rule, a gain or loss of sodium is accompanied by a gain or loss of water. Therefore, the extracellular fluid volume (ECFV) increases with positive sodium balances and decreases with negative sodium balance. The ECFV is important in supporting the circulation, including circulation to the kidneys, and, thus, the excretion of water and of sodium.

Several derangements of sodium and water balance can occur (4):

1. *Isotonic dehydration (water loss in isotonic proportions to sodium loss)* results in depletion of the ECFV. It occurs in gastrointestinal fluid losses, burns, chronic renal failure, osmotic diuresis, and excess sweating. Signs and symptoms include hypotension, tachycardia, weak pulse, poor skin turgor, cool extremities, and increases in hematocrit and hemoglobin. In treatment, both water and sodium are given.

2. *Hypertonic dehydration (hyperosmolality; hypernatremia; water deficit)* indicates water loss greater than sodium loss resulting in serum sodium concentration greater than 145 mEq/L. These losses can be the consequence of inadequate water intake in impaired consciousness, impaired thirst, or in severely weak or restrained patients. Losses can also result from losses of solute-free water from the gastrointestinal or respiratory system, severe sweating, or in renal loss when there is a concentrating defect. Signs and symptoms include confusion, stupor, decreased intravascular volume, and intracellular dehydration. Treatment consists of hypotonic solutions, isotonic nonelectrolyte solutions, or oral low-electrolyte solutions if the patient can take fluids by mouth.

The size of the water deficit can be calculated as follows:

$$\text{H}_2\text{O deficit (L)} = 0.6 \times \text{BW} \times \frac{(\text{Na} - 140)}{\text{Na}} \quad \textbf{(4-4)}$$

where BW = body weight in kg

    0.6 = proportion of adult male body weight, which is water (use 0.5 for adult females)
    Na = serum Na concentration in mEq/L
    140 = normal serum sodium concentration in mEq/L

3. *Hypotonic dehydration (hypo-osmolality, hyponatremia)* occurs when there is excess water relative to the solute content of body fluids. It occurs when sodium loss is greater than water loss and may be associated with low, normal, or high ECFV.

Clinical manifestations include hypovolemia, low serum sodium, and low serum osmolality. This condition can occur in excess use of diuretics, adrenal insufficiency, gastrointestinal suctioning, and renal tubular disease (low ECFV), in hyperglycemia, administration of excess free water, inappropriate ADH secretion (normal ECFV), and in congestive heart failure, nephrotic syndrome, renal failure, and cirrhosis of the liver (high ECFV). If the low sodium concentration is the result of dilution with excess water, the extent of the excess can be calculated as follows:

$$H_2O \text{ excess} = 0.6 \times BW \times \frac{140 - Na}{140} \quad \textbf{(4-5)}$$

See Eq. (4-4) for the meaning of the symbols.

4. *Salt and water excess* results in expansion of the extracellular space. Clinical manifestations include sudden weight gain, edema, ascites, oliguria, hypertension, distended neck veins, and pulmonary congestion. An underlying cardiac, renal, or hepatic disease is usually present. Patients are often treated with diuretics and fluid restriction.

Sodium, Potassium, and Energy Metabolism

The sodium pump (Na-K-ATPase pump) is important in maintaining cell volume. When the pump is inadequate, the intracellular fluid becomes hypertonic, and the cell could swell and burst as fluid moves in. The sodium pump exchanges sodium for potassium, pumping sodium out of the ICF in exchange for potassium. The pump also maintains transmembrane electric potential and participates in the transport of glucose and nitrogen across the cell membrane.

The sodium pump has a high-energy need, estimated to be as much as 40 percent of basal metabolic rate. Thus, in conditions where membrane permeability to sodium increases (e.g., traumatic injury), increased energy expenditure is required to maintain the sodium gradient across the membrane.

Energy is also required for renal function which, in time, regulates whole-body water, sodium and potassium. Malnutrition reduces glomerular filtration rate, renal blood flow, renal concentrating ability, and acid excretion.

TABLE 4-4   Sodium

	Hypernatremia	Hyponatremia

Functions:	Regulates body fluid:
	    Water retention
	    Maintenance of fluid volumes, including blood volume and circulation
	    Maintenance of osmotic pressure
	    Water excretion
	Regulates acid-based balance
	Irritability of nerves	

Imbalances	Hypernatremia	Hyponatremia
	(Usually same as hyperosmolality with water deficit)	(Usually same as hypoosmolality with water excess)
Causes and contributing factors	Inadequate water intake Excess administration of salt (oral or IV) Watery diarrhea Osmotic diuresis High-protein diet with inadequate water Cushing's disease Primary hyperaldosteronism	Diuretic therapy excess Acute or chronic renal failure Adrenal failure ECF depletion Major burns Fistula drainage ECF excess and edema Hypoaldosteronism SIADH (syndrome of inappropriate antidiuretic hormone) Sickle cell syndrome

Manifestation	Thirst
	    blood osmolality
	    plasma Na^+, plasma Cl^-
	Hypertension, tachycardia
	Confusion, obtundation
	Agitation, coma
	Dry, sticky mucus membranes
	Flushed skin
	Excess weight gain
	Dyspnea
	Pitting edema
		Plasma Na^+, plasma Cl^-
		Anorexia
		Nausea, vomiting, diarrhea
		ECF contraction, shock, circulatory failure
		Lethargy, stupor, coma
		Abdominal cramps

TABLE 4-5 Potassium

Functions:	Major intracellular cation
	Catalyst for energy production, cofactor in metabolism
	Synthesis of protein, glycogen
	Maintain fluid, electrolyte, acid-base balance, and osmotic pressure
	Determine resting membrane potential
	Transmission of nerve impulse, maintain muscle activity.

Imbalances	Hypokalemia	Hyperkalemia
Causes and contributing factors	Deficient intake: anorexia, alcoholism Diuretic therapy Glucocorticoid Renal: K^+-losing nephritis, pyelonephritis, renal tubular acidosis Surgery, wound healing, lean body mass, and glycogen synthesis and storage Gastrointestinal: suction, diarrhea, nausea, vomiting, fistulas, pancreatic drainage Sweat, fever, fluid overhydration, K^+-free IV fluids, excessive enemas Leukemia Shift into cells: alkalosis, excess insulin, hyperalimentation Cushing's syndrome, hyperaldosteronism, K^+-exchange resins Osmotic diuresis Large Na^+ intake Ingestion of licorice	K shift out of cells Fever, burns, crushing injury, thyrotoxicosis, acidosis, glycogenolysis, hyperglycemia, uncontrolled diabetes mellitus, digitalis toxicity Shock, dehydration, hypovolemia Excess intake, blood transfusions, K-containing medications Sodium deficiency Renal: acute or chronic failure, diuretic therapy Addison's disease
Manifestation	Low serum K^+ Low plasma Cl^- High plasma HCO_3^- Muscular weakness/paralysis, cyanosis, apnea, respiratory arrest Tachycardia, EKG abnormality, cardiac arrest, hypotension Anorexia, nausea, vomiting, abdominal distension Paralytic ileus Reflexes decreased or absent Metabolic alkalosis Digitalis toxicity Apathy, drowsiness, irritability, paresthesias, tetany, coma	Intraventricular conduction disturbances, bradycardia Cardiac arrest in diastole Muscle weakness Oliguria, anuria Diarrhea, nausea, intestinal colic Apathy, confusion, paresthesias of face, tongue, scalp, extremities Respiratory paralysis

ACID-BASE BALANCE

Normal cell function requires that the hydrogen ion concentration in the extracellular fluid be maintained within very narrow limits. Death occurs if these limits are violated.

ACIDS, BASES, AND BUFFERS: SOME DEFINITIONS

As a quick review, some definitions will be provided here. Greater detail is available in elementary biochemistry tests.

Acid, a substance that contains hydrogen ions (H^+) that can be released

Base, a substance that is able to accept hydrogen ions from acids

Buffer, a mixture of an acid and a base that acts to moderate changes in H^+ concentration

pH, the negative logarithm of the hydrogen ion concentration. A pH <7 indicates an acid; pH 7.0 is neutral, and pH >7 indicates a base.

TABLE 4-6   Chloride

Functions:	Major anion in ECF
	Maintenance of osmotic pressure and acid-based balance
	Conservation of K +
	Component of gastrointestinal secretion; synthesis of HCl in stomach
	Component of cerebral spinal fluid
	Chloride shift in RBC to increase CO_2 carrying capacity

Imbalances	Hyperchloremia	Hypochloremia
Causes and contributing factors	Acidosis	Water excess
	Iatrogenic-normal saline in nonalkalotic pts.	Wasting diseases
		Alkalosis 2° to HCO_3^-
		Persistent vomiting or suctioning without replacement
		Low-salt diet
		Salt-losing nephritis
		Diuretic use
		Prolonged sweating
Manifestation	Metabolic acidosis	Metabolic alkalosis
	Increased serum chloride	

NORMAL BLOOD PH

The optimum pH range in the ECF is from 7.35 to 7.45. Death occurs if the pH of the ECF is less than 6.8 or more than 7.8. Yet there are many circumstances that have the potential to change the pH of the ECF.

TABLE 4-7   Calcium

Functions:	Major component of bones and teeth
	Muscle contraction
	Nerve irritability
	Enzyme activator
	Blood coagulation

Imbalances	Hypercalcemia	Hypocalcemia
Causes and contributing factors	Hyperthyroidism	Malabsorption
	Immobilization	Bowel restriction
	Malignancies	Vitamin D deficiency
	Thiazide medication	Hypoparathyroidism
	Vitamin D and/or A intoxication	Acute pancreatitis
	Ionic exchange resins	Hypomagnesemia
	Parenteral nutrition	Uremia
		Massive transfusion
		IV Plasma expanders, phosphate
Manifestation	Depressed nerve function	Numbness and tingling of fingers, toes, around mouth
	Drowsiness, confusion, loss of memory, decreased reflexes	Hyperactive reflexes
	Muscle weakness, hypotonia	Muscle cramps
	Soft tissue calcification	Chvostek's and Trousseau's signs
	Thirst, polydipsia, anorexia, nausea, vomiting, constipation	Convulsions
	Pancreatitis	Cardiac arrhythmias
	Peptic ulcer disease	Bone pain, fragility, deformities, fractures
	Polyuria, renal calculi, hypertension, renal failure	

TABLE 4-8   Phosphorus

Functions:	Major anion in cells, organic form in carbohydrate, fat, protein inorganic for generation of ATP
	Essential for synthesis of phospholipids in cell membranes, nucleic acids, and nucleoproteins, ATP, creatine phosphate
	Oxygen delivery to tissues with ATP and diphosphoglycerate
	In renal buffering system

Imbalances	Hyperphosphatemia	Hypophosphaternia
Causes and contributing factors	Renal disease	Hyperaldosteronism
	Hypoparathyroidism	Hyperparathyroidism
	Increased intake, e.g., as in antacids, laxatives, enemas, oral agents	Volume expansion; glucose administration
		Gram-negative bacteremia
		Alcoholism
		Hypocalcemia, hypokalemia, hypomagnesemia
		Malabsorption, starvation
		Refeeding syndrome
		Pregnancy
		Hemodialysis
		Administration of fructose, glycerol, lactate, bicarbonate, diuretics, insulin, glucagon, gastrin, phosphate binders
Manifestations	Neuroexcitability	Decreased ATP
	Tetany	Malaise, ataxia, encephalopathy seizures, coma
	Convulsions	Muscle weakness, cardiac and respiratory failure
		Red blood cell hemolysis
		Acute liver failure
		Proximal renal tubule dysfunction
		Metabolic acidosis
		Increased parathyroid hormone
		Calcium resorption from bone
		Bone pain

SOURCES OF ACID IN THE BODY

Diet and tissue metabolism are the primary sources of acid in the body. These acids are categorized as (1) *volatile acids*, (2) *inorganic acids*, and (3) *organic acids*.

The greatest source of *volatile acids* is carbon dioxide (CO_2), produced via metabolic processes. It reacts with water to form carbonic acid in a reversible equation:

$$CO_2 + H_2O \leftrightarrow H_2CO_3 \leftrightarrow H^+ + HCO_3^- \qquad \textbf{(4-6)}$$
$$\text{(acid)} \qquad\qquad\qquad \text{(base)}$$

Inorganic acids include sulfuric and phosphoric acids. Sulfuric acid is produced from metabolism of methionine and cystine from protein in the diet. Phosphoric acid is produced from metabolism of organic phosphorus compounds.

Organic acids include lactic acid and uric acid. In addition, β-hydroxybutyric and acetoacetic acids are produced in incomplete metabolism of carbohydrate and fat. These acids are especially important in diabetes mellitus (see Chapter 19).

REGULATION OF THE ACID-BASE BALANCE

The regulation of acid-base balance within very narrow limits is provided by three "systems" of control: (1) chemical buffers in body fluids, (2) the respiratory system, and (3) the kidneys.

The Chemical Buffer System
The buffers in the body fluids act at the cellular level to accept or donate electrons. The most important example is given in Eq. 4-6 above in which CO_2 reacting with water, is the acid, and bicarbonate (HCO_3^-) is the base in the acid-base pair.

Other buffers include: (1) the phosphate system and (2) the blood proteins, including hemoglobin. The buffer pair in the phosphate system consists of NaH_2PO_4 (the acid or hydrogen donor) and Na_2HPO_4 (the base or hydrogen acceptor), the relative amounts depending on the pH of the environment. The phosphate buffer acts primarily within cells. It is especially important in red blood cells and in tubule cells of the kidney. Protein also acts in the tissue cells and in the plasma. Hemoglobin: oxyhemoglobin is an important protein buffer pair in the red blood cells.

The chemical buffer system is the most rapid regulator. It functions within a fraction of a second.

The Respiratory System
The respiratory system controls the hydrogen ion concentration by affecting the CO_2 content of the plasma. As Eq. 4-6 shows, the amount of hydrogen ion is

TABLE 4-9 Magnesium

Functions:	Hormone secretion	
	Protein secretion	
	Bone mineralization	
	Enzyme reactions	
	Calcium and potassium balance	

Imbalances	Hypermagnesemia	Hypomagnesemia
Cause and contributing factors	Rare: Hyperparathyroidism Aldosteronism Antacid ingestion in renal failure	Decreased intake: malnutrition, chronic alcoholism, prolonged IV therapy Decreased absorption: malabsorption syndrome, short-bowel syndrome Gastrointestinal losses: laxative use, nasogastric suction, biliary and intestinal fistulas Urinary losses: renal tubule disorders, diuretics, diabetic ketoacidosis Acute pancreatitis Multiple transfusions Osmotic diuresis Drug toxicity Congenital syndromes: Bartter's, Welt's
Manifestation	Transient hypotension arrhythmias Muscle weakness Respiratory depression Depression, paralysis, loss of deep tendon reflexes, coma	Hypokalemia, hypophosphatemia, hypocalcemia, metabolic alkalosis Anorexia, nausea, weakness Vertigo, tetany Irritability, depression, psychoses EKG changes, cardiac arrhythmias, cardiac arrest Tumors

directly related to the amount of CO_2 produced. When H^+ concentration is high, it acts on the respiratory center in the brain to increase the rate of respiration, removing CO_2 and thus reducing H^+ concentration. The pH then rises. For example, if a patient has a normal respiratory rate of 20 breaths per minute and a blood pH of 7.4, doubling the respiratory rate to 40 can raise the blood pH to 7.63.

Conversely, when H^+ concentration is low, the respiratory rate decreases and CO_2 is retained. The pH then falls. For example, reducing a respiratory rate of 20 to 5 breaths per minute can reduce blood pH to 7.0. This system is slower than chemical buffering but responds within minutes.

The Renal System

The kidneys affect the H^+ concentration primarily by manipulating the blood bicarbonate concentration. CO_2 combines to form carbonic acid and then bicarbonate—Eq.4-6, again!—in the renal tubule cells. The H^+ is secreted into the glomerular filtrate, and a sodium ion is reabsorbed in exchange. The bicarbonate ion in the tubule cell combines with the sodium and diffuses back into the ECF, making a greater amount of base available.

Renal action provides the slowest control of H^+ concentration. It acts within a few hours to more than a day.

ACID-BASE IMBALANCES

Four major imbalances are the consequences of decreases in the body's ability to regulate hydrogen ion concentration. These are (1) respiratory acidosis, (2) respiratory alkalosis, (3) metabolic acidosis, and (4) metabolic alkalosis. The respiratory imbalances involve primarily alterations in carbon dioxide control, while metabolic imbalances involve bicarbonate control. These may be acute or chronic. In addition, mixtures of these may occur.

Table 4-10 gives the primary disturbance, compensatory mechanisms, causes and contributing factors, and the signs and symptoms of each of these conditions.

INTERPRETING LABORATORY VALUES

The patient's acid-base status is determined from arterial blood gases (ABGs) measured in blood obtained from the radial, brachial, or femoral arteries. Blood bicarbonate concentration is measured at the same time. These values are used to assess the degree of acidosis or alkalosis.

The values for blood gases are given for oxygen and carbon dioxide as partial pressures, indicated as pO_2 and pCO_2. The mean and normal ranges of blood pH and ABG values are as follows:

TABLE 4-10　Summary of Hydrogen Ion Concentration Imbalances *

Type of Imbalance	Causes and Contributors	Signs and Symptoms	Primary Disturbance	Compensated Action
Respiratory Acidosis (or hypercapnia)	Airway obstruction Chronic lung disease Depressed respiratory center Cardiopulmonary failure Neuromuscular disorders (trauma, infection, drugs, metabolic or degenerative disease)	Blood pH < normal Serum Na and K may be >normal Decreased rate and depth of respiration Ventricular fibrillation; Tachycardia Dyspnea Headache Confusion Somnolence Hyperphosphatemia	↑pCO_2	↑ HCO_3^- concentration via: ↑ renal acid excretion and ↑ renal HCO_3^- generation
Respiratory alkalosis (or hypocapnia)	Lung disease Central nervous system disease Congestive heart failure Liver failure Sepsis Hypoxia Salicylate toxicity Anxiety Fever Mechanical ventilator-related condition	Blood pH > normal ↑ Chloride ↓ serum phosphate ↓ serum potassium Depressed mentation Seizures Tetany Paresthesias Hypotension ↓ Cardiac output ↓ Cardiac arrhythmias	↓ pCO_2	↓ HCO_3^- concentration via ↓ renal acid excretion and ↑ HCO_3^- excretion in urine
Metabolic acidosis	*With increased anion gap (> 16 mEq/L):* 　Uremia 　Ketoacidosis 　　e.g. diabetes, alcoholic starvation 　Lactic acidosis 　Toxicity 　　e.g, salicylate, methyl alcohol *Hyperchloremia (with normal anion gap):* 　Diarrhea 　Adrenal insufficiency 　Pancreatic drainage 　Biliary drainage 　Hyperalimentation 　Renal tubular acidosis 　Treatment with NH_4Cl, $CaCl_2$, amino acids chloride salts, cholestyramine 　Uretoenteric diversion	Blood pH < normal Hyperkalemia Anorexia Nausea Lethargy Tachycardia Pulmonary edema Ventricular fibrillation Hyperkalemia Deep respirations	↓ HCO_3^-	↓ pCO_2 via hyperventilation
Metabolic Alkalosis	Vomiting Gastric suction Diuretics Villous adenoma Congenital chloride diarrhea Primary hyperaldosteronism Cushing's syndrome Bartter's syndrome Severe hypokalemia	↑ Blood pH CO_2 normal ↓ K and Cl Lethargy Confusion Agitation Twitching Cardiac arrhythmias Hypoxemia Hypokalemia	↑ HCO_3^- concentration	↑ pCO_2 via hypoventilation

* ↑ = increased;.　↓ = decreased;　HCO_3^- = bicarbonate;　pCO_2 = carbon dioxide tension.

pH	7.4 (7.35–7.45)
pO_2	90 (80–100) mm Hg
pCO_2	40 (35–45) mm Hg
HCO_3^-	24 (22–26) mEq/L

The first three of these are reported in the medical record in the following form:

$$ABG = 7.40/90/40$$

where pH, pO_2, and pCO_2 are given in sequence.

These values and serum bicarbonate are used, not only to determine the patient's acid-base status, but also to differentiate among the four types of disturbances in acid-base balance.

Some general guidelines may be used for interpretation of these laboratory values. To simplify the examples, we will use the mean values just given and ignore the ranges.

First, determine the direction of the change from normal by comparing the patient's blood pH to the normal value. It is increased in alkalosis and decreased in acidosis. Thus, a pH of 7.2 indicates acidosis; 7.5 indicates alkalosis.

Then, determine the type of acidosis or alkalosis by identifying the parameter that is predominantly abnormal. The value for pCO_2 represents the respiratory effect on pH. An increase contributes to acidosis and indicates hypoventilaton. A decrease contributes to alkalosis and indicates hyperventilation. The pO_2 is not used in assessment of acid-base balance but is an indicator of oxygenation.

The bicarbonate represents the metabolic (nonrespiratory) effect on acid-base balance. A high value indicates alkalosis, while a low value is associated with acidosis.

Interpretation can be confirmed and quantified as follows: Determine the difference between the patient's pCO_2 and the normal value. Let us assume, for example, that the medical record gives the values 7.32/90/50. Then, $50 - 40 = 10$. Next, calculate the theoretical pH, assuming that *each change of 10 mm Hg in pCO_2 causes a change in pH of 0.08 units in the opposite direction.* If pCO_2 increases, pH will decrease (become more acid); if pCO_2 decreases, pH will increase (become more alkaline). Note carefully that the carbon dioxide represents the acid, and the bicarbonate represents the base in acid-base balance calculations. Thus, continuing the calculation:

$$7.4 - 0.08 = 7.32$$

If calculated and measured pH are very similar, the changes are caused by alterations in pCO_2; thus the changes are respiratory. In this example, the results indicate *respiratory* acidosis.

Another useful distinction is the differentiation between acute and chronic respiratory conditions. As a general rule of thumb, if the *change* in pH is of the order of 0.08 units, the respiratory acidosis or alkalosis is acute, while if the change is 0.2 to 0.3 units, the condition is chronic. The patient in the example, then, has acute respiratory acidosis.

In *metabolic* acidosis or alkalosis, a change in serum pH results from a change in serum bicarbonate. Bicarbonate values and pH vary from normal in the same direction, while the patient's pCO_2 changes from normal in a direction to compensate for the change in bicarbonate.

A patient who presents with an elevated pH resulting from increased bicarbonate (a base) will have a partially compensatory increase in pCO_2 (an acid). This patient is in metabolic alkalosis, a condition often referred to as *base excess.* For example, if values are ABG = 7.62/90/50, and serum bicarbonate is 50 mEq/L, the patient is in metabolic alkalosis. Since the base (bicarbonate) has increased more—from 24 to 50, or > 100 percent—than the pCO_2 (acid—from 40 to 50, or 20 percent— the patient is considered to have a base excess.

On the other hand, a patient who presents with a depressed pH resulting from bicarbonate loss will have a partially compensatory decrease in pCO_2. This patient is in metabolic acidosis, often referred to as *base deficit.* For example, if the record states that ABG = 7.20/90/25 and blood bicarbonate is 10 mEq/L, the patient has metabolic acidosis. Since the base (bicarbonate) has decreased more than pCO_2 (acid), the patient is considered to have a base deficit.

Metabolic acidosis can be caused by the addition of a strong acid or by the loss of base (via the GI tract or kidney). In order to distinguish between these two causes, the *anion gap* (AG) is calculated from concentrations of Na^+, K^+, Cl^-, and HCO_3^-:

$$AG = (Na^+ + K^+) - (Cl^- + HCO_3^-) \qquad (4\text{-}7)$$

where all values are stated in mEq/L. Normal anion gap is 12 to 16 mEq/L.

If the anion gap is greater than 16, there is a decrease in bicarbonate balanced by an increase in unmeasured H^+, instead of an increase in Cl^-. The patient has *normochloremic acidosis*, also called *anion gap acidosis*. This may occur in *diabetic ketoacidosis* (DKA), in other conditions causing increased acid production or decreased acid excretion, or when certain toxic materials have been ingested.

If the patient loses bicarbonate, balanced by an increase in chloride, the result is *nonanion gap (hyperchloremic) acidosis*. This condition may result from gastrointestinal or renal loss of bicarbonate.

SUMMARY

Disorders of fluid, electrolyte, and acid-base balances are common to a great many pathological conditions. The material in this chapter will be applied in most of the chapters which follow.

TOPICS FOR FURTHER DISCUSSION

1. Food sources of selected electrolytes.

REFERENCES

1. **Young, D.S**. Implementation of SI units for clinical laboratory data. *Ann. Int. Med.* 106: (1987)114—129.

2. **Fomon, S.J.**, and **E.E. Ziegler**. Water and renal solute load. In *Nutrition of Normal Infant*, St. Louis: Mosby, 1993, 91.

3. **Ganong, W.F.** *Review of Medical Physiology*, 16th ed. Norwalk, CT: Appleton Lange, 1993.

4. **Goldberger, E.** *A Primer of Water, Electrolyte and Acid-Base Syndromes*, 7th ed. Philadelphia: Lea & Febiger, 1986.

ADDITIONAL SOURCES OF INFORMATION

Arieff, A.I., and **R.A. De Fronzo**. *Fluid, Electrolyte and Acid-Base Disorders*. New York: Churchill Livingstone, 1985.

Cogan, M.G. *Fluid and Electrolyte—Physiology and Pathophysiology*. Norwalk, CT: Appleton & Lange, 1991.

Collins, R.D. *Illustrated Manual of Fluid and Electrolyte Disorders*, 2nd ed. Philadelphia: Lippincott, 1983.

Groer, M.W. *Physiology and Pathophysiology of the Body Fluids*, 2d ed. St. Louis: Mosby, 1981.

Halperin, M.L. and **M.B. Goldstein**. *Fluid, Electrolyte and Acid-Base Physiology*, 2d ed. Philadelphia: Saunders, 1994.

Kokko, J.P. and **R.L. Tannen**, eds. *Fluids and Electrolytes* 2d ed. Philadelphia: Saunders, 1990.

Drieger, J.N. and **D.S. Sherrard**. *Practical Fluids and Electrolytes*. Norwalk, CT: Appleton & Lange, 1991.

Metheny, N.M. *Fluid and Electrolyte Balance. Nursing Considerations*. Philadelphia: Lippincott, 1992.

Rose, B.D. *Clinical Physiology of Acid-Base and Electrolyte Disorders*, 4th ed. New York: McGraw-Hill, 1994.

Stroot, V.R., **C.A.B. Lee** and **C.A. Barrett**. *Fluids and Electrolytes— A Practical Approach*, 3d ed. Philadelphia: Davis, 1984.

☑ TO TEST YOUR UNDERSTANDING

1. a. Estimate the total water available to the following patient. 20 y.o. active adult male. 75 kg total body weight.
Diet: 100 g protein, 80 g fat, 250 g carbohydrate, and containing 1,550 ml preformed water.
Fluids: 1,500 ml in water, fruit juice, soup, and soft drinks.
b. Estimate this man's normal fluid needs. Show your calculations.

2. In the list below, number the substances in order of their osmolality when each is mixed in the same quantity of water. Number the most osmotically active material as 1 and the least active as 7.

—— NaCl, 1 mmol
—— MgCl$_2$, 1 mmol
—— Glucose, 180 mg
—— Sucrose, 180 mg
—— Dextrin, 180 mg
—— Glycine, 100 mg
—— Casein, 100 mg

3. Calculate the osmolality of a solution consisting of 1 g NaCl in 1,000 g H$_2$O. Show your calculations.

4. A patient has a serum Na level of 142 mEq/L, a BUN of 14 mg/dL, and blood glucose level of 100 mg/dL. Estimate the serum osmolality. Show your calculations. Compare the values given and your results with normal values.

5. If tube-feeding solutions with the following osmolalities are fed into the jejunum, give the net direction of fluid movement for each:
a. 600 mOsm/kg ——
b. 294 mOsm/kg ——
c. 176 mOsm/kg ——

6. Estimate the renal solute load of 2,000 ml of a feeding formula for an adult, providing 1 kcal/mL, 4.6 g crystalline amino acids/dL, and 20.3 g carbohydrate/dL. The formula contains, in addition, the following electrolytes: 3.3 mEq Na/dL, 1.79 mEq K/dL, and 5.24 mEq Cl/dL of formula. Show your calculations.

7. a. Calculate the obligatory fluid necessary for excretion when intake is 92.6 g protein and 2,320 mg NaCl. Show your calculations.
b. What fluid volume would provide maximum renal excretory efficiency?

8. The items in the list that follows may be found in formula feedings. In the spaces provided, write the letter *O* for any material that would have a significant effect on the osmolality of a tube feeding. Write an *R* before any material that would contribute significantly to renal solute load.

—— a. Casein   —— g. Disaccharides
—— b. Hydrolyzed Casein —— h. Monosaccharides
—— c. Crystalline   —— i. Triglycerides
　　　amino acids
—— d. Cornstarch   —— j. NaCl
—— e. Tapioca starch   —— k. NaHCO$_3$
—— f. Starch   —— l. KCl
　　　hydrolysates

9. Mrs. J.W. became dehydrated as a result of a urinary tract infection. Her body weight was 55 kg. Serum sodium value was 146 mEq/L.
a. List the symptoms you would expect to see in this patient.
b. Calculate the fluid deficit.

10. The following values are given for a patient:

	Patient	Normal
Blood glucose, mg/dL	504	——
Urine glucose (by test strip)	+++	——
ABG:　pH	7.21	——
pCO$_2$, mm Hg	2.7	——
HCO$_3$, mEq/L	11.2	——
Electrolytes:　Na$^+$, mEq/L	133	——
K$^+$, mEq/L	5.3	——
Cl$^-$, mEq/L	100	——
BUN	35	——

a. Fill in normal values in the spaces provided above.
b. Calculate the anion gap. Show your calculations.
c. Calculate the patient's serum osmolality. Show your calculations.
d. Circle the conditions indicated by these results and give the values that indicate the conditions you circle.

Respiratory acidosis   Dehydration
Metabolic acidosis   Normal hydration
Respiratory alkalosis   Normochloremic acidosis
Metabolic alkalosis   Hyperchloremic acidosis

5 Evaluating Nutritional Status

Nutritional assessment consists of the gathering and interpretation of data to (1) identify individuals who require specialized nutritional care, (2) determine the cause and degree of malnutrition, and (3) determine the potential risk for development of malnutrition or related complications. It serves as a basis for planning nutritional therapy and evaluating an individual's response to that therapy. In order to complete a comprehensive nutritional assessment, the nutritional care specialist must be skilled in anthropometric, biochemical, clinical, and dietary methods of evaluating nutritional status. This chapter discusses procedures for evaluating nutritional status in adults, including the elderly. Diet evaluation is described in Chapter 6, and nutritional assessment in children is discussed in Chapter 9. You will find it helpful to review the related material in your text before you begin. You will have an opportunity to practice the skills described in this chapter. In order to complete the practice exercises, you should have access to the following equipment:

1. Calipers for measuring skinfolds
2. Tape measure (or Inser-Tape from Ross Laboratories, Columbus, OH)

EVALUATION OF PROTEIN ENERGY STATUS

Protein energy status is evaluated primarily by anthropometric and biochemical methods.

ANTHROPOMETRIC MEASUREMENTS

Anthropometry is the measurement (*-ometry*) of man (*anthro-*). In clinical situations, anthropometry is used to estimate body energy stores and protein mass.

Anthropometric data usually consist of height, weight, skinfold measurements, and measurements of circumferences of various body parts.

Height and Weight

For most patients, height and weight measurements are obtained on admission and are useful for a rapid preliminary assessment of energy and protein stores. They are useful in combination with other observations but are of limited value when used alone, since they do not provide information on changes in body composition and are subject to alterations by disease processes unrelated to nutrition.

Measurement. Height and weight, which are measured by the nursing staff when the patient's condition permits, are recorded in the patient's medical record. Weight may be recorded in pounds or kilograms (1 kg = 2.2#). Height may be recorded in feet and inches or in centimeters (1 in = 2.54 cm). Height is ordinarily based on the patient's stature when standing. Tables of standard values may assume either that the subject is barefoot or that the subject is wearing shoes, in which case the height of the heel is indicated. To use such a table, therefore, the heel height must be added to the height of the barefoot patient. For example, to use a table based on the assumption that the subject is wearing shoes with 1-inch heels, a patient who is 5 feet, 5 inches tall without shoes must be considered to be 5 feet, 6 inches tall when using the table. For patients who are unable to stand, *sitting height*, or *crown-rump length*, may be measured, but this is considered less accurate. The total length of a recumbent patient is the *crown-heel length*, or *recumbent bed height*. It is approximately 3.68 cm greater than standing height (1).

Knee height can be used to indicate stature in patients who are bedfast, are confined to a wheelchair, or have curvature of the spine. This method is particularly useful with the elderly (2). The patient lies supine (on his back) and bends his left knee to a 90-degree angle. Measurement is made, with an especially large caliper, from under the heel of the foot to the anterior surface of the thigh at the knee. Knee height plus age and sex are used to compute stature using the following equations:

For men
$$\text{Height in cm} = 64.19 - (0.04 \times \text{age in years}) + (2.02 \times \text{knee height in cm}) \quad \textbf{(5-1)}$$

For women
$$\text{Height in cm} = 84.88 - (0.24 \times \text{age in years}) + (1.83 \times \text{knee height in cm}) \quad \textbf{(5-2)}$$

If necessary, stature may also be calculated from measurement of *arm span*, the distance between the tips of the middle fingers when both arms are maximally extended to the side at shoulder height. Arm span and stature are almost equal in the young adult. Since arm span does not change significantly as the patient ages, this method is useful in determining maximum mature stature (2, 3). Measurement of arm span can be difficult because of deformity of an arm, osteoporosis, kyphosis or lung disease. In such cases, it may be useful to double the measure from the notch at the top of the sternum to the fingertips of one arm (4, 5).

Bed scales may be available to weigh a recumbent patient who is unable to sit or stand on a scale. If measurements of height and weight are not available, the patient may be asked for this information, but information from a patient is notoriously inaccurate.

Some adjustments make these or other height-weight tables more suitable in reference to any individual. Adjustments for frame size, age, and amputations are common.

Frame Size Adjustments
The values in Tables F-1 and F-2 in Appendix F are categorized according to sex, age, and stature. However, body build (muscularity, bone thickness, and body proportions) also affect body weight. In order to adjust for these factors, it is necessary to adjust for an individual's frame size. Body frame size may be estimated in one of two ways:

a. Measurement of Wrist Circumference
Procedure:

Step.1: Measure the wrist circumference just distal (toward the hand) to the styloid process at the wrist crease of the left hand (see Fig. 5-1).

Step 2: Calculate the ratio (*r*) of height (ht) to wrist circumference with this equation:

$$r = \frac{\text{ht(cm)}}{\text{wrist circumference (cm)}} \quad \textbf{(5-3)}$$

Step 3: Determine frame size by comparing the *r* value with the following:

	Small	Medium	Large
Men	> 10.4	10.4 – 9.6	< 9.6
Women	>11	10.1 – 11.0	< 10.1

b. Measurement of Elbow Breadth
Procedure:

Step 1: The patient extends one arm and bends the forearm up at the 90-degree angle. The palm faces away from the body, and the fingers are straight.

Step 2: Measure the distance between the two prominent bones on each side of the elbow (the epicondyles of the humerus) with calipers.

Step 3: Consult Appendix Table F-3 for a range of elbow breadth measurements of medium-frame persons of various heights. Measurements lower than these values indicate a small frame; those higher than these values indicate a large frame.

In this manual, we will use the combined values obtained from the National Health and Nutrition Examination Surveys in 1971 to 1974 (NHANES I) and 1976 to 1980 (NHANES II). In total, the data are based on a sample size of 44,130 (6). Tables F-1 and F-2 in the appendix give the mean weights for heights and standard deviations for males and females for ages 2 to 74 years in this sample population. Weight for selected percentiles are also given. Note that procedures for nutritional assessments in children are given in Chapter 9.

If height-weight tables are not available as guidelines, "ideal" body weight (IBW) may be estimated by using the following equations:

For men
$$\text{IBW} = 106\# + 6\# \text{ for each inch} > 60 \text{ inches} \quad \textbf{(5-4)}$$

For women
$$\text{IBW} = 100\# + 5\# \text{ for each inch} > 60 \text{ inches} \quad \textbf{(5-5)}$$

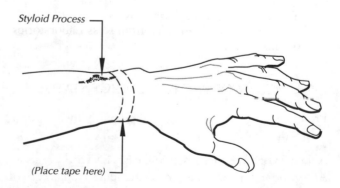

Styloid Process

(Place tape here)

FIGURE 5-1 Estimating Frame Size

In Eq. (5-4) and (5-5), adjustments for frame size are made by subtracting 10 percent for small frames and adding 10 percent for large frames.

Tables F-4 and F-5 give means, standard deviations, and percentiles of weights and ages for males and females, respectively, with small, medium and large frames.

Adjustment for Age

The age span of subjects included in Tables F-1, F-2, F-4, and F-5 is 36 years. However, there are age-related changes within the groupings given. Therefore, an age correction equation has been provided (7).

Adjusted weight standard = unadjusted weight
standard + (age correction factor × deviation
from median age) **(5-6)**

As an example, assume a medium-frame female patient, aged 60, height 154 cm, weight 65 kg. Her adjusted weight standard is 60.7 kg at the 50th pecentile (see Table F-2). Age correction factors and median weights are given in Table F-6. In the example given, the calculations would be:

Adjusted weight = 65 + (− 0.196)(60−66)
= 65 + (− 0.196)(−6)
= 65 + 1.206 = 66.2

Thus the patient's weight is 6.2 kg above the median.

Adjustment must also be made for the patient with an amputated extremity. An estimated weight of the amputated part should be subtracted from the standard of reference body weight to arrive at the adjusted body weight for the amputee. Following are some estimated weights:

Extremity	% of Total Body Weight
Hand	0.3
Forearm and hand	2.6
Entire arm	6.2
Foot	1.7
Below-knee amputation	7.0
Above-knee amputation	11.0
Entire leg	18.6

For example, a woman 5 feet, 4 inches tall as an estimated body weight of 120 pounds. If she were to have an above knee amputation,

$$120 - (120 \times 0.11) = 120 - 13 = 107$$

Adjusted body weight would then be 107 ± 11 pounds.

Interpretation. After consultation with a height-weight table and applying the corrections described above, a body weight value is obtained which has been described as "optimal," "ideal," or "desirable." In the interests of brevity, we will use the term *optimal body weight* (OBW).

Body weight either much greater or lower than OBW are risk factors. Body weight at the 85th percentile or more is associated with hypertension; hypercholesterolemia; diabetes; coronary heart disease; colon, rectal, and prostate cancers; and breast, uterine, endometrial, cervical, ovarian, and biliary system cancers (8). These studies found minimum mortality in subjects with relative weights at 75 to 105 percent. Relative weight (RW) is calculated:

$$RW = \frac{\text{actual weight}}{\text{midpoint of medium frame}} \times 100 \quad \textbf{(5-7)}$$

Relative weight corresponding to the 85th percentile is 120 percent..

An alternative method of evaluation uses the *body-mass index* (BMI) or Quetelet's index. The BMI is calculated from body weight in kilograms divided by the stature in meters squared:

$$BMI = \frac{\text{weight (kg)}}{[\text{stature (m)}]^2} \text{ or } \frac{w}{s^2} \quad \textbf{(5-8)}$$

For example, a woman who weighs 92.5 kg with a height of 162.5 cm or 1.625 m would have a BMI of $92.5/1.625^2 = 92.5/2.64 = 35$. Means and percentile are given in Table F - 7. The BMI corresponding to the 85th percentiles are 27.8 for men and 27.3 for women. Minimum mortality has been reported to be at a BMI of 22 to 25 (9) or 10 percent below the U.S. average (10).

Another classification of the BMI suggests overall risks (11):

BMI < 20: may be associated with health problems in some individuals.

BMI 20–25: associated with lowest risks for most

BMI 25–27: May be associated with health problems such as cardiovascular disease and diabetes.

The height-weight tables are often used to establish goals for weight loss in healthy individuals. For patients who are ill, however, the tables are often used to determine goals for weight gain or weight maintenance. When the patient has lost weight, other calculations are useful in evaluation. The proportion of weight loss may be calculated:

$$\text{Weight loss (\%)} = \frac{\text{UBW} - \text{CBW}}{\text{UBW}} \times 100 \quad \textbf{(5-9)}$$

where UBW = usual body weight
CBW = current body weight.

Alternatively, the proportion remaining of the usual weight is calculated by:

$$\text{Remaining usual weight } (\%) = \frac{\text{CBW}}{\text{UBW}} \times 100$$

$$(5\text{-}10)$$

At the high end of the scale, recall that values above the 85th percentile are also considered to indicate moderate risk, and those above the 95th percentile at high risk. Similar equations may be used to compare the patient's body weight to IBW, admission weight, weight at previous assessment, or weight prior to a specific course of treatment. One word of caution: If the patient is dehydrated or edematous, the weight data will be misleading.

An additional consideration is the rate at which weight loss occurred. One basis for interpretation, including both amount and rate of loss, is given in Appendix F, Table F-8.

An alternative method uses percentiles to show the position of the patient's measurements within the chosen population. A measurement at the 5th percentile, for example, is lower than the same measurement seen in 95 percent of that population. In these tables, measurements below the 5th percentile are considered depleted, while those between the 5th and 15th percentiles are considered to be at risk of becoming depleted. This method does not consider the rate at which the weight was lost, however.

Figure 5-2 diagrams a normal curve and the relationships of the percentiles and standard deviations, each of which may be used in interpretation of risk related to body weight. As a general rule of thumb, the mean ±1 standard deviation is within normal range. Values between 1 and 2 standard deviations from normal are "at risk," or "at risk of becoming..." or "at moderate risk." Values between 2 and 3 standard deviations from normal are "depleted," or "at high risk."

Body Fat Stores

Height and weight measurements are useful, but do not give information on the type of tissue that is gained or lost as weight changes. For this purpose, other measurements are necessary.

Skinfold thicknesses, which include the subcutaneous fat layer, are measured to indicate the body's calorie reserve. Sites, often used in combination, are the skinfolds over the biceps and triceps muscles and in the sub scapular and suprailiac area.

Triceps Skinfold (TSF). The most commonly used site is over the triceps muscle. Depending on the institution, the accepted procedure may be to use either the nondominant arm or the right arm. When sequential measurements are made, they must be done in exactly the same way. Fat distribution varies with location; therefore, techniques must be precise in order to be reproducible.

Procedure

Step 1: Take the measurement on the bare arm with the patient standing or sitting erect if possible. The arm should be hanging down at the side. Alternatively, a supine patient may be asked to lift the arm so that the elbow is pointing to the ceiling. The arm is bent at a 90-degree angle, and the hand is in a fist with palm facing up.

Step 2: Locate the olecranon process of the ulna and the acromial process of the scapula, and mark each point on the skin with a pen or adhesive label.

Step 3: Place a tape measure between the two points, and mark the midpoint in line with the olecranon process. (The Inser-Tape is useful for this purpose for practice in class but should not be used clinically. See Fig. 5-3).

Step 4: Pick up, between thumb and forefinger, a vertical fold of skin and fat 1 cm above the midpoint, in line with the point of the olecranon process. The fold should be pulled carefully away from the underlying muscle. Ask the patient to contract the underlying muscle to be sure muscle and fascia are not included in the skinfold.

Step 5: Place the caliper jaws perpendicular to the fatfold at the midpoint, and release the spring-loaded lever, but not the pinch (see Fig. 5-4).

Step 6: Read the measurement in about 2 seconds.

Step 7: Repeat the measurement in Step 5 twice more, and average the three results.

Interpretation: Means, standard deviations, and percentiles for triceps skinfolds are given in Table F-9 for males and females for ages 1 to 74 years. As in the interpretation of weight data, both the lower and upper ends of the curve are considered to indicate risk:

Percentile	Fat Status
0.0–5.0	Lean
5.1–15.0	Below average
15.1–75.0	Average
75.1–85.0	Above average
85.1–100.0	Excess Fat

Since fat deposits are not evenly distributed, measurements of skinfolds at multiple sites is believed to improve the accuracy of these measurements. Therefore, other measures are sometimes used. The mean and percentile values for subscapular skinfolds, for example, are contained in Table F-10. Interpretations of values on the table are the same as those used for the TSF.

Combined data from multiple sites are generally considered to be more accurate and informative than measurement at one site. However, there is disagreement on which sites should be used, how results should be weighted, and the effects of genetics, gender, and specific disease states (12).

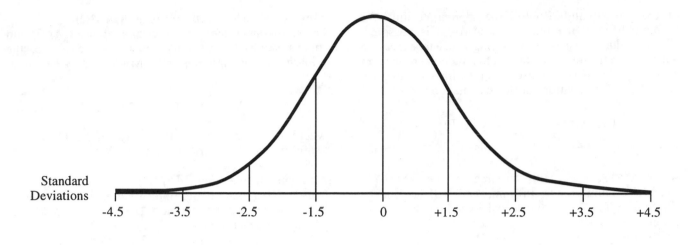

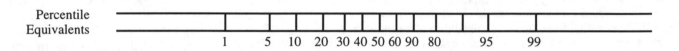

FIGURE 5-2 Relationship between standard deviations and percentiles.

Waist-Hip Circumference Ratio. The ratio of the circumference of the waist and the hips is calculated with the equation:

$$R = \frac{W}{H} \qquad (5\text{-}11)$$

Where R = ratio and W and H are waist and hip circumferences, respectively, in millimeters.

Increased cardiovascular disease and mortality are associated with a ratio greater than 1.0 in men and 0.8 in women (13, 14). Increased ratio is correlated with increased intraabdominal fat.

Limb Fat Area
Skinfold thickness and the circumference of a limb may be used to calculate limb fat area. This provides an indication of total body fat. In addition to measurement

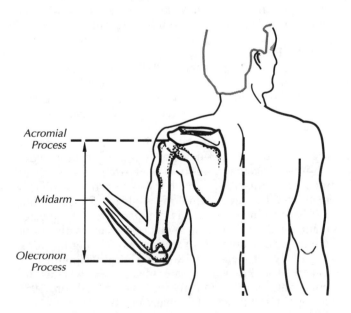

FIGURE 5-3 Finding the midpoint

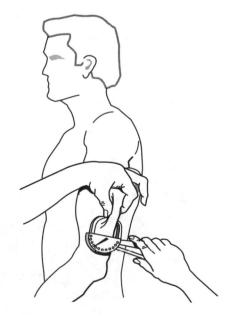

FIGURE 5-4 Measuring triceps skinfold

of TSF, the circumference of the appropriate limb, for example the midarm circumference (MAC), is measured. The procedure consists of measuring with a tape measure aligned with the top of the tape at the midpoint of the arm (Fig. 5-5). MAC is then used, along with TSF, to arrive at fat area. The equation for this calculation is:

$$MAFA = \frac{TSF \times MAC}{2} - \frac{3.14 \times (TSF)^2}{4} \quad \text{(5-12)}$$

where MAFA is midarm fat area in mm², MAC is midarm circumference in mm, and TSF is triceps skinfold in mm. Results are calculated to the nearest 0.1 cm.

Interpretation. Means and percentile values for midarm fat areas are given in Table F-11. Percentile values interpreted on the same scale are described above for TSF. This method should not be used for patients with edema or ascites or for those who are extremely obese. Although percentage of body fat can be calculated from MAFA, its predictive value is no better than using TSF (15).

Somatic Protein

The somatic protein (skeletal protein mass) serves as the major protein "store." Assessment of muscle protein therefore serves as an indication of the protein reserves in the body. The muscle circumference and muscle area in mid-upper arm, at the same site used for TSF and MAFA, are correlated with total muscle mass. Therefore, this midarm muscle circumference MAMC and midarm muscle area (MAMA) are used to monitor protein nutritional status.

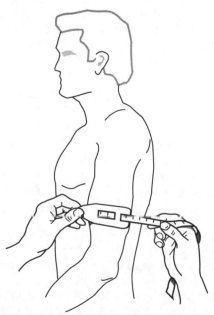

FIGURE 5-5 Measuring midarm circumference

Midarm Muscle Circumference (MAMC)

Having obtained the midarm circumference (MAC) and triceps skinfold (TSF) data as described above, the midarm muscle circumference (MAMC) may be calculated as follows:

$$MAMC = MAC - (3.14 \times TSF) \quad \text{(5-13)}$$

where all values are in cm. However, MAC is more useful for calculation of area measures.

Midarm Muscle Area (MAMA)

Muscle area data better indicate changes in muscle tissue than does circumference. The midarm muscle area is calculated as follows:

$$MAMA = \frac{[MAC - (3.14\ TSF)]^2}{4 \times 3.14} \quad \text{(5-14)}$$

where MAMA is in mm², and MAC and TSF are in mm.

Standards of comparison are given for age in Table F-12 and in Table F-13 for men and women of small, medium, and large frames.

Heymsfield (16) found that Eq. (5-14) overestimates the muscle area. Thus, it would tend to mask partly the extent of muscle atrophy. A correction factor of -10.0 cm² for men and -6.5 cm² for women was suggested to adjust for the presence of bone. These correction factors have been applied to the data in Tables F-12 and F-13.

LABORATORY MEASUREMENTS

Laboratory measurements are used in nutritional assessments primarily to evaluate visceral (nonstructural) protein. They may also be used to indicate somatic protein, vitamin, and mineral status.

Somatic Protein

The *creatinine-height index* (CHI) is occasionally used as a biochemical method for assessment of somatic protein. Creatinine is released from muscle tissue at a relatively constant rate; therefore, urinary creatinine is proportional to muscle mass.

In this method, a 24- hour urine collection is necessary. Sometimes, a 3-day collection is recommended for greater accuracy. Also, a meat-free diet is given, since the muscle of meat would provide dietary creatinine. The urine sample is analyzed for creatinine, and the creatinine content is compared to the expected creatinine excretion in a man or woman of the same height. The expected excretion is 23 mg/kg ideal weight/day for men, and 18 mg/kg ideal weight/day for women. The kg weights are ideal body weights for appropriate height and frame size, based on 1959 Metropolitan Insurance Company tables.

The creatinine-height index is calculated with the following equation:

% CHI =

$$\frac{\text{Actual 24 hr creatinine excretion}}{\text{Expected 24 hr creatine excretion for height}} \times 100$$

(5-15)

Various standards have been established for interpretation. These may show expected creatinine excretion per cm height, per cm height for age, per cm height divided into small, medium, and large frames. A simplified table, sufficient for the purposes of this text, is given in Table F-14. From 80 to 90 percent of expected CHI is considered a mild deficit; 60 to 80 percent, a moderate deficit; and less than 60 percent is a severe deficit. Results are not valid in patients with acute renal dysfunction, amputations, advanced age, emotional stress, sepsis, trauma, or fever, or those who eat a high-meat diet or take steroids, methadone hydrochloride, tobramycin sulfate, or Mandol.

Visceral Proteins

Serum Proteins. Serum proteins have varying half-lives and differing sensitivities to nutritional depletion and repletion.

Serum albumin is usually recorded in the patient's medical record as part of the admission laboratory workup; because of its availability, therefore, this is the value most frequently used. The range of normal values is considered to be 40 to 60 g/L. Half-life is 14 to 20 days. Depletion is interpreted as mild at 30 to 35 g/L, moderate at 21 to 30 g/L, and severe at 21 g/L or less.

Serum transferrin (TF) may be determined directly; however, it is more common to estimate it from a laboratory determination of total iron-binding capacity (TIBC). Several equations are currently used for this purpose. The equation we will use is

$$\text{TF (g/L)} = 0.8 \text{ TIBC (μmol/L)} - 43 \qquad \textbf{(5-16)}$$

This value, however, has been reported to overestimate serum transferrin by 10 to 20 percent. An alternative equation has recently been suggested and is used in some institutions:

$$\text{TF(g/L)} = 0.68 \text{ TIBC (μmol/L)} + 21 \qquad \textbf{(5-17)}$$

Half-life is 8 to 10.5 days. Normal TF range is 1.7 to 3.7 g/L. Mild depletion is interpreted as 1.5 to 1.7 g/L, moderate depletion at 1.0 to 1.5 g/L, and severe depletion at less than 1.0 g/L. Normal TIBC is 45 to 82 mmol/L.

Ranges of normal values are given because abnormal increases, as well as decreases, may occur. Fluctuations in serum albumin levels may be the result of factors other than nutritional depletion, Nonnutritional causes of low serum albumin include any factors that result in increased loss, increased degradation, or decreased synthesis, such as may occur in liver disease, kidney disease, some forms of gastrointestinal disease, congenital heart disease, some endocrine disorders, trauma, stress, sepsis, and pregnancy. Increased serum albumin levels may be seen in dehydrated patients. Low transferrin (or TIBC) levels may occur in chronic infection or in liver or kidney disease. In the patient with any of these conditions, serum albumin and transferrin data must be interpreted with caution. Additional diagnostic tests are often necessary.

FUNCTION TESTS

Function tests may also be used to assess protein nutriture. Immunological function and muscle function are most frequently used.

Immune Function. Currently used estimates of cell-mediated immune function (CMI) are based on total lymphocyte count (TLC) and measures of delayed cutaneous hypersensitivity (DCH).

Total lymphocyte count. To obtain the TLC, note the *total white blood cell* (WBC) count, which is obtained during the admission laboratory workup and is recorded in the patient's chart. In addition, the *differential count* gives the percentage of each of the five types of white blood cells. *Total lymphocyte count* (TLC) is then obtained by applying the following equation:

$$\text{TLC} = \text{total WBC/mm}^3 \times (\% \text{ lymphocytes/100}) \quad \textbf{(5-18)}$$

For example, a patient whose total WBC count is 10,000/mm^3 and who has 25 percent lymphocytes would have a TLC of

$$10,000 \times 0.25 = 2500/\text{mm}^3$$

Normal WBC count is usually 5, 000 to 10,000 cells/mm^3, and lymphocytes are 20 to 35 percent of these. There is some variation in the lymphocyte counts, which is considered normal. Normal values are 2,000 to 3,500 cells/mm^3. Mild depletion is at 1,500 to 1,800 cells/mm^3; 900 to 1,500 is moderate depletion; and less than 900 is severe. These data must be interpreted with caution, since other factors, including injury, radiotherapy, surgery, and immunosuppressive medication, also influence the TLC. In addition, depressed total WBC count and resulting lower TLC may be the result of some medications or viral infection, even if the patient's nutritional status is normal.

Delayed cutaneous hypersensitivity (DCH). Some institutions test for failure of the cell-mediated immune system (anergy) by testing the response to a battery of skin antigens. The antigens used vary among institutions but are usually chosen from Candida albicans, trychophyton, mumps, purified protein derivative (PPD), or dinitro-chlorobenzene (DNCB).

In this procedure, 0.1 ml of each of the chosen antigens is injected, usually by a nurse, subcutaneously in the inner aspect of the forearm. The area of the injection is examined for a reaction in 24 hours, and then again in 48 hours. A reaction consists of a "wheal and flare," that is, a raised and hardened area of skin (*induration*) surrounded by a reddened area (*erythema*).

A patient who has an induration of 5 mm or more in at least one dimension is considered reactive. If the induration measures 1 to 4 mm, the result is considered "relative anergy," a suboptimal response, while lack of response indicates anergy. The area of the erythema is not usually considered relevant.

There is controversy concerning the number and choice of antigens, the necessity to read the results at both 24 and 48 hours, and the number of responses necessary to be considered a positive response.

While anergy may result from malnutrition, other nonnutritional conditions may interfere with the immune response and should be considered in interpretation. These include various infections, renal and hepatic disease, inflammatory bowel disease, sarcoidosis, neoplastic disease, and primary disorders of the immune system. In addition, treatments affecting the immune response include radiation therapy, anesthesia, and drug therapy with steroids, immunosuppressants, antineoplastic drugs, cimetidine, and aspirin. These factors must be taken into account in interpretation of results.

Muscle Function. Several methods of testing muscle function are currently under investigation. Grip strength, relaxation rate, and fatigue rate may be affected by malnutrition, but adequate standards are not available.

CLINICAL EVALUATION OF PROTEIN-ENERGY MALNUTRITION

Clinical findings indicating protein-energy malnutrition (PEM) generally occur when the deficiency is advanced and already evident by the methods just described. Clinical evaluation of nutritional status is summarized in Table F-15.

Clinical findings in PEM may include the following:

Decreased head circumference

Dry, wiry, brittle, sparse, depigmented, and easily pluckable hair

Hypertrophy of fungiform papillae of tongue

Possible parotid gland enlargement

Bilateral edema in legs and feet

Growth retardation and fat loss

The existence of these conditions may not be diagnostic of nutritional deficiency; other disorders associated with these conditions are also listed in Table F-15.

Conversely, the diet history sometimes provides evidence of nutrient deficiency or excess. When this is the case, certain clinical conditions may occur; these are listed in Table F-16.

OVERALL EVALUATION OF PROTEIN AND ENERGY NUTRITIONAL STATUS

Assessment may determine current status or predict risk factors.

Evaluation of Current Status
Patients may be evaluated to be normally nourished or to be depleted of protein, energy, or both to a mild, moderate, or severe degree. Indications for each type of deficit are as follows:

Type of deficit	Body weight	Body fat	Somatic protein	Serum protein	Immune function
Energy (Marasmus)	Decreased	Decreased	Decreased	Moderate or Normal	Decreased
Protein (Kwashiorkor)	Decreased	Normal	Normal	Decreased	Decreased
Protein-energy (Marasmic-kwashiorkor)	Decreased	Decreased	Decreased	Decreased	Decreased

Evaluation of Risk Factors
Calculations of energy and nitrogen balance may be used to predict risk of malnutrition, to measure the severity of deficits, and to evaluate the adequacy of intake. These calculations are therefore useful for planning therapy.

Energy Balance. Protein nutrition must be considered in concert with an estimate of energy expenditure. Basal energy expenditure (BEE) may be calculated from anthropometric data using the Harris-Benedict equations (17):

For men
$$BEE = 66 + 13.7W + 5H - 6.8A \quad \textbf{(5-19)}$$

For women
$$BEE = 655 + 9.6W + 1.8H - 4.7A \quad \textbf{(5-20)}$$

where W = body weight in kg, H = height in cm, and A = age in years.

In order to more accurately assess total energy expenditure and, thus, the maintenance energy needs of patients, factors must be included for activity and injury.

Activity factors are as follows:

1.2	for patient confined to bed
1.3	for ambulatory patients
1.5–1.75	for most normally active persons
2.0	for extremely active persons

Injury factors are as follows:

1.2	for patients who have undergone minor surgery
1.35	for patients with skeletal trauma
1.44	for patients who have undergone elective surgery
1.6–1.9	for patients with major sepsis
1.88	for trauma plus steroids
2.1–2.5	for patients with severe thermal burns

The total daily energy expenditure (TDE) for a male would thus be obtained from this adaptation of Eq. (5-19):

$$TDE = (66 + 13.7W + 5H - 6.8A)(AF)(IF) \quad \textbf{(5-21)}$$

where AF = the activity factor and IF = the injury factor. For example, a male ambulatory patient's total maintenance energy need following elective surgery would be estimated as follows:

$$TDE = (66 + 13.7W + 5H - 6.8A)(1.3)(1.44)$$

Similarly, if the patient were female:

$$TDE = (655 + 9.6W + 1.8H - 4.7A)(1.3)(1.44)$$

Estimates of current or future energy needs may be used to:

1. Evaluate current intake relative to need
2. Plan for future nutritional support
3. Plan weight-reduction diets

This formula might be used, for example, to plan support of a patient currently of normal weight who is to undergo major surgery. If the patient is already underweight, an additional factor must be used to compensate for that deficit.

Nitrogen Balance. Two procedures are useful in estimating nitrogen balance in clinical situations. Normally, adults are in nitrogen balance, that is, nitrogen balance is approximately zero. Negative nitrogen balance is an abnormal condition, occurring when protein breakdown exceeds formation. Individuals in persistent negative nitrogen balance are at risk of developing protein malnutrition. Positive nitrogen balance occurs during growth in children, during pregnancy, and in wound healing. The goal in nutritional support of the depleted patient is a positive nitrogen balance of 4 to 6 g/day. A preliminary estimate of requirement for *anabolism* is sometimes obtained by using 1.2 to 1.5 g protein/kg actual body weight. This should then be adjusted, as will be described next.

Calculations based on nitrogen excretion. Urinary urea nitrogen (UUN) may be used to estimate a patient's nitrogen balance. Like CHI, the use of this method is limited by the need to collect a 24-hour urine sample.

The results are sometimes of particular value to the nutritional care specialist, however, so it is important to understand the method.

Step 1: UUN is measured in an aliquot from a 24-hour urine sample.

Step 2: Use the concentration of UUN and the 24-hour urine volume to calculate the total UUN per day using the equation

$$Total\ UUN = \frac{(UUN)\ (urine\ volume)}{100} \quad \textbf{(5-22)}$$

where total UUN is in mg, urinary UUN is in mg/dL, and urine volume is in mL.

Step 3: Estimate the patient's protein intake for the day.

(See Chapter 6 if you did not learn how to do this in your Normal Nutrition course.)

Step 4: Calculate the patient's nitrogen balance (N) using the equation:

$$N\ (g/day) = \frac{protein\ intake}{6.25} - (UUN + 3) \quad \textbf{(5-23)}$$

where 6.25 converts protein intake to nitrogen intake (since protein is 16 percent nitrogen); protein intake and UUN are given in grams; and 3 represents grams of nitrogen excretion by routes other than urinary, plus urinary nitrogen other than in urea.

Here is an example: A patient has a protein intake of 62.5 g/day and a urinary excretion of 500 mg UUN/dL in 2,000 ml of urine.

$$UUN = 500 \times \frac{2,000}{100} = 10,000\ mg\ or\ 10g$$

$$N(g/day) = \frac{62.5}{6.25} - (10.0 + 3)$$

$$= 10.0 - 13.0$$

$$= -3.0$$

Thus, current protein intake is inadequate and should be increased to allow for current needs plus repletion.

Calculations based on estimated energy requirement. Nitrogen balance may also be estimated by comparing a patient's intake with a calculation of estimated need.

Procedure

Step 1: Obtain an estimate of the patient's energy needs as described in Equation 5-21.

Step 2: Estimate desired ratio of kcal/g of dietary nitrogen. This varies with the patient's condition and will be discussed in later chapters. For the present, use 150:1 for anabolism and 200:1 for maintenance.

Step 3: Calculate the nitrogen requirement from the following equations:

$$\text{N required (g)} = \frac{\text{kcal}}{\text{kcal:N ratio}} \qquad \textbf{(5-24)}$$

For example, assume a patient's estimated energy need is 2,250 kcal/day, and her needed kcal/nitrogen ratio is estimated to be 150:1. Nitrogen need is estimated to be

$$\text{N required} = \frac{2,250}{150} = 15 \text{ g nitrogen}$$

Step 4: Using this equation, calculate the amount of protein that would contain 15 g nitrogen:

$$\text{Pro (g)} = \text{nitrogen (g)} \times 6.25 \qquad \textbf{(5-25)}$$

In our example, the needed 15 g nitrogen would be supplied in 15 x 6.25 = 93.75 g protein.

OTHER INDICATORS OF NUTRITIONAL STATUS

A number of other biochemical tests are used to evaluate the patient's status related to nutrients other than protein and energy when circumstances indicate that these values are necessary. Although these tests are less frequently used, they are helpful in certain clinical situations, some of which will be demonstrated in coming chapters.

HEMATOLOGICAL ASSESSMENT

The purposes of hematological assessment are to:

1. Detect the presence of anemia and characterize its type
2. Detect related nutritional deficiency, if any
3. Indicate appropriate nutritional intervention
4. Screen selected patients for excess alcohol intake (sometimes indicated by megaloblastic anemia secondary to folate deficiency)

Iron deficiency can result not only from insufficient intake but also from impaired absorption, increased loss, or increased requirements.

The initial screening for anemia usually includes hemoglobin (Hgb) and hematocrit (Hct) or packed-cell volume (PVC). *Hematocrit* is the proportion of the total volume of blood that is blood cells. Normal values are given in Table F-17. In addition, the number of red blood cells are counted and reported as the number per mm^3. (See Table E-3). These values will appear in the patient's medical record when a CBC, or complete blood count, has been ordered. This is a routine procedure on hospital admission.

The blood cells may be examined under a microscope and classified according to

Size: microcytic (small); normocytic (normal); or macrocytic (large)

Color: hypochromic (pale) or normochromic (normal)

Shape: normocytosis (homogeneous, normal shape) or poikilocytosis (irregular in shape)

Additional calculations, sometimes reported in the medical record, include the following:

Mean corpuscular volume (MCV) indicates the size of the red blood cell.

$$\text{MCV (fL)} = \frac{\text{Hct} \times 1000}{\text{number of RBC} \times 10^{12}/\text{L}} \qquad \textbf{(5-26)}$$

MCV is increased in megaloblastic anemia and reduced in microcytic anemia.

Mean corpuscular hemoglobin (MCH) indicates the Hgb content per cell. MCH is obtained with this equation:

$$\text{MCH (pg)} = \frac{\text{Hgb(g/L} \times 10)}{\text{number of RBC} \times 10^{12}/\text{L}} \qquad \textbf{(5-27)}$$

Results may be given in picograms (pg). A low value would be found if cells were hypochromic. MCH is low in iron deficiency; the RBCs are small. It is high in megaloblastic anemia; the RBCs are larger.

Mean corpuscular hemoglobin concentration (MCHC) indicates the hemoglobin content per volume of RBC. A low value is obtained when hemoglobin is decreased more than is Hct. MCHC is obtained with the following equation:

$$\text{MCHC (g/L)} = \frac{\text{Hgb (g/L)}}{\text{Hct}} \times 100 \qquad \textbf{(5-28)}$$

Normal values are given in Table E-3.

In iron-deficiency anemia, MCV, MCH, and MCHC are low. In the macrocytic anemias of vitamin B_{12} or folate deficiency, they may be high or normal. A patient with both a macrocytic and microcytic cause for anemia, such as both a folate deficiency and an iron deficiency, may have normal indices because the effects have averaged out, but the cell morphology will be mixed.

Other values used in evaluation of nutritional anemias are serum iron, folate, and vitamin B_{12} and transferrin saturation. Guidelines for evaluation are given in Table F-17. Since anemia may be caused by other conditions, data for differential diagnosis are given in Table F-18.

HYDRATION STATUS

Serum osmolality may be estimated to give an indication of the patient's hydration status. The procedure for evaluation of serum osmolality is discussed in Chapter 4.

Interpretation

Normal values = 275–295 mOsm/kg for adults
270–285 mOsm/kg for children

Variations from normal are usually the result of changes in serum sodium concentration. Osmolality and the significance of its value in relation to specific diseases will be discussed further in later chapters. At low concentrations, such as in body fluids, olmolarity and osmolality are approximately the same. At high concentrations, they differ. The significance of these differences will be discussed in Chapters 13 and 14.

IDENTIFICATION OF OTHER RISK FACTORS

Even individuals who are currently well nourished can be at risk of developing malnutrition. During nutritional assessment, these risk factors must be identified in order to provide a basis for prevention or treatment, including education. Among these risk factors are medications, some treatments, physiological status, including extremes of age, some chronic diseases, and social, psychological, and economic conditions.

MEDICATIONS AND TREATMENTS

Drugs may interfere with food intake, digestive and absorption, or utilization of nutrients. They may also increase nutrient losses and raise requirements. The nutritional care specialist should have references available for consultation when encountering unfamiliar drugs in the patient's medical record. Table 5-1 provides a list of possible nutrition-related effects on nutrition and Table 5-2 gives examples of drugs that fit into each category. Generally, drug effects are considered only if the patient will be taking the drug for 7 days or more.

In addition to the action of the prescribed drugs on food intake and on specific nutrients, the following questions should be explored:

TABLE 5-1 Nutrient-Drug Interactions

Effects of drugs on nutrition
    Alterations in tests and odor perceptions
    Increase or decrease in taste activity
    Induce bad taste
    Increase or depress appetite
    Gastrointestinal upsets: nausea, vomiting, diarrhea
    Primary or secondary malabsorption
    Alterations in nutrient metabolism
    Stimulation of protein synthesis
    Depression of protein synthesis
    Increase or decrease in plasma or cholesterol levels
    Increase or decrease in serum blood glucose levels
    Chelation of some minerals
    Interference with tissue distributuion, enzyme action
    Increased excretion of some nutrients
Effects of food and nutrition on drugs
    Increase or decrease in drug absorption
    Increase or decrease in protein bonding
    Increase or decrease in metabolism, excretion

TABLE 5-2 Nutrition-Related Drugs

Drug Effect	Examples of Specific Drugs	Classifications
Alter taste sensations	Benzocaine	Anesthetic
	Amphetamines	Anorectic
	Penicillin	Antibiotic
	Furosemide	Diuretic
	Cholestyramine	Hypolipemic
	Chlorpromazine	Tranquilizer
Cause nausea, vomiting, anorexia	Digitalis	Antiarrhythmic
	Phenobarbital	Anticonvulsant
	Griseofulvin	Antifungal
	Tetracycline	Anti-infective
	Cis-platin	Antineoplastic
Cause intestinal absorption defects	Phenytoin	Anticonvulsant
	Methotrexate	Antineoplastic
	Cholestyramine	Hypolipemic
	Milk of magnesia	Laxative
Affect nutrient metabolism	Tetracyclines	Inhibits synthesis
Protein	Anabolic steroids	Stimulate synthesis
Lipids	Carbamazepine	Decreases serum level
	Corticosteroids	Increases serum level
Carbohydrate	Phenytoin, thiazides	Hyperglycemic
Vitamins and minerals	Aspirin	Analgesic
	Aluminum hydroxide	Antacid
	Digoxin	Antiarrhythmic
	Phenytoin	Anticonvulsant
Cause gastric irritation	Aspirin	Analgesic
	Coumarin	Anticoagulant
	Hydrochlorothiazide	Diuretic

1. Does the diet affect the absorption, action, or excretion of the drug? Would change in diet and food habits enhance drug action?
2. Does the patient chronically use self-prescribed non-prescription ("over the counter") drugs? Identify the drugs. What are the effects?
3. Does the patient take nutrient supplements? Quantity? Frequency? Content?
4. Is *polypharmacy* a consideration? (*Polypharmacy* refers to taking several or many drugs. The combination of these may have negative effects.)

PHYSIOLOGICAL STATUS

During the periods of pregnancy and lactation, childhood, and advanced age, special needs must be considered in assessment.

Considerations in pregnancy and lactation are described in Chapter 8, and in childhood, in Chapter 9. Percentile values for anthropometric measurements in children and in advanced age are included in Appendix F.

SOCIAL, PSYCHOLOGICAL, AND ECONOMIC FACTORS

The patient's living conditions, economic status, and psychological state have great potential for affecting his or her nutritional status and future risk. Information on some of these matters may be found in the patient's medical record. Other information must be elicited by patient interview.

Table 5-3 lists factors that may need to be considered, particularly as they apply to the elderly. In this area, the nutritional care specialist's background in sociology, psychology, and economics will be put to use.

TABLE 5-3 Psychological and Economic Factors Affecting Nutritional Status

Economic Status	Source and adequacy of income
	Frequency and steadiness of employment
	Reliance on economic assistance: welfare; food stamps–cost of stamps
	Amount of income spent for food
	Adequacy of heating or cooling
	Availability of stove, refrigerator, kitchen space, storage space
Social Isolation	Lives alone? With others? Eat together?
	Availabiltiy of support systems
	Transportation; shopping facilities
Physical abilities and disabilities	Occupation: type, hrs./wk., shift, amount of effort
	Exercise: type, amount of effort and time, frequency, seasonality
	Sleep: hours/day, interruption?
	Inactivity, immobility
	Disabling/handicapping condition
	Manual dexterity
	Strength
	Use of assistive devices
	Functional status
	Competency in activities of daily living (ADLs)*

Bathing	Transportation
Dressing	Transferring
Toileting	Continence
Ambulation	Food prepreation
	Eating

Competency in instrumental activities of daily living (IADLs)*

Ability to use telephone	Mode of transportation
Shopping	Responsibility for own medication
Housekeeping	Ability to handle finances
Laundry	

Ethnic and Cultural Background	Religion
	Education
	Ethnicity
	Influences on eating habits

(continued)

TABLE 5-3 *(continued)*

Diseases and Other Abnormal Conditions	Abnormal body weight (deficient or excess)
	Loss or gain? Over what time? Involuntary?'
	Dental or oral problems
	Problems with swallowing? Salivation? "Stick in throat?"
	Loss of teeth? Dentures?
	Foods that cannot be eaten
	Appetite: Good? Poor? Changes?
	Taste and smell perception changes?
	Factors affecting appetite
	Allergies, intolerances, avoidances
	Description of problems with foods
	Food avoided? Reasons? Length of time?
	Gastrointestinal disorders
	Nausea? Vomiting? Diarrhea? Bloating? Flatulence?
	Distention? Constipation? Constant? Sporadic? Frequency?
	Antacid, laxative, or other home remedy use?
	Cognitive or emotional impairment
	Depression? Dementia? Retardation?
	Psychiatric or neurologic disorder?
	Sensory impairment: vision? hearing?
	Chronic infection
	Tendency to pressure sores
	Chronic cardiovascular, renal, hepatic, skeletal, endocrine, gastrointestinal disorders?
	Diet modifications prescribed
Chronic Medications/ drug use	Medications: type, amount, frequency, length of time taken
	Prescribed? Self-prescribed?
	Nutritional supplements: type, amount, frequency
	Polypharmacy?
	Quantity?
	Illicit drug use?
Age	Advanced age (80 years and up)
Recent traumatic events	Retirement
	Bereavement
	Loss of income

* Important for elderly or handicapped.
Compiled from L.K. Mahan and M. Arlin, *Krause's Food Nutrition and Diet Therapy*, 8th ed. Philadelphia: Saunders, 1992, and Nutritional Screening Initiative. *Report of Nutrition Screening 1: Toward a Common View*. Washington DC: Nutrition Screening Initiative, 1992.

TOPICS FOR FURTHER DISCUSSION

1. Differentiate a "screening" from an "in-depth" nutritional assessment. What data would constitute a "screening assessment"?
2. How often should nutritional status be assessed? Which procedures should be used?
3. Discuss the advantages and disadvantages of using each of the following as the standard by which a patient's body weight is evaluated:

a. Weight at the 50th percentile of a person of the same height, sex, and age

b. Desirable body weight of a person of the same height, sex, and age

c. The patient's usual weight

4. What are hemosiderin, sideroblasts, and reticulocytes? What is their significance in nutritional assessment?

REFERENCES

1. **Gray, D., J.B. Cricker, C. Kelley,** and **L.C. Dickerson.** Accuracy of recumbent height measurement. *JPEN* 9:(1985)712.

2. **Chumlea, W.C., A.F. Roche,** and **D. Mukerjee.** *Nutritional Assessment of the Elderly Through Anthropometry.* Columbus: Ross Laboratories, 1984.

3. **Dequeker, J.V., J.P. Baeyens,** and **J. Claessens.** The significance of stature as a clinical measurement of aging. *J.Am. Geriatr. Soc.* 17:(1969)169.

4. **Lohman, T., A.F. Roche,** and **R. Martorell.** *Anthropometric Standardization Reference Manual.* Champaign, IL: Human Kinetics Books, 1988.

5. **Mitchell, C.** and **D. Lipschitz.** Arm length measurement as an alternative to height in nutritional assessment of the elderly. *JPEN* 6:(1982)226.

6. **Frisancho, A.R.** *Anthropometric Standards for the Assessment of Growth and Nutritional Status.* Ann Arbor: University of Michigan Press, 1990.

7. ——. New standards of weight and body composition by frame size and height for assessment of nutritional status of adults and the elderly. *Am. J. Clin. Nutr.* 40:(1984)808.

8. National Institute of Health. *Consensus Development Conferences Statement,* Vol. 5, No. 9, 1985.

9. **Bray, G.** Obesity. *Disease-a-Month.* July 1989.

10. **Manson, J.E., M.J. Stampfer, C.H. Hennekins** and W.C. **Willett.** Body weight and longevity, a reassessment. *J. Amer. Med. Assoc.* 257:(1987)353.

11. Health and Welfare Canada. *Promoting Healthy Weights: A discussion paper.* Ottawa: Health Services and Promotion Branch, Health and Welfare, 1988.

12. **Gibson, R.** *Principles of Nutritional Assessment.* New York: Oxford University Press, 1990.

13. **Bjorntorp, P.** Regional patterns of fat distribution: health implications. *Am. J. Int. Med.* 103:(1985).

14. ——. Classification of obese patients and complications related to the distribution of obese fat. *Am J. Clin. Nutr.* 45:(1987)1120.

15. **Himes, J. H., A.F. Roche,** and **P.** Webb. Fat areas as estimates of total body fat. *Am. J. Clin. Nutr.* 33:(1980)2093.

16. **Heymsfield, S.B., C.B. McManus, J. Smith, V. Stephens** and **D.W. Nixon.** Anthropometric measurement of muscle mass: revised equations for calculating bone-free arm muscle area. *Am. J. Clin. Nutr.* 36 :(1982)680.

17. **Bistrian, B., G.L. Blackburn, M. Sherman** and **N.S. Scrimshaw.** Therapeutic index of nutritional depletion in hospitalized patients. *Surg., Gynecol, and Obstet.* 141:(1973)512.

ADDITIONAL SOURCES OF INFORMATION

Grant, A and **S. Dehoog.** *Nutritional Assessment and Support,* 4th ed. Seattle, WA: Anne Grant/Susan DeHoog, 1991.

☑ TO TEST YOUR UNDERSTANDING

1. List methods of measuring or estimating body height (length).

2. How would you determine or estimate the height of the following patients:
    a. A patient who has a leg in traction and cannot get out of bed?
    b. A patient whose legs have been amputated?
    c. An elderly woman with osteoporosis and spinal curvature?

3. Estimate the height or a 68-year-old male patient who has a knee height of 54 cm. Show your calculations.

4. With a tape measure or Inser-Tape, measure the wrist circumference of a classmate and state the frame size indicated. With calipers or a tape measure, measure the elbow breadth of the same classmate and state the frame size indicated. Compare the results of these two methods.

5. A patient's height is 5 feet, 5 inches. What is her height in centimeters?

6. A patient's weight is 132 pounds. How many kilograms does she weigh?

7. An adult female patient is 5 feet, 6 inches tall and weighs 112 pounds. Giving specific figures, how does this patient's body weight compare with the following:
    a. Optimal body weight at the 50th percentile for height?
    b. "Ideal" body weight estimated from a formula?

8. A male patient, age 45, is 5 feet, 9 inches tall with a medium frame. He states that his usual weight is 165 pounds. He recently lost 35 pounds because of illness. How would you evaluate his body weight? Would you consider him at nutritional risk? Why?

9. A male patient, age 70, has a height of 180.9 cm and weighs 80.2 kg. Four weeks ago, he weighed 85 kg. Would you consider this patient to be at risk? Explain your answer.

10. A 67-year-old female patient has an amputation of the right leg above the knee. Knee height obtained from the left leg is 48.75 cm. Calculate
    a. Estimated height
    b. Optimal body weight prior to amputation
    c. Optimal body weight following amputation

11. Measure the triceps skinfold of a classmate. Repeat the measurement twice more and compare the three results. How reproducible are your results?

12. A female patient, age 40, is 5 feet, 3 inches tall and weighs 194 pounds.
    a. Calculate her BMI.
    b. What do you conclude about this patient's body fat?

13. A 40-year-old female patient has a midarm circumference of 27.3 cm and a triceps skinfold of 1.25 cm.
    a. Calculate the MAMA of the patient described in the previous question.
    b. How would you interpret your results?

14. Using the Heymsfield correction factor,
    a. Calculate the MAMA for the same patient.
    b. How would you interpret the result?

15. The medical record of a 65-year-old male patient provides the following information:

Serum albumin	30 g/L
TIBC	165 μmol/L
WBC	4,500 cells/mm^3
Differential	
Neutrophils	70%
Lymphocytes	20%
Eosinophils	3%
Basophils	2%
Monocytes	5%
DCH response	
Candida	2 mm in 24 hr
PPD	2 mm in 24 hr
Mumps	none

    a. Calculate the total lymphocyte count (TLC)
    b. Fill in the following form:

	Normal	*Patient's value*
Serum albumin		
White blood cells		
Total lymphocyte count		

    c. Evaluate the patient's visceral protein status

16. A female patient is 40 years old and is 5 feet, 3 inches tall, with a heavy frame. She has lost 25 pounds in the last 2 months and now weighs 130 pounds. Other assessment values for this patient include the following:

TSF	24.0 mm
MAC	24.5 cm
WBC	4,000 (25% lymphocytes)
DCH	3 mm induration in 48 hours for two antigens of three tested
Serum albumin	30 g/L

(continued)

☑ **TO TEST YOUR UNDERSTANDING** (*continued*)

How would you evaluate this patient's nutritional status? Explain your reasoning.

17. List procedures for assessing:
   a. Somatic protein
   b. Visceral protein
   c. Cell-mediated immunity

18. A male patient, age 62, is 5 feet, 10 inches tall and weighs 150 pounds. He has a protein intake of 70 g/day. The patient is confined to bed with multiple bone fractures. Laboratory results include the following:

UUN	600 mg/dL
Urine volume	1,950 mL
Serum sodium	138 μmol/L
SUN	9.9 mmol/L
Blood glucose	100 mg/dL

   a. Calculate the patient's basal energy expenditure (BEE).
   b. Calculate the patient's total daily energy expenditure (TDE).
   c. What is the patient's nitrogen balance?
   d. How would you interpret these results?

19. How might the patient's nitrogen balance and energy expenditure be interrelated?

20. A preliminary screening by your assistant reveals that patient Mr. L has very limited variety in his diet. You suspect that his diet may be deficient in iron or folate.
   a. What nutritional assessment test would help distinguish between these two possibilities and what results would you expect in each case?
   b. You plan to interview Mr. L in greater depth concerning his previous diet. What foods would you question him about in some detail? Iron sources? Folate sources?

21. a. Explain how, in Eq. (5-27) for serum osmolality, the values for sodium can be given in mEq and the values for glucose and urea in mg, yet the result is in mmol.
   b. Why are mEq of Na doubled?

22. a. Estimate the serum osmolality in a patient whose laboratory values are as follows:

Na	138 mEq/L
BUN	9.24 mg/dL
Blood glucose	90 mg/dL

   b. Interpret your results.

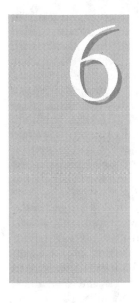

6 Evaluating the Patient's Diet

An important part of a comprehensive nutritional status evaluation is the assessment of the patient's nutrient intake and identification of risk factors affecting intake. This chapter will be limited to those methods most frequently used in evaluating the diets of individuals, rather than of groups or populations.

The most commonly used procedure consists of three steps: (1) Information is obtained on the intake of food and fluid and on factors affecting this intake. This step usually requires the use of interviewing techniques you learned in Chapter 3. (2) The nutrient content of the foods specified is determined. (3) These results are then compared with the patient's nutrient requirements. Each of these steps will be described in turn, and you will be given an opportunity to use these methods.

In addition to evaluation of nutritional status and identification of risk factors at the time the patient seeks care, the information obtained by these methods is also used in planning for nutritional care and evaluating its effectiveness. These procedures are described in subsequent chapters.

METHODS FOR COLLECTING INTAKE INFORMATION

The methods of collecting information vary in their accuracy and ease of use. Only those that are practical in clinical situations will be described here.

24-HOUR RECALL

The 24-hour recall is one of the easiest methods for collecting information on the patient's intake, but the method is prone to important errors. It consists essentially of obtaining information on food and fluid intake for the previous day or for the previous 24 hours and is based on the assumption that the intake described is typical of daily intake. The information is usually obtained by interviewing the patient or a family member. Interviewing skill (see Chapter 3) can improve the accuracy of the information obtained, but the interviewer should be aware of the following sources of error and seek to avoid them if possible:

1. The patient may not be able to recall the foods eaten. It is often helpful to base questioning on the sequence of activities, beginning with questions such as "What time did you get up in the morning?" "What did you eat first?" and then proceeding methodically in similar fashion through the next 24 hours. Alternatively, you might start with the present and work back through the previous 24 hours. There is a tendency to forget snack foods, fruits, and gravies and sauces in particular, but skillful questioning can jog the patient's memory on these as well as other points.
2. The patient may not be able to estimate the amounts of each food eaten. It is helpful to have food models or illustrations of usual portion sizes on hand to provide a basis for comparison.
3. The information given may not be sufficiently specific without skillful questioning. A list of some of the types of information that are needed to provide greater accuracy is given in Table 6-1.
4. The patient may not be telling the truth. The interviewer must be careful to avoid suggesting the answers expected and must not appear judgmental.
5. The intake during the previous 24 hours may not be typical. The patient should be asked about this and, and if necessary, questioned about a more typical day's intake.

TABLE 6-1 Checklist for Diet Records

Type of Food	Information Needed
All	Portion size: Cups, bottles, cans? Length, width, thickness, diameter, shape compared to a model?
Milk and nondairy substitutes	% fat, powder, liquid? Evaporated? Dairy or nondairy? Type of fat? Added sweetening? Unsweetened? Chocolate?
Eggs and egg substitutes	Fresh? Frozen? Size? How prepared? Added fat? Milk? Other? Powder? Liquid? Frozen? Brand?
Meat, fish, poultry	Cut? Fat trimmed? Bone in or out? Cooked weight? How prepared? Added fat, amount, kind? % fat (ground meat)?
Vegetables	Cooked or raw? Fresh, frozen, canned? Added sauce or fat? Kind of fat or sauce? Size of serving?
Fruit and juice	Cooked or raw? Fresh, frozen, canned, dried? Sweetened? Heavy, medium, light syrup? Unsweetened? Size of serving (piece or cup)?
Cereals	Ready-to-eat? Cooked? Brand? Additions such as raisins, sugar, milk? How much? Size of servings?
Baked products	Homemade or commercial? Brand? From scratch or mix? Single or double crust (pie)? Meringue, frosting, topping? Yeast or quick bread (sweet rolls, muffins, and so on)? Dimensions of servings? Weight or number (crackers)?
Fats and oils	Margarine: Major oil? Stick, tub, squeeze, or liquid? Brand? P/S ratio? Diet? Whipped? Oil and shortening: Brand? Major oil? Solid? Salad dressing: Homemade or commercial? Type of oil or brand name? Creamy? Clear? Additions (cheese, bacon)?
Mixed dishes	Homemade: Ingredients and amounts? Cooking methods? Commercial: Brand? Cooking method?
Gravies and sauces	Type of fat? Amount? Liquid, milk or other? Other additions? Amount used?
Beverages	Diet, low-cal, sweetened? Brand? Caffeine? Decaf? Added sugar, milk, cream? Cola or noncola? Alcohol content? Type of alcoholic beverage? Amount?
Snacks and candies	Brand? Size? Weight?
Restaurant meals	Name of restaurant? Price range?

Many institutions have a form suggesting the line of questioning and providing space for recording information. An example is Form A found in the Sample Forms section in Appendix M.

FOOD-FREQUENCY QUESTIONNAIRE

The food-frequency questionnaire is often used in combination with the 24-hour recall. It provides a list of foods or food groups, and the patient answers with information on the frequency with which the food is eaten. Common choices of answers are *never, rarely, occasionally,* or *frequently.* When these terms are used, it is important to define very specifically the terms *occasionally* and *frequently.* In order to avoid this problem, some forms give choices *never, daily, weekly, monthly,* and *less than monthly.*

The foods on the questionnaire may be listed in a few broad categories or may be categorized in more detail to provide a larger number of groups and more precise definition. For example, a simple grouping might consist of the following four categories: meat and meat substitutes, milk and milk products, fruits and vegetables, breads and cereals. In a more detailed listing, the fruit and vegetable group might be subdivided into deep green and leafy vegetables, dark yellow fruits and vegetables, other vegetables, potatoes, legumes, and others. In any case, the food-frequency questionnaire does not provide information on quantities, but it is useful for checking the accuracy of the 24-hour recall. The form may be general, including all food groups, or it may be specialized for certain categories of patients, providing information on intake of specific nutrients. For example, a special form inquiring about intake of foods containing appreciable amounts of protein, sodium, potassium, and fluid might be used when interviewing patients with certain forms of renal disease. Form B in the Sample Forms section, is an example of a general food-frequency questionnaire.

FOOD DIARY

It is sometimes useful to have the patient keep a record of food and drink intake for a specified period. Three days, often 2 weekdays and 1 weekend day, are most commonly used. A longer period is necessary if the daily food intake is highly variable because it will take more time to obtain an overview of the patient's usual intake.

OBSERVATION OF FOOD INTAKE

Direct observation of food intake may be practical for hospitalized patients or individuals in residential facilities, and it may be required for those unable to provide the necessary information. Very frequently, information on a patient's total energy intake is required. This "calorie count" is obtained by observing the difference between the amounts served on the patient's tray and the amount not eaten. The protein content of the diet eaten is usually also reported.

NUTRITION HISTORY

The nutrition history is used to collect information on the general pattern of food intake and on other factors influencing the patient's food habits. It is a much more thorough and comprehensive procedure and usually includes a 24-hour recall, a food frequency list, and an extensive interview, as well as a thorough reading of the patient's medical record. A list of factors that may be considered is shown in Table 5-3. It should be obvious from the length of that list that obtaining a nutrition history is time-consuming. In addition, it tends to overestimate food intake. You can see that many of the factors to be considered are included in Forms A and B. This procedure will detect risk factors not evident with more abbreviated methods.

ESTIMATING NUTRIENT CONTENT OF THE DIET

Once you have information on the patient's food intake, you must translate this information into estimation of the amount of each nutrient under consideration that those foods contain. The method you choose will depend on the degree of precision you require. If, for example, the patient is the subject of a research program, it may even be necessary to have a chemical analysis of an aliquot of the food. In most clinical situations, however, such precision is impractical and unnecessary. The methods more commonly used are more approximate but faster and thus less expensive in labor cost.

CALCULATION WITH EXCHANGE LISTS

Instead of detailed calculations, diets may be evaluated using an appropriate food-grouping system. Such a system is established by grouping together foods that are similar in nutritive value and, to some extent, on their use in the meal. The use of food groups is based on the assumption that eating appropriate amounts of foods in each group will provide proper amounts of protein, calcium, iron, and the vitamins A, ascorbic acid, thiamin, riboflavin, and niacin. It is further assumed that if a wide variety of foods within the groups are consumed, the other nutrients will be obtained in sufficient quantities.

A number of these grouping systems are available, and several are useful in clinical situations. One of those most commonly used in an initial diet assessment is described here. Others, used in planning modified diets, will be described in later chapters.

The most commonly used grouping is based on lists of foods called *exchanges* (1). It is assumed that all foods in an exchange list have approximately the same content of protein, fat, and carbohydrate, and thus can be "exchanged" one for another without making a substantial alteration in the average nutrient intake. The lists of exchanges were originally established for use in diets for diabetic patients, but have since been found useful for other purposes. The protein, fat, and carbohydrate content of each exchange list is given in the tables in Appendix C. Values in Parts I or II of this appendix may be used. They do not differ greatly.

Additional values that are sometimes useful when the exchanges are used for diet evaluation for nondiabetics include the following:

1 t (teaspoon) sugar	contains	5.0 g carbohydrate
1 t jam or jelly	contains	5.0 g carbohydrate
1 serving fruit in heavy syrup	contains	50.0 g carbohydrate
1 serving sweetened gelatin dessert (5 servings/pkg)	contains	1.6 g protein and 15.0 g carbohydrate

The protein, fat, and carbohydrate contents of a diet may be calculated using these values. For example, let us assume that a patient's daily intake consists of the following items:

Breakfast	Lunch	Dinner
1/2 grapefruit	1/2 c tomato jc.	4 oz. roast beef
3/4 cup (c) cornflakes	Cheese sandwich:	1/2 c mashed potatoes
1/2 c milk, nonfat	2 slices bread	1/2 c carrots
1 t sugar	2 oz. cheddar cheese	1 c tossed green salad
1 poached egg	1/2 c milk, non-fat	1 T French dressing
1 slice toast	1 1/4 c fresh strawberries	1/2 c fresh fruit
1 t butter		1 c milk, nonfat

This menu contains the following exchanges, summarized, with the protein, fat, and carbohydrate content indicated, based on Appendix C, Part II:

		Pro (g)	Fat (g)	CHO (g)
2	Milk exchanges, nonfat (1/2 + 1/2 + 1)	16		24
2	Vegetable exchanges (1/2 c tomato, 1/2 c carrots, 1 c tossed salad)	6		15
3	Fruit exchanges (1/2 grapefruit, 1 1/4 c strawberries, ½c fresh fruit cup)			45
5	Starch/bread exchanges (3/4 c conflakes, 1/2 c potatoes, 3 slices bread)	15		75
7	Meat exchanges 1 egg (medium fat) 2 cheese, 4 beef (high fat)	7 42	5 48	
2	Fat exchanges (1 t butter, 1 T French dressing)		10	
1	Other foods (1 t sugar)			5
	TOTAL	86	63	164

The values obtained may be used to evaluate the adequacy of protein and energy intake. The adequacy of vitamin and mineral intake may be estimated by comparing intakes with one of the guides described in the next section or by using the vitamin and mineral exchanges in Table B-1.

If you do not have information on common food sources of nutrients, it is important that you develop a store of this knowledge. In this and succeeding chapters, you will be given an opportunity to do so. The vitamin and mineral contents of major food groups are summarized in Table 6-2.

ANALYSIS FROM TABLES OF FOOD VALUES

Tables of food values may be used to calculate nutrient content of diets when more detailed information is necessary. This method is time-consuming when done manually but can be quite rapid when computer analysis is available. The values in the database for the computer may be those from the United States Department of Agriculture's (USDA) Handbook 8 (2) or other currently available tables (3-6). Some patients eat large quantities of "fast foods." Detailed information on the nutrient content of fast foods can be obtained from the headquarters of the fast food franchise or from other published sources (3-7). The more detailed food composition values have some specific uses in clinical situations:

1. For calculation of nutrient content of foods with greater precision than that provided by using exchange lists
2. For calculation of intake of nutrients not included in exchange lists—for example, the vitamins and minerals
3. To provide information on nutrient content of foods not included in exchange lists—for example, the nutritional value of a variety of baked desserts
4. As a source of information of food sources of a specific nutrient—for example, the best food sources of riboflavin.

USING INFORMATION FROM PACKAGE LABELS

In May 1994, new government regulations, the National Labeling and Educational Act of 1990 (NLEA), specifying nutritional information on packaged food took effect. These regulations provide recent, more accurate, and more understandable information on nutrient content.

The information may be used to expand and up date data in the tables of food values described in the previous section. These labels can be expected to help health professionals and consumers make better judgments on food intake. Therefore, it is essential that they be understood in detail.

An illustration of the label is shown in Fig. 6-1, entitled "Nutrition Facts." Directly beneath the title, the serving size and numbers of servings per container are given. The serving sizes are based on the amount

TABLE 6-2.   Nutrient Content in Major Food Groups

Nutrient	Milk Group	Bread & Cereals Group	Fruits & Vegetables Group	Meat Group
Protein	x	x		x
Fat	x			x
Carbohydrate	x	x	x	
Thiamin		x	x	x
Riboflavin	x	x		x
Niacin	x	x		x
Folate	x	x	x	
Vitamin B$_{12}$	x			x
Ascorbic Acid			x	
Vitamin A	x		x	x
Vitamin D	x			
Calcium	x		x	
Iron		x	x	x
Fiber		x	x	x

that people usually eat. Thus, it is less likely that a manufacturer can mislead the consumer by stating unrealistic serving sizes. For example, it will no longer be possible to give a serving size of 2 tablespoons for a food ordinarily eaten in 1 cup servings. In addition, similar foods have similar serving sizes, making it easier to compare similar foods.

The nutrients required to be listed on the label are those considered to be most important to consumer health. As seen on the illustration, the number of calories and calories from fat are given. The next section provides information on the content of fats, cholesterol, sodium, carbohydrate, including fiber, and protein. The right hand column shows how these nutrients contribute to a 2,000-calorie reference diet. The "% Daily Value" is set by the government and is based on current recommendations (e.g., the RDA). When an individual's energy needs vary from 2,000-calories, it is necessary to adjust the "% Daily Value" proportionately. Translation of "% Daily Values" may be given in grams and milligrams, in a footnote.

Among the vitamins and minerals, vitamin A, vitamin C, calcium, and iron are required on the label. Others can be included voluntarily. A footnote gives calories per gram of protein, fat, and carbohydrate. The regulations

Nutrition Facts

Serving Size 1 cup (228 g)
Servings Per Container 2

Amount Per Serving

Calories 90	Calories from Fat 30

	% Daily Value*
Total Fat 3 g	5%
Saturated Fat 0 g	0%
Cholesterol 0 mg	0%
Sodium 300 mg	13%
Total Carbohydrates 13 g	4%
Dietary Fiber 3 g	12%
Sugars 3 g	
Protein 3 g	

Vitamin A 80%	Vitamin C 60%
Calcium 4%	Iron 4%

*Percent Daily Values are based on a 2,000 calorie diet. Your daily values may be higher or lower depending on your calorie needs:

	Calories	2,000	2,500
Total Fat	Less than	65 g	80 g
Sat Fat	Less than	20 g	25 g
Cholesterol	Less than	300 mg	300 mg
Sodium	Less than	2,400 mg	2,400 mg
Total Carbohydrate		300 g	375 g
Dietary Fiber		25 g	30 g

Calories per gram:
Fat 9 • Carbohydrates 4 • Protein 4

FIGURE 6-1 Nutrition Facts Chart (Source: Food and Drug Administration)

also control the use of label claims such as "low," "high," "light" or "lite," and "-free." Definitions are based on reference amounts.

These claims must meet the following definitions per reference amount, that is, per standard serving size.

Calories:	*Defined as:*
Calorie-free	< 5 kcals
Low calorie	40 kcal or less
Light or Lite	1/3 fewer kcalories or 50% less fat

Fat	
Fat-free	< 0.5 g fat
Low fat	3 g or less fat; not more than 1 g saturated fat; not more than 15% kcalories from saturated fat
Light or Lite	50% less fat if > 50% kcalories from fat

Cholesterol	
Cholesterol-free	< 2 mg cholesterol and 2 g or less saturated fat
Low cholesterol	20 mg or less cholesterol and 2 g or less saturated fat

Sodium	
Sodium-free	Less than 5 mg sodium
Very low sodium	35 mg or less sodium
Low sodium	140 mg or less sodium
Light in sodium	50% less sodium than in comparable products

Sugar	
Sugar-free	Less than 0.5 g sugar

Fiber	
High fiber	5 g or more fiber

Other definitions include the following:

Lean (usually refers to meat or seafood):	< 10 g total fat/100 g serving < 4 g saturated fat < 95 mg of cholesterol
Extra lean (meat and fish	< 5 g fat/100 g serving < 2 g saturated fat, and < 95 mg cholesterol
High (for desirable nutrients, e.g., vitamins and fiber)	20% or more of the Daily Value
Good source	Contains 10-19% of the Daily Value
Reduced, fewer or less	Contains 24% less than similar food
More or added (e.g., fiber)	Contains at least 10% more of the Daily Value of a nutrient than in a reference food. Applies also to fortified and enriched. 2.5 g more fiber than a reference food
Healthy	Can be used if food is low in fat, low in saturated fat, contains 480 mg or less of sodium, or 60 mg or less of cholesterol per 100 g of the food (FDA regulations) or Meets definition of lean and has < 480 mg sodium per serving.
Light	In addition to nutrition information, may be used to describe properties such as texture and color

Health claims (that is, description of a relationship between nutrients and diseases or health-related conditions) have been carried in the past. The new regulations now allow claims of only seven of these relationships:

High calcium	Osteoporosis
High in fruits, vegetables, and fiber-containing grain products	Cancer
High in fruits or vegetables (high in dietary fiber or vitamins A or C)	Cancer
Low in fat	Cancer
Low in sodium	Hypertension
Low in saturated fat and cholesterol	Heart disease
High in fiber from fruits, vegetables and grain products	Heart disease

The law also calls for "voluntary" nutritional labeling of fresh fruits and vegetables and seafood. If a survey shows that 60 percent of a representative sample of retailers comply by labeling 90 percent of the most commonly used fruits, vegetables, and seafoods, the program will remain voluntary. Otherwise, the law requires the Food and Drug Administration to make the program mandatory.

The Food Safety and Inspection Service (FSIS) of the Department of Agriculture has a voluntary program providing nutrition information for the 45 best-selling cuts of raw meats and poultry. The information may be placed on the product itself or on nearby posters or brochures.

The items must contain the following information:

Name of the cut

Serving size (raw or cooked weight)

Calories per servings

Calories from total fat and saturated fat per serving

Amount by weight per serving of total fat, saturated fat, cholesterol, and sodium, and % Daily Value of each

Amount of protein by weight

% Daily Values per serving for calcium and iron

Some packages are allowed exceptions to the FDA labeling requirements:

1. Packages with < 12 square inches of surface area (Information must be available by mail or telephone on request).
2. Foods with no nutritional significance (< 5 calories, < 5 mg sodium; < 0.5 g total carbohydrate; < 0.5 g dietary fiber; < 0.5 g protein; and < 2% of recommended dietary intake of vitamins A and C, iron, and calcium).
3. Cartons of eggs if size doesn't accommodate the label (Information can be included before sale. If sold in bulk, information must be made available on request).
4. Bulk shipments repacked before sale (If sold in bulk, information must be made available).
5. Gift packages (can put the label on an insert).
6. Food made by small businesses, e.g., delicatessens, bakeries, take-outs (Nutritional information must be available on demand if health claims are made).

COMPARISON WITH THE DAILY FOOD GUIDE

It is not usually necessary to evaluate the patient's intake in great detail. Instead, if the patient can eat normal foods and does not have a condition that markedly increases nutrient needs, it is often sufficient to compare the intake with one or more of the "food guides" intended primarily for consumer education. One of these guides may be used clinically as the basis for a rough estimate of diet adequacy.

A 24-hour recall can be evaluated by comparing its contents with the items on one of these guides. This system has been criticized as superficial and insensitive; however, a study of results of this method compared to results of the use of an abbreviated food composition table demonstrated that scoring with a food guide was sufficiently sensitive to dietary adequacy (10).

When such guides were originally established, the recommendations were focused primarily on promoting adequacy of intake. More recently, recommendations were added that are designed to limit nutrients frequently in excess in the diet, such as fat, salt, and sweets.

The recommendations most recently issued provide the following general guidelines for meal planning for consumers and can be used to evaluate a diet for healthy persons aged 2 years and up (11):

Eat a variety of foods.

Maintain healthy weight.

Choose a diet low in fat, saturated fat, and cholesterol.

Choose a diet with plenty of vegetables, fruits and grain products.

Use sugars only in moderation.

Use salt and sodium only in moderation.

If you drink alcoholic beverages, do so in moderation.

These guidelines and the RDA were then used as a basis for development of a general outline of foods to eat each day known as the *Food Guide Pyramid* (12). The Pyramid, shown in Figure 6-2 recommends:

6–11 servings	Bread, cereals, rice, and pasta
3–5 servings	Vegetables
2–4 servings	Fruits
2–3 servings	Milk, yogurt, and cheese
2–3 servings	Meat, poultry, fish, dry beans, eggs, and nuts
Use sparingly	Naturally occurring and added fats and oil and added sweets

When using this guide, further adjustments are necessary to apply the plan for an individual diet. A decision must be made on the number of servings within the range recommended. In the pyramid, if the lowest number in each category is used, total kilocalories are about 1,600. If the largest number of servings are used, kilocalories total about 2,800 (12). Thus, the total caloric need can be used to suggest the number of servings.

Next, the definition of a "serving" must be considered. The serving sizes used in formulating the Food Guide Pyramid (Fig. 6-2) are listed in Table 6-3. If more guidance is needed, the diabetic exchange lists (Appendix C) may be consulted. However, one must take care to observe that, in the meat group in particular, a serving and an exchange are not identical. For example, *one 2–3 oz, serving* is equivalent to 2 or 3 exchanges. Some other recommendations on choices within the food groups are also given in Table 6-3.

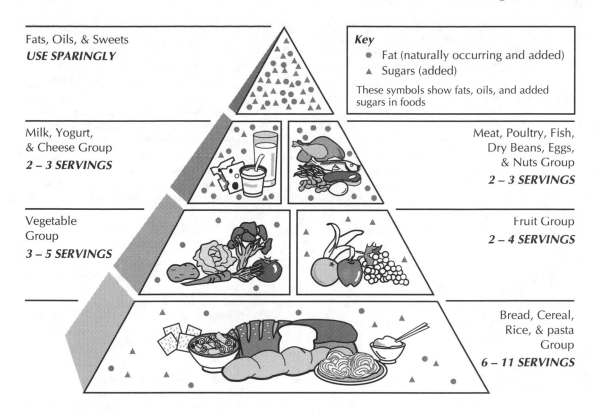

FIGURE 6-2 Food Guide Pyramid: A Guide to Daily Food Choices

In addition to the Food Guide Pyramid, a variety of other plans have been suggested (13). Some of these are designed for preventive purposes. Depending on their focus, they may recommend more fiber, less cholesterol, less saturated fat, less sodium, and less alcohol. These will be discussed in later chapters describing diseases for which these modifications are appropriate.

EVALUATING THE ADEQUACY OF THE DIET

Once the nutrient content of the patient's intake is determined, the nutritionist must evaluate the adequacy of the intake compared to the patient's nutritional requirements

COMPARISON WITH THE RECOMMENDED DIETARY ALLOWANCES

The Recommended Dietary Allowances (RDA) may be used when it is necessary to evaluate the intake of many nutrients. For your convenience, the RDA from the Food and Nutrition Board of the National Research Council (8) is given in Tables A-1 to A-4. The Canadian standards (9) are given in Table A-5.

When you are using the RDA (8), it is important to keep in mind several facts that you learned from your courses in Normal Nutrition:

1. The recommendations are set at a level to provide for the needs of most members of the population group, *not* for specific individuals; they therefore exceed requirements of many individuals (except for the energy requirement).
2. The recommendations are designed to apply to healthy populations and do not cover special needs. Thus, the nutritionist must apply professional judgment when evaluating patients' diets compared to these recommendations. An individual who does not receive the amounts recommended each day is not necessarily malnourished. On the other hand, those with increased needs may be deficient even if recommended amounts are obtained. Conditions in which special needs occur will be described in the chapters that follow.

COMPARISON TO CALCULATED REQUIREMENTS

As discussed in Chapter 5, estimates of an individual patient's nutritional requirements may be calculated. This estimate may then be used as a basis for evaluation of the patient's intake. For example, let us assume that a patient's intake is 1,250 kcal and 70 g protein, but the calculated total daily expenditure (TDE) is 1,550 kcal with a 70-g protein requirement. It should be clear that the patient needs supplementation of her energy intake.

TABLE 6-3. Definition of a Serving in the Food Guide Pyramid

Food	Amount	Further Suggestions
Bread, cereal, rice, pasta		
Bread	1 slice	Choose several servings of whole grain
Ready-to-eat cereal	1 oz (3/4 c).	Choose mostly products with little fat or sugar
Cooked cereal, rice, pasta	1/2 c	Limit fat and sugars as spreads, seasonings or toppings
Vegetables		
Raw leafy	1 c	Use several times weekly.
Others, cooked or chopped raw	1/2 c	Use deep-yellow and starchy vegetables often
Vegetable juice	3/4 c	Use legumes several times per week or use in place of meat
		Use low fat salad dressings
Fruit		
Medium whole	One	Eat whole fruits often
(e.g., apple, orange)		Include citrus fruits, melons, and berries.
Chopped, cooked, or canned	1/2 c	
Fruit juice	3/4 c	Count any 100% fruit juices;
		punches, ades, and fruit "drinks" do not qualify
		Limit sweetened juice and fruit canned or frozen in heavy syrup unless energy need is high
Milk, Yogurt, Cheese		
Milk or yogurt	1 c	Choose skim milk or nonfat yogurt often.
Natural cheese	1 1/2 oz	Limit high fat cheese and ice cream
Process cheese	2 oz	Prefer "part skim" or nonfat cheese and lower fat milk desserts
		Use 3 servings for pregnancy, lactation, adolescents and adults to age 24
Meat, poultry, fish, dry beans, eggs, nuts		
Cooked lean meat, poultry, fish	2–3 oz	Choose lean meat, fish, poultry without skin
		Trim all visible fat and cook by broiling, roasting, boiling, not frying
Cooked dry beans	1/2 c	Use dried beans and peas often
Egg	One=1 oz lean meat or 1/3 sv	Limit use of egg yolks to 3-4/week
Peanut butter	2 T= 1 oz lean meat or 1/3 sv	Eat nuts and seeds in moderation
Other items		
Fat	Limit to 30% of cals	Lowest fat choices in each will give half of the recommended amount
Saturated fat	Limit to 10% or 1/3 of total above	Found in meats, dairy products and nut oils
Monounsaturated fat		Found mostly in olive, peanut, and canola oils.
Polyunsaturated fat		Found mostly in safflower, sunflower, corn, soy, and cotton seed oils and some fish
Cholesterol	300 mg or less/day[1]	Found in animal fats
Salt and sodium	2,400 to 3,000 mg/day[2]	Found in salt, cured meats, luncheon meats, some cheeses, canned soups and vegetables, prepared foods, soy sauces
Sugars	Limit to 6 tsp for 1,600 kcal diet; 18 tsp for 2,800 kcal diet[3]	Found in candy, soft drinks, jam, jelly, desserts, and other highly sweetened foods
Alcohol	Limit to 1–2 drinks per day "if you choose to drink"	Equivalent "drinks" are 12 oz beer, 5 oz dry wine, or 1 1/2 oz liquor

[1] See Chapter 20.
[2] See Chapter 20, 21.
[3] See Chapter 19..

REFERENCES

1. *Exchange Lists for Meal Planning*. Washington, DC: American Diabetes Association, 1995, Chicago: American Dietetic Association, 1995.

2. *Composition of Foods*. Agricultural Handbooks No. 8-1 to 8-16. Washington, DC: Consumer and Food Economics Institute, USDA, 1976–82.

3. **Pennington, J.A.T.** *Bowes and Church's Food Values of Portions Commonly Used*, 16th ed. New York: Lippincott, 1994.

4. United States Department of Agriculture, Science and Education Administration. *Nutritive Value of Foods*. Home and Garden Bulletin No. 72. Washington, DC: USDA, 1981.

5. **Leveille, G.A., M.E. Zabick, and K.J. Morgan.** *Nutrients in Foods*. Cambridge, MA: Nutrition Guild, 1983.

6. **Paul, A., and D.A.T. Southgate.** *McCance and Widdowson's The Composition of Foods*, 4th ed., New York: Elsevier/North Holland. 1978 (with supplements: Boca Raton, FL: CRC Press, 1944).

7. **Young, E.A., E.H. Brennan, and G.L. Irving.** Update: nutritional analysis of fast foods. *Dietetic Currents* 8(2):(1981)1–12.

8. Food and Nutrition Board, National Research Council. *Recommended Dietary Allowances*, 10th ed. Washington, DC: National Academy Press, 1990.

9. Committee for Revision of the Canadian Dietary Standard, Bureau of Nutritional Sciences, Health and Welfare, Canada. *Recommended Nutrient Intakes for Canadians*. Ottawa: Information Canada, 1975.

10. **Guthrie, H.A., and J.C. Scheer.** Validity of a dietary score for assessing nutrient adequacy. *J. Am. Dietet. Assoc.* 78:(1981)240..

11. U.S. Department of Agriculture and U.S. Department of Health and Human Services. *Nutrition and Your Health: Diet Guidelines for Americans*. Washington, DC: Home and Garden Bulletin, No. 232, 1990.

12. ———.*The Food Guide Pyramid*. Washington, DC: Home and Garden Bulletin, No. 252, 1992.

13. **Cronin, F.J., and A.M. Shaw.** Summary of dietary recommendations for healthy Americans. *Nutrition Today* 23:(1988) 26–34.

 ## TO TEST YOUR UNDERSTANDING

1. During your interview with a patient, she lists the following items eaten the previous day. In order to make the 24-hour recall as accurate as possible, list the further information you would seek on each item, exclusive of serving size.

Coffee
Cornflakes
Chicken salad sandwich
Milk
Canned peaches
Filet of sole
Toast
Mashed potatoes
Buttered broccoli
Tossed salad

2. If a patient mentioned the following items, suggest some procedures you might use to increase the accuracy of the patient's estimate of portion size. (Use your ingenuity and imagination. You will not find the answers in this volume.)

Pork chop
Fruit juice
Buttered frozen peas
Cooked breakfast cereal

3. Revise the following questions or statements to improve the interviewing technique, and increase the accuracy of the information obtained. Explain your reasons for the changes you make. (Consult Chapter 3 if necessary.)

a. "What kind of vegetable did you have with your steak dinner?"
b. "Now that we have information on your breakfast, tell me what you had for lunch."
c. "Do you drink this much beer every day?"

4. Which methods of collecting information on food intake would you choose for each of the following? Why?
a. Mr. M., a traveling salesman, was admitted this morning for elective minor surgery. He is alert and cooperative. His surgery is scheduled for tomorrow.
b. Susan L., age 3, and her mother were involved in an automobile accident. Susan has two fractured legs. Her mother is in a coma with head injuries.

5. You are asked to report a patient's protein and kcal intake. After observing her food intake and the uneaten food on her tray, you compile the following list of food which she ate in 1 day. Using the exchange lists in Appendix C, calculate the values requested and show your calculations on Form C from Appendix M.

1/2 c orange juice	tea with lemon
1/4 c farina	1 c bouillon
1/2 c skim milk	6 saltines
coffee	5 oz chicken (no bone or skin)
1 t sugar	1/2 c green beans
2-egg omelet	1 large tomato, sliced
1 t margarine	1 T French dressing
2 t butter	1/2 c ice cream

(continued)

TO TEST YOUR UNDERSTANDING *(continued)*

6. In the menu given in the previous question, what are the major sources of:

calcium?
iron?
ascorbic acid?
thiamin?
riboflavin?
niacin?
vitamin A?

7. Given the degree of accuracy of the information obtained in a 24-hour recall and the time required for calculation, which method do you think is most likely to be useful and practical in most clinical situations?

8. You interview a 22-year-old male patient who is hospitalized for tooth extraction. He is in good health with body weight 5 percent below the 50th percentile for his height. Your analysis of the patient's 24-hour recall indicates that he has an intake of ascorbic acid that is 10 percent below the RDA. Give your evaluation of his diet.

9. Six months later, you see the same patient. He has been in a motorcycle accident and has multiple fractures. You know that his injuries result in an increase in his metabolic rate.

   a. What effect would the healing process have on his ascorbic acid requirement?

   b. Assuming his diet had not changed in the 6 months prior to his injuries, what effect would his injuries have on the adequacy of his diet in kcals? ascorbic acid?

10. Write a SOAP note concerning the adequacy of the patient's diet to meet his present needs.

11. Ms. J.C. gives you the following 24-hour recall, which she says is typical of her daily diet.

Breakfast:
1/2 c orange juice
1 fried egg
2 slices white toast, buttered, enriched
coffee, black

Lunch:
tuna fish salad sandwich (enriched bread)
Sliced tomatoes with French dressing
1 fresh peach
1 c milk

Dinner:
1 c beef stew with vegetables on 1 c buttered noodles
1/2 c spinach
1/8 head lettuce wedge/Thousand Island dressing
1/2 c serving of cherry cobbler
1 c milk
Tea with lemon

   a. Does this day's intake contain all the food groups recommended by the Food Guide Pyramid? If not, what is lacking?

   b. Ms. J. C., age 48, is 5 feet, 8 inches tall and weighs 110 pounds. What would you conclude about the adequacy of her diet?

   c. Is your conclusion in question *b* confirmed if you calculate the energy content of the diet using exchange lists? (Show your calculations.)

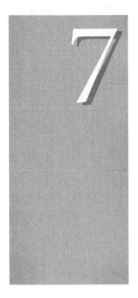

7 Counseling the Patient

Betsy B. Holli, Ed.D., R.D.

The information obtained in the nutrition interview and used in evaluating the individual's current food intake and nutritional status is the basis for nutrition counseling. In comparing the patient's current diet with the dietary prescription for a diabetic diet, for example, or in evaluating the nutritional status of a pregnant woman, it is obvious to the nutrition care specialist, but not to the client, that some changes need to be made. These changes are the basis for counseling.

Like interviewing, counseling is a communication skill. Repeated practice is needed to improve the skill. Nutrition counseling may be defined as a process that assists individuals in understanding and learning about their dietary habits or behaviors as part of their lifestyle and total environment and in solving problems related to necessary changes that need to be made (1). Counseling is concerned primarily with the building of personal competencies in order for individuals to cope better with their life situation. Self-care and self-management are the ultimate goals.

COMPONENTS OF COMMUNICATION

There are three major components in the communication process: verbal communication, nonverbal communication, and listening. The understanding of all three is useful to the nutrition care specialist.

VERBAL COMMUNICATION

Good communication skills are essential for competent professional practice. Communication is important to the development of the interpersonal relationship between the counselor and the client or patient. Good communication skills are not ends in themselves but are the basis

for effective treatment in which the individual needs to make dietary and behavioral changes. Poor communication skills may result in obtaining inadequate dietary information as a basis for treatment, inadequate nutrition care plans, poor patient satisfaction, and possible lack of adherence to the dietary regimen.

Some of the essential communication skills were already discussed in the chapter on interviewing. These same skills of developing rapport; using open, closed, primary, secondary, and neutral questions; and using understanding, probing, and confrontational responses are also used in counseling and should be reviewed. In addition, paraphrasing is an important skill in counseling.

To be sure that the client is understood, the counselor needs to stop periodically to summarize and paraphrase what the individual is saying or feeling in order to confirm that one is understanding correctly. For example:

"I want to be sure that I understand. You are saying that you have been on diets twice before. Each time you lost weight, but after 2 weeks, you felt weak and tired and went off the diet."

Paraphrasing periodically tells the client verbally that the counselor is listening, caring, and trying to understand. In addition, the individual can verify whether or not the counselor is correct.

NONVERBAL COMMUNICATION

During the communication process, both parties are aware of nonverbal communication, sometimes called *body language*. Nonverbal communication includes facial expression, tone of voice, gestures, posture, and body movements. Even the clothing one wears and office furniture arrangements convey a message. As a result, counselors need to be sure that their nonverbal messages are not only appropriate but also congruent with their verbal communication.

Appropriate nonverbal communication includes smiling or a pleasant facial expression, eye contact, a moderate tone of voice, and leaning slightly forward in the chair to show interest. Counselors realize that nonverbal communication varies among different ethnic groups. In some groups, for example, eye contact is avoided. Appropriate professional clothing with a conservative hair style, and limited jewelry and cosmetics make a favorable impression. On the other hand, slouching, frowning, constant looking at a watch, clock, or papers, constant writing or other failure to pay attention to the client, all create negative impressions and interfere with the interpersonal relationship one is trying to establish. Besides being aware of one's own nonverbal communication, counselors need to observe and interpret the nonverbal communication of their clients.

Furniture arrangements also communicate a message. Chairs should be arranged close enough to hear well. If standing, an arm's length away is considered appropriate. In group counseling, a circular arrangement of chairs so that everyone has eye contact promotes the best interaction. In an office, a chair alongside a desk is less formal and more "equal" when one is trying to establish a helping relationship with the client participating. A chair situated across from the counselor's desk suggests that the professional is an expert or authority figure.

LISTENING

Attentive listening suggests a counselor who is concerned and caring. Good listening skills need to be practiced and developed. Counselors must respond verbally and nonverbally in a way that shows that they listen to and understand clients and what they are saying.

Inexperienced counselors may have other thoughts on their minds that interfere with listening. Instead of concentrating on the individual's story, they may be thinking about what questions to ask next or pondering previous responses. Or the mind may wander to earlier events or to one's plans for later in the day, as it does when we are in school or meetings.

Needless to say, taking notes disrupts one's concentration on the person's conversation. If notes are necessary, they should be kept to an absolute minimum. Preferably, notes are written or dictated at the conclusion of the counseling session. Full undivided attention must be given to what the individual is saying.

THE HELPING RELATIONSHIP

One of the keys to successful nutrition counseling depends on the relationship established between the counselor and the client. Counseling assumes an ongoing relationship over time, not merely one appointment. The clinical dietitian in the hospital who has the opportunity to see a patient only once and then just prior to discharge cannot expect much of the patient as far as dietary adherence. Additional referral to an outpatient dietitian or dietitian in private practice who can have a continuing relationship in promoting dietary change is advisable.

Influencing others to change should be based on caring, understanding, and collaboration. The assumption is that individuals learn the skills they need to improve their dietary practices and health through the counseling process.

An autocratic relationship based on the premise that the counselor is the expert who knows what to do and tells the passive patient the necessary changes to make is seldom effective. If I tell you what to do, you are likely to think I do not understand you and likely to tell me why you cannot do it. For example:

"You've got to eat breakfast every day."

"But I am never hungry in the morning, and I don't have time."

Instead the counselor needs to develop a relationship in which the two parties are equal partners in solving problems. The counselor is a helper, but the decisions about solving dietary problems and making dietary changes belong to the client. Solutions that the individual comes up with are far more likely to be implemented, while solutions that others give seldom work. The counselor can guide the change and help clients explore both their dietary behaviors and their feelings. Certainly the counselor will provide information, resources, and alternatives. But then the client must decide whether or not to accept. The individual must become an active, not passive, participant in the counseling and problem-solving process. Self-care, self-management, and self-control are necessary. The nutrition care specialist will not be there every day to see that the dietary regimen is followed. Individuals eventually have to learn to solve their own problems.

The counselor should create an environment of respect and trust. Clients must perceive that they are accepted, valued, and understood, faults and all. Avoiding judgments that what the person eats is "right" or "wrong," "nutritious" or "ridiculous," "good for him" or "bad for him," is very important. Trust must be earned. Any indication that the counselor is judging the person tends to inhibit the relationship and rapport and to decrease the self-disclosure so necessary for helping. Credibility may be strained when the counselor is unable to project warmth, respect, empathy, and concern.

ASSESSMENT, TREATMENT, AND CHANGE

Prior to counseling, the nutrition care specialist needs to collect and assess data that bear on the client's eating problems. Some of the data may be found on the medical record, such as height, weight, age, diagnosis, family status, occupation, and the like. Information on current eating habits is obtained by using the nutrition interview described in Chapter 3. All factors in the environment that impact on eating behavior, whether physical, social, or cognitive, need to be explored.

The assessment identifies dietary behaviors that need to be changed. The difference between what should be eaten, according to the diet prescription, and what is currently being eaten suggests the areas of change.

Since a number of changes which can be discouraging to individuals, may be needed, it is preferable to discuss first what does not need changing. For example:

"Your breakfast and lunch are great, Mr. Smith. I don't see any problems with them. You can continue eating what you're eating now."

Afterwards the problems may be discussed. The counselor examines with clients the changes they think they are able to make easily. And with the more difficult changes, one can discuss how the individual can fit the change into his or her lifestyle. The client making the changes has to find the solutions and make these decisions, not the counselor. We avoid giving advice, such as "I think you should…" or "I would suggest that you…" Instead, we assist in the problem-solving process.

SETTING GOALS

When eating changes are identified, the client is encouraged to set goals for change. The counselor may ask: "What one or two changes can you make now?" There are limits on the number of changes (one or two) that can be made at any one time. It is preferable to start with a limited number of goals, and to select those at which the individual is most likely to be successful. When these are accomplished, other goals can be set.

Goals should be stated positively, very specifically, and in terms of food behaviors to change (1). For example:

"I will eat fresh fruit instead of cookies this week."
"I will use pepper and onion in place of salt."
"I will eat prepared cereal with skim milk every morning for breakfast."

The following goals are less well stated:

"I will lose 3 pounds this week" (not a food behavior).
"I will not use salt anymore" (negative goal).
"I will eat breakfast every day" (vague goal).

Helping others to set goals has several advantages. Goals are guides to action and commitment. They are also a self-motivation tool as well as a standard against which to measure performance.

The dietary changes required sound simple enough. Eat this, but don't eat that. Cook your food differently. Limit the quantity of food you eat. Read food labels at the grocery store. Purchase different foods. Select different foods when you eat in restaurants. The educated professional, steeped in the knowledge of nutrition, knows just what the individual needs to do.

PROMOTING COMPLIANCE

Some clients are referred back to the nutrition care specialist because they are having problems following the dietary regimen. Knowing what to do, and doing it, are not the same. Studies on dietary compliance show that adherence rates are low (2). Of all the lifestyle changes that individuals need to make to improve their health—such as increasing exercise, stopping smoking, taking medications and the like—making dietary changes seems to be the most difficult. Yet some people are successful. Information on per-capita consumption of foods, for example, show that Americans now eat fewer eggs, less beef, and more chicken and fish (3). The nutrition care specialist needs to recognize that change is difficult, but possible. Effective counseling strategies help to promote change.

Why is dietary change so difficult? There are a number of reasons. People's current eating habits are long-standing and firmly embedded in lifestyle practices. Many eating practices and preferences date back to childhood and to what mother served us. Did your mother serve broccoli, for example? If not, you may not eat it either. And food is associated with love and with pleasure. Observing a baby enjoying a bottle or the breast should leave no doubt that the association between food, love, and happiness starts early in life (1).

People do not just eat because they are hungry. They eat when they are lonely, depressed, worried, tired, upset, or bored. And they eat when they are happy, socializing, and celebrating events, such as birthdays, anniversaries, graduations, and promotions. Besides being associated with both positive and negative emotions, food is associated with physiological feelings, such as hunger and fatigue. One's dietary changes may be easily postponed in favor of eating to satisfy a more immediate emotional or physiological need.

There are a number of suggestions for making changes easier for others. Make the changes as simple and easy as possible, for example. Complex changes are more difficult to follow. Help the person fit the change into his or her current lifestyle and values as far as time, cost, and family or personal situation. See that there are still pleasurable foods that the individual can eat (1). An unpleasant, restrictive diet is less likely to be followed. The very term *diet* has negative connotations. Also, one needs to examine the person's motivation for change.

COUNSELING THEORIES AND APPROACHES

The practice of counseling is based on theories of learning and behavioral change. There are a number of different approaches, and certain approaches may work better with one individual or dietary problem than with another. Thus it is well for the nutrition care specialist to be familiar with and able to use several of the theories. In this chapter, client-centered, behavioral/learning, imitative learning, and cognitive counseling theories and strategies are discussed.

Counseling is really a learning experience in which a person's behavior is changed, although theories disagree on how the learning takes place, whether in the nature of the counseling relationship or in positive reinforcement, for example. Theories also differ somewhat in the role of the counselor and how much control is exercised.

CLIENT-CENTERED COUNSELING

Client-centered counseling is associated most frequently with Dr. Carl Rogers, a psychologist. According to his theory, the emphasis is almost exclusively on the relationship between the counselor and the client rather than on techniques (4). To develop the relationship, counselors must be genuine or congruent with patients and accept them unconditionally and nonjudgmentally regardless of their behaviors. An empathic understanding of the patient's internal frame of reference is essential. Counselors try to understand as if they were that individual. The counselor's unconditional positive regard as well as the empathic understanding must be communicated to the patient both verbally and nonverbally. In this supportive, threat-free, accepting atmosphere, the individual is comfortable in revealing all thoughts and feelings both freely and openly (4,5).

Under the proper counseling conditions, it is assumed that the client will be able to gain self-insight and perceive and evaluate his or her experiences accurately. As problems are explored, individuals begin to understand themselves. Rather than providing answers, the counselor assists while individuals find their own solutions to their problems, set goals, and change their behaviors. The emphasis is on releasing the client's potential and ability to direct his or her own life.

BEHAVIORAL/LEARNING THEORY

Behavioral/learning theory is based on the premise that most behaviors, whether maladaptive or effective, are learned (4). If learned, they can be changed, and other behaviors can be learned instead. Behavioral techniques are applied frequently in the treatment of obesity, eating disorders, cardiovascular diseases, and other medical problems (6–9).

Behavioral/learning theory also recognizes the importance of the relationship between the client and the counselor. But the counselor takes a somewhat more active role in guiding the treatment to alter eating behaviors, using a combination of techniques in terms of specific maladaptive behaviors to be changed. These approaches are based on principles of learning.

People learn in different ways. Behavior is often the result of some environmental or stimulus situation, such as eating in response to hunger or boredom. The eating behavior results in some type of consequence, such as feeling better, happier, less bored, or less hungry. Positive consequences are rewarding to the individual, making it more likely that if the same stimulus situation occurs in the future (boredom or hunger), it will be followed by the same response behavior (eating), which is a learned or conditioned response. Other terms describing positive consequences are positive reinforcement or reward.

In addition to learning taking place in stimulus-response-consequences associations, learning takes place through the observation and imitation of others. Children, for example, exhibit behaviors similar to those of a significant person in their lives, and are positively reinforced for doing so.

A third type of learning is influenced by cognitions. Learning may result from thinking things over, for example. Cognitions or thoughts influence eating in positive as well as negative ways. Counseling for modification of eating behaviors, as described in this section, examines the influence of learned eating behaviors, how they can be analyzed, and how maladaptive responses may be modified.

Behavioral theory sees people mainly as products of their interactions with their environments. Behaviors are shaped according to stimulus-response associations and the process of conditioning (4). There are two types of conditioning: (1) classical or respondent conditioning and (2) operant or instrumental conditioning (10).

Most people are familiar with classical conditioning as described with Ivan Pavlov's dogs. When food (unconditioned stimulus) was presented, the dogs salivated (unconditioned response). The researchers added a bell (conditioned stimulus) when food was presented. Over time, the dogs were conditioned to salivate at only the sound of a bell in the absence of food. People also become conditioned to respond to certain stimuli, for example, to like certain foods and dislike others due to previous associations and conditioning.

CUES TO EATING

The counselor and the client need to identify, analyze, and discuss the undesirable stimuli or cues to eating in the person's physical and social environments. Examples of environmental situations that cue eating are arriving home; walking through the kitchen; certain times of day; watching television; attending movies; social events; emotions such as boredom, loneliness, and happiness; and physiological feelings of hunger or fatigue. Table 7-1 summarizes some possible cues to eating that counselors may identify with clients. Over a period of time many situations become associated with eating food and thus cue eating (1, 12).

After identifying the individual's cues to eating, the client and counselor approach each undesirable one with one of several strategies. Alternatives are: (1) to decrease the number of times the person is exposed to the cue

TABLE 7-1   Cues to Eating

Emotional : boredom, loneliness, happiness

Celebrations: birthdays, parties

Watching movies, television

Time of day

Certain rooms in the house

Driving in the car

Sight of food at the store or at home

Certain friends, family members, or coworkers

Cognitions or thoughts about food

Physiological feelings: hunger, fatigue

(watch less television, for example), (2) remove negative cues (avoid buying improper foods), (3) introduce new cues (exercise or phone a friend instead of eating), and (4) restrict behavior to one set of cues (eat only at designated times and only while seated at one place designated for eating).

REINFORCEMENT

While behavior in classical conditioning is controlled by its antecedents, behavior in operant conditioning is controlled by its consequences (10). Operant conditioning depends on the use of reinforcement or rewards after a behavior. There are two kinds of reinforcement, positive and negative (4).

Both positive and negative reinforcement increase the future likelihood or probability of a response in the presence of the same or a similar stimulus (5). Positive reinforcement is satisfying. Verbal praise received after eating the right foods, for example, strengthens the probability of eating right in the future.

Negative reinforcement is due to the removal of an aversive or unpleasant stimulus condition, and is also satisfying. Behaviors that reduce or eliminate unpleasant conditions in our lives are often reinforced since the results are gratifying. Having learned to eat food (response) to relieve anxiety or fatigue (stimulus) is an example of negative reinforcement. The food is pleasant (reinforcement) as it assists in removing the unpleasant stimulus of anxiety or fatigue. Thus eating tends to occur again in the presence of the same stimulus. In the long run, however, these can be maladaptive, undesirable, and self-defeating responses (4). They may be considered "escape" or "avoidance" behaviors (11).

It is possible to use negative reinforcement to strengthen healthy behaviors (11). For example, a verbal commitment or written contract to eat differently and lose weight presumably serves as a negative reinforcer in that weight is lost at least in part to "avoid" the social consequences of not living up to one's recorded commitment.

Behaviors are also subject to extinction. Extinction may occur when a response is never reinforced. If a person is never praised for eating the right foods, for example, the proper response may weaken and become extinct.

After discussing eating cues, the client and the counselor can explore what is reinforcing or rewarding current eating behaviors, since behaviors are more likely to reoccur with positive reinforcement. It is very possible that current eating, since it is pleasurable, is its own reward. As a result, any recommended changes in eating should also be pleasurable. In addition, new nonfood reinforcers can be identified, such as those in Table 7-2.

To determine what else besides eating the person finds pleasurable, the counselor may ask a number of questions, such as the following (13):

> Whom do you like to spend time with?
> What do you like to do with your spare time?
> What do you like to spend money on?
> What do you do for fun? For relaxation?

New activities, when identified, can be used to positively reinforce new eating behaviors. If the dietary regimen is followed, for example, clients reward themselves with a small purchase, a phone call to a friend, or other reward.

Scheduling reinforcement is also necessary. At first almost every new eating change should be reinforced. However, continuous reinforcement tends to lose its effectiveness, and later a schedule of intermittent reinforcement is preferable.

In behavioral/learning theory, the counselor takes a more active role in helping people to identify behaviors that need changing, recognize and change the stimuli or cues to eating, understand the use of reinforcers or rewards, and plan strategies to strengthen proper eating and weaken improper eating which may lead eventually to its extinction.

TABLE 7-2   Positive Reinforcers

Walking or exercising

Telephoning a friend

Writing a letter

Listening to favorite music

Reading favorite materials

Setting aside a sum of money for a future purchase

Attending movies, theatre, musical or sporting events

Hobbies

Spending time doing favorite activities

Praise from others

Self-praise

Shopping

SELF-MONITORING

Frequently we ask clients to keep daily records of their food intake, such as the example in Table 7-3. In addition to food, we like to know about the time and place of eating, others present, concurrent activities such as reading or watching television, and moods or feelings, such as fatigue or boredom. Examination and discussion of these records may help identify both cues to eating and reinforcers. Needless to say, one cannot change a behavior until one recognizes what it is. Clients become much more aware of their own eating problems as they keep records, which lead to better self-understanding (13).

IMITATIVE LEARNING

Although some behaviors may be shaped by controlling the reinforcement, other behaviors are learned by observation and imitation of others who serve as role models. Albert Bandura has stressed the influence of modeling on learning (4).

In modeling, an individual observes the behavior of another person vicariously, assesses the other's behavior, and imitates it. For example, Johnny imitates what his dad eats while Suzie imitates what her mother eats and how she behaves. A great deal of learning takes place through modeling after others whom we contact personally or through symbolic representations, such as in films or on television.

Not everyone serves as a model for others, however. Many people model their behaviors after those they admire or with whom they can identify. The counselor may want to present counselees with live or filmed models who demonstrate the desired behavioral outcomes, as for example eating changes that result in weight loss. The closer the identification with the model, the more likely that imitative learning will take place (4, 5). The counselor also should be a good role model.

COGNITIONS

Besides the influence of eating cues, positive reinforcement, and imitative learning, eating behaviors are influenced by one's cognitions. Cognitions may be defined as conscious thoughts at a particular moment in time. They are also referred to as *internal dialogue* or *self-talk* (1).

This self-talk may be positive, negative, or neutral. A positive cognition is: "I think that I can change what I am eating." Positive cognitions support behaviors, while negative ones inhibit them. An example of a negative cognition is: "This new diet looks very difficult." Obese people are reported to have negative cognitions (14). Cognitive distortions are also problems in those with eating disorders (5, 15).

Since cognitions are also learned responses, the counselor and client can collaborate to identify the current cognitions and to restructure those that are negative into more constructive, coping thoughts. The first step is to help people become aware of what they are thinking.

TABLE 7-3   Self-Monitoring Record

Date/Time	Place	Food/Amount	Thoughts	Others Present	Mood	Other Activity
Example:						
9/27 6:15	Kitchen	Baked chicken Baked potato Broccoli Tossed salad Apple Iced tea	"I feel hungry and tired"	Spouse	Upset	Talking

This may be done with verbal questions ("What do you think about…?" or "How do you feel about…?"), and by asking the client to keep self-monitoring records of thoughts before and after eating. Before eating, for example, a depressed patient may be thinking: "I'll feel better if I eat a piece of cake." After eating the cake, the self-talk may be: "Now I do feel better." It is rare for people to recognize that thoughts are part of their eating problems. The client needs to discover this.

The second step is to examine the negative and self-defeating thoughts and implement cognitive restructuring. The client can learn to ask:

> Is that really true? What is the evidence?
> What can I say instead which is more positive and coping?
> How do these thoughts affect what I eat?

Together the client and counselor can explore the negative thoughts and their influence on eating. Rather than providing answers, the counselor asks questions that promote client self-discovery and eventually more positive and coping responses. "Thought-stopping" techniques may also be helpful. Clients are taught to say "stop" mentally whenever they recognize that they are having negative cognitions.

EVALUATION AND FOLLOW-UP

Records of the patient's problems and goals for change are kept for future counseling sessions. At follow-up, the initial conversation should emphasize the successes, i.e., what went well and what goals were reached, with the counselor providing positive reinforcement. Problems may then be discussed. Eating problems should be viewed as opportunities for new learning, not as uncooperative behavior. Then new goals for change should be set using the goal-setting process.

REFERENCES

1. **Holli, B.B., and R.J. Calabrese.** *Communication and Education Skills: The Dietitian's Guide*, 2d ed. Philadelphia: Lea & Febiger, 1991.

2. **Glanz, K.** *Trends in Patient Compliance.* Chicago: American Dietetic Association, 1981.

3. **Putnam, J.J.** Food consumption, 1970–1990. *National Food Review* 14: (1991) 2–12.

4. **Avenshine, C.D., and A.L. Noffsinger.** *Counseling: An Introduction for the Health and Human Services.* Baltimore: University Park Press, 1984.

5. **Corey, Gerald.** *Theory and Practice of Counseling and Psychotherapy.* Pacific Grove, CA: Brooks/Cole, 1991.

6. **Storlie J., and H.A. Jordan.** *Behavioral Management of Obesity.* New York: Medical & Scientific Books, 1984.

7. **Agras, W.S.** *Eating Disorders: Management of Obesity, Bulimia, and Anorexia Nervosa.* New York: Pergamon Press, 1987.

8. **Zwann M., and J. Mitchell.** Bulimia nervosa. *Clin. Appl. Nutr.* 1 (2): (1991) 40–48.

9. **Remmell, P.S., D.D. Gorder, Y. Hall, and J.L. Tillotson.** Assessing dietary adherence in the Multiple Risk Factor Intervention Trial (MRFIT). *J. Am. Dietet. Assoc.* 76: (1980) 351–60.

10. **George, R.L., and T.S. Cristiani.** *Counseling Theory and Practice,* 3d ed.. Englewood Cliffs, NJ: Prentice Hall, 1990.

11. **Elder, J.P., M.F. Hovell, T.M. Lasater, B.L. Wells, and R.A. Carleton.** Applications of behavior modification to community health education: The case of heart disease prevention. *Health Educ. Q.* 12: (1985) 151–68.

12. **Stunkard, A.J. and H.C. Berthold.** What is behavior therapy? *Am.J. Clin. Nutr.* 41: (1985) 821–23.

13. **Holli, B.B.** Using behavior modification in nutrition counseling. *J. Am. Dietet. Assoc.* 88: (1988) 1530–38.

14. **Stunkard, A.J.** Conservative treatments for obesity. *Am. J. Clin. Nutr.* 45: (1987) 1142–54.

15. **Hoffman, L. and K.A. Halmi.** Recent developments in anorexia nervosa. *Clin. Appl. Nutr.* 1 (2): (1991) 49–54.

ADDITIONAL SOURCES OF INFORMATION

Aronson, V., Fitzgerald, B., and L.V. Hewes. Guidebook for Nutrition Counselors, 2d ed. Englewood Cliffs, NJ: Prentice Hall, 1990.

Curry, K.R., and S.P. Himburg. *Establishing an Effective Nutrition Education/Counseling Program: Skills for the RD.* Study Kit 11. Chicago: American Dietetic Association, 1988.

Frankle, R.T., and M.U. Yang. *Obesity and Weight Control: The Health Professional's Guide to Understanding and Treatment.* Rockville, MD: Aspen Publishers, 1988.

Hodges, P.A.M., and C.E. Vickery. *Effective Counseling: Strategies for Dietary Management.* Rockville, MD: Aspen Publishers, 1989.

Muldary, T.W. *Interpersonal Relations for Health Professionals: A Social Skills Approach.* New York: Macmillan, 1983.

Snetselaar, L.G. *Nutrition Counseling Skills: Assessment, Treatment, and Evaluation,* 2d ed. Rockville, MD: Aspen Publishers, 1988.

Storlie, J., and H.A. Jordan. *Behavioral Management of Obesity.* New York: Spectrum, 1984.

☑ TO TEST YOUR UNDERSTANDING

1. Paraphrase either the thought or the feelings expressed in the following statements:

a. "The doctor says that I need to lose weight because of my blood pressure. I don't know how I can do it eating in restaurants all the time."

b. "At my age of 75, I don't feel like doing a lot of cooking. I live alone and don't have the energy that I used to have."

c. "They told me that I have diabetes and that I will have to follow a diet, take insulin, and do a lot of other things I have never done before."

d. "Since my heart attack, I have tried to eat less cholesterol and fatty foods. I have had to give up a lot of my favorite foods, such as cheese, ice cream, bacon, and eggs."

2. Describe the optimum kind of helping relationship to establish with a client or patient.

3. List the kinds of information that should be obtained in assessing an individual's eating practices or behaviors.

4. Write examples of appropriate goals for dietary change for a pregnant woman, teenager, elderly person, and for individuals with obesity, diabetes mellitus, and cardiovascular disease.

5. Discuss the reasons why dietary changes are difficult for people and what can be done to make them easier to follow.

6. Restructure these negative cognitions into ones that are more positive and coping:

a. "I never could follow a diet. I'm a failure."

b. "I ate the whole bag of cookies. I'm a pig."

c. "I've had such a hard day. A candy bar will make me feel better."

Nutritional Assessment

To The Learner

This case study provides you with an opportunity to integrate and summarize the material and skills you learned in Chapters 1 through 6. Read the material given here carefully, and use only the information given when forming your answers.

Mrs. C. is a 73-year-old woman who lives alone in a walk-up apartment. She has been a widow for 2 years and has no children. She has a very limited income. Mrs. C. was visited by the police when a neighbor reported that she had not been seen for several days. Finding her weak, bedridden, and unattended, the police brought Mrs. C. to the hospital emergency room, from which she was admitted to the internal medicine service.

For your initial nutritional assessment, the patient's medical record provided the following information:

Height		5 ft, 4 in
Present weight		100#
Serum albumin, g/L		26
Total leukocyte count, 10^9/L		4.0
Differential:	Lymphocytes, %	25
	Neutrophils, %	70
	Eosinophils, %	1
	Basophils, %	0.5
	Monocytes, %	3.5
Total RBC count, $\times 10^{12}$/L		4.6
Hct		0.25
Hgb, g/L		76

The in-depth nutritional assessment yielded the following additional information:

Triceps skinfold, mm	11.0
Midarm circumference, cm	20.4
Wrist measurement, in	6
Cell-mediated immunity in 48 hrs:	
PPD, mm	3.0
Mumps, mm	4.0
Candida, mm	2.5
Urinary urea nitrogen, mmol/d UREA	450
Total iron-binding capacity, μmol/L	40

Mrs. C. has arthritis and poorly fitting dentures. She stated that she does not have "enough money to buy more food." In addition, she said she is afraid to walk alone to the supermarket, which is a mile away, and has no other means of transportation. Instead she sometimes shops at a small convenience store nearby, where prices are higher. A neighbor occasionally brings her groceries. Mrs. C. further states that she has no allergies. She likes and is willing to eat any food except those that are too hard to chew, because of her ill-fitting dentures. She says that she weighed "about 125 pounds" for many years, but has been losing weight since her husband died.

Her typical intake, which you obtained in an interview, is represented by a 24-hour recall:

Breakfast	4 oz canned orange juice
	1/2 c oatmeal, 1 t sugar
	1/2 c evaporated whole milk
	Coffee, 1 t sugar
Lunch	1 c chicken broth with 1/2 c rice
	6 saltines
	1 oz sliced cold cuts
	1 slice white bread, enriched
	1 t butter
	Tea with 1 t sugar
	1 T evaporated whole milk
Supper	2 oz ground-beef patty
	1/2 c macaroni
	1 small banana
	Tea with 1 t sugar
	1 T evaporated whole milk

Mrs. C. said that she does not eat between meals and that food "doesn't have much taste any more." She reported that she takes one "multivitamin-with-iron tablet" daily, and takes "a lot" of aspirin for her arthritis. She denied taking any other medication, drinking alcoholic beverages, or smoking. There is no evidence of disease to account for her condition.

(continued)

Nutritional Assessment *(continued)*

QUESTIONS

1. Using Form C, summarize Mrs. C.'s protein, fat, carbohydrate and caloric intake from the 24-hr recall. On the lower part of Form C, indicate the major vitamin and mineral content of foods listed in the 24-hr recall. What nutrients are likely to be deficient in Mrs. C.'s diet?

2. Your hospital uses Form D for recording the results of nutritional assessments. Fill in the form for Mrs. C.'s assessment, using the information given and *performing any necessary calculations. Hint:* Be careful of units in calculations.

3. Explain the basis for your evaluation of nutritional status given at the end of Form D.

4. a. Hematological data suggest that the patient has anemia that is (circle all that apply)

    microcytic, normocytic, macrocytic

    hypochromic, normochromic, hyperchromic

b. Based on your calculations of hematological data in form D, a deficiency of _____ is suggested by depressed _____ and normal _____. The deficiency could be made more severe by _____ 2° to the high aspirin intake.

5. List five factors, *other than* the height, weight, and laboratory data, that suggest the patient is at nutritional risk.

6. For three of the factors listed in question 5, identify a goal and at least one measurable objective for each.

7. According to the problem list, problem 1 is primary malnutrition and problem 2 is degenerative arthritis. The attending physician has ordered "diet as tolerated" and has asked for the dietitian's recommendation both for hospital feeding and for diet after discharge. Write the SOAP note you would record in the patient's medical record.

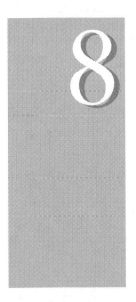

8 Nutrition During Pregnancy and Lactation

Adequate nutrition during pregnancy and lactation is extremely important to both maternal and fetal health (1, 2). In this chapter we will discuss the monitoring of pregnancy, nutritional requirements for pregnancy and lactation, maternal nutritional assessment, and complications of pregnancy. You may wish to use one of the suggested references to provide additional background information.

MONITORING PREGNANCY

The normal human gestation period is approximately 40 weeks. Gestational age, or the maturity of a pregnancy, is calculated from the first day of the last menstrual period (LMP). The estimated date of delivery (EDD), ± 2 weeks, can be arrived at by using the following equation (3):

$$EDD = \text{1st day of LMP} - 3 \text{ months} +$$
$$(1 \text{ year} + 7 \text{ days}) \qquad \textbf{(8-1)}$$

Detection of human chorionic gonadotropin (HCG) in urine is considered indicative of pregnancy. Commonly used urine tests for pregnancy are sensitive enough to detect HCG at levels normally found at 4 weeks from the LMP, or approximately 2 weeks after conception. A blood test is also available.

TERMINOLOGY

In obtaining information from the medical record, you will need to become familiar with specific terminology that is used to describe obstetrical history. *Gravidity* refers to the total number of pregnancies. A *primigravida* is a woman who is pregnant for the first time, and a *multigravida* is a woman who has been pregnant more

than once. These may be written in the medical records as *gravida I* or *gravida II* for increasing numbers of pregnancies, or abbreviated as G_1 or G_2. *Parity* is the state of having given birth to an infant or infants weighing at least 500 g or having an estimated gestational age of at least 24 weeks. A woman who has been pregnant 3 times, has two living children, and had a miscarriage at 12 weeks is described as G_3P_2, whereas a woman who has been pregnant 3 times and has two living children and one stillborn is G_3, P_3. A current pregnancy is also included, so a woman pregnant for the first time is G_1P_0.

In addition to gravidity and parity, the number of *abortions* (Ab), either spontaneous or therapeutic, and *living children* (LC) are summarized in a woman's obstetrical history. An abortion or miscarriage occurs when a baby is lost prior to 24 weeks of gestation. A nonpregnant woman who is $G_5P_4Ab_1LC_3$ has been pregnant 5 times, delivered four children weighing at least 500 g, lost one baby prior to 24 weeks gestation, either through miscarriage or abortion, lost another child in some way, such as accident or illness, and has three living children. The number of premature births, if any, is usually also noted.

ROUTINE PRENATAL CARE

For low-risk gravidas, the usual frequency of visits for prenatal care is monthly until 28 to 30 weeks, every 2 weeks until 36 weeks, and then weekly. Clinical data routinely obtained and recorded at these visits include gestational age, blood pressure, weight, presence of glucose or protein in urine, fetal heart sounds and movement, fetal presentation, and presence or absence of edema (3). In addition to these parameters, *fundal height*, or the distance from the top of the symphysis pubis to the top of the uterine fundus, is measured at prenatal visits.

Fundal height in centimeters demonstrates a one-to-one correlation with gestational age after 16 weeks gestation. Gestational age can also be determined prior to 20 weeks gestation by ultrasound measurement of the fetal biparietal diameter. The biparietal diameter is the measurement between the most distant opposite points of the two parietal bones in the fetal skull.

Nutritional education is a routine part of prenatal care, and in general, pregnant women are highly motivated to follow health care advice. The setting and organization of prenatal nutritional education programs vary. Counseling may take place on an individual basis, in a classroom or group setting, using closed-circuit television or an interactive computer program, or via printed education materials.

GESTATIONAL WEIGHT GAIN

Weight gain during pregnancy, or gestational weight gain, reflects growth of both fetal and maternal tissues as outlined in Table 8-1. The weight of the fetus and associated tissues, including the placenta, enlarged uterus, and amniotic fluid, contributes approximately half the weight gain associated with pregnancy. The increase in weight of various maternal tissues is needed for maintenance of pregnancy and is largely composed of increases in subcutaneous body fat, distributed over the abdomen, back, and upper thighs (4). The action of progesterone in the pregnant woman mediates the formation of this fat pad to serve as a calorie reserve for fetal growth and lactation. The pregnant woman can restrict weight gain to avoid development of the fat pad, but this may also affect to some degree the normal development of the fetus. Low gestational weight gain is associated with an increased risk of giving birth to a growth-retarded infant and an increased risk of fetal and infant mortality (1).

Women giving birth to healthy optimally grown infants demonstrate a large variation in gestational weight gain. For example, in the United States in 1980, the 15th and 85th percentiles of weight gain were 16 and 40 pounds (7.3 and 18.2 kg), respectively, for normal-weight women who delivered full-term babies weighing 6.6 to 8.8 pounds (3 to 4 kg) (1).

TABLE 8-1 Average Composition of Pregnancy Weight Gain

Tissue	Weight (lb)	
Fetus	7.5	
Placenta	1.0	Fetal = 13 lb
Amniotic fluid	2.0	
Uterus*	2.5	
Breast tissue*	3.0	
Blood volume*	4.0 (1,500 ml)	Maternal = 11–15 lb
Maternal stores	4.0–8.0	
Total		24–28 lb

Adapted from: Maternal nutrition and the course of pregnancry NAS, 1970.
* Weight increase.

A woman's prepregnancy weight for height is an important determinant of the effect of gestational weight gain on fetal growth, as illustrated in Fig. 8-1. An underweight woman will show a greater response in infant birth weight compared to a heavier woman with the same weight gain. Underweight or thin women, however, have smaller babies than heavier women with the same gestational weight gain. Infant birth weight is independent of gestational weight gain in overweight women who tend to have heavier babies (5).

An evaluation of a woman's prepregnancy weight for height is needed to determine the recommended gestational weight gain. Recommended gestational weight gains for underweight women are higher than those for women of normal weight, whereas desirable weight gains for overweight and obese women are lower, as summarized in Table 8-2 (1). These recommendations reflect data on pregnancy outcome (6) and the important correlation between birth weight and infant health. To evaluate prepregnancy weight for height, it is necessary to calculate a woman's prepregnancy body mass index (BMI) or to compare the prepregnancy weight for height to a weight-for-height reference standard, as discussed in Chapter 5. The Subcommittee on Nutrtional Status and Weight Gain During Pregnancy of the National Academy of Science's Institute of Medicine (1) has established arbitrary cutoff points to classify prepregnancy BMI, as shown in Table 8-2. Additional research will be needed to validate these categories for pregnancy outcome.

Epidemiologic evidence suggests that other maternal characteristics may modify the effect of gestational weight gain on fetal growth. For example, adolescents who are less than 2 years postmenarche may give birth to smaller infants for a given weight gain than older women. In addition black infants tend to be smaller than white infants for the same gestational weight gain. Thus, young adolescents and black women should strive for weight gains toward the upper end of the ranges recommended for women with a similar BMI (1). Short women, i.e., less than 62 inches (157 cm), may have more obstetrical complications associated with a large gestational weight gain and delivery of an infant weighing over 8.8 pounds (4 kg). Thus, short women should strive toward the lower end of the ranges recommended for women with similar BMIs. The recommended total gestational weight gain for women carrying twins is 35 to 45 pounds (16 to 20.5 kg) (1).

The optimal *pattern* of weight gain during pregnancy also depends on an evaluation of the prepregnancy BMI with a higher recommended rate of weight gain in underweight than normal or overweight women. A weight gain of 2 to 5 pounds (0.9 to 2.3 kg) is recommended during the first trimester of pregnancy, with a linear gain of 0.67 to 1.07 pounds (0.30 to 0.49 kg) during the second and third trimesters (Table 8-2). Because most of the fetal weight gain occurs during the last trimester, it is especially important to avoid restricting weight gain during this period.

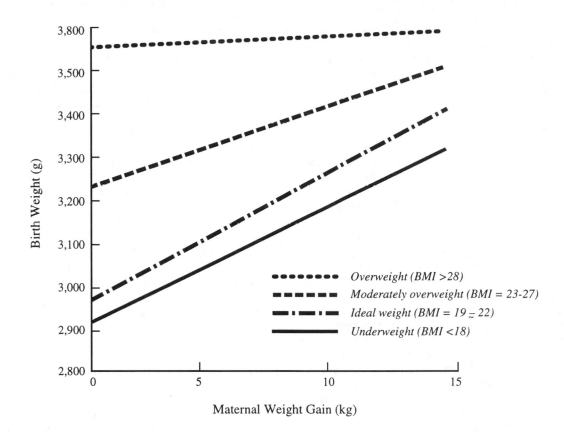

FIGURE 8-1 Birth weight of live-born infants at term by prepregnancy body mass index (BMI) and weight gain. Data were adjusted for maternal age, race, parity, socioeconomic status, cigarette consumption, and gestational age (*n* = 2,964). From B.F. Abrams and R.K. Laros, *Am J. Obstet. Gynecol.* 154:(1986)503. Published with permission.

TABLE 8-2 Recommended Total Weight Gain Ranges for Pregnant Women[*] By Pregnancy Body Mass Index (BMI)[†]

Weight-for-height category[‡]	Recommended Total Gain		Usual Rate of Gain	
	kg	lb	1st trimester, kg (lb)	2d and 3d trimesters kg (lb) per week
Underweight (BMI < 19.8)	12.5–18.0	28–40	2.3 (5.0)	0.49 (1.07)
Normal (BMI of 19.8–26.0)	11.5–16.0	25–35	1.6 (3.5)	0.44 (0.97)
Overweight[§] (BMI > 26.0–29.0)	7.5–11.5	15–25	0.9 (2.0)	0.30 (0.67)

[*]Young adolescents and black women should strive for gains at the upper end of the recommended range. Short women (< 157 cm, or 62 in.) should strive for gains at the lower end of the range.
[†]BMI is calculated using metric units.
[‡]The ranges for BMI generally correspond to 90, 120, and 135% of the 1959 Metropolitan Life Insurance Company's weight-for-height standards.
[§]The recommended target weight gain for obese women (BMI >29.0) is at least 6.0 kg (15 lb)
Adapted from *Nutrition During Pregnancy*. National Academy Press. Washington, D.C., 1990.

NUTRITIONAL REQUIREMENTS

Nutrient intake recommendations for nonpregnant, pregnant, and lactating adolescents and adult women are given in the 1989 edition of the Recommended Dietary Allowances (7). The RDAs are listed in Appendix A, and the increments in the RDAs for selected nutrients during pregnancy and lactation are shown in Table 8-3.

PREGNANCY

The total energy cost of pregnancy in healthy, well-nourished women is controversial and the focus of debate among nutritionists. The World Health Organization (WHO) (8) and the U.S. Food and Nutrition Board in the 1989 edition of the RDAs (7) estimate a total energy cost of 80,000 kcal for a full-term pregnancy during which the mother gains 27.5 pounds (12.5 kg) and gives birth to a 7.26 pound (3.3 kg) baby. The National Academy of Science's Institute of Medicine states in *Nutrition During Pregnancy* that the total energy cost of pregnancy is now believed to be 55,000 kcal (1). The large difference in these estimates of energy expenditure reflect assumptions regarding the composition of weight gain, the usual energy intake of pregnant women, and measurement of the different components of energy expenditure. Current research using whole-body calorimetry to measure energy expenditure in pregnant women has demonstrated a large interindividual variation in the energy cost of pregnancy (9).

The 1989 RDAs recommend an additional 300 kcal/day during only the second and third trimesters of pregnancy and an additional 10 g of high-quality protein/day throughout pregnancy, an amount even lower than previous estimates. The increase in energy needs reflects greater energy requirements for maintenance due to a larger tissue mass, the energy equivalent of new maternal and fetal tissues, and the cost of synthesizing these new tissues. The current RDA for protein during pregnancy reflects a decrease in the protein requirement from 30 to 10 g/day compared to the 1980 RDAs. The need for additional protein during pregnancy has been overemphasized, in part, because of the use of nitrogen balance data rather than the factorial method to estimate protein retention during pregnancy. Most American women routinely consume the total protein allowance of 60 g/day currently recommended during pregnancy.

All vitamins and minerals are needed in increased amounts during pregnancy. Requirements for vitamin B_6, folate, calcium, magnesium, iron, and zinc, however, increase substantially. According to the United States Department of Agriculture 1977–1978 and 1987–1988 Nationwide Food Consumption Surveys (10, 11) and the 1986 Continuing Survey of Food Intake of low-income women and their children (12), vitamin B_6, calcium, iron, and zinc are the nutrients most likely to be consumed in inadequate amounts by America women.. Information on the vitamin and mineral content of foods can be found in Appendix B.

The increase in energy needs during pregnancy is not large in comparison to the greater requirements for protein, vitamins, and minerals. Consequently, the *quality* of the diet, that is, the ratio of nutrients to energy intake, must be very high during pregnancy.

LACTATION

The production of high-quality milk is a major physiological priority during lactation. Women who consume diets with different amounts of carbohydrate, protein, and fat still produce breast milk with similar macronutrient composition. The average composition of 3.6 oz (100 ml) of breast milk is 70 kcal, 0.9 g protein, 7 g lactose, and 4 g fat (13). The distribution of fatty acids in breast milk varies with the type of fat eaten by the mother. For example, women who adhere to vegetarian diets will usually produce milk with a greater proportion of unsaturated fatty acids than women who consume larger amounts of saturated animal fats.

The fat and water-soluble vitamin content of human milk may vary depending on the mother's current vitamin intake and her vitamin stores. The concentrations

TABLE 8-3 Increments in Recommended Dietary Allowances for Selected Nutrients During Pregnancy and Lactation*

	Energy (kcal/day)	Protein (g)	Vitamin B_6 (mg)	Folate (μg)	Calcium (mg)	Magnesium (mg)	Iron (mg)	Zinc (mg)
Pregnant	+300[†]	+10	+0.6	+400[**]	1200[‡]	+40	+15	+3
Lactating								
1st 6 months	+500	+15	+0.5	+400[**]	1200[‡]	+75	+0	+7
2nd 6 months	+500	+12	+0.5	+400[**]	1200[‡]	+60	+0	+4

* Adapted from: *Recommended Dietary Allowances.* Food and Nutrition Board, National Academy of Sciences—National Research Council, 1989.
** The U.S. Public Health Service recommends that all women of childbearing age who are capable of becoming pregnant should consume 400 μg of folate per day for the purpose of reducing their risk of having a pregnancy affected with a neural tube defect, see Ref. 18.
† Refers only to the second and third trimesters of pregnancy; the first trimester does not require an increase in energy intake.
‡ Absorption of calcium increases during pregnancy and lactation. A total calcium intake of 1200 mg/day is recommended throughout pregnancy and lactation. Pregnant adolescents with a gynecological age of ≤3 should consume an additional 400 mg calcium for a total calcium intake of 1600 mg/day.

of major minerals (calcium, phosphorus, magnesium, sodium, and potassium) in human milk are not affected by maternal diet (2). Evidence suggests that maternal stores of calcium, magnesium, zinc, folate, and vitamin B_6 may be depleted to provide for adequate levels in human milk, if maternal intake of these nutrients is not adequate (2). Maternal intakes of nutrients above the RDA usually do not result in elevated levels of the nutrients in human milk, with the possible exception of vitamins B_6, and D, iodine, and selenium.

The lactating woman requires some nutrients at the same level recommended during pregnancy, others at a higher level because of greater energy needs and content of these nutrients in the milk being produced, and others, such as iron, at a lower level. Requirements for energy, protein, zinc, magnesium, and fluid increase to a greater extent during lactation than during pregnancy, as shown in Table 8-3. The additional protein required for lactation is estimated from the protein concentration of human milk, the mean volume of milk produced, and the efficiency of converting dietary protein to milk protein. Average milk production during the first 6 months of lactation is 750 mL/day, which corresponds to an increment in the RDA for protein of 15 g. During the second 6 months of lactation, milk production averages 600 mL/day, with an increment in the RDA for protein of 12 g. Fluid needs are usually satisfied by consuming fluids to alleviate natural thirst, usually 2.5 to 3.5 quarts of fluid per day.

Energy requirements for lactation, like protein requirements, are proportional to the quantity of milk produced. Approximately 85 kcal are required for every 100 mL of milk produced (7). Thus, the average woman would require an additional 640 kcal per day and 510 kcal per day in the first and second 6 months of lactation, respectively. The RDA of only an additional 500 kcal per day is based on the assumption that 2 to 4 kg of body fat are stored during pregnancy to provide energy reserves for lactation. These fat stores can theoretically provide 100 to 150 kcal per day during the first 6 months of lactation. Thus, lactating women typically lose 1 to 2 pounds per month (0.5 to 1 kg) and some women lose as much as 4 pounds (2 kg) per month while successfully maintaining milk volume (2). The recommended energy allowance for women whose gestational weight gain is subnormal, or whose weight during lactation falls below the standard for their height and age, is an additional 650 kcal per day during the first 6 months of lactation (7). While these energy recommendations are based on sound data, recent evidence suggests that the current RDA may overestimate energy needs during lactation (14). An energy intake of at least 1,800 kcal per day should be encouraged during lactation. Intakes below 1,500 kcal per day are not recommended at any time during lactation (2).

Because most compounds that enter the mother's body are secreted into breast milk, attention should be given to the mother's intake of drugs and alcohol and to her smoking habits.

PLANNING TO MEET NUTRITIONAL REQUIREMENTS

The Daily Food Guide for Women (15) can be used for planning and evaluating adequate maternal dietary intakes, as outlined in Table 8-4.

NUTRIENT SUPPLEMENTATION

Iron is the only nutrient for which the National Academy of Science's Institute of Medicine recommends routine supplementation during pregnancy (1). Supplemental iron is not recommended during lactation because losses of iron in milk are less than menstrual loss, which is often absent during lactation. Routine vitamin-mineral supplementation during lactation is not recommended (2). Special circumstances during pregnancy and lactation increase the risk of developing nutrient deficiencies and may require vitamin or mineral supplementation, as outlined in Table 8-5. These special circumstances include adherence to a complete or strict vegetarian diet, which excludes all animal products, limited intake of dairy products, and circumstances often associated with a history of inadequate dietary intake such as alcohol or drug abuse. During lactation, ingestion of less than 1800 kcal per day often results in inadequate nutrient intake and the need for a multiple vitamin-mineral supplement (2).

For the general population of pregnant women, an intake of 30 mg ferrous iron is recommended during the second and third trimesters. The typical American diet provides only about 6 mg of iron per 1,000 calories. Thus, the pregnancy RDA of 30 mg of iron is difficult to achieve with a daily intake of 2,000 to 2,400 calories. Absorption of dietary iron, however, increases during pregnancy to meet increased needs, and some investigators suggest that women who enter pregnancy with sufficient iron stores do not require iron supplementation (16). Assessment of iron status during pregnancy, as discussed later in this chapter, is useful for identifying women who are at risk for iron depletion.

Iron supplementation may interfere with absorption of other minerals from the diet. To enhance absorption of iron and minimize interference with the absorption of other minerals, iron supplements should be taken on an empty stomach, at bedtime or between meals.

Supplementation with more than 30 mg iron/day has been associated with a decrease in maternal plasma zinc levels (17) due to decreased absorption of zinc. Zinc supplementation may also decrease the absorption of copper. For this reason, zinc and copper supplementation are recommended for women taking therapeutic doses of iron (>30 mg/day) to treat anemia, as outlined in Table 8-5. Calcium may interfere with the absorption of both iron and zinc, and if a calcium supplement is needed, it should be taken at mealtimes to minimize interference with iron supplements (1).

Large doses of vitamin supplements many cause birth defects, especially when taken during the first trimester

TABLE 8.4 Daily Food Guide for Women

Food Groups	One Serving Equals		Recommended Minimum Servings		
			Nonpregnant		Pregnant/ lactating
			11–24 yrs	25 + yrs	
Protein foods: Provide protein, iron, zinc, and B vitamins for growth of muscles, bone, blood, and nerves. Vegetable protein provides fiber to prevent constipation.	Animal protein: 1 oz cooked chicken or turkey 1 oz cooked lean beef, lamb, or pork 1 oz or 1/4 cup fish or other seafood 1 egg 2 fish sticks or hot dogs 2 slices luncheon meat	Vegetable protein: 1/2 cup cooked dry beans, lentils, or split peas 3 oz tofu 1 oz or 1/4 cup peanuts, pumpkin, or sunflower seeds 1 1/2 oz or 1/3 cup other nuts 2 tbsp peanut butter	5 A half serving of vegetable protein daily	5	7 One serving of vegetable protein daily
Milk Products: Provide some protein and calcium to build strong bones, teeth, healthy nerves and muscles, and to promote normal blood clotting.	8 oz milk 8 oz yogurt 1 cup milk shake 1 1/2 cups cream soup (made with milk) 1 1/2 oz or 1/3 cup grated cheese (like cheddar, monterey, mozzerella, or swiss.)	1 1/2 –2 slices presliced American cheese 4 tbsp parmesan cheese 2 cups cottage cheese 1 cup pudding 1 cup custard or flan 1 1/2 cups ice milk, ice cream, or frozen yogurt	3	2	3
Breads, cereals, grains: Provide carbohydrates and B vitamins for energy and healthy nerves. Also provide iron for healthy blood. Whole grains provide fiber to prevent constipation.	1 slice bread 1 dinner roll 1/2 bun or bagel 1/2 English muffin or pita 1 small tortilla 3/4 cup dry cereal 1/2 cup granola 1/2 cup cooked cereal	1/2 cup rice 1/2 cup noodles or spaghetti 1/4 cup wheat germ 1 4-inch pancake or waffle 1 small muffin 8 medium crackers 4 graham cracker squares 3 cups popcorn	7 Four servings of whole-grain product daily	6	7
Vitamin C-rich fruits and vegetables: Provide vitamin C to prevent infection and to promote healing and iron absorption. Also provide fiber to prevent constipation.	6 oz orange, grapefruit, or fruit juice enriched with vitamin C 6 oz tomato juice or vegetable juice cocktail 1 orange, kiwi, mango 1/2 grapefruit, canteloupe 1/2 cup papaya 2 tangerines	1/2 cup strawberries 1/2 cup cooked or 1 cup raw cabbage 1/2 cup broccoli, Brussels sprouts, or cauliflower 1/2 cup snow peas, sweet peppers, or tomato puree 2 tomatoes	1	1	1
Vitamin A-rich fruits and vegetables: Provide beta-carotene and vitamin A to prevent infection and to promote wound healing and night vision. Also provide fiber to prevent constipation.	6 oz apricot nectar or vegetable juice cocktail 3 raw or 1/4 cup dried apricots 1/4 cantaloupe or mango 1 small or 1/2 cup sliced carrots 2 tomatoes	1/2 cup cooked or 1 cup raw spinach 1/2 cup cooked greens (beet, chard, collards, dandelion, kale, mustard) 1/2 cup pumpkin, sweet potato, winter squash, or yams	1	1	1

(continued)

TABLE 8.4 (*continued*)			Recommended Minimum Servings		
Food Groups	One Serving Equals		Nonpregnant		Pregnant/ lactating
			11–24 yrs	25 + yrs	
Other fruits and vegetables: Provide carbohydrates for energy and fiber to prevent constipation.	6 oz fruit juice (if not listed above) 1 medium or 1/2 cup sliced fruit (apple, banana, peach, pear) 1/2 cup berries (other than strawberries) 1/2 cup cherries or grapes 1/2 cup pineapple 1/2 cup watermelon	1/4 cup dried fruit 1/2 cup sliced vegetable (asparagus, beets, green beans, celery, corn, eggplant, mushrooms, onion, peas, potato, summer squash, zucchini 1/2 artichoke 1 cup lettuce	3	3	3
Unsaturated fats: Provide vitamin E to protect tissue	1/8 medium avocado 1 tsp margarine 1 tsp mayonnaise 1 tsp vegetable oil	2 tsp salad dressing (mayonnaise-based) 1 tbsp salad dressing (oil-based)	3	3	3

Note: The Daily Food Guide for Women may not provide all the calories you require. The best way to increase your intake is to include more than the minimum servings recommended.

* From Maternal and Child Health Branch. WIC Supplemental Food Branch. California Department of Health Sciences June 1990.

of pregnancy. Birth defects have been reported in women taking large doses of vitamin A and the acne medication Acutane, which contains a vitamin A analog, 13-cis-retinoic acid (13). Available data suggest that vitamin A supplements to pregnant women should not exceed 8,000 IU daily. Carotene intake need not be restricted during pregnancy. Large doses of vitamin D have also been linked with birth defects, and supplemental intake of vitamin D should not exceed 400 IU daily during pregnancy.

New evidence suggests that folic acid or folate may help reduce the number of infants born with neural tube defects, such as spina bifida and anencephaly. In order to reduce the frequency of neural tube defects the United States Public Health Service currently recommends that all the women of childbearing age who are capable of becoming pregnant should consume 400 µg (0.4 mg) of folic acid per day (18). An intake of folic acid greater than 1 mg per day is not routinely recommended because this may complicate the diagnosis of vitamin B_{12} deficiency and have other possiblly deleterious effects. One special circumstance which justifies a higher intake of folic acid is for women who have had a prior pregnancy affected by a neural tube defect. These women should consult their physician who may recommend a supplement of 4.0 mg daily of folic acid from at least one month before conception through the first three months of pregnancy (18).

An intake of folic acid of 400 µg per day can be obtained through careful selection of foods. However, most women don't consume the recommended amount of folate as the average consumption of dietary folate is estimated to be about 200 µg per day in the United States (1). Folate is a generic term for food compounds that have the biologic activity of folic acid; in general, folates obtained from foods are not as well absorbed as is folic acid. Important food sources of folate include: fortified breakfast cereals, orange juice, broccoli and other green leafy vegetables, beans, lentils, beets, and some nuts.

ABSORPTION OF NONHEME AND HEME IRON FROM FOOD

Many women are intolerant of iron supplements because of abdominal discomfort and constipation. Dietary measures may help to increase the absorption or bioavailability of dietary iron. The principal dietary sources of iron include meat, eggs, vegetables, and cereals, especially fortified cereal products. Iron is found in two main forms in food, nonheme iron, which is found principally in plant products, and heme iron, which is found mainly in animal tissues. Most of the iron in the diet is present as nonheme iron and consists primarily of iron salts. The absorption of nonheme iron is strongly affected by its solubility in the upper part of the small intestine, which in turn depends on the composition of the meal as a whole (19). Heme iron is highly absorbable in comparison to nonheme iron, and its absorption is relatively unaffected by other dietary constituents.

The absorption of nonheme iron from a meal can be increased by ingesting a small amount of meat and vitamin C–containing foods with the meal. In contrast, meals that contain large amounts of legumes, phytate from wheat bran and unleavened whole grain products, and

TABLE 8-5   Recommendations for Vitamin–Mineral Supplementation During Pregnancy*

Nutrient	Indication for Supplementation
Iron: 30 mg of ferrous iron[†] daily, taken between meals or at bedtime on an empty stomach	General population of pregnant women during the second and third trimesters
	Special Circumstances
Folate: 400 µg daily (4 mg daily)	Women whose dietary folate intake is marginal due to limited intake of fruits, green vegetables, legumes, peas, and whole-grained or fortified cereals (Women who have previously given birth to an infant with a neural tube defect)
Calcium: 600 mg daily, taken at mealtime to limit interaction with iron supplements	Women under age 25 whose daily dietary calcium intake is less than 600 mg·[‡]
Vitamin D: 10 µg (400 IU) daily	Women who are complete[§] vegetarians, consume limited amounts of Vitamin D-fortified milk or have minimal exposure to sunlight[‡]
Zinc and Copper: 15 mg zinc and 2 mg copper daily	Women who are taking theraputic levels of iron (> 30 mg/day) to treat anemia
Vitamin B-12: 2.0 µg daily	Women who are complete vegetarians·[‡]
Multivitamin Mineral Supplement	Women who are at high-risk for nutrient deficiencies because of: multiple gestation, heavy cigarette smoking, alcohol or drug abuse, or history of limited dietary intake.[‡]

Iron, 30 mg	Vitamin B$_6$, 2 mg
Zinc, 15 mg	Folate, 400 µg
Copper, 2 mg	Vitamin C, 50 mg
Calcium, 250 mg	Vitamin D, 5 µg

The supplement should be taken daily
between meals or at bedtime.

---

*Adapted from National Academy of Sciences Nutrition During Pregnancy, 1990. See reference 1 and Centers for Disease Control, recommendations for the use of folic acid to reduce the number of cases of spina bifide and other neural tube defects, *Morbidity and Mortality Weekly Report* (Supp), 41 (rr–14): 1–7, Sept. 1992.

[†]Provided by 150 mg of ferrous sulfate, 300 mg of ferrous gluconate or 100 mg of ferrous fumarate. Simultaneous ingestion of ascorbic acid and supplements containing ferrous iron does not enhance iron absorption.

[‡]Also applies to lactation especially if total energy intake is <1800 kcal per day.

[§]Those who consume no animal products.

---

tannin from tea tend to reduce iron absorption by decreasing the intestinal solubility of nonheme iron (1). Ingestion of coffee and calcium phosphate supplements with a meal will also reduce iron absorption. Thus, women may enhance their absorption of dietary iron by including red meats and vitamin C–rich fruits and vegetables with meals and by avoiding tea and coffee at mealtimes. Ingestion of vitamin C with supplements containing ferrous iron, however, does not enhance iron absorption (1).

ALCOHOL AND CAFFEINE

Excessive consumption of alcohol during pregnancy is associated with the fetal alcohol syndrome and a spec-

trum of adverse effects on fetal development. Fetal alcohol syndrome is estimated to affect one to two infants per 1,000 live births in the United States and is characterized by growth retardation, distinct facial anomalies, and mental deficiency (1). Evidence concerning the effects of low levels of alcohol consumption is both limited and inconsistent. Based on present data, total abstinence from alcohol is recommended during pregnancy (20).

There is no convincing evidence that ingestion of caffeine or coffee is associated with birth defects in humans. However, studies have demonstrated that heavy caffeine consumption (more than 300 mg/day or 3 cups of coffee) during pregnancy may lower infant birth weight without increasing the incidence of premature birth (21) and may increase the risk of fetal loss (22). Additional evidence suggests that caffeine may adversely affect mineral status, in particular, calcium, zinc, and iron in nonpregnant populations. The current recommendation is for pregnant women to use caffeine in moderation, no more than 2 cups of a caffeine-containing beverage per day.

NUTRITIONAL ASSESSMENT

Nutritional assessment during pregnancy includes an evaluation of pertinent clinical risk factors and consideration of dietary, anthropometric, and biochemical data. A form for recording pertinent nutritional assessment data, Nutritional Assessment for Pregnant Women, is provided in appendix Table G-1.

RISK FACTORS

Every pregnant woman needs an individual assessment of nutritional status. The assessment should begin with an examination of certain key nutritional risk factors, which will help to identify those women in need of in-depth nutritional counseling. These risk factors include a consideration of age, body weight, parity, previous reproductive performance, economic status, weight gain during pregnancy, preconception nutrition and social habits, and medical history. Table 8-6 gives an outline of the nutritional risk factors whose consideration will assist with nutritional assessment during pregnancy. A form for recording information related to nutritional risk factors during pregnancy, the Nutritional Questionnaire for Pregnant Women, is provided in appendix Table G-2.

DIETARY ASSESSMENT

The Daily Food Guide for Women (Table 8-4) provides a quick and easy means for evaluating the adequacy of dietary intake as it was developed to insure a minimum average intake of at least 90 percent of the RDA for nonpregnant, pregnant, and lactating women of average height and weight. Comparing the number of servings eaten with the recommended number of servings in each of the seven food groups shown in Table 8-4 can help identify nutrient shortages and imbalances. The Daily Food Guide for Women can also be used by counselors to demonstrate how to make wise food choices and how to plan nutritionally adequate diets. This food guide system differs from earlier versions in that it reflects currently available information about nutrient composition, dietary recommendations for disease prevention, and food consumption patterns for women during their reproductive years (15).

Sometimes it is useful to provide information about foods rich in the nutrients needed in substantially greater amounts during pregnancy and lactation. These nutrients include vitamin B_6, folate, magnesium, iron, calcium, and zinc, as outlined in Table 8-3. Tables of food values are provided in Appendix B.

The practice of pica during pregnancy should also be assessed. Pica is the compulsive eating of nonfood substances having little or no nutritional value—such as dirt, clay, laundry starch, paint chips, plaster, chalk or ice. Starch and clay eating is frequently reported by African American women, while clay eating alone is more common among other cultural groups (15). The medical implications of pica are unclear. Pica substances may displace essential nutrients in the diet, provide excess calories as in the case of starch, contain toxic substances such as lead, and provide compounds that interfere with the absorption of minerals, in particular, iron. Microbial contamination may also be a problem with pica substances.

Dietary assessment of lactating women must often be done very quickly by nurses and other health care personnel. Simple questions which can help screen for nutritional adequacy include (2):

Are dairy products eaten regularly?

Does the diet include vitamin D fortified milk or cereal, or is there adequate exposure to sunlight?

Are fruits and vegetables eaten regularly?

Does the mother follow a complete or strict vegetarian diet?

Is the mother restricting her food intake severely in an attempt to lose weight?

Are there life circumstances such as poverty or abuse of drugs or alcohol that might interfere with an adequate diet?

Dietary assessment should also address common problems during pregnancy including nausea, constipation, and heartburn. General nutritional guidance during pregnancy will often help alleviate these common discomforts.

Nausea

Nausea and vomiting usually occur during the first trimester of pregnancy. Because these symptoms often occur on arising, the term *morning sickness* is commonly used. Simple dietary practices may improve food tolerance during this time. Small, frequent, dry meals consisting chiefly of high-carbohydrate foods are more readily tolerated. Fluid should be taken between meals. It is important not to skip meals but to avoid greasy or spicy food or caffeinated drinks that may worsen symptoms. Occasionally, hyperemesis, or severe, prolonged, and persistent vomiting, will develop. Hyperemesis requires medical attention to prevent dehydration.

Constipation

Constipation is common during pregnancy due both to hormonal changes that tend to increase relaxation of the gastrointestinal muscles and to the pressure of the enlarging uterus on the colon. Iron supplementation is also associated with constipation in pregnancy. Increased fluid intake and use of naturally laxative foods such as whole grains with added bran, fibrous fruits and vegetables, dried fruits, and other fruits and juices

TABLE 8-6   Nutritional Risk Factors During Pregnancy

Nutritional Risk Factors at the Onset of Pregnancy

1. 17 years of age or less

2. Economically deprived (an income less than the poverty line or a recipient of local, state, or federal assistance, such as Medicaid or the USDA Food Programs, such as WIC)

3. Food faddism (ingestion of nutritionally restrictive diet)

4. Heavy smoking

5. Drug abuse

6. Alcoholism

7. Prepregnancy body mass index (BMI) of <20 or >26

8. High parity and short interpregnancy interval (five or more previous deliveries and 12 months or less between termination of pregnancy and conception)

9. History of poor obstetrical or fetal performance including delivery of a low birth weight infant

10. Presence of a chronic systemic disease such as diabetes or hypertension

Risk Factors During Prenatal Care

11. Inadequate weight gain (gain of <1 pound (0.5 kg) per month for obese women and <2 pounds (1 kg) per month for women of normal weight)

12. Excessive weight gain (gain of >6.5 pounds (3 kg) per month)

13. Anemia as suggested by a hemoglobin of <110 g/L during the first and third trimesters and <105 g/L during the second trimester

14. Hypovolemia as suggested by a hemoglobin above 139 g/L or a hematocrit above 0.419 between 24–34 weeks gestation

15. Twins or triplets

generally help maintain regularity. A regular pattern of exercise may also help.

Heartburn

Heartburn may occur after meals, especially during the later stages of pregnancy. Estrogen and progesterone reduce pressure of the lower esophageal sphincter, possibly by decreasing the response to gastrin. Crowding of the stomach by the enlarging uterus may also contribute. The symptoms of heartburn are usually reduced by eating smaller, more frequent meals. Wearing loose-fitting clothing, eating slowly, avoiding reclining after meals, and elevating the head of the bed may also help.

ANTHROPOMETRIC ASSESSMENT

The two most important tools for anthropometric assessment during pregnancy are evaluation of prepregnancy weight for height and determination of weight gain throughout the course of pregnancy by plotting weight gain on a prenatal weight gain grid. In order to accomplish this assessment, the woman's height and weight must be measured at her first prenatal visit, and her weight at every prenatal visit thereafter. Evaluation of prepregnancy weight for height allows determination of an appropriate total weight gain target, as outlined in Table 8-2.

Many prenatal weight gain grids are available, although few have been validated based on the reproductive outcomes of large groups of pregnant women. Prenatal weight gain grids are provided (1, 15) for women classified as underweight, normal weight, or overweight based on their prepregnancy weight for height (see Appendix G, Figures 1 to 3). These weight gain grids show the recommended target gain as the end points and the recommended gain as the slope. A notation should be made if gestational age is uncertain, since this will affect placement of weight gain on the chart. Plotting a prenatal weight gain grid provides a visual impression of the progress of weight gain and simplifies detection of an abnormal change in weight over time. Deviations from the expected rate of gain should be investigated to determine if they are related to nutrient intake or other physiological changes. Inadequate weight gain may be related to restricted dietary intake or extenuating social circumstances. A sudden sharp increase in weight after the 20th week of pregnancy may indicate water retention and the onset of preeclampsia, as will be discussed later.

BIOCHEMICAL ASSESSMENT

Normal gestation is associated with changes from the nonpregnant state in various laboratory indices of nutritional metabolic status. Expansion of the plasma volume during pregnancy results in dilution of the plasma proteins. A serum albumin level of 30 g/L and a total serum protein value of 60 g/L are normal for pregnancy but would be considered low-normal for the nonpregnant state. Limited information is currently available regarding the vitamin and mineral status of pregnant and lactating women. However, whenever possible, values for pregnant women should be compared with "normal" values derived from pregnant women. Selected normal laboratory values for pregnancy are included in Appendix E, Tables E-6 and E-7.

Women are at increased risk for developing carbohydrate intolerance during pregnancy because of alterations in metabolism mediated by the production of placental hormones. Changes in glucose tolerance normally accompany pregnancy and include lower fasting plasma glucose values and higher postprandial plasma glucose levels in pregnant compared to nonpregnant women. The American Diabetes Association currently recommends that all women be screened for glucose intolerance during the 24th to 28th week of gestation, as discussed in Chapter 19.

Assessment of hematological status is the most common type of biochemical assessment conducted during routine prenatal care. Deficiencies of iron, folate, and vitamin B_{12} are the most common causes of nonphysiological anemias in pregnancy. Anemia caused by vitamin B_{12} deficiency is unlikely except in women who are strict vegetarians consuming no animal products. Iron deficiency accounts for the majority of anemias in pregnancy although folate deficiency anemia is not uncommon. Risk factors for folate deficiency include multiple pregnancy, restricted dietary intake, anticonvulsant therapy, malabsorption syndromes, or hematologic disorders such as hemoglobinopathies (15).

Iron Deficiency Anemia

Iron deficiency anemia is the most common nutritional complication of pregnancy. This reflects the modest iron content of typical diets and the additional need of approximately 1,000 mg of iron during pregnancy to supply the growing fetus and placenta and to increase the maternal red blood cell mass. Factors associated with an increased risk of iron deficiency include low socioeconomic status, low level of education, black or Hispanic background, high parity, the second two trimesters of pregnancy, menorrhagia (loss of more than 80 ml of blood per month), ingestion of diets low in both meat and ascorbic acid, blood donation more than 3 times per year, and chronic use of aspirin (1).

Anemia is defined as a hemoglobin concentration that is more than 2 standard deviations below the mean or below the fifth percentile for the same age, sex, and stage of pregnancy (1). Normal hemoglobin values fluctuate during pregnancy, as shown in Fig. 8-2. The fall in hemoglobin concentration and hematocrit observed during pregnancy in healthy women reflects a relatively greater expansion of plasma volume compared to the increase in hemoglobin mass and red blood cell volume. During pregnancy, the blood volume increases by approximately 50 percent, and the red blood cell mass by about 25 percent. During the second trimester of pregnancy, the increase in plasma volume relative to red blood cell mass is greater than during the third trimester when plasma expansion ceases and hemoglobin mass continues to increase. This is reflected in a mean hemoglobin concentration of 116 g/L during the second trimester of pregnancy and of 125 g/L during the third trimester of pregnancy (1). Screening for anemia is often done at the first visit, again at 28 to 32 weeks' gestation, and once more at 36 to 38 weeks' gestation.

Iron depletion is often described as progressing in three stages, depletion of storage iron, impairment of hemoglobin production, and iron deficiency anemia as evidenced by a decrease in hemoglobin concentration. In the non pregnant population there are useful hematological indices to assess these three stages of iron depletion. For example, low serum ferritin levels are a very sensitive indicator of the first stage, depletion of storage iron. For pregnancy, however, the normal ranges for these laboratory indices are not adequately characterized, and responses in laboratory indices to iron deficiency may differ from that in nonpregnant women. For example, a decrease in mean corpuscular volume (MCV) is observed with iron deficiency anemia in the nonpregnant population but, during pregnancy, the MCV normally rises by about 5 percent, which makes it of little use for diagnosing anemia during pregnancy. The difficulty of predicting the subsequent development of iron deficiency from laboratory tests during pregnancy supports routine iron supplementation during pregnancy (1).

The Centers for Disease Control established guidelines for screening pregnant women for anemia as outlined in Table 8-7 (23). They established cutoff values for hemoglobin concentrations of 110, 105, and 110 g/L blood for the first, second, and third trimesters of pregnancy, respectively. In addition, if these criteria for hemoglobin concentration are met and a serum ferritin concentration of <12 µg/L is noted, the cause of the anemia can be assumed to be iron deficiency, because other causes of anemia are not associated with a low serum ferritin level (1). The World Health Organization defines anemia in nonpregnant women based on a hemoglobin concentration of <120 g/L, and in pregnant women based on a uniform hemoglobin concentration of <110 g/L.

Hypovolemia, or inadequate expansion of the plasma volume, is a risk factor associated with preeclampsia, fetal growth retardation, and premature labor (15). There is an inverse relationship between high hemoglobin levels and plasma volume in pregnant women. A pregnant woman with a hemoglobin above 139 g/L or a hematocrit above 41.9 percent between 24 to 34 weeks gestation may be at risk for hypovolemia and should receive nutritional assessment and intervention. Research indicates that an inadequate intake of food or fluids may restrict the expansion of plasma volume during pregnancy.

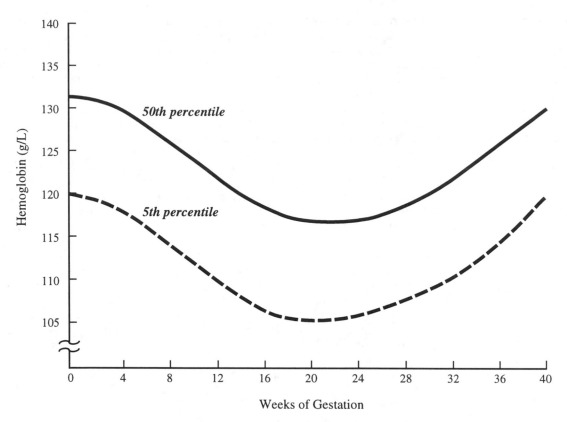

FIGURE 8-2   Normal hemoglobin values during pregnancy. From Institute of Medicine, *Nutrition During Pregnancy*, Washington DC: National Academy Press, 1990. Published with permission.

NUTRITIONAL COUNSELING

The nutrtional care specialist should view maternal nutritional counseling as a special opportunity to impart nutritional information. The influence of counseling often extends beyond the pregnancy and may benefit the health of every family member. Successful counseling includes individual assessment and education, as discussed more fully in Chapter 7. The counseling process should ultimately change the woman's behavior to enhance her health and the well-being of her developing child (15).

Appropriate counseling consistent with a woman's ethnic, cultural, and financial considerations should be provided to help a woman achieve her weight gain goal. Discussions of cultural influences on nutritional care and considerations for planning vegetarian diets are provided in Chapters 10 and 11. Referral to a social worker and to public assistance programs may be needed if income is limited or there are extenuating psychosocial circumstances. Public assistance programs that may be helpful include food stamps, the special supplemental food program for Women, Infants and Children (WIC), or the Expanded Food and Nutrition Education Program (EFNEP).

Early in pregnancy a weight gain goal should be set with the pregnant woman and an explanation of why weight gain is important, should be provided (1). The weight gain goal should be identified as a *range* of total desirable gestational weight gain. For example, women with normal prepregnancy weight for height are recommended to gain 25 to 35 pounds. All women should be encouraged to gain enough weight to achieve at least the lower limit of weight specified for their weight-for-height category in Table 8-2.

TABLE 8-7   Guidelines for Laboratory Evaluation of Anemia in Women Based on Hemoglobin Concentration (g/L in blood)*

	Not Acceptable	Mean
Nonpregnant	<120	135
Pregnant +		
1st trimester	<110	—
2d trimester	<105	116
3d trimester	<110	125

*Adapted from Centers for Disease Control, Department of Health and Human Services. CDC criteria for anemia in children and childbearing-age women. *Morbia Mortal Wkly Rep.* 38 (22): (1989), 400–04.

+A pregnant women can be assumed to have iron deficiency anemia if the above criteria are met *and* the serum ferritin concentration is <12 µg/L. Hemoglobin values >139 g/L suggest inadequate expansion of plasma volume.

The monitoring of weight gain is a key part of follow-up prenatal care. The pattern of weight gain should be assessed relative to the established weight gain goal. Reasons for marked or persistent deviations from the expected pattern of gain should be investigated. In particular, gains of less than 1 pound (0.5 kg) per month for obese women and less than 2 pounds (1 kg) per month for women of normal weight require further evaluation (1).

Gains greater than 6.5 pounds (3 kg) per month may also need further evaluation. If dietary factors contribute to the abnormal pattern of weight gain, changes in eating habits should be discussed with the woman. It is very important to assume a positive, nonjudgmental attitude during this process and to reinforce the positive aspects of the woman's diet.

Assessment of the adequacy of dietary intake should be conducted using the Daily Food Guide for Women in parallel with monitoring of prenatal weight gain. Evaluation of the hematological status should also be conducted by checking hemoglobin levels throughout pregnancy. A summary of considerations in prenatal nutritional counseling is provided in Table 8-8.

COMPLICATIONS OF PREGNANCY

Complications of pregnancy with nutritional and dietary implications may occur if the pregnant woman is overweight, is an adolescent, or demonstrates an elevation in blood pressure.

THE OVERWEIGHT PREGNANT WOMAN

Women who are overweight (BMI >26–29) or obese (BMI >29) at conception need individualized dietary assessment and nutritional counseling. These women are the most likely to develop gestational diabetes, which is discussed in Chapter 19. Another consideration is that a lower total weight gain of 15 to 25 pounds is recommended for the moderately overweight women, and a minimum gain of 15 pounds is recommended for the obese woman. Dietary counseling is important to ensure an adequate diet while limiting weight gain, because these women often consume excessive energy from foods low in nutrients.

The energy needs of obese pregnant women are unclear. Energy intakes recommended for normal weight women may be excessive for the overweight woman. Energy needs of the obese pregnant woman may be more accurately calculated using *ideal,* rather than *actual,* body weight. A modest caloric restriction of 1700 to 1800 kcal per day or 25 kcal per kg ideal prepregnancy weight was not associated with ketonuria or negative effects in obese women or their infants (24). Infants born to obese mothers, however, were significantly heavier than infants born to a control group in spite of the lower gestational weight gain associated with the modest caloric restriction. In counseling the obese pregnant woman, the best approach to assessment of energy needs is to monitor the pattern of weight gain and to adjust the dietary energy intake accordingly. Energy intake should not be less than 25 kcal per kg of ideal prepregnancy body weight in order to ensure that weight loss does not occur during pregnancy.

HYPERTENSIVE DISORDERS ASSOCIATED WITH PREGNANCY

High blood pressure complicates almost 10 percent of all pregnancies and may be caused by many factors. Hypertension during pregnancy is classified into four categories (25): chronic hypertension (see Chapter 20), preeclampsia-eclampsia, which is unique to pregnancy, preeclampsia superimposed on chronic hypertension, and transient hypertension. Pregnancy-specific preeclampsia and preeclampsia superimposed on chronic hypertension represent the greatest risk to the mother and fetus and comprise the majority of the hypertensive disorders in pregnancy. Preeclampsia-eclampsia occurs most frequently in primigravidae and women carrying more than one fetus.

The term *pregnancy-induced hypertension* (PIH) is often used to denote pregnancy-specific preeclampsia with progression of symptoms to eclampsia (26). The term *toxemia* was previously used to denote preeclampsia-eclampsia, but it is actually a misnomer. *Toxemia* means "toxins in the blood," which doesn't apply to preeclampsia.

Chronic Hypertension
Hypertension is defined as a blood pressure equal to or greater than 140/90 mm Hg. Elevated blood pressure is the primary pathophysiological feature of chronic hypertension that is present and observable before pregnancy. Women with chronic hypertension often experience a drop in blood pressure during the early weeks of pregnancy, a small rise after the 20th week, which accompanies the expansion of plasma volume, and a persistent elevation in blood pressure after delivery. Women with chronic hypertension prior to pregnancy are at higher risk for the development of preeclampsia, which may progress to eclampsia if untreated. Black women in the childbearing age have 2 to 3 times the prevalence of essential hypertension as do white women. They also demonstrate a greater incidence of preeclampsia superimposed on chronic hypertension, which is often misdiagnosed as pregnancy-specific preeclampsia (25). Women with chronic hypertension who develop preeclampsia during pregnancy are more likely to have a recurrence of hypertension with subsequent pregnancies as women who develop the pregnancy-specific form of preeclampsia.

Preeclampsia-Eclampsia
The pregnancy-specific condition is termed *preeclampsia* in the American College of Obstetricians and Gynecologists classification and usually occurs after 20

TABLE 8-8   Considerations in Prenatal Nutirtional Counseling

Initial Visit

Assessment

1. Screen for risk factors and dietary practices with Nutritional Questionaire*.

2. Evaluate usual dietary intake using Daily Food Guide for Women (Table 8-4) and Dietary Intake* form. Identify need for vitamin-mineral supplementation (Table 8-5).

3. Determine prepregnancy weight and height. Calculate prepregnancy BMI, and identify total weight gain goal (Table 8-2). Record anthropometric information on Prenatal Weight Gain Grid*.

Education

1. Discuss importance of nutrition during pregnancy and lactation.

2. Explain use of Daily Food Guide for Women.

3. Establish a total weight gain goal with the pregnant woman, and explain why weight gain is important.

4. Advise about vitamin-mineral supplementation, and discuss the bioavailability of dietary iron.

5. Discuss dietary practices which can alleviate common gastrointestinal problems associated with pregnancy.

Follow-Up Care

Assessment

1. Identify any abnormal pattern of weight gain using Prenatal Weight Gain Grid*.

2. Reevaluate dietary intake.

3. Check hemoglobin values (Table 8-7).

Education

1. Discuss diet related problems.

2. Provide positive reinforcement regarding dietary intake in relation to Daily Food Guide for Women, and discuss opportunities for improving dietary habits.

3. Discuss diet and lactation.

4. Discuss infant feeding.

*These forms are provided in Appendix G. The form Nutritional Assessment for Pregnant Women in Appendix G can be used to summarize information obtained from the initia prenatal visit.

weeks gestation (25). It is characterized by poor perfusion of many organs, including the placenta, and usually has increased blood pressure accompanied by proteinuria, edema, or both. Expansion of the plasma volume, a normal part of pregnancy, does not occur or is reduced significantly in women with preeclampsia-eclampsia. Thus, hypovolemia as evidenced by a hemoglobin concentration of >139 g/L is often observed in preeclampsia.

Eclampsia comes from the Greek word *eclampsis,* meaning a "sudden flash" or a "sudden development." Eclampsia is defined as the occurrence of seizures in a patient with preeclampsia that cannot be attributed to other causes. These seizures may occur when the blood pressure is only mildly increased (25), thus justifying the aggressive treatment of preeclampsia.

The etiology of preeclampsia-eclampsia is poorly understood, although the tendency for preeclampsia is thought to be inherited. There is some evidence that suggests that preeclampsia involves interaction between nutritional intake and the physiologic adjustments associated with pregnancy (13). However, most of the studies linking maternal nutrition and preeclampsia were

conducted over 20 years ago when diagnostic criteria for preeclampsia were not well defined.

A major pathophysiological feature of preeclampsia-eclampsia is a marked increase in peripheral vascular resistance. Vascular constriction or vasospasm increases the resistance to blood flow and promotes arterial hypertension and reduced blood perfusion to various organs, including the placenta and kidney. Proteinuria results from reduced blood flow through the kidney. The vasospasm is due, in part, to increased vascular responsiveness to circulating angiotensin II and catecholamines. Other evidence suggests that preeclampsia may be associated with inappropriately increased production of a prostaglandin with vasoconstrictor properties. Alternatively, it may be related to increased inactiviaton or diminished synthesis or release of another prostaglandin compound with vasodilator properties (25).

Symptoms

The symptoms associated with preeclampsia-eclampsia usually occur after the 20th week of gestation and include hypertension, proteinuria, and edema. Table 8-9 summarizes the symptoms associated with the progression from preeclampsia to eclampsia.

Hypertension. A blood pressure greater than 140/90 is used to diagnose hypertension in the nonpregnant population. This value is not useful during pregnancy because many younger females have normal blood pressures of less than 120/80, and use of the 140/90 diagnostic value will often miss their hypertension. Hypertension associated with pregnancy is best assessed by comparison with individuals' usual blood pressure levels (26). The diagnosis of hypertension in pregnancy is indicated by repeated blood pressure measurements of 140/90 or by an elevation of 30 mm Hg systolic or 15 mm Hg diastolic from previous blood pressure measurements during pregnancy.

Proteinuria. Proteinuria usually develops later in the course of preeclampsia. The degree of proteinuria varies with the progression from preeclampsia to eclampsia. With preeclampsia, a 24-hour urine collection may include 300 mg of protein; with progression to severe preeclampsia, the collection may contain at least 5 g of protein.

Edema. The majority of pregnant women develop a certain amount of edema in the extremities during the last trimester of pregnancy. This is a normal consequence of the expansion of the plasma volume, decrease in plasma albumin, and the pressure exerted on the venous vasculature by an enlarging uterus. The edema associated with preeclampsia is much more severe. It is usually evident in the hands, face, feet, and legs and may be associated with dizziness, headache, visual disturbances, nausea, and vomiting.

Treatment

A major goal in the management of preeclampsia is the prevention of eclampsia, which can be life threatening. Medications and induction of labor may be necessary, although nonpharmacologic treatment is the mainstay of management of pregnant women with hypertension. The strategies for nonpharmacologic treatment of hypertension during pregnancy differ from those in nonpregnant individuals. Whereas weight reduction and exercise might benefit a nonpregnant individual, these measures are not encouraged during pregnancy (25). Bed rest is a good means of maximizing uteroplacental blood flow during pregnancy and is considered established therapy in preeclampsia.

Sodium restriction is generally not recommended during pregnancy because of the need to expand the plasma volume. If, however, a pregnant woman with chronic hypertension is known to have salt-sensitive hypertension and has been treated successfully with a low-sodium diet before pregnancy, restriction of sodium intake to not less than 3 grams per day may be continued during pregnancy. At the onset of edema, a moderate sodium restriction of 4 to 5 grams per day is often recommended. This can be easily achieved by elimination of added salt at the table and by avoiding obviously salty foods such as chips, pickles, most fast foods, and canned soups. Sodium-restricted diets are discussed in Chapter 20.

Preliminary studies have shown that dietary calcium supplementation lowers blood pressure in pregnant and nonpregnant individuals (27). The implications of these findings for the treatment of preeclampsia are unclear.

TABLE 8-9 Symptoms of Preeclampsia–Eclampsia

Stage	Symptom
Preeclampsia	*Hypertension:* 140/90 or increase of 30 mm Hg systolic or 15 mm Hg diastolic above woman's usual baseline; at least two observations 6 or more hours apart. *Proteinuria:* 300 mg or more in 24-hour urine collection or random 1+ protein; develops later. *Edema:* significant; usually in face and hands or rapid increase in weight without evident swelling.
Severe preeclampsia	One or more of the following symptoms: *Hypertension:* systolic pressure 160 mm Hg or diastolic 110 mm Hg on two observations 6 or more hours apart at bed rest. *Proteinuria:* 5 g or more of protein per 24 hours or random 3+ to 4+ protein. *Edema:* pulmonary edema. *Clinical:* blurred vision, headache, altered consciousness. *Advancing disease:* epigastric or upper-quadrant pain, impaired liver function, thrombocytopenia.
Eclampsia	Extension of preeclampsia with grand mal seizure occurring near time of labor.

THE PREGNANT ADOLESCENT

Adolescent pregnancy refers to gestation which occurs between the maternal ages of 11 and 18 years. In the United States, approximately 13 percent of all babies are born to adolescent mothers, and the birth rate is increasing among adolescents who are less than 16 years of age (28). By their 18th birthday, 26 percent of black teens and 7 percent of white teens will have had a pregnancy carried to term. Pregnant adolescents are viewed as a high-risk population susceptible to suboptimal pregnancy outcome. However, current evidence suggests that adolescent mothers can have healthy pregnancies with proper nutritional intake, weight gain, and prenatal care.

Adolescence is the state or process of maturing physically and psychosocially from a child into an adult. For the pregnant adolescent, the nutritional demands of pregnancy are superimposed on those required for physiological and psychosocial maturation. Biologic immaturity and a variety of psychosocial circumstances contribute to the problems experienced by the pregnant adolescent. Nutritional risk factors for pregnant adolescents are generally the same as those listed in Table 8-6, although gynecological age should also be evaluated. Interviewing and counseling skills for the population need to be appropriate for the adolescent's stage of psychosocial development, as reviewed elsewhere (28).

Gynecological Age

Gynecological age or biological age is defined as the number of years that have passed since menarche, or the onset of menses. For example, a 16-year-old who started menstruating at age 11 years would have gynecological age of 5 years. The average age of menarche in the United States is now 12.9 years (28). A consideration of gynecological age can be used as an indirect measure of biologic maturity and growth potential, thus reflecting the nutritional needs of the pregnant adolescent.

The onset of the adolescent growth spurt is quite variable but usually occurs by 10.5 years of age in females, with a range of 9.5 to 14.5 years (28). Peak height velocity usually occurs at age 12, and peak weight velocity usually occurs about 6 months later. The growth spurt typically lasts 24 to 36 months, with menarche occurring when growth velocity is beginning to slow down. After menarche, height increases very little, usually only 2 to 4 inches, most of which occurs in the first 2 years past menarche. Growth is generally complete 4 years. after menarche. Thus, adolescents who become pregnant as a gynecological age of less than 2 to 3 years have greater nutritional needs and are at greater risk because they are more biologically immature. Recent evidence demonstrates that adolescent mothers continue to grow during and after their pregnancy (29). However, there may be competition for nutrients between mother and fetus (28).

Associated Risks

Pregnancy during adolescence places the young woman at increased risk for medical, economic, and psychoso-cial problems when compared to a more mature woman. Maternal health risks associated with adolescent pregnancy include preeclampsia, anemia, maternal mortality, and increased incidence of cephalopelvic disproportion.

Neonatal risks associated with adolescent pregnancy include: increased mortality, prematurity, intrauterine growth retardation, and poor parenting skill. Low birth weight and prematurity pose the most significant medical risks for infants born to adolescent mothers, because prematurity is the leading cause of perinatal morbidity and mortality in the United States. Data collected by both the National Center for Health Statistics and the Collaborative Perinatal Project show that the risk of low birth weight (<2,500 g) is significantly higher for adolescent mothers, especially those 16 years or younger (28). It is interesting that even with a similar gestational weight gain, the weight of the infant and placenta are usually less in adolescents compared to mature women.

Recommendations for total gestational weight gain for pregnant adolescents are largely based on empirical information. Gains at the upper end of the recommended ranges in Table 8-2 are recommended for underweight, normal weight, and overweight pregnant adolescents based on BMI. Unfortunately, good reference data for assessing the weight status of adolescents are lacking. Use of the National Center for Health Statistics growth charts for ages 12 to 17 years will give a rough indication of how the adolescent compares to other young women her age (30).

Nutritional Requirements

Data regarding nutrient requirements during both adolescence and adolescent pregnancy are very limited (1). In general, nutrient needs parallel the rate of growth, with the greatest needs occurring at the time of the adolescent growth spurt, which can be assessed indirectly by gynecological age. The RDAs for pregnancy as listed in Appendix A apply to all pregnant women regardless of age. This expression of the RDAs may underestimate total pregnancy needs for the very young adolescent. Alternatively, one can estimate the nutrient needs of pregnant adolescents by using the increments in the RDAs for pregnancy shown in Table 8-3 and adding them to the RDAs specified for adolescents ages 11 to 14 and 15 to 18 years.

Population surveys suggest that adolescents generally consume limited amounts of vitamins A, B_6, folate, and riboflavin, and the minerals calcium, iron, and zinc. Total energy intake is often low as adolescents are often preoccupied with achieving a thin appearance. Snacking is a common eating pattern for adolescents, as is frequent consumption of fast foods. Prenatal vitamin-mineral supplement is often recommended. In general, energy intake should not fall below 2,000 kcal per day for the pregnant adolescent. A calcium intake of 1,200 to 1,500 mg per day is probably adequate for the adolescent with a gynecological age of greater than 3, whereas 1,600 mg of calcium per day are suggested for the very young pregnant adolescent.

TOPICS FOR FURTHER DISCUSSION

1. What are the recommendations for exercise during pregnancy? Discuss some of the advantages of an exercise program during pregnancy.
2. What are some of the nutritional effects associated with the use of oral contraceptive agents?
3. As nutritional care specialist, you present an informal prenatal class on breast feeding. Briefly outline the main topics that you will discuss.
4. Discuss the Women, Infants and Children (WIC) supplemental feeding program. What are its requirements to qualify? What does it provide? What have been its effects?
5. What opportunities are available for the maternal-infant population as part of the Expanded Food and Nutrition Education Program (EFNEP)?

REFERENCES

1. Institute of Medicine. *Nutrition During Pregnancy: Part 1—weight gain; Part II—nutrient supplements.* Washington, DC: National Academy Press, 1990.
2. ———*Nutrition During Lactation.* Washington, DC: National Academy Press, 1991.
3. **Cunningham, F.G., P.C MacDonald, and N.F. Grant, K.J. Levend, and L.C. Gilstrap.** Antepartum: management of normal pregnancy. In *Williams Obstetrics,* 19th ed. Norwalk, CT: Appleton & Lange, 1993, 247–271.
4. **Taggart, N.R., R.M.. Holliday, W.Z.. Billewicz, F.E. Hy Hen, and A.M. Thomsom.** Changes in skinfolds during pregnancy. *Br. J. Nutr.,* 21:(1967) 439–51.
5. **Abrams B.F. and R.K. Laros.** Prepregnancy weight, weight gain, and birth weight. *Am. J. Obstet. Gynecol.,* 154:(1986) 503–09.
6. **Naeye, R.L.** Weight gain and the outcome of pregnancy. *Am J. Obstet. Gynecol.,* 135: (1979) 3–9.
7. Food and Nutrition Board, Commission on Life Sciences, National Research Council. *Recommended Dietary Allowances,* 10th ed. Washington, DC: National Academy Press, 1989.
8. WHO (World Health Organization). *Energy and Protein Requirements.* Report of a Joint FAO/WHO/UNU Expert Consultation. Technical Report Series 724. World Health Organization, Geneva, 206 pp. 1985.
9. **Prentice, A.M., G.R.Goldberg, H.L.Davis, P.R.Murgatroyd, W. Scott.** Energy adaptations in human pregnancy assessed by whole body calorimetry. *Br. J. Nutr.* 62:(1989) 5–22.
10. **Cleveland, L.E. and A.B. Pfeffer.** Planning diets to meet the National Research Council's guidelines for reducing cancer risk. *J. Am. Dietet. Assoc.* 87:(1987)162–68.
11. **Wright, H.S., H.A.Guthrie, M.Q.Wang, V. Bernado.** The 1987–88 Nationwide Food Consumption Survey: an update on the nutrient intake of respondents. *Nutr. Today,* 26: (1991) 21-27.
12. Nutrition Monitoring Division. Human Nutrition Information Service. Nationwide Food Consumption Survey: CSFI/II–1986. **Nutr. Today,** 24: (1989) 35–38.
13. **Worthington-Roberts, B.S.** Prenatal nutrition-general issues. In: Worthington-Roberts, B.S. ,and S.R. Williams, eds. *Nutrition in Pregnancy and Lactation.* 5th ed. St. Louis: Times Mirror/Mosby, (1993) 91-155.
14. **Van Raaij, J.M.A., C.M. Schonk, S.H.Vermoat-Miedema, M.E.M. Peck, J.G.A.J. Hautvast.** Energy cost of lactation, and

energy balances of well-nourished Dutch lactating women: reappraisal of the extra energy requirements of lactation. *Am. J. Clin. Nutr.,* 53:(1991) 612–19.
15. Maternal and Child Health Branch. WIC Supplemental Food Branch, California Department of Health Services. *Nutrition During Pregnancy and the Postpartum Period; a Manual for Health Care Professionals.* June 1990.
16. **Lind, T.** Iron supplementation during pregnancy. In: D.M. Campbell, M.D.G. Gilmer, eds. *Proceedings of the Tenth Study Group of the Royal College of Obstetricians and Gynaecologists,* September 1982. The Royal College of Obstetricians and Gynaecologists, London, 1983, 181–91.
17. **Hambridge, K.M., N.F. Krebs, L. Sibley, J. English.** Acute effects of iron therapy on zinc status during pregnancy. *Am. J. Obstet. Gynecol.* 70: (1987) 593–96.
18. Centers for Disease Control, Department of Health and Human Services. Recommendations for the use of folic acid to reduce the number of cases of spina bifida and other neural tube defects. *Morbid Mortal Wkly Rept.* Vol 4 41(RR-14):1-7(1992).
19. **Monson, R.T.** Iron nutriture and absorption: dietary factors which impact iron bioavailability. *J. Am. Dietet. Assoc.* 88: (1988) 786–95.
20. Council on Scientific Affairs. Fetal effects of maternal alcohol use. *JAMA.* 249: (1983) 2517–2521.
21. **Fenster, L., B. Eskenazi, G.C. Windham, S.H. Swan.** Caffeine consumption during pregnancy and fetal growth. *Am. J. Public Health,* 81:(1991) 458-461.
22. **Infante-Rivard, C.A. Fernandez, R. Gauthier, M. David and G.E. Rivard.** Fetal loss associated with caffeine intake before and during pregnancy. *J.A.M.A.* 270: (1993) 2940-2943.
23. Centers For Disease Control, Department of Health & Human Services. CDC criteria for anemia in children and childbearing-age women. *Morbid Mortal Wkly Rep.* 38 (22): (1989) 400–04.
24. **Algert, S., P. Shragg, D.R. Hollingsworth.** Moderate caloric restriction in obese women with gestational diabetes. *Am. J. Obstet. Gynecol.* 65: (1985) 487–91.
25. National Heart, Lung and Blood Institute. Consensus Report - National High Blood Pressure Education Program Working Group Report on High Blood Pressure in Pregnancy. *Am. J. Obstet. Gynecol.* 163: (1990) 1689–712.
26. **Willis, S.E.** Hypertension in pregnancy. *Am. J. Nurs.* 82:(1982)792–808.
27. **Repke, J.T. and J. Villar.** Pregnancy - Induced hypertension and low birth weight: the role of calcium. *Am. J. Clin. Nutr.* 54: (1991) 2375–415.
28. March of Dimes Birth Defects Foundation, U.S. Dept. of Health & Human Services and U.S. Dept. of Agriculture. *Nutrition Management of the Pregnant Adolescent.* Story, M., ed. National Clearinghouse, Washington, DC, 1990.
29. **Scholl, T.O., M.L. Hediger, and I.G. Ances.** Maternal growth during pregnancy and decreased infant birth weight. *Am J. Clin Nutr* 51: (1990) 790–793.
30. National Center for Health Statistics. *Height and Weight of Youths 12–17 Years, United States.* Vital and Health Statistics, Series II, No. 124. Health Services and Mental Administrations, Washington, DC: U.S. Government Printing Office, 1973.

ADDITIONAL SOURCES OF INFORMATION

American Dietetic Association. Position of the American Dietetic Association: Nutrition Care for Pregnant Adolescents. *J. Am. Dietet. Assoc.* 94: (1994) 449.
Bobak, I.M., M.D. Jensen, and M.K. Zalar, *Maternity and Gynecological Care: The Nurse and the Family,* (4th ed) St. Louis: Mosby, 1989

Eden, R.D. and F.H. Boehm. *Assessment and Care of the Fetus: Physiological, Clinical, and Medicolegal Principles*. Norwalk, CT: Appleton and Lange, 1990.

Lawrence, R. *Breastfeeding: A Guide for the Medical Profession*, 4th ed. St. Louis: Mosby, 1994.

Nilsson, L. *A Child is Born*. New York: Delacorte Press/Seymour Lawrence, 1990.

Rosenfield, A. and Fathalla, C. *The FICO Manual of Human Reproduction*. Park Ridge, NJ: Parthenon, 1990.

 ## TO TEST YOUR UNDERSTANDING

11. You are working in a prenatal program associated with a clinic. You prepare to speak with a woman who has just received the results of a positive pregnancy test. The following information is noted in the medical record:

$G_3P_1Ab_1LC_0$

first day of LMP = 9/1/95

present date = 11/1/95

a. Describe the woman's obstetrical history.

b. What is the approximate gestational age in weeks?

c. What is the EDD?

2. A primigravida at 25 weeks gestation tells you that she is concerned about the extra fat around her thighs and back. She has decided to reduce her food intake because this extra fat has nothing to do with her baby's growth. How would you counsel this woman?

3. a. Using the RDAs in Appendix A, list nutrients that are needed in increased and decreased amounts during lactation compared to pregnancy.

b. Explain why these differences in nutrient requirements occur when comparing needs in lactation to those during pregnancy.

4. A woman has been exclusively breast feeding her infant for 4 months. She has attained her prepregnancy weight and is continuing to lose weight.

a. Explain the nature of the weight loss.

b. What would you recommend to maintain present body weight?

5. Provide a list of foods that could supply a total daily intake of the following nutrients. (Use a handbook of food composition or consult Table B-1:

Iron, 30 mg

Calcium, 1,200 mg

Folate, 400 µg

6. A pregnant Mexican-American patient tells you that she will not drink milk. What suggestions would you make to her to improve the calcium content of her diet?

7. A woman's prepregnancy height and weight are 5 feet, 4 inches and 115 pounds, respectively. She demonstrates the following pattern of weight gain throughout her pregnancy:

Week of gestation	Weight (#)
0	115
12	116
18	118
22	120
24	122
26	125
28	130
30	136
32	142

a. What is the woman's prepregnancy BMI?

b. Suggest an appropriate range for total gestational weight gain for this woman.

c. How does the above rate of gain compare with the recommended pattern?

d. What problems are suggested by the pattern of gain after 26 weeks?

8. A lacto-ovo-vegetarian patient who has not taken a prenatal supplement has a Hgb value of 100 g/L, a transferrin saturation of <15 percent, an MCV of 80 fL, and a serum folate value of 6 µg/L at 30 weeks gestation.

a. Suggest what nutrient might be deficient in her diet.

b. How could her intake of this nutrient be improved?

c. What suggestions could be made to improve the bioavailability of nonheme iron in this woman's diet?

9. A young pregnant woman tells you that her mother has suggested that she avoid salt and carefully watch her weight gain during pregnancy in order to prevent the development of "toxemia." How would you advise the young woman?

10. Amy is a 14-year-old pregnant adolescent who has been referred to you for prenatal nutrition counseling. Her prepregnancy height and weight are 5 feet, 6 inches, and 120 pounds, respectively. She began menstruating at age 12.

a. What is Amy's gynecological age? Estimate at what age Amy achieved peak growth with respect to height velocity.

b. Suggest an appropriate range for total gestational weight gain for Amy.

c. Suggest what nutrients may be limiting in her diet.

Nutrition During Pregnancy and Lactation

Part I: Presentation

Present illness: Juanita is a 32 year old G_8P_6, Mexican American mother of five who requests a pregnancy test at the local public health clinic (LMP = 4/1, approximately 12 weeks ago). The pregnancy test is positive (G_9P_6).

Previous obstetrical history $G_9P_6Ab_2LC_5$. She has had two early spontaneous abortions and delivered one stillborn. Her living children are ages 14, 12, 5, 2, and about 1. Her last two liveborn children were born 1 and 2 years ago and weighed 9 1/2 pounds and 10 pounds, respectively, at birth. All her children were breast fed and Juanita plans to nurse this child. She gained 35 pounds with her last pregnancy and lost about 25 pounds before this conception.

Family history: Her mother died of influenza and her father died at age 55 from complications resulting from diabetes.

Social history: Lives with husband who works as a gardener; does housekeeping work to earn extra money. The family receives $200 per month in Food Stamps.

Physical exam: Ht 5 ft, 2 in, prepregnancy wt 160#, present wt 163#, BP = 120/80.

Laboratory: Hct 0.35, Hgb 110g/L.

Impression: Intrauterine pregnancy at 12 weeks.

QUESTIONS

You speak with Juanita at the public health clinic after she receives the positive results of her pregnancy test. The results of a brief diet history indicate that the family diet consists mainly of rice, beans, tortillas, chilies, eggs, and occasionally, meat. Juanita likes milk but usually drinks soft drinks with her meals. You help Juanita apply for the special supplementary food program for Women, Infants, and Children (WIC). The WIC program provides vouchers for the purchase of foods high in those nutrients needed in increased amounts during pregnancy. These foods may include eggs, fruit and vegetable juices, milk, cheese, iron-fortified cereals, or infant formulas. You also schedule Juanita to attend the clinic's prenatal nutrition class, which is held once a month for an hour.

1. List four nutritional risk factors for pregnancy that this patient displays (see Table 8-4).

2. In what nutrients is her diet likely to be deficient?

3. Assuming that Juanita is eligible for the WIC program, suggest four changes that she could make in her diet.

4. You are responsible for teaching the public health clinic prenatal nutrition class. Describe four areas you will cover in your class.

Part II Excessive Weight Gain in the First Two Trimesters

Juanita's pregnancy progresses without difficulty, but at 30 weeks the physician becomes concerned because Juanita has already gained 30 pounds and the fetus appears to be large. The physician suspects that the EDD may have been incorrectly calculated because the fundal height is consistent with a gestational age of closer to 34 weeks. An ultrasound test is performed to get a better idea of gestational age; the results suggest an age of 33 weeks.

Because of Juanita's history of delivering large infants and family history of diabetes, gestational diabetes is another concern. An oral, nonfasting, loading test for gestational diabetes, using a 50 g glucose load, is given. The 1-hour plasma glucose value is 7.2 mmol/dL, which is also within normal limits (WNL), suggesting normal gestational carbohydrate tolerance.

Laboratory determinations at 33 weeks are as follows: BP 125/85, wt 195#, Hgb 10 g/dL, Hct 0.30, MCV 82 fL, serum albumin 30 g/L, and urine is negative for protein and sugar.

The physical examination indicates a fundal height of 34 cm, a trace of edema, the presence of fetal heart sounds, and a vertex fetal position.

The physician asks you to counsel Juanita regarding her dietary intake.

(continued)

QUESTIONS

5. a. Calculate Juanita's prepregnancy BMI and state the recommended range of total gestational weight gain based on prepregnancy BMI, Table 8-2.

b. Plot Juanita's weight gain on the appropriate prenatal weight-gain grid in Appendix G using the values given here.

Weeks of gestation	Weight (#)
0	160
12	163
18	173
24	185
33	195

c. What does the pattern of weight gain suggest?

d. Would you recommend holding weight stable for the remainder of pregnancy? Explain why. If not, what pattern of weight gain would you recommend for the remainder of pregnancy?

6. What is suggested by the change in hematological values between 12 and 33 weeks gestation?

7. You obtain a 24-hour recall from Juanita as follows:

1 c nonfat milk	1 c refried beans	1 c nonfat milk
1 fried egg	2 oz cheese	1 c refried beans
2 doughnuts	2 c rice	2 flour tortillas
2 c orange juice	2 flour tortillas	2 c vegetable soup
3 slices bacon	12 oz cola	with 1 oz meat
		1 2-oz candy bar

She also comments that she does not take a prenatal iron supplement.

a. Using the 1993 Pregnancy Diet Intake form (in Appendix G), evaluate the diet. List the food groups being consumed in inadequate amounts and the nutrients that are limiting in the diet due to this eating pattern. Also, suggest appropriate foods to include in the diet from the food groups that are being consumed in inadequate amounts.

b. What correlation can you make between dietary intake and hematological status? Should a prenatal vitamin- mineral supplement be recommended? If so, what kind?

c. Using the 1995 ADA exchange system, list the number of exchanges consumed and estimate the daily calorie intake.

d. How many kcal per day are coming from empty calorie foods, which provide energy but are low in proteins, vitamins, and minerals?

e. What daily calorie intake would you estimate is required for Juanita to achieve an optimal weight gain for the remainder of pregnancy? Explain your answer.

8. Assume that you will use the Pregnancy Diet Intake form as a teaching tool to show Juanita how she should modify her diet.

a. List those foods that she should eliminate from her diet. Explain why she should eliminate these foods.

b. What alterations in food preparation might help to control Juanita's caloric intake?

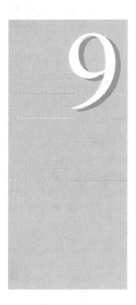

Pediatric Nutrition

The pediatric population comprises individuals who are from newborn to 18 years of age. The population can be divided into the following age groups: infants (0–12 months), preschoolers (1–5 years), school-age children (5–11 years), and adolescents (11–18 years). This chapter will focus on nutritional requirements, feeding patterns, and nutritional assessment for the pediatric population. A knowledge of normal pediatric feeding patterns forms the basis of diet modification for specific pediatric disease states.

Nutritional requirements for the pediatric population are a function of the child's age, size, activity, and rate of growth. Because there is considerable individual variation in growth rate and size, the RDAs are expressed per kg of body weight for the infant. In general, nutritional requirements are the greatest during the two periods of peak growth rate—infancy and adolescence. (The RDAs for the pediatric population can be found in Table A-1. Daily fluid requirements are discussed in Chapter 4.)

INFANT FEEDING

Breast milk or infant formula is the basis of an infant's diet. For developmental and nutritional reasons, solid foods are usually not needed in the diet until 4 to 6 months of age. The need for supplementation of specific vitamins and minerals during infancy depends on whether the infant receives human milk or other milk feeding. This section reviews breast feeding, bottle feeding, introduction of solid food to the diet, and infant formulas.

The guidelines for normal infant feeding presented in this chapter represent the opinions of various well-regarded pediatric nutrition groups (1–3), including the American Academy of Pediatrics (4). You should be aware that there are no firm data to support specific infant feeding recommendations and that a wide variety of feeding practices have been shown to result in healthy babies.

Breast Feeding

Human milk is considered the optimal sole food for an infant's first 4 to 6 months of life. The decision to breast feed should be made during the prenatal period. Because breast feeding is a learned skill, health professionals need to be prepared to assist new mothers in the techniques of successful breast feeding. Several useful references on this topic are listed at the end of this chapter.

Data from the National Survey of Family Growth for 1987 indicate that 56.3 percent of infants in the United States are breast fed for some period of time (5). The prevalence of breast feeding is not uniform throughout the United States. The highest incidence of breast feeding is noted in women who are white, older in age, college educated, and living in urban and western regions of the United states. The lowest rates of breast feeding are noted among women who are black, with less than a college education, residing in rural and southern regions of the United States, and younger in age. Low birthweight infants are less likely to be breast fed than infants of normal birth weight.

Advantages. Breast feeding has advantages for both mother and infant (2, 4). Breast milk provides the infant with immunological protection from gastroenteritis, respiratory infection and allergic reactions. Breast feeding also promotes facial and muscular development and thus assists with the development of speech. Breast feeding helps the mother lose weight gained during pregnancy and also helps the uterus return to its normal size. It is also the most economical method of feeding.

The adequately breast-fed infant of a well-nourished mother does not require vitamin and mineral supplementation, with the possible exception of fluoride, and vitamin D in those areas where the infant may not receive sufficient sunlight (4).

Frequency and Duration of Feedings.

Breast feeding should be initiated as soon after delivery as possible. During the first weeks of life, infants usually require feeding every 2 to 3 hours, with a minimum of 8 to 10 feedings every 24 hours. The infant should nurse from both breasts at each feeding to empty the initial side and stimulate production in the alternate breast. Generally, 15 minutes on the first breast plus 5 to 10 minutes on the other side are appropriate.

A baby is usually getting enough breast milk if he or she is sleeping 2 to 3 hours between feedings, has 6 to 8 wet diapers each day, has frequent bowel movements during the first 6 weeks of life, and is gaining weight. Failure to regain birth weight by 3 weeks of age or continued weight loss after 10 days of life suggests that the intake of breast milk is inadequate.

Supplemental Feedings.

Routine supplemental feedings of water or formula should be discouraged during the first 2 weeks of breast feeding. Adequate breast feeding provides the infant's fluid needs. An infant given water or supplements is less likely to provide adequate suckling stimulation for the mother to produce an appropriate quantity of milk. Also, bottle feeding may result in nipple confusion, as standard nipples promote a suckling action different from that needed for successful breast feeding.

Once lactation is well established, generally after 4 weeks, replacement bottles of breast milk or formula can be used. For the working mother who wishes to continue to feed her infant breast milk, it is suggested that the separated mother pump her breast at about the same time the infant feeds and then store the milk in the refrigerator to use as a replacement feeding within 24 to 48 hours. If she does this in addition to frequent feedings when they are together, she should maintain her milk supply. Alternatively, the mother may wish to nurse her child when she is not at work and then use commercial formula for the remainder of the day's feedings. This will result in reduction of the mother's milk volume but may allow the working mother to partially breast feed her infant.

Cup Introduction and Weaning.

The breast-fed infant can be weaned directly to a cup, omitting the use of a bottle. The infant can usually begin drinking from a cup at 5 to 6 months of age. A small plastic cup with a top and spout works well to start. To accomplish weaning, the quantity of fluid consumed by cup should be gradually increased as the number of breast feedings is reduced. While drinking from a cup should be introduced between 5 and 6 months, breast feeding may continue until 12 months of age or longer.

Bottle Feeding

Bottle feeding of infant formulas provides the best alternative to breast feeding to meet nutritional needs during the first year. Because there is increasing social pressure to breast feed, it is important to avoid making a woman feel guilty if she decides to bottle feed. Various aspects of good bottle-feeding techniques are discussed in this section.

Number and Volume of Bottle Feedings.

At birth the full-term infant's stomach holds between 30 and 90 ml. As the infant grows, the stomach enlarges and its rate of emptying slows. During the first week of life, an infant usually consumes 6 to 10 feedings of 30 to 90 mL each per day. Recommendations for number and volume of bottle feedings for a normal infant are shown in Table 9-1. Fifteen or twenty minutes is an adequate bottle-feeding time for most infants.

Good Feeding Technique.

Infants should be held when bottle fed; the bottle should never be propped up. Putting an infant to bed with a bottle should be discouraged because the practice can cause dental caries and may be associated with a high incidence of otitis media and a psychological dependence on the bottle.

The bottle should be held and tilted so that the nipple is always filled with formula, not air. Many styles of bottles are available. The disposable plastic-bag bottles generally decrease the amount of air that is swallowed during feedings. Bottles should only be used for formula or water feeding, not for introduction of juices or solids such as cereal.

Weaning from the Bottle.

Weaning from the bottle is usually started between 5 and 8 months of age. At this age, the infant usually receives four 8-oz bottles per day, often corresponding to three bottles during the day and one before bedtime. Weaning is usually accomplished by eliminating one bottle feeding at a time and substituting a cup. During this time, the infant is also being offered an increased amount and variety of solid foods. This makes it practical to plan a three-meal-a-day-plus-snacks pattern with the rest of the family. Usually, the infant can take 3 to 4 oz of fluid by cup with a meal and the same amount between meals.

Children 1 to 2 years of age or older should not be taking a daily or nightly bottle. Bottle feeding in the toddler can lead to an excessive intake of milk or other sweetened liquids, which may interfere with recommended nutrient intake or lead to excessive calorie intake.

TABLE 9-1 Dietary Evaluation Guidelines for Infants (0–12 months)

Age (months)	0	1	2	3	4	5	6	7	8	9	10	11	12
50th percentile of weight in kg (#)	3.3 (7.3)	4.1 (9.0)	5.0 (11.0)	5.7 (12.5)	6.4 (14.1)	7.0 (15.4)	7.5 (16.5)	8.0 (17.6)	8.5 (18.7)	8.9 (19.6)	9.2 (20.2)	9.6 (21.1)	9.9 (21.8)
kcal per 24 hr range	108 kcal/kg (95–145 kcal/kg) 49 kcal/# (43–66 kcal/#)				98 kcal/kg (80–135 kcal/kg) 45 kcal/# (36–61 kcal/#)								
Fluid per 24 hr (oz)	125–145 mL/kg (4–4.8 oz/kg; 2–2 1/2 oz/#)												
No. of milk feedings per 24 hr *	8 or more	7 or 8	6 or 7		4 or 5				3 or 4			3	
Oz formula per feedings †	2 1/2–4	3 1/2–5	4–6	5–7			6–8					6–7	
Solids ‡					Strained (pureed) foods					Junior (chopped) foods		Table foods §	
Breads and cereals					Iron-fortified cereal, rice		Teething biscuit			Iron-fortified mixed-grain cereals			
Vegetables						Carrots, squash, beans, peas							
Fruits §							Applesauce, pears, peaches, bananas						
Meat group and meat alternates								Strained meats, cheese, yogurt, cooked beans, egg yolk					
Age (months)	0	1	2	3	4	5	6	7	8	9	10	11	12

* Milk is breast milk or formula, with the possible introduction of whole cow milk after 6–7 months of age See footnote †
† Formula is preferred to whole milk during the first year of life.
‡ No solid foods should be introduced until the infant is 4–6 months of age or has reached 6–7 kg of weight.
§ Whole eggs, orange juice, and citrus fruits should not be introduced until the enfant is 12 months old.
Copyright 1983 Denise Ney, R.D. and Elizabeth G. Jones R.D.

Introduction of Cow Milk. Breast milk or commercial formula is the recommended feeding from birth through 12 months of age (6). The feeding of skim or low fat milk during infancy is not recommended because the lower calorie density of these milks does not meet energy needs, and contributes to a high renal solute load and increased risk of dehydration (1). Whole cow milk is also not recommended because recent evidence suggests that healthy infants fed cow milk during the second 6 months of life are at greater risk for iron deficiency than infants fed iron-fortified formula (6). Other concerns regarding the early introduction of whole cow milk include a high renal solute load, low intakes of essential nutrients, especially iron, linoleic acid, and vitamins E and C, and allergy to cow milk protein. Whole cow milk is usually offered to a child between 1 and 2 years of age (1, 4).

Solid Foods, or Beikost

The introduction of beikost, or foods other than milk, into an infant's diet should be withheld until 4 to 6 months of age. The rationale for this recommendation is based on the developmental readiness of the infant to consume solids, the increased probability of the infant's developing allergies with early introduction of solids, the lack of sound data to suggest that early feeding of solids helps the infant sleep though the night, and the fact that, until 4 to 6 months of age, breast milk or formula best meets the infant's nutritional needs. The order of introduction of solid foods is usually iron-fortified cereal, followed by vegetables, fruit, meat, and egg yolk. Table 9-2 summarizes recommendations for the introduction of solid foods, including the rationale and the stage of feeding development.

As the infant starts eating greater amounts of solid foods, the volume of formula or milk consumed will decrease. After 9 months of age, infants generally do not need more than 32 oz of formula per day. By the age of one year, most babies take approximately 16 to 24 oz of formula per day plus solids equal to 4 to 6 jars (2 to 3 cups) of baby food. Portion sizes for solid foods in the infant aged 4 to 12 months are summarized in Table 9-3.

Foods to Avoid in Infancy

It is wise to avoid feeding certain foods to infants. Nuts, potato chips, fruits with seeds, popcorn, celery, grapes, wieners, carrots, fish with bones, tough meat, and small or hard candies may cause choking in children until 3 years of age. Daily intake of cookies, pastry, sugar-coated cereals, candy, soft drinks, and artificially flavored fruit drinks may replace more nutritious foods and encourage a desire for sweets. Honey and corn syrup should be avoided in the child under one year of age. Evidence shows that these sweeteners may be contaminated with *Clostridium botulinum* spores (7). Chapter 15 discusses the foods most likely to cause allergic reactions in atopic children. Sensitization can sometimes be prevented in atopic children by introducing these foods only after one year of age.

INFANT FORMULAS

Commercial formulas can meet the nutritional needs of infants when the mother cannot or chooses not to breast feed. The major goal in preparing infant formulas or human milk substitutes is to formulate an acceptable product that mimics the nutritional profile of human milk as closely as possible. The Infant Formula Act of 1980 and subsequent amendments specify quality assurance testing and procedures, labeling requirements, and guidelines for the nutrient requirements for infant formulas (8). The guidelines for nutrient requirements reflect recommendations from the Committee on Nutrition, American Academy of Pediatrics (9), as summarized in Table 9-4. Commercial infant formulas can be divided into four categories: standard formulas for full-term infants, formulas for preterm and low birth-weight infants, formulas for infants with unusual medical and dietary problems, and formulas for infants with metabolic disorders. The Food and Drug Administration has exempted some types of infant formulas from meeting the nutrient requirements specified in Table 9-4, recognizing that standard infant formula profiles would be inappropriate and medically contraindicated for some infants (8). Categories of exempt infant formulas include the formulas for preterm and low birthweight infants, infants with unusual medical or dietary problems and infants with metabolic disorders.

A less expensive, homemade version of infant formula can be prepared using evaporated whole milk. This type of formula is not commonly recommended, but it is less expensive than commercial formulas and superior to unmodified whole milk. The protein content and renal solute load of evaporated whole-milk formula are higher, and the fat is not as well absorbed compared with breast milk or commercial infant formula. Supplemental vitamin C and iron must be provided when feeding this formula. A common recipe for this formula consists of one can of vitamin D fortified evaporated whole milk (12 oz), 18 oz of water, and 2 tablespoons of sugar.

This section contains a general discussion of the characteristics of three categories of infant formulas: standard infant formulas for full-term infants, formulas for preterm and low birth-weight infants, and special indication formulas for infants with unusual medical and dietary problems. Appendix H provides tables that outline the nutrient profile of representative formulas from these three categories of infant formulas.

Standard Formulas for Full-Term Infants

The standard formulas for full-term infants fall into two groups: those based on cow milk protein and those based on soy protein. Cow milk-based infant formulas are the formula of first choice and comprise approximately 80 percent of total infant formula sales in the United States. Soy protein-based formulas, which are lactose free, are recommended for infants with cow's milk protein allergy, galactosemia, primary lactase deficiency, and secondary lactose intolerance such as occurs after an

TABLE 9-2   Introduction to Solid Foods (Beikost)

Age	Introduction of New Foods	Reasons for Introduction	Development
Birth–12 months	Breast milk or formula.	Meets the infant's nutritional needs for the first 4-6 months or 6–7 kg of weight.	Rooting reflex, suck-swallow pattern, extension tongue movement.
4–6 months (6–7 kg)	Iron-fortified cereal (rice, oats, barley)	Provides a dietary source of iron at the age when body stores from birth are depleting. Cereal is hypoallergenic.	Lips have muscular control to seal oral cavity. Tongue can move back and forth. Infant can begin to draw in lower lip as spoon is removed.
5–7 months	Strained or pureed vegetables and fruits. Unsweetened fruit juice (except orange juice) may be introduced by cup.	Provides dietary sources of vitamins, minerals, and calories. Introduces new food flavors. Starts setting basis for good eating habits. Introduce vegetables first to reduce the tendency to develop a taste for sweets.	Up-and-down movement begins (beginning of chewing process). (This does not begin until the biting reflex fades at 3 to 5 months.) Controls sucking impulse. Opens mouth to accept spoon. Turns head freely.
6–8 months	Cottage cheese, plain yogurt, egg yolk, strained meats (start with lamb), poultry, and meat alternates (purees of beans and lentils), dried breads.	Provides additional protein, vitamins, and iron for rapid growth. Encourages chewing when teeth erupt. (Note: To avoid allergies, egg white is not suggested until 12 months.)	Infant has ability to grasp and route food from hand to mouth, and can sit with support. Teeth begin to come in.
7–9 months	Junior meats, poultry, or cooked fish, mashed vegetables and fruits, mild cheese, other infant cereals (wheat, mixed grain, and high protein).	Adds variety and additional protein, minerals, and vitamins for rapid growth.	Infant can sit alone, has mobility of shoulders, can reach, grasp, and transfer items. Infant has more tongue maturity for spoon feeding. Can suck from a cup. Can tolerate harder-to-masticate foods (junior types).
8–10 months	Chewy finger foods, bite-size meat, poultry, and fish. Soft-cooked vegetables in strips or slices.	Encourages the development of hand-to-mouth coordination and proper chewing.	Infant has concept of spoon and its use. Has increased hand and eye control, and can drink from a cup.
9–12 months	Variety of regular table foods. Meat, poultry, fish, and cheese. Mild casserole dishes, beans, fruits, vegetables, cereal, and breads.	Infant can feed self.	Infant develops pincer grasp. Has rotary chewing movements, holds and transfers food to mouth. Tries to feed self.
12 months	Whole egg, orange juice, cow milk.	Infant can drink from a cup. Infant should be weaned from a bottle, and may be weaned from the breast.	Infant is able to spit and stick out tongue. Is more interested in feeding self and is quieter at meals.

Adapted from material developed by Elizabeth G. Jones, pediatric nutrition consultant, San Diego, CA

episode of acute diarrhea (10). Infants from vegetarian families where animal proteins are not eaten may also select soy protein-based formulas. Soy protein-based formulas are not recommended for routine management of colic (10). About 15 percent of formula-fed infants receive a formula based on soy protein. In accordance with the Infant Formula Act, standard cow milk or soy-based formulas provide a caloric density of 20 kcal/oz (67 kcal/100 mL), an osmolality of 300 to 400 mOsm/L, and a caloric distribution of 7.2 to 18 percent protein, 30 to 54 percent fat, and 40 to 50 percent carbohydrate (9). Cow milk-based formula has a potential renal solute load of 133 mOsm/L; soy formula, of 177 mOsm/L; and human milk, of 93 mOsm/L (11). Vitamins

TABLE 9-3 Portion Sizes for the Infant Aged 4–12 Months

4–6 months	6–8 months	8–10 months	10–12 months
Breast milk or formula			
24–32 oz in 5—6 feedings	24–32 oz in 4–5 feedings in a cup	24–32 oz in 3–4 feedings in a cup	24 oz in 3 feedings in a cup
cereal (dry)			
2–4 T	4 T	4 T or more	4 T or more
vegetables			
——	4 T or 1/2 jar	4 T or more	4 T bite-size pieces
Fruit			
——	4 T or 1/2 jar	4 T or more	4 T bite-size pieces
Meat			
——	strained—up to 4 T or 1/2 jar	Junior—up to 4 T or 1/2 jar	4-6 T bite-size pieces
Water			
——	3-4 oz if, desired	As needed	As needed
Other			
Dilute cereal with breast milk or formula and feed with a spoon.	Teething foods—dry toast, crackers, cottage cheese, and plain yogurt— 2–4 T	Fruit juice, 3–4 oz/day, teething foods; start introducing finger and table foods	Fruit juice, 4 oz/day, teething foods, variety of table foods, including mild casserole dishes

and minerals are supplemented to provide for infant needs, as specified in Table 9-5. Some of the formulas are supplemented with approximately 12 mg/L of iron, while others are not and require that the infant receive an additional iron source by 4 to 6 months of age, when iron stores may be depleted. A summary is given in Appendix H, Table 1.

Three forms of formula are available:

1. Powder—The powder comes in 1-pound cans and requires dilution with water. The usual dilution is 1 T or 1 measure (included in each can) to 2 oz water. The formula should be refrigerated and prepared fresh daily. Powder is the least expensive form of formula.
2. Liquid concentrate—Concentrates come in 13-oz cans and are prepared by diluting 1 oz water to 1 oz concentrate.
3. Ready-to-feed—This form comes in various size cans and needs no dilution. It is the most expensive type of formula.

The most commonly used cow milk-based formulas are Enfamil (Mead Johnson Nutritionals), Similac (Ross Laboratories), and SMA (Wyeth-Ayerst Laboratories). These proprietary, or exclusively manufacturer-protected, formulas are prepared by one of two methods. The first includes a blending of nonfat cow milk, a mixture of vegetable oils or vegetable and monounsaturated (oleo) oils, lactose, vitamins, minerals, and the amino acid taurine. This produces a whey:casein ratio of 20:80. The other method blends partially demineralized whey, nonfat cow milk, vegetable oils or vegetable and monounsaturated (oleo) oils, lactose, vitamins, minerals, and taurine to achieve a whey:casein ratio of 60:40, which more closely approximates the 70:30 to 80:20 whey:casein ratio of human milk. There may be advantages of the whey-predominant formulas for preterm infants, although there is no evidence to suggest that either the casein- or whey-predominant formulas are superior for full-term infants.

Taurine can be synthesized from the sulfur-containing amino acid cysteine, although the rate of synthesis may be low in newborns, especially preterm infants. Human milk is a good source of taurine, whereas casein has a lower cysteine content than whey protein. Taurine is currently added to many infant formulas because of its important role in the development of retinal and nervous tissue.

The most commonly used soy-based infant formulas are Prosobee (Mead Johnson Nutritionals), Isomil (Ross Laboratories), and Nursoy (Wyeth-Ayerst Laboratories). These formulas consist of methionine-fortified isolated soy protein, a mixture of vegetable oils or vegetable and oleo oils, carbohydrate as a blend of sucrose, corn syrup, or glucose polymers, vitamins, minerals, taurine, and carnitine. All soy protein-based infant formulas are fortified with iron. Clinical data show that 10 to 20 percent of the infants who exhibit clinical symptoms of cow milk intolerance also develop soy protein-based intolerance (4).

Formulas for Preterm and Low Birth-weight Infants
Feeding practices for preterm (born before 37 weeks gestation) and low birth-weight (<2,500 g) infants vary but are based primarily on the birth-weight of the infant. Formulas for preterm infants reflect the estimated nutrient requirement of the low birthweight infant and take into consideration the immature infant's limited ability to digest, absorb, and metabolize the formula. They are manufactured to provide 20 or 24 kcal/oz (67 to 80 kcal/100 mL) at normal dilution and are usually fed at a level of 120 kcal/kg body weight. This provides the low birth-weight infant with a fluid intake of 150 mL/kg body weight and a potential renal solute load of 160 to 220 mOsm/L (31 mOsm/kg/day). Renal solute load is discussed in Chapter 4. The section on low birth-weight infants later in this chapter includes a discussion of the nutritional needs of premature and low birth-weight infants.

Formulas for preterm and low birth-weight infants generally contain whey-predominant proteins (60:40 whey:casein ratio) with added taurine, a mixture of

TABLE 9-4 Nutrient Content of Cow Milk and Human Milk and Nutrient Specifications for Infant Formula Compositions

Constituent	Cow Milk (per liter)	Human Milk (per liter)	Infant Formulas[*] (per liter)	Nutrient Specifications[*] (per 100 kcal)
Energy (kcal)	660	690	670	—
Protein (gm)	35	9	12.1–30	1.8–4.5
Fat (gm)	38	40	22.1–40.2[†]	3.3–6.0[†]
Lactose (gm)	49	70	—	—
Vitamins:				
Vitamin A (IU)	1,025	1,898	1,675–5,025	250–750
Vitamin D (activity)	14	40	268–670	40–100
Vitamin E (U)	0.4	3.2	20.1[‡]	0.7
Vitamin K(µg)	10–20	2.1	26.8	4.0
Thiamin (µg)	370	160	268	40
Riboflavin (µg)	1,700	350	402	60
Niacin (mg)	0.9	2.0	1,675	250
Pyridoxine (µg)	460	280	234.5[§]	35
Folic Acid (µg)	2.9–68	41–84.6	26.8	4
Cobalamine (µg)	4	0.26	1.0	0.15
Ascorbic acid (µg)	17	40	53.6	8
Biotin (µg)	30	60	10.7	1.5
Minerals:				
Calcium (mg)	1,200	241–340	335[‖]	60
Phosphorus (mg)	920	150	167[‖]	30
Sodium (mg)	506	150	134–402[**]	20–60
Potassium (mg)	1,570	580	536–1340[**]	80–200
Chlorine (mg)	1,028	400	368–1005[**]	55–150
Magnesium (mg)	120	30	40.2	6
Sulfur (mg)	300	140[††]	—	—
Iron (mg)	0.5	0.3–1.0	1.0–20	0.15–3.0
Iodine (µg)	80	70	33–503	5–75
Manganese (µg)	20–40	4–15	33.5	5
Copper (µg)	110	350	402	60
Zinc (mg)	3–5	1.66	3.35	0.5
Selenium (µg)	5–50	20	—	—
Fluoride (mg)	0.03–0.1	0.05	—	—

Adapted from *Pediatrics,* A.M. Rudolph, ed, 19th ed.,. Norwalk, CT: Appleton and Lange, 1991.
[*] From Committee on Nutrition, American Academy of Pediatrics, *Pediatr.* 57(2):(1976) 278. Copyright American Academy of Pediatrics 1976, and Food and Drug Administration, Rules and Regulations. Nutrient requirements for infant formulas. *Fed. Regist* 50:(1985) 45106-8 (21 CFR Part 107).
[†] Minimum 300 mg linoleate
[‡] 0.7 IU/g linoleate
[§] 15µg/g protein. In addition, non-milk-based formulas require 7 mg choline and 4 mg inositol per 100 kcal.
[‖] Calcium to phosphorus ratio must be no less than 1.1 but no more than 2.0
[**] The molar ratios of Na:K should be in the range of 0.5:1 to 1:1, and the molar ratios of (Na +K)/Cl should be in the range of 2.0-2.5, as occurs in human milk.
[‡‡] Median values at 2 weeks and 5 months of lactation.

lactose and glucose polymers, a fat mixture of medium-chain triglycerides (MCT), and relatively unsaturated long-chain triglycerides (see Chapter 17) and, in some cases, added carnitine. Soy protein-based infant formulas are not recommended for low birth-weight infants because of reports of hypophosphatemia and rickets in very low birth-weight infants receiving soy-based formulas (4). Preterm formulas have significantly greater levels of protein, vitamins A, C, D, and K, folate, calcium, phosphorus, magnesium, and zinc than standard infant formulas. Some preterm formulas must be supplemented with vitamin D, iron, and fluoride, while others contain adequate levels of vitamin D and iron. These formulas are available only by prescription, and company instructions should be followed carefully. (see appendix Table H-2.)

Breast milk may also be used for the preterm infant, although evidence suggests that the protein and mineral content and caloric density of human milk is not sufficient for the rapidly growing preterm infant. A common practice is to supplement breast milk with lactose, vitamins, minerals, and energy from glucose polymers or MCT. Special products have been developed to fortify human milk for this purpose.

Special Indication Formulas

Nutrition management is an important factor for infants with unusual medical or dietary problems, and specialized infant formulas are often required for these infants to achieve an optimal growth rate. Formulas for children with metabolic disorders pose especially challenging circumstances. The formulas are discussed in Chapter 23.

Characteristics of special indication formulas may include the following (12):

Hypercaloric to meet increased energy requirements in a limited volume

Low electrolytes for renal disorders

Protein hydrolysates for protein malabsorption disorders and/or food allergies

Modified fat for fat malabsorption disorders

An alternate carbohydrate source for infants with disaccharidase deficiencies

The nutrient profile of representative special indication formulas is given in Appendix H, Table 2. A brief discussion of the primary indication for some of these formulas follows, although individual companies should be consulted for more detailed information. Nutramigen is a lactose-free, casein hydrolysate formula that contains supplemental amino acids. It is appropriate for oral or tube feedings for infants and children with severe or multiple food allergies, colic, galactosemia, persistent diarrhea, or other gastrointestinal disturbances. Pregestimil is similar in composition to Nutramigen, except that it contains less carbohydrate and more fat from a mixture of MCT and vegetable oils. It is appropriate for infants with impaired fat absorption or sensitivity to intact proteins of milk and other foods. Portagen contains a greater proportion of MCT than Pregestimil and is used for infants, children, and adults who do not efficiently digest conventional food fat or absorb the resulting long-chain fatty acids. Nutramigen, Pregestimal, and Portagen are all manufactured by Mead Johnson Nutritionals.

Alimentum Protein Hydrolysate formula by Ross Laboratories contains MCT, and amino acids and peptides from a casein hydrolysate. It is free of lactose and corn and contains low levels of fructose and glucose. Infants with conditions similar to those described for Pregestimil and Portagen may benefit from Alimentum Protein Hydrolysate formula. Calcilo XD is a vitamin D–free low-calcium formula that is used for the dietary management of infants with hypercalcemia. ProViMin is a nutritionally incomplete protein base containing *only* a blend of casein, minerals, and vitamins, with added taurine and carnitine. It is useful in liquid diets of infants and children with chronic diarrhea and other malabsorptive disorders that require restriction of fat and carbohydrate. RCF (Ross Carbohydrate-Free) is a nutritionally incomplete, carbohydrate-free, soy-formula base with added taurine, methionine, and carnitine. It is useful for persons unable to tolerate carbohydrate.

The Wyeth-Ayerst Laboratories formulas, S-14, S-29, and S-44 are nutritionally incomplete formulas useful for infants with leucine-sensitive hypoglycemia (S-14), infants who need an extremely low renal solute load (S-29), and for infants who need an extremely low renal solute load and who have idiopathic hypercalcemia or hypervitaminosis D (S-44).

Vitamin and Mineral Supplementation

Guidelines for vitamin and mineral supplementation in healthy, full-term infants are summarized in Table 9-5. In addition, infants usually receive 1 mg of vitamin K at birth. Supplementation with most nutrients is not generally needed for full-term infants fed breast milk or commercial formula supplemented with iron. Nutrients that *may* need to be supplemented include both vitamin D in the breast-fed infant not exposed to sunlight, and fluoride.

The importance of supplementing a breast-fed infant's diet with vitamin D is less than previously thought. This reflects evidence that the concentration of vitamin D in human milk is affected by the mother's intake of vitamin D (13) and, to a lesser extent, her exposure to sunlight. The most important source of vitamin D in the breast-fed infant comes with exposure of the infant to sunlight. Light-skinned infants probably need less than 1 hour per week of exposure of head, forearms, and hands to permit adequate synthesis of vitamin D (14). Dark-skinned infants require greater exposure to sunlight than light-skinned infants to provide for their vitamin D requirements.

The American Academy of Pediatrics (4) recommends that supplementation with fluoride in the breast-fed infant be initiated shortly after birth or at least by 6 months of age, since fluoride is not thought to pass into breast milk in significant amounts. If powdered or

TABLE 9-5 Guidelines for Vitamin-Mineral Supplementation in Healthy Full-Term Infants

Alimentation	A	C	D	E	Folic Acid	Iron	Fluoride
Human milk	−	−	±	−	−'	−	±
Commercial formula without iron	−	−	−	−	−	+	±
Commercial formula, iron-fortified	−	−	−	−	−	−	±
Cow milk, evaporated	±	+	±	−	−	+	±
Goat milk, evaporated	±	+	±	−	++	+	±

++ = Supplementation strongly recommended;
+ = supplementation recommended;
− = supplementation not recommended;
± = supplementation may be required.

concentrated commercial formulas are used, fluoride supplements should be administered only if the community water supply contains less than 0.3 µg/g of fluoride. Ready-to-use formulas contain little fluoride, so fluoride supplementation should begin shortly after birth. Recommendations for fluoride supplementation are included in Table 9-6.

Iron stores for the term infant may be depleted by 4 to 6 months of age. Infants fed breast milk or infant formula not fortified with iron should start to receive an iron supplement by 6 months of age. This may be in the form of iron-fortified infant cereal or iron sulfate drops. Current evidence suggests that the iron in infant cereals has a low bioavailability and is of limited use in meeting the iron requirements of infants (15).

Liquid multivitamin preparations are available with or without iron or fluoride for infants. Generally, they contain either vitamins A, C, and D, with or without iron or vitamins A, C, D, E, thiamin, riboflavin, niacin, and vitamin B_6 with or without iron. Folic acid is omitted from liquid dietary supplements because it is relatively unstable in liquid preparations. Preparations with fluoride are available only with a prescription.

THE LOW BIRTH WEIGHT INFANT

The normal, full-term infant is born between 37 and 42 weeks' gestation and weighs approximately 3,500 g (7.7 pounds). Infants weighing less than 2,500 g (5 1/2 pounds) are defined as *low birth weight* (LBW), those weighing less than 1,500 g (3 1/2 pounds), as *very low birth weight* (VLBW), and those weighing less than 1,000 g (2 1/4 pounds), as extremely low birth weight (16). Infants have low birth weights, most commonly, for one of two reasons. Either they may be born before 37 weeks' gestation, in which case they are *premature,* or they may exhibit a retarded rate of intrauterine growth, which makes them *small for gestational age* (SGA).

Because LBW infants may have a variety of clinical problems in the postnatal period, their management frequently involves care in tertiary-care hospitals with neonatal intensive care units (NICUs). Recent advances in neonatology are increasing the survival rate of LBW infants, although those born before 23 weeks' gestation still rarely survive. This increase in survival rate has resulted in a great interest in providing optimal nutritional support for these infants and, consequently, in an increased use of the nutritional care specialist. Skills required of the nutrition care specialist as a member of a NICU nutrition support team include: screening for various nutrition problems, development and implementation of a nutrition care plan, and monitoring and assessment of the nutrition care plan.

Premature infants are born with small metabolic reserves that make them particularly vulnerable to interruption of the influx of water, energy, and nutrients that occurs at birth. At the same time, immature development of the respiratory, cardiovascular, and gastrointestinal systems results in a wide range of medical problems that pose challenges for the delivery of fluids and nutrients to the infant. Enteral tube feeding, parenteral nutrition, or a combination of enteral and parenteral feeding are frequently necessary (see Chapters 13 and 14). Parenteral feedings are usually needed in infants weighing less than 1,600 g. When the infant gains weight and the gastrointestinal tract develops more fully, enteral feedings can begin, although a gradual transition from parenteral to enteral feeding is needed. A detailed discussion of parenteral nutrition in pediatrics is provided by Kerner (17), and information on protocols for enteral feeding of premature infants is provided by O'Leary (16).

Nutritional requirements and optimal growth for the LBW infant are poorly understood and are the subject of current research. One commonly used approach is to estimate nutritional requirements based on the goal of having the LBW infant continue a rate of growth similar to that which would have occurred in utero. The goal of mimicking growth in utero has been criticized based on differences in the intrauterine and extrauterine environment. For example, delivery of nutrients by the placenta is very different than administration via the enteral or

TABLE 9-6 Recommended Daily Fluoride Supplementation (mg/day) as Influenced by Fluoride Concentration in the Drinking Water

Fluoride concentration in drinking water (µg/g)	Age		
	2 weeks–2 years	2–3 years	3–16 years
<0.3	0.25	0.50	1.00
0.3–0.7	0	0.25	0.50
>0.7	0	0	0

Adapted from Committee on Nutrition, American Academy of Pediatrics. Fluorid supplementation 77:(1986) 758.

parenteral route and, whereas glucose is the primary nutrient for the fetus, fat usually provides approximately 50 percent of the energy in human milk or infant formulas. During the last 10 weeks of gestation, infant weight doubles, length increases by 25 percent, and two-thirds of the mineral deposition in the fetal skeleton occurs (4).

Energy, Protein, and Mineral Needs

The energy, protein, and mineral needs of premature infants are higher than those of full-term infants, although the exact amounts needed are still being defined. A greater proportion of the total nutrient intake of premature infants is needed for synthesis of new tissue to support a more rapid growth rate. In addition, low nutrient stores due to shortened gestation, decreased retention and utilization of nutrients related to physiological and metabolic limitations, and increased needs associated with stress, illness, and use of certain medications all contribute to greater nutrient needs in the premature infant.

The enterally fed preterm infant is estimated to require 120–130 kcal/kg/day to provide adequate energy for growth and 75 kcal/kg/day to meet maintenance energy needs as summarized in Table 9-7 (18). Greater heat losses due to a lack of insulating subcutaneous fat and a large body surface area relative to mass contribute to greater energy expenditure in preterm than in full-term infants. The energy needs of premature infants receiving parenteral nutrition are less than those of preterm infants who are enterally fed, because absorptive or fecal losses do not occur when nutritional intake bypasses the gastrointestinal tract. Premature neonates demonstrate adequate growth with parenteral energy intakes of 70 to 90 kcal/kg/day (19). In estimating the energy needs of individual infants, it is important to monitor the infants' growth process and to *individualize* energy intake to match the growth rate. The range of energy needs of premature infants is 110 to 150 kcal/kg/day (4). Nutritional requirements for premature infants are summarized in Table 9-8.

In infants born after 26 weeks' gestation, protein digestion and absorption are generally adequate, although several enzymes of amino acid metabolism are immature, resulting in possible essentiality of the amino acids cysteine, tyrosine, and taurine. For cysteine and taurine, low hepatic cystathionase activity may result in inadequate conversion of methionine to cysteine, and since taurine is formed from cysteine, it may also be conditionally essential for the premature infant. The protein requirements of preterm infants is a controversial subject because of basic questions about optimal postnatal growth and changes in tissue composition. The advisable protein intake for enterally fed infants is 3.5 to 4 g/kg/day, and for parenterally fed infants, it is 2 to 2.5 g/kg/day (4, 16). Whey-predominant proteins are tolerated better than casein-based proteins, as suggested by less frequent metabolic acidosis and more normal plasma amino acid patterns. Current amino acid solutions for

TABLE 9-7 Estimated Energy Requirementws for Growth of a Premature Infant

	kcal/kg/day
Resting energy expenditure	50
Growth	25
Activity	15
Fecal loses	12
Cold stress	10
Diet-induaced thermogenesis	8
Total	120

Adapted from American Academy of Pediatrics, Committee on Nutrition. Nutritional needs of low-birth-weight infants. *Pediatr.* 75:(1985) 976–86.

parenteral nutrition in preterm infants are not considered to provide optimal amounts of amino acids, and efforts are being made to develop new solutions.

Increased intakes of calcium, phosphorus, and vitamin D are required for optimal bone mineralization in growing premature infants. During the final weeks of gestation the fetus accumulates 120 to 160 mg calcium/kg/day and about 75 mg phosphorus/kg/day; the premature infant is deprived of this intrauterine mineralization (17). Inadequate dietary intakes can result in osteopenia or "rickets of prematurity." This disorder appears to be caused by a deficiency of calcium and phosphorus rather than by a defect in vitamin D metabolism (17). Premature infants with bronchopulmonary dysplasia and those fed unsupplemented human milk have a high incidence of osteopenia. Human milk does not contain sufficient quantities of calcium and phosphorus to meet the needs of preterm infants. Low mineral intakes due to parenteral nutrition and high urinary mineral losses secondary to furosemide diuretic therapy contribute to osteopenia in infants with bronchopulmonary dysplasia. For preterm infants, recommended enteral intakes of calcium are 120 to 230 mg/kg/day; of phosphorus, 60 to 140 mg/kg/day; and of vitamin D, 400 to 600 IU per day until the infant reaches a postnatal weight of 2 to 2.5 kg (4, 20). This assumes an average calcium retention of 64 percent and a phosphorus retention of 71 percent (20). Addition of sufficient amounts of calcium and phosphorus to parenteral nutrition solutions for preterm infants has been difficult because of precipitation of the minerals. Special precautions in the formulation of preterm parenteral nutrition solutions have shown that up to 120 mg calcium/kg/day and 55 mg phosphorus/kg/day can be administered parenterally.

Preterm infants are especially susceptible to iron deficiency because they have reduced iron stores associated with preterm birth. The iron intake currently recommended for preterm infants is 2 mg/kg/day, twice that recommended for full-term infants. Certain types of premature infant formulas may contain adequate levels of iron (see Table H-2). Iron supplements of 2 mg/kg/day are recommended starting as early as 2 weeks of age or

TABLE 9.8   Summary of Nutritional Recommendations for Preterm Infants

Nutrient	Recommendation	Nutritional consideration
Energy	Enteral: 120–130 kcal/kg/day 75 kcal/kg/day maintenance Parenteral: 70–90- kcal/kg/day growth 50–60 kcal/kg/day maintenance	LBW formulas providing 24 kcal/oz are recommended for infants weighing <2 kg
Protein	Enteral: 3.5–4 g/kg/day; 7–16% energy from protein Parenteral: 2–2.5 g/kg/day	Whey-based enteral formulas (60:40 whey: casein ratio) are recommended; cysteine, taurine and tyrosine may be essential
Carbohydrate	Enteral formulas providing a mixture of lactose and either glucose polymers or sucrose are preferred	Lactase activity is not usually fully developed until the end of a full-term gestation
Fat	30–55% of enteral kcal as fat with 4–12% of total kcal as linoleic acid and 1–2% of total kcal as linolenic acid	LBW formulas providing unsaturated vegetable oils plus MCT are well absorbed; human milk fat is also well absorbed
Minerals (enteral) Calcium	120–230 mg/kg/day 3.0–5.63 mmol/kg/day	Ca: P ratio by weight of ~2:1 is recommended
Phosphorus	60–140 mg/kg/day 1.94–4.52 mmol/kg/day	LBW formulas provide adequate amounts of minerals whereas human milk provides inadequate amounts of Ca and P
Iron	2 mg/kg/day starting at 2 weeks to 2 months, or at 2 kg body weight	Preterm infants are susceptible to iron deficiency because of low iron stores. LBW formulas are available with or without iron
Vitamins (enteral) Vitamin D Vitamin E Vitamin C Folic Acid	400–600 IU per day 5–25 IU per day 35 mg per day 50 µg per day	

Adapted from American Academy of Pediatrics. Committee on Nutrition. W.W.K Koo, & R.C. Tsang, Nutritional needs of low birth-weight infants. *Pediatr* 75: (1985) 976–86. Calcium, magnesium, and phosphorus. In R.C. Tsang, A. Lucas, R. Uauy, and S. Zlotkin, (eds) *Nutritional Needs of the Preterm Infant,* Baltimore: Williams & Wilkins, 1993. 148–150; and M.J. O'Leary, and J. Zerzan Nourishing the premature and low birth-weight infant. In P.L. Pipes, (ed) *Nutrition in Infancy and Childhood,* 5th ed. St. Louis: Times Mirror/Mosby, (1993) 309–333.

at least by 2 months of age when body weight usually doubles or reaches 2 kg (4).

Methods of Enteral Feeding

Most infants of less than 32 to 34 weeks' gestational age have poor coordination of sucking, swallowing, and respiration, and immature development of the gastrointestinal and respiratory systems. Both these factors result in the preterm infant's frequently being unable to nipple feed until at least 34 weeks gestational age. Enteral tube feeding of the premature infant reduces energy expenditure compared to nipple feeding. Continuous orogastric tube feeding is usually used in LBW infants who are unable to suck because most newborns are obligate nose breathers, and orogastric feeding interferes less with breathing than does nasogastric feeding. Continuous, rather than bolus or intermittent, tube feeding is preferred because gastric capacity is very small in these infants. Transpyloric feeding such as orojejunal feeding is now rarely used to feed LBW infants because of problems with decreased fat absorption and intestinal perforation.

The formulas available for feeding LBW infants include standard infant formulas, human milk from the infant's mother (preterm human milk or PTHM), or special formulas designed for LBW or preterm infants. The previous section on infant formulas reviews the general characteristics of these formulas, and Appendix H summarizes their nutrient profiles. Standard infant formulas may be used for LBW infants who weigh at least 2 kg, while PTHM or special LBW formulas should be used for infants weighing less than 2 kg. PTHM has several advantages compared with mature human milk, which is not recommended for a preterm infant (4). PTHM has a similar calorie content as mature human milk but contains more protein, sodium, chloride, magnesium, and iron (21). Even so, PTHM does not contain adequate amounts of protein, calcium, and phosphorus for the rapidly growing premature infant, and fortification of PTHM as discussed under the infant formula section is recommended. The specialized LBW formulas contain adequate amounts of nutrients for the preterm infant but do not provide the immunological protection available from fresh PTHM. Choice of an optimal feeding for an LBW infant is complicated by the fact that no ideal feeding is known (16).

Assessment of Growth

All neonates lose weight after birth because of losses of extracellular fluid. Growth in the preterm infant usually begins by the second week after birth once the infant has stabilized and adjusted to enteral or parenteral feeding. When full nutrient intake is possible, many preterm infants will gain 20 to 30 g per day. Specialized growth charts (22) may be used initially to assess weight gain in the infant born prematurely. The growth charts for full-term infants from birth to 3 years of age from the National Center for Health Statistics, as discussed later in this chapter, can also be used for preterm infants after 40 weeks' gestation if age is corrected or adjusted for prematurity. For example, at 3 months postnatal age, the growth parameters of a premature infant born at 32 weeks of gestation can be compared with those of a 1-month baby born at term (16). Premature infants often catch up to the growth of full-term babies by 2 years of age.

THE PRESCHOOL CHILD

The growth rate slows after the first year of life, resulting in both a decrease in nutrient requirements per unit of body weight and a decrease in appetite. Irregular weight gain is not unusual for the preschool child. Average growth for the group is 12 cm during the second year, 8 to 9 cm during the third year, and 7 cm per year thereafter. The average weight gain during those years is 2 to 2 1/2 kg per year.

During these years, children learn to walk and speak; they also develop the fine motor skills which allow them to learn to feed themselves. Children learn to feed themselves independently between 1 and 2 years of age. Messiness is common between 10 and 18 months, but by 2 years of age most children spill very little.

Feeding the preschool child can be frustrating. At this age, food jags and rituals are common, as are strong food preferences and dislikes and, at times, an apparent lack of interest in eating. It is important to realize that a decrease in appetite is expected during these years because of the decreased growth rate; in addition, many of the food behaviors common in this age group are related to the child's developing sense of independence. Children should not be forced to eat, nor should food be used as a reward. The development of good eating patterns in a child should allow the child to stop eating whenever satiety is reached.

It is important to be familiar with the appropriate portion sizes for the preschool child (see Table 9-9). In general it is better to offer a child less to eat, and thus to allow for success, than to overwhelm the child with large portions. In general children will self-regulate their food intake. Most children in the age group eat five to six small meals per day.

Several generalizations can be made about the food preferences of the preschool child. Fibrous meats are not well accepted because rotary chewing motion is not well established until 2 1/2 years of age. Before this age, fish, chicken, ground meats, and cheese are usually preferred. Single foods are more popular than combination dishes. Finger foods are especially popular because children are interested in the texture of food. Color and variety are also important. Raw vegetables are often more popular than cooked ones. Dry foods are usually hard for a preschool child to swallow and should be combined with moister food. A final consideration is the ease with which a food can be manipulated. For example, soup or peas might not be good choices for a 2-year-old child. Warm, rather than hot, foods are usually preferred.

THE SCHOOL- AGE CHILD

Growth of the school-age child tends to be more stable, and there are generally fewer apparent feeding problems compared with the preschool child. Height usually increases by 5 to 6 cm each year, and the average weight increase is 2 kg each year for the first 2 to 3 years and 4.0 to 4.5 kg per year as the child approaches puberty. School-age children usually eat four to five times per day on school days and generally eat after-school snacks which they prepare themselves.

THE ADOLESCENT

After a slow rate of growth during the childhood years, adolescence is characterized by an increase in the velocity of physical growth similar to that seen during infancy. Up to the age of approximately 9 years, males and females grow in height and weight at about the same rate. The growth spurt preceding puberty, or the initial ability to reproduce, begins between 10 and 12 years of age in girls and about 2 years later in boys. The ages at which average peak growth velocity is achieved in males is 14.1 years for height and 14.3 years for weight (23). In females, average peak velocities of height and weight increases are observed at 12.1 and 12.9 years, respectively (23). Menarche occurs at the end of the growth spurt, approximately 9 to 12 months after peak height velocity is attained.

TABLE 9-9 Dietary Evaluation Guidelines for Children 1–15 Years Old

Food Group	Recommended Number of Servings per Day	Average Size of Servings					
		1 yr. (1.000 kcal/day)	2–3 yr (1,300 kcal/day)	4–5 yr (1,700 kcal/day)	6–9 yr. (2,100 kcal/day)	10–12 yr. (2,500 kcal/day)	13–15 yr. (2.600–3,000 kcal/day)
Milk and Cheese	4						
Milk		1/2 c	1/2–3/4 c	1/2–3/4 c	3/4–1 c	1 c	1 c
Cheese		3/4 oz	3/4–1 1/8 oz	3/4–1 1/8 oz	3/4–1 1/2 oz	1 1/2 oz	1 1/2 c
Ice Cream		3/4 c	3/4–1 1/8 c	3/4—1 1/8 c	3/4–1 1/2 c	1 1/2 c	1 1/2 c
Yogurt		1/2 c	1/2–3/4 c	1/2–3/4 c	3/4–1 c	1 c	1 c
Meat and meat alternatives	2 or 3						
Egg		1	1	1	1	1	1 or more
Meat, poultry, fish		2 T	2 T	4 T (2 oz)	2–3 oz	3–4 oz	4–5 oz
Peanut butter		—	1 T	2 T	2–3 T	3 T	3 T
Dried beans, peas		4 T	4 T	1/2 c	3/4 c	1 c	1–1 1/2 c
Fruits and vegetables	4						
Vitamin C sources (citrus fruits, berries, tomatoes, etc)	1	4 T (1/4 c)	8 T (1/2 c)	1/2 c	1 c	1 c	1 c
Vitamin A sources (e.g., green or yellow fruits and vegetables)	1	2 T	3 T	1/4 c	1/4 c	1/4 c	1/2 c
Others	2	2 T	3 T	1/2 c	1/2 c	1/2 c	3/4 c
Bread and cereals	4						
Bread		1/2 slice	1 slice	1–1 1/2 slices	1 or 2 slices	2 slices	2 slices
Cold cereal		1/2 c	3/4 c	1 c	1 c	1–1 1/2c	1–1 1/2 c
Cooked cereal or pasta		4 T	5 T (1/3 c)	1/2 c	1/2 c	3/4 c	1 c or more
Fats and carbohydrates	to meet caloric needs						
Butter, margarine, mayonnaise, or oil (100 kcal/T)		1 T	1 T	1 T	2 T	2 T	2–4 T

Reproduced with permission from *Manual of Pediatric Nutrition*, D.G. Kelts and E.G. Jones, eds. Boston: Little, Brown. 1984

Nutrient requirements in the adolescent population parallel the growth rate, with the greatest need occurring at the peak velocity of growth. The RDAs for energy in the adolescent population are expressed as ranges of kcals for two age periods—11 to 14 years and 15 to 18 years of age. Ranges are used because the individual rate of growth is quite variable during adolescence. Most of the allowances for nutrients are extrapolations from data on young children and adults, and are therefore only estimates of nutritional needs. Rate of growth, as determined by rate of increase in height, and activity level are key factors in estimating energy needs for adolescents.

There are several general nutritional concerns in the adolescent population. Eating patterns tend to be erratic, with frequent skipping of meals, adherence to various fad weight-reduction diets, snacking, and reliance on "fast foods." Nutrients that are frequently limiting in the diet include zinc, iron, and vitamins A, D, B_6, and folate (24). Many females become preoccupied with slimness during the adolescent years, resulting in marginally adequate dietary intakes and a high incidence of eating disorders such as bulimia and anorexia nervosa (25). Pregnancy in adolescence is also of nutritional relevance, as discussed in Chapter 8.

NUTRITIONAL ASSESSMENT

Nutritional assessment for the pediatric population, as for adults, includes an evaluation of pertinent dietary, biochemical, and anthropometric data. Evaluation of the progress of physical growth is a unique and powerful additional tool for the assessment of nutritional status in children.

DIETARY

Evaluation of the adequacy of dietary intake in the pediatric population requires a knowledge of nutritional requirements, normal feeding patterns, including appropriate portion sizes, and normal development of feeding skills. Tables 9-1, 9-2, and 9-3 provide a summary of information needed to evaluate the diet of an infant, and Table 9-9 provides a summary of information relevant to assessing dietary intake in the older child.

Children's dietary intake of fat and cholesterol is currently of great interest as evidence suggests that the origin of atherosclerosis in genetically predisposed individuals is in childhood (26). The population approach to the prevention of cardiovascular disease suggests that all children over 2 years of age should consume a low-cholesterol, low-saturated fat or Step 1 diet (26). Many pediatricians and nutritionists disagree with this universal recommendation because of insufficient evidence demonstrating that such diets provide adequate energy and essential nutrients for normal growth and development (27). However, the American Academy of Pediatrics has recently endorsed use of the Step 1 diet for all children over 2 years of age (28). The Step 1 diet includes an average daily intake of 30 percent of total calories from fat, less than 10 percent of total calories from saturated fat, and less than 300 mg of cholesterol per day (26). United States Department of Agriculture food consumption surveys indicate that children ages 1-19 years consume 14 percent of total calories from saturated fatty acids, 35-36 percent of total calories from fat and 233 to 305 mg of cholesterol per day (28).

BIOCHEMICAL

Determination of various biochemical parameters is a useful part of nutritional status assessment in the pediatric population. The procedures and calculations necessary to assess these parameters are similar for children and adults, and are discussed in detail in Chapter 4. Normal laboratory values for both children and adults can be found in Appendix Tables E-3 and E-4, and also in Appendix F.

The calculation of nitrogen balance differs slightly in children compared to the method used for adults (24). Instead of a value of 4 g to account for nonurinary nitrogen losses, a value of 1.2 g is more appropriate for children. The adjusted equation is

$$\Delta N \text{ (g/day)} = \frac{\text{protein intake}}{6.25} - (\text{UUN} + 1.2) \quad \textbf{(9-1)}$$

where UUN is urinary urea nitrogen and all values are given in g. Total urinary nitrogen excretion is more accurate than UUN and should be used if available.

Normal children are in positive nitrogen balance which reflects growth. Values for ranges of nitrogen balance in healthy children include (29):

0–4 months	+180 to +90 mg N/kg body weight
4–17 months	+90 mg N/kg body weight
17 months–3 years	+70 mg N/kg body weight
3–7 years	+40 mg N/kg body weight

Cholesterol testing is currently recommended by the American Academy of Pediatrics (30) and the National Institutes of Health (26) for children over age 2 who are at risk for the development of atherosclerosis. Children should have blood cholesterol screening if their parents or grandparents have been diagnosed as having cardiovascular disease or have experienced a cardiac event before age 55, or if one or both parents have serum cholesterol levels over 240 mg/dL. Dietary treatment is recommended for children with borderline low-density lipoprotein (LDL), cholesterol levels of 110 to 129 mg/dL, and drug therapy is recommended for children over 10 years of age who have serum cholesterol levels over 200 mg/dL or LDL cholesterol levels over 130 mg/dL that do not respond to diet (26). (see

Table 9-10.) Diet and cardiovascular disease is discussed further in Chapter 20.

EVALUATION OF GROWTH

Growth standards for height (or length), weight, and head circumference make it possible to evaluate a child's growth. Evaluation of growth using *growth charts* is considered the most useful nutritional assessment tool for children. If the growth chart indicates that growth is not proceeding normally, additional assessment methods, such as measurement of skinfold thickness and determination of bone age, may be useful. Determinations of skinfold thickness and arm circumference provide a basis for assessing adiposity, as discussed in Chapter 5. Standards for bone age permit an estimate of a child's physiologic maturity.

Growth Charts

Growth charts have been constructed from repeated measurements of height and weight obtained from large-scale studies of healthy children from a cross section of ethnic and economic backgrounds. The height and weight measurements are ranked in percentiles based on a scale of 100. For example, if a child is at the 30th percentile for height, 70 percent of children of the same age and sex are taller, and 29 percent are shorter. At a specific age, 95 percent of the population of children, or the mean ± 2 standard deviations, are between the 2.5th and 97.5th percentile. The most commonly used growth charts are those provided by the National Center for Health Statistics (NCHS) (31).

NCHS growth charts for the pediatric population appear in Appendix I. Separate grids are available for boys and girls from birth to 36 months of age. These growth charts allow both determination of age-specific percentiles for length, weight, and head circumference and evaluation of weight for length. The NCHS growth charts include data on head circumference only from birth to 36 months of age. Head circumference in children over 36 months of age can be evaluated using graphs prepared by Nellhaus (32). For children aged 2 to 18 years, NCHS graphs are available to evaluate height and weight and weight for stature.

Measurement Techniques. Weight values for the child of less than 36 months of age should be obtained while the child is nude, using calibrated beam-balance scales. Stature is measured as recumbent length, not height, when using the birth-to-36-month chart. Recumbent length can be determined using a wooden length board. The charts for children between 2 and 18 years of age use measurements of children in stocking feet and standard clothing worn during examination. Weight is recorded to the nearest 0.1 kg or 1.0 oz and length to the nearest 0.5 cm or 0.125 in.

Interpretation. When undernutrition exists, gain in weight is affected earlier and to a greater degree than gain in height. If malnutrition persists, height will eventually be retarded or halted and/or pubertal maturation and epiphyseal closure will be delayed. In general, weight gain is decreased when energy intake is deficient, while linear growth is more delayed when protein intake is inadequate. Over nutrition usually results in taller, heavier, more physically mature children.

Growth charts are used to evaluate growth in height and weight by determination of either single or repeated measurements. Plotting of height and weight for a child at a *single age* gives information of the relationship of weight to height compared with other children of the same age and sex. Alternatively, *repeated* measurements of height and weight plotted on a growth grid at different ages in the same child allow determination of the pattern of growth in comparison with that of healthy children. An evaluation of weight without comparison to length has little meaning other than in a statistical sense.

Single measurements. Single measurements of weight and height can be interpreted in two ways: (1) height, and (2) weight for length or height. These approaches give the same information—that is, weight relative to height—but use different growth charts.

We will use an example of a single measurement of height and weight in one child to illustrate how these data can be interpreted in each of the two ways just described. Consider a boy who is 24 months old and weighs 25 pounds, 8 ounces and measures 34.5 inches in length. Fig. 9-1 demonstrates that the child is at the 25th percentile for weight and at the 50th percentile for length

---

TABLE 9-10   Treatment Recommendations Based on Cholesterol Testing in High-Risk Children Over Age 2*

Category	Total Cholesterol		Low-Density Lipoprotein (LDL) Cholesterol		Recommended Treatment
	(mmol/L)	(mg/dL)	(mmol/L)	(mg/dL)	
Acceptable	<4.4	<170	<2.8	<110	None
Borderline	4.4–5.1	170–199	2.8–3.3	110–129	Step 1 diet
High	≥5.2	≥200	≥3.4	≥130	Step 1, then Step 2 diet; drug therapy if not responsive to diet

Adapted from The National Cholesterol Education Program, Report of the Expert Panel on Blood Cholesterol Levels in Children and Adolescents, Bethesda, MD, 1991, National Heartt, Lung and Blood Institute.
* Values are for serum; plasma values × 1.03 = serum value.

and that the child is at approximately the 25th percentile *weight for length*.(see Appendix I.) We can interpret these single measurements using the two methods as follows:

1. Compared to children his age, the child's weight at the 25th percentile does not correlate with the weight of other children who are his length. In other words, 50th percentile for weight and 50th percentile for length are the usual values observed. This suggests that calorie intake may be low or that the child is genetically leaner in comparison to his height than the majority of children his age. If the child is healthy and eating an adequate diet, it probably indicates normal growth.

2. A 25th percentile *weight for length* indicates the same information as the weight-for-height method but uses a different growth chart. Measurements that fall within the 50th percentile of weight for length indicate median weight for height. Values over the 50 percentile suggest above-average weight for stature and values under the 50th percentile suggest below-average weight for stature.

Since both methods actually give the same information, you may choose to use the growth chart you find easiest to work with. However, it is important to understand the terminology used in each approach.

An evaluation of *weight for stature* in adolescents (males taller than 145 cm and females taller than 138 cm) using growth charts is not useful because of individual variation in the rate of maturation. If single measurements are used in adolescents, it is most useful to evaluate body weight and height by comparison with age-specific height and weight values.

Repeated measurements. If possible, it is generally better to evaluate growth by plotting repeated measures of height, weight, and head circumference on an appropriate growth chart. This allows one to visualize how a child's growth is proceeding and also highlights certain growth patterns. In evaluating growth curves, it should be recognized that growth does not always proceed in a smooth curve, as the charts depict. In general, however, children will grow along approximately the same percentile track and, if there is a substantial change in the percentile of growth, nutritional or clinical factors need to be further evaluated.

For example, consider the pattern of growth shown in Figure 9-1, for child A. The child is near the 75th percentile for both length and weight at birth. Weight drops to the 50th percentile by 3 months of age and continues along the 50th percentile until about 9 months of age, when the rate of weight gain again falls off. By 24 months of age, weight has dropped to the 25th percentile. Length also drops from the 75th percentile from birth but lags behind the drop in weight percentile. By 24 months, length is at the 50th percentile. One would project that this child would normally grow along a curve between the 75th and 50th percentiles for both weight and length.

The drop in percentile growth may suggest interference with growth potential due to poor food intake secondary to irregular eating habits, which are particularly common in the second year of life, increased activity, a disease process, or any combination of these factors. A clinical evaluation if the child is symptomatic or a careful dietary evaluation if the child is asymptomatic will help clarify the nature of the growth pattern. In the asymptomatic child, this growth pattern is most likely to be a temporary result of poor eating habits, which will probably improve as the child ages.

As an example of a clearly abnormal growth curve, consider Fig. 9-1 for child B. Growth in weight and length practically ceases, or flattens, between 12 and 24 months of age. This type of curve indicates interference in growth potential due to a disease process or inadequate nutrition, or both. A child with this type of growth curve would need a careful clinical evaluation to rule out an underlying disease process. Children with conditions such as chronic renal failure commonly display growth patterns similar to the curve for child B.

During adolescence, growth patterns may change in percentiles due to differences in maturation rates. The early maturer may jump to a higher percentile, and the late maturer may be at a lower percentile at the same age point. Both patterns usually return to the original percentiles by the time growth is completed.

Head Circumference

Changes in head circumference reflect brain growth but are not a sensitive indicator of nutritional status. After 36 months of age, there is little relationship between nutrition and head circumference because maximum head circumference is usually attained by this age (32).

Bone Age

Bone, or skeletal, age can be determined by evaluation of the degree of fusion on the epiphyses using roentgenographic studies. Epiphyseal closure is a measure of how far the bones have progressed toward maturity. Once the epiphyses have closed, there is no further growth in height. Estimation of bone age, or degree of epiphyseal closure, allows for an estimation of the potential for catch-up growth in children with growth retardation. Bone age is generally retarded in any condition in which growth in height is slowed secondary to malnutrition, but the percent of retardation may be less for epiphyseal closure than for height. As an example, consider a 10-year-old child who is growth retarded and of a height comparable with that of a 6-year-old. The bone age would also most likely be retarded and fall somewhere between 6 and 10 years. Knowing the bone age would thus give an indication of how many years remained for promotion of "catch-up growth" before epiphyseal closure. Roentgenograms of the hand and wrist are generally used to assess epiphyseal closure, or bone age, in comparison to standards (33).

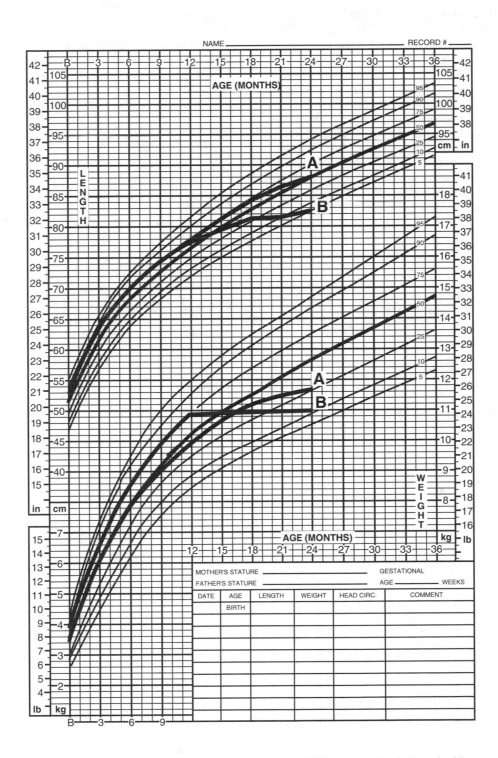

FIGURE 9-1   Boys: Birth to 36 months' physical growth, NCHS percentiles. (Adapted with permission from P.V.V. Hamill, T.A. Drizd, C.L. Johnson, R.B. Reed, A.F. Roche, and W.M. Moore. Physical growth: National Center for Health Statistics percentiles. *A. J. Clin. Nutr.* 32:(1979) 607–29. Data from the Fels Research Institute, Wright State University School of Medicine, Yellow Springs, OH.

TOPICS FOR FURTHER DISCUSSION

1. Discuss proper breast-feeding techniques, including positioning and latching on.
2. Assume that you are planning a class on infant feeding to be given to women who are in their last trimester of pregnancy. List the major topics you might include in your class and outline the major points you would discuss in relation to each topic.
3. Discuss the incidence, etiology, and treatment of bulimia and anorexia nervosa.
4. Visit a grocery store and observe the variety, cost, and content of the various baby foods. Outline how you would instruct mothers to prepare their own baby foods.
5. Compare the cost of the various forms of infant formulas.
6. Discuss the advantages and potential problems of human milk as the sole feeding for a premature infant.
7. Investigate the long-term prognosis for growth and development of premature infants.

REFERENCES

1. **Foman, S.J., L.J. Filer, T.A. Anderson, and E.E. Ziegler.** Recommendations for feeding normal infants. *Pediatrics* 63:(1979) 52–59.
2. **Jones, E.G.** Normal infant feeding. In D.G. Kelts and E.G. Jones, eds., *Manual of Pediatric Nutrition*, Boston: Little, Brown, 1985, 21–48.
3. **Fomon, S.J..** Reflections on infant feeding in the 1970s and 1980s. *Am. J. Clin. Nutr.* 46:(1987) 171–182.
4. Committee on Nutrition. *Pediatric Nutrition Handbook* 3d ed., Elk Grove Village, Ill.: American Academy of Pediatrics, 1993.
5. **Ryan, A.S., W.F., Pratt, J.L Wysong, G., Lewandowski, J.W McNally, and F.W. Krieger.** A comparison of breast-feeding data from the national surveys of family growth and the Ross laboratories mothers survey. *Am. J. Public Health* 81:(1991) 1049–52.
6. Committee on Nutrition, American Academy of Pediatrics. The use of whole cow's milk in infancy. *Pediatrics* 89:(1992) 1105–09.
7. **Kautter, D.A., T. Lilly, H.M. Solomon, and R.K. Lynt.** Clostridium botulinum spores in infant foods: a survey. *J. of Food Protection* 45:(1982) 1028–29.
8. Food and Drug Administration. Rules and regulations. Nutrient requirements for infant formulas. *Fed Regist.* 50:(1985) 45106-8 (21 CFR Part 107).
9. Committee on Nutrition, American Academy of Pediatrics. Commentary of breast feeding and infant formulas, including proposed standards for formulas. *Pediatrics* 57:(1976)278-285.
10. ———Soy-protein formulas: recommendations for use in infant feeding. *Pediatrics* 72:(1983) 359–63.
11. **Ziegler, E. and S.J. Fomon,** Potential renal solute load of infant formulas. *J. Nutr.* 119:(1989) 1785–88.
12. United States Department of Agriculture Food and Nutrition Service. Infant Formulas. Exempt Infant Formulas, and Medical Foods Eligible for Use in WIC. U.S. Government Printing Office. Sept. 1990.
13. **Specker, B.L., R.C. Tsang, and B.W. Hollis,** Effect of race and diet on human-milk vitamin D and 25-hydroxyvitamin D. *Am.J. Dis. Child* 139:(1985)1134–7.
14. **Fomon, S.J.** Breast-feeding and evolution. *J. Am. Dietet. Assoc.* 86:(1986) 317–18.
15. ———Bioavailability of supplemental iron in commercially prepared dry infant cereals. *J. Pediatr.* 110:(1987) 660–61.
16. **O'Leary, M.J. and J. Zerzan,** Nourishing the premature and low birth weight infant. In P.L. Pipes, (ed) *Nutrition in Infancy and Childhood*, 5th ed., St. Louis: Times Mirror/Mosby, 1993.
17. **Kerner, J. A.** In J.A. Kerner, (ed): *Manual of Pediatric Parenteral Nutrition.* New York: John Wiley & Sons, Inc., 1983.
18. American Academy of Pediatrics Committee on Nutrition. Nutritional needs of the low-birth-weight infants. *Pediatr.* 75:(1985) 976–86.
19. **Cashore W.J., J.R. Sedaghatian, and R.H. Usher.** Nutritional supplements with intravenously administered lipid, protein hydrolysate, and glucose in small premature infants. *Pediatr.* 56:(1975) 8–16.
20. **Koo, W.W.K. and R.C. Tsang.** Calcium, magnesium, phosphorus and vitamin D. (In): R.C. Tsang, (ed) *Nutritional Needs of the Preterm Infant.* Baltimore: Williams & Wilkins, 1993, 135–55.
21. **Lemons, J.A. , L. Moye, D. Hall, and M. Simmons.** Differences in the composition of preterm and term human milk during early lactation. *Pediat. Res.* 16:(1983) 113–17.
22. **Dancis, J., J.R. O'Connell, and L.E. Holt.** A grid for recording the age of premature infants. *J. Pediatr.* 33:(1948) 570–72.
23. **Tanner, J.M., R.H. Whitehouse, and M. Takaishi.** Standards from birth to maturity for height, weight, height velocity, and weight velocity: British children, 1965. *Arch. Dis. Childh.* 41:(1966) 454–71.
24. **Greger, J. L., M.M. Higgins, R.P. Abernathy, A. Kirksey, M.B. Delcorso, and P. Baligar.** Nutritional status of adolescent girls in regard to zinc, copper, and iron. *Am. J. Clin. Nutr.* 31:(1978) 269–75.
25. Position of the American Dietetic Association: Nutrition intervention in the treatment of anorexia nervosa, bulimia nervosa, and binge eating. J. Am. Dietet. Assoc. 94:(1994) 902-907.
26. Department of Health and Human Services, National Heart, Lung, and Blood Institute, *The National Cholesterol Education Program. Report of the Expert Panel on Blood Cholesterol Levels in Children and Adolescents.* Bethesda, MD: National Heart, Lung, and Blood Institute. 1991.
27. American Academy of Pediatrics. Committee on Nutrition. Prudent lifestyles for children—dietary fats and cholesterol. *Pediatr.* 78:(1986) 521–25.
28. American Academy of Pediatrics. Committee on Nutrition. Statement on Cholesterol. *Pediatr.* 90: (1992) 469–73
29. **Ney, D., C. Bay, J.-M. Saudubray, D.G. Kelts, S. Kulovich, L. Sweetman and W.L. Nyhan.** An evaluation of protein requirements in methylmalonic acidaemia. *J. Inher. Metab. Dis.* 8:(1985) 132–42.
30. American Academy of Pediatrics. Committee on Nutrition. Indications for cholesterol testing in children. *Pediatr.* 83: (1989) 141–42.
31. **Hamill, P.V.V., T.A. Drizd, C.L. Johnson, et. al.,**NCHS Growth Charts. 1976. Rockville, Md.: *Monthly Vital Statistics Report* (HBS) 25(3):(1976)76-1120 (Suppl.).
32. **Nellhaus, G.** Head circumference from birth to 18 years. *Pediatr.* 41:(1968)106–114.
33. **Greulich, W.W. and S.I. Pyle.** *Radiographic Atlas of Skeletal Development of the Hand and Wrist* 2d ed. Stanford: Stanford University Press, 1959.

Additional Sources of Information

Tsang, R.C. and B.L. Nichols. *Nutrition During Infancy*. Palo Alto, CA: Hanley and Belfus, Inc., 1988.

Satter, E. *Child of Mine: Feeding with Love and Good Sense*. Palo Alto, CA: Bull Publishing Co., 1988.

Behrman, R.E. (ed) *Nelson Textbook of Pediatrics*, 14th ed. Philadelphia: W.B. Saunders Co., 1992.

Suskind, R.M. and L. Lewinter-Suskind. *Textbook of Pediatric Nutrition* 2d ed.. New York: Raven Press, 1993.

Tsang, R.C., A. Lucas, R. Uauy, and S. Zlotkin (ed), *Nutritional Needs of the Preterm Infant*. Baltimore: Wiiliams & Wilkins, 1993.

Nettleton, J.A. Are n-3 fatty acids essential nutrients for fetal and infant development? *J Am. Dietet. Assoc.* 93:(1993) 58–64.

Lawrence, R.A. *Breastfeeding: A Guide for the Medical Profession*, 4th ed. St. Louis: Times Mirror/Mosby, 1994.

 ## TO TEST YOUR UNDERSTANDING

1. a. A new mother is concerned that her baby may not be receiving enough breast milk. What clues can you tell her to watch for?

b. Another new mother is concerned that her 2-day-old baby does not consume much of the 4-oz bottle of formula which the nurses on the obstetrics floor gave her at each feeding. How would you advise the mother?

2. Patty is exclusively breast-fed until 3 months of age. At this point her mother returns to work and weans Patty to Enfamil with iron formula. Approximately how many feedings of Enfamil will Patty require each day and how much formula will she consume at each feeding?

3. How would you respond to the following question from a young mother? "My baby is 2 months old, and I'm nursing him, but my mother tells me that I need to start giving him solids. The nurse who gave my baby his immunizations said not to start any solid food until the baby is 4 months old. Why should I wait to start solid foods for so long?"

4. Under what circumstances would vitamin D and fluoride supplementation be required for an infant given breast milk, evaporated milk formula, or iron-fortified full-term infant formula?

5. A list of snacks for infants ranging in age from 6 to 12 months follows. Circle those snacks that would not be a good choice for an infant and explain why these snacks should be avoided

Snack	Reason to Avoid
Cooked Egg white	
Popcorn	
Fruit juice in a bottle	
Fruit juice in a cup	
Raw celery and carrot sticks	
Hard candy	
Banana	
Toast with honey	
Yogurt	

6. Suggest appropriate specific infant formula(s) for the following situations.

Infant Description	Recommended Formula
Allergy to cow milk protein	
Infant has cystic fibrosis, which affects fat digestion and absorption	
Lactose intolerance without fat malabsorption	
Persistent diarrhea with tolerance to fat but intolerance to intact protein-containing formulas	
Normal full-term infant	

7. Compare the energy, protein, and fluid requirements for a term (3.5 kg) infant and an LBW (1.8 kg) infant. How much of the formulas listed below would the LBW infant (1.8 kg) have to consume to meet her protein needs?

	mL/day
Mature human milk	
Enfamil	
Enfamil Premature 24	

8. Why do formulas for LBW infants contain more energy, protein, and calcium per unit volume than do formulas for full-term infants?

9. The following nutritional assessment data is obtained from a 5-year-old girl who has a history of multiple allergies, chronic emesis, and diarrhea:

At birth:	Weight	3.6 kg
	Length	51.0 cm
	Head circumference	34.5 cm
At 5 years:	Weight	15.0 kg
	Length	105.0 cm
	Head circumference	50.0 cm
	MAC	15.7 cm
	TSF	7.0 mm
	Average daily protein intake	35.0 g
	24-hr urine volume	700.0 mL
	Urine total N	0.61 g/dL

continued

TO TEST YOUR UNDERSTANDING *(continued)*

a. What are the patient's percentiles for age at birth and at 5 years for the following parameters?

	Birth	5 years
Weight	—————	—————
Length/height	—————	—————
Head circumference	—————	—————
Weight for length	—————	—————

Provide an interpretation of the child's growth pattern.

b. Determine the percentile for TSF _____

Calculate MAMA _____cm² and percentile for MAMA _____

c. Calculate N balance (mg N/kg) using Equation 9-1.

_____mg N/kg

d. Discuss how the information in parts *b* and *c* of this question relates to the parameters of growth that were evaluated in part *a*.

e. Assume that the child is referred to you for dietary counseling for a milk-free, wheat-free diet. Her usual dietary intake is as follows: 6 oz Isomil formula, 1 egg, 1 c rice, 3 oz meat, 1 c juice, 1/2 c vegetables, and one 3.5 oz bag of corn chips. Write a SOAP note summarizing her nutritional status and your recommendations for energy and protein intake.

Infant Nutrition

Mrs. Johnson has been feeding Enfamil formula to 12-month-old Jack since the age of three months. Prior to then he was breastfed. Jack's growth record is shown below:

	Height	Weight
Birth	21.5 in	9 # 2 oz
3 months	25.5 in	16 # 0 oz
12 months	32.0 in	27 # 0 oz

Numzit, for teething pain, is the only medication he receives. The food record for a typical daily intake is shown below. A computerized nutritional analysis of this food record is shown on the next page.

Breakfast	Lunch	Dinner
6 oz oatmeal prep with whole milk	1 jar jr chicken/ veg dinner	1 jar jr Macaroni/ tomato/ beef dinner
1 jar jr bananas with tapioca	1 jar jr peaches	1 jar jr carrots
8 oz Enfamil	8 oz Enfamil	1 jar Dutch apple dessert
		8 oz Enfamil

Snacks
8 oz. Enfamil in a bottle at bedtime
8 oz. fruit punch in a bottle at naptime
6 Ritz crackers

Refer to the above case study to answer the following questions.

1. Comment on the following aspects of Jack's diet:
   a. amount and type of formula consumed
   b. age appropriateness of the foods and feeding methods
   c. bedtime bottles
   d. choking risk

2. Mrs. Johnson plans to stop using infant formula and start using cow milk. Discuss the appropriateness of this action and indicate the possible problems of changing to whole cow milk? Skim milk?

3. Assess Jack's growth data with respect to weight for length, weight percentile, and length percentile. What can be said about his weight and length in relation to other children of his age? Does he demonstrate a case of failure to thrive? Explain your answer.

4. Calculate Jack's total fluid intake and renal solute load. Is his fluid intake acceptable assuming normal renal function? Explain your answer.

5. Compare Jack's protein and energy intake with the 1989 RDAs. Discuss any needed changes in his diet.

6. Discuss Jack's need for nutritional supplement(s)? How does this differ from his need for supplementation when he was breastfed?

(continued)

Jack Johnson

- 6 oz oatmeal prep w/whole milk
- 1 ea jr bananas w/tapioca
- 1 ea jr chix/veg/ dinner
- 1 ea jr peaches
- 1 ea jr tomato/mac/beef dinner
- 1 ea jr carrots
- 1 ea jr Dutch apple dessert
- 6 ea Ritz crackers
- 8 oz fruit punch
- 32 oz Enfamil formula

Weight	2,356 g	*Water Weight*	2159 g
Calories	1,634	Vitamin B_6	1.09 mg
Protein	33.6 g	Vitamin B_{12}	2.31 µg
Carbohydrates	268.0 g	Folacin	168.0 µg
Dietary fiber	6.42 g	Pantothenic Acid	4.62 mg
Fat, total	54 g	Vitamin C	293 mg
Fat, saturated	2.56 g	Vitamin E	19.2 mg
Fat, mono	2.4 g	Calcium	727 mg
Fat, poly	0.581g	Copper	1.15 mg
Cholesterol	1.4 mg	Iron	9.59 mg
Vitamin A-carotene	2.27 RE	Magnesium	170 mg
Vitamin A-preformed	0 RE	Phosphorus	639 mg
Vitamin A-total	3,595 RE	Potassium	2164 mg
Thiamin	1.18 mg	Selenium	1.53 µg
Riboflavin	1.67 mg	Sodium	608 mg
Niacin	18.1 mg	Zinc	8.53 mg

Calories from protein:	8%	Poly/Sat 0.2:1	
Calories from carbohydrate:	63 %	Sod/Pot 0.3:1	
Calories from fats:	29%	Ca/Phos 1.1:1	

(Food Processor II computer program analysis)

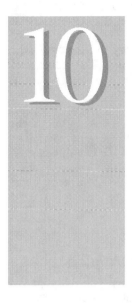

10 Nutritional Care of the Vegetarian Patient

The number of people who adhere to some form of vegetarian diet has grown in recent years. Vegetarians now number about 7 million in the United States. In addition to their increased numbers, their motivations and the types of vegetarian diets they follow are more varied. A person may become a vegetarian because of religion. Seventh-Day Adventists and adherents to various Eastern religions and philosophical groups follow vegetarian diets; others become vegetarians because of opposition to killing animals or concern about the purity of the food supply and a desire to maintain and improve health. In many parts of the world, populations are wholly or partially vegetarian because of poverty and unavailability of animal foods. In the more prosperous, developed countries, this is less often the case. Instead, people *choose* to be vegetarians. In this country the cost of a vegetarian diet is not markedly different from the cost of a diet containing meat.

Vegetarians are widely distributed geographically; it is highly probable, therefore, that you will have opportunities to provide nutritional care to vegetarians. It is thus important to understand the types of vegetarian diets and their advantages and disadvantages, and to be skilled in planning diets for, and counseling, these patients.

TYPES OF VEGETARIANS

Vegetarians are often classified according to either the extent of restriction of meat products in their diets or, conversely, the types of meat products they are willing to eat. A person whose diet includes plant foods and all categories of animal foods is an *omnivore*. However, most, if not all, societies refuse to eat some animal foods. In the United States and Canada, for example, insects, dogs,

cats, and horses are generally not considered acceptable food, although these are prized in some societies. *Partial vegetarians*, or semivegetarians, avoid some animal foods but not others. For example, some avoid red meats only. The *pollovegetarian* will eat poultry in addition to plant foods, while the *pescovegetarian* eats fish plus plant foods. *Lacto-ovo-vegetarians* accept milk, milk products, and eggs; more restricted versions are *lactovegetarians* (milk and milk products, but no eggs or meat) and *ovo-vegetarians* (eggs, but no milk or milk products or meat.) The *total*, *pure*, or *strict vegetarian*, or *vegan*, will not accept any animal products, but eats only plant foods. The *fruitarian*, who eats a diet largely composed of fruits, nuts, honey, and olive oil, is rare (1,2).

Vegetarians can also be categorized into traditional and new vegetarians. *Traditional vegetarians* are members of religions or cultures traditionally associated with vegetarian diets. Seventh-Day Adventists, one of the traditional vegetarian groups, are a denomination with about a half million members. The church recommends a lacto-ovo-vegetarian diet, and about half of the members adhere to this diet. Most members abstain from eating pork products, caffeine-containing products, hot condiments and spices, and alcoholic beverages. Some abstain from highly refined foods. Most do not smoke.

The *new vegetarians* are a heterogeneous group whose diets often include avoidance of other foods and are accompanied by life-styles and philosophical beliefs different from those previously followed (1, 3). Some groups among the new vegetarians can be identified; there are other individuals whose diets can be described only after obtaining a careful diet history.

The *Zen macrobiotic philosophy*, described in the 1960s by Ohsawa (4), advanced the concept that the path to health and happiness consisted of four parts: no medicine, no surgery, no inactivity, and a diet of natural food. The stated objective was to maintain a good balance of *yin* and *yang*.

The "yin-yang" theory goes by different names in other cultural groups, such as the Chinese and some Spanish-speaking groups, but the basic beliefs are similar. Adherents to this theory believe that their health depends on a balance between opposing forces known as yin and yang. *Yin* (or *lyang*) is described as "female," negative, introverted, empty, dark, or cold, while *yang* (or *bou*) is "male," positive, extroverted, full, warm, or light. The classification applies to other aspects of life as well as to food.

Foods may be classified as yin or yang depending on the effects that a food is believed to have on the body. The classification is not dependent upon color, texture, flavor, or temperature. Rather, foods are classified according to five "flavors"—acid, salt, sweet, bitter, or pungent—and according to seasons and other factors. Meat is a yang food and its use is discouraged.

Too much or too little yin or yang is believed by adherents to be the cause of certain diseases. In groups that adhere to these beliefs, a folk healer might use yang foods or herbs to treat a disease caused by an overabundance of yin. Nutritional counseling of patients with these beliefs may be more effective if suggestions are in accordance with the yin-yang classification.

In the macrobiotic diet, there are ten levels of diets, numbered from -3 to$+7$, with progressively greater restriction (4). Avoidance of preservatives and processed foods is emphasized, in addition to maintenance of the balance of yin and yang. Fluid intake is restricted. Diets from -3 to$+3$ may be made nutritionally adequate with care, but may be deficient in calcium, iron, ascorbic acid, and vitamin B_{12}. The more restricted diets have resulted in cases of scurvy, hypocalcemia, hypoproteinemia, anemia, and emaciation. The final level ($+7$) consists only of grain, usually brown rice, and boiled herb tea. This diet was believed to have the proper balance of yin and yang, but several deaths have resulted from its use. More recently, adherents to this philosophy have been encouraged to "eat more widely"—that is, to eat a greater variety of foods, including dairy products, eggs, and fish (5).

RISKS AND BENEFITS OF VEGETARIAN DIETS

Certain groups who may be particularly at risk are pregnant and lactating women, infants, children, and those with problems such as lactose intolerance and diabetes. For any person, the risks of malnutrition from poorly planned vegetarian diets increase with greater restrictions on varieties of foods eaten. Thus the risk of malnutrition is greater for a vegan than for a lacto-ovo-vegetarian. The vegan may risk inadequacies in protein, calcium, iron, zinc, and vitamins B_{12}, D, and riboflavin.

Among vegans, those who are members of traditional vegetarian groups are not likely to have deficient diets. On the other hand, some "new" vegetarians may lack expertise in planning adequate diets. They may also have more restricted diets because many reject "refined," "processed" or "unnatural" foods (6). The nutritional care specialist must develop expertise in diet planning and counseling for these high-risk groups.

Studies of various vegetarian groups have indicated some health benefits. Different groups vary in the extent to which differences in habits of exercise, smoking, alcohol and caffeine consumption, affect the health benefits. Among the suggested benefits are decreases in body weight, hypertension, blood lipid levels, coronary heart disease, osteoporosis, urinary stones, gallstones, and some cancers.

SPECIAL FOODS USED IN VEGETARIAN DIETS

When interviewing patients, you may encounter references to unfamiliar foods. Some foods used by vegetarians, often unfamiliar to omnivores, are described here.

SOY PRODUCTS

Soy flour contains about 40 percent protein, or 50 percent if defatted. *Soy protein concentrate* (SPC) is 60 percent protein, while *isolated soy protein* (IPC, or *isolated protein concentrate*) is 90 percent protein. *Soy grits* are partially cooked and cracked soy beans. All soy products should be cooked or roasted. This process destroys the enzyme *phytohemagglutinin*, an antitrypsin factor that impairs intestinal protein digestion.

Tofu, a curd, or "cheese," prepared from fresh soybeans, and *miso*, a paste of soybeans, wheat or barley, salt, and water, have been common ingredients in oriental foods. They are now used as source of protein in Western diets. Miso is high in sodium and cannot be used by patients requiring a low-sodium diet. Tofu may be a good source of calcium, depending upon the coagulant used. Sea salt as a coagulant is high in magnesium.

Tempeh (pronounced *tem-pay*) is an Indonesian dish which is growing in popularity. It is usually made from soybeans, but may be prepared from other beans or from grains or seeds. It is prepared by culturing with *Rhizopus oblgosporus* by a method analogous to those used to prepare cheese or yogurt. It may be steamed, fried, grated, or mixed in salads, appetizers, and main dishes.

Four ounces of tempeh contain 169 kcal, 21 g protein, 4.5 g fat, 9.5 g carbohydrate, 1,471 mg calcium, 175 mg phosphorus, and 11 mg iron. The culture is reported to synthesize niacin, riboflavin, and vitamin B_6 as it grows. These vitamins are thus increased while thiamin decreases. The bacteria Klebsiella, found on many plant materials, grows during the culturing of tempeh. Klebsiella produces vitamin B_{12}, but the amount produced depends on the number of bacteria. Since the amount is variable, tempeh should not be relied upon as a sole source of the vitamin (7).

VEGETABLE PROTEIN PRODUCTS

Textured vegetable proteins, often called *TVP*, are usually made from beans and are available in dried form. They may be used in casseroles, stews, sausages, and hamburger-type dishes.

"Meat analogs" or "meat alternates" are foods designed to look and taste like meat. They are made primarily of plant foods, usually soy, wheat gluten, or nuts, and then canned or frozen. Many are made from soy spun protein. They may be flavored to resemble beef, poultry, bacon, or sausage. The vitamin and mineral contents often vary from those of the meats they resemble, and labels should be read carefully. Since these products are processed foods, they are not acceptable to individuals who eat only unprocessed foods. Some of these products contain egg albumin or dried milk and are not acceptable to vegans.

Recipes, catalogs, and nutritional analyses of meat analogs may be obtained from the manufacturers. As the number of vegetarians has increased, these products have become available in larger supermarkets. Detailed information on their contents is contained in the diet manual from the Seventh-Day Adventist Dietetic Association (8).

NUTRITIONAL, OR FOOD, YEAST

Nutritional yeast was formerly a by-product of brewing of beer and was known as *brewer's yeast*. Now, it is cultured separately and may be known either as *nutritional yeast*, *food yeast*, or *brewer's yeast*. It may serve as a good source of B vitamins, particularly thiamin and folate, and also iron and protein. One tablespoon contains 3 g of protein.

MILK SUBSTITUTES

Milk substitutes may be commercially prepared or homemade. Most commercially prepared products have soy protein as a base. Sesame seeds and almonds may also be used. These milks are usually fortified with calcium and vitamins A, D, B_{12}, and sometimes K.

Homemade products are usually soy based and not fortified. They may be deficient in calcium and vitamin B_{12}. If they are not heated to destroy the antitrypsin factor in raw soybeans, their available protein can be highly variable. Homemade soy milk may be fortified by the addition of a scant teaspoon of calcium carbonate per quart and a ground 25-mg vitamin B_{12} tablet in each 2 quarts.

Kokkoh is sometimes prepared and used by vegans as an infant formula. It is prepared with 30 percent brown rice, 30 percent sesame seeds, 20 percent sweet brown rice, and 10 percent azuki beans. The remaining 10 percent consists of equal parts by weight of soybeans, wheat, and oats. It has been used in infant feeding, with unfortunate results. The protein is of high quality, but kokkoh has been used in very dilute form, and the total volume necessary to meet infants' energy and protein needs exceeds their capacity.

SELECTED CHEESES

Rennin, the enzyme used in processing many hard or semihard cheeses, is an animal product. It is thus unacceptable to some vegetarians. Among domestic cheeses, only ricotta cheese is never made with rennin. Rennin is not used in all cottage cheeses; the processor can identify those in which rennin is not used.

SEAWEED AND ALGAE PRODUCTS

Sea products are sometimes used as food by vegetarians. *Agar-agar*, for example, is a gelatin which has been used in puddings and soups. Seaweed and algae may have some vitamin B_{12} from contamination with plankton, but the amount is variable and thus unreliable. *Kombu* is a seaweed found in deep sea water.

MISCELLANEOUS PRODUCTS

Several other products, not usually familiar to an omnivore, are sometimes encountered when interviewing vegetarian patients:

> *gosamasio*—roasted sesame seeds ground with sea salt, high in sodium, and used as a condiment on grains
> *mochi*—a glutinous rice
> *hummus*—a spread for bread made from chick peas and sesame seeds
> *tahini*—a paste made from sesame seeds

CONSIDERATIONS RELATIVE TO SPECIFIC NUTRIENTS

ENERGY

The first consideration in planning an adequate vegetarian diet is the provision of sufficient energy. Energy may be limited because most foods acceptable for vegetarian diets are low in fat. In addition, the foods tend to be high in bulk resulting in reduced total intake. If the energy content is inadequate, protein will then be metabolized to provide energy.

PROTEIN

Vegetarian diets which contain a source of complete protein, such as milk or eggs, can be planned for nutritional adequacy with relative ease. In contrast, diets containing only plant proteins must be planned with great care to ensure nutritional adequacy.

The plant proteins, which are sources of protein in the diet of vegans, are *incomplete*—that is, deficient in one or more essential amino acids. The essential amino acid that is present in least amount in proportion to the requirement is the *limiting amino acid*. The most limiting amino acids from plant proteins are lysine, methionine, threonine, and tryptophan. In general, grains are low in lysine and high in methionine, while legumes are low in methionine and tryptophan and high in lysine. Most nuts and seeds are lysine deficient. Thus, if a high-lysine, low-methionine food is combined with a high-methionine, low-lysine food, the two sources will compensate for each other's deficiencies. Adequate amounts of all amino acids may be obtained by including a combination of different foods, called complementary proteins, that provide all the necessary amino acids. This process, called *mutual supplementation*, is effective only if the foods providing all the essential amino acids are provided over the course of a day (9). The foods do not need to be provided at the same meal except in the case of rapidly growing infants. For your assistance in planning, Table 10-1 gives the limiting and abundant amino acids in foods that are especially useful in planning for protein intake on vegetarian diets (10).

Three types of combinations have been described to provide the essential amino acids: (1) grains and legumes, (2) grains and a small amount of milk products, and (3) seeds and legumes: however, not all items in each group contribute equally. Examples of complementary proteins are given in Table 10-2. In counseling, you need to advise patients to use plant foods in combinations as indicated in the table. In addition, the quantities used must provide the necessary proportions of amino acids. Some useful proportions, given as dry measures, are as follows

1 c grain + 1/8 c soy grits (granules)
1 c grain + 1/3 c sesame or sunflower seeds + 2 T soy
1 1/3 c grain + 1/2 c beans
1/2 c seeds + 1/3 c beans
1 c seeds + 3/4 c peanuts

IRON

Iron exists in foods as easily absorbed heme iron and as nonheme iron. *Heme iron* constitutes 40 percent of the total iron in animal foods. *Nonheme iron* is 60 percent of the iron in animal foods and all the iron in plant foods, iron-fortified foods, and eggs. Absorption of nonheme iron is reduced by phytic and oxalic acids and large amounts of fiber in plants, tannic acid in tea, and phosvitin in egg yolk. Absorption of nonheme, but not heme, iron is increased by ascorbic acid. In counseling and menu planning for vegetarians, foods high in iron and ascorbic acid should be recommended to be included in *each meal*. In general, foods high in iron are dark green, leafy vegetables, winter squash, sweet

TABLE 10-1 Limiting and Abundant Amino Acids in Selected Foods

	Limiting Amino Acids	Abundant Amino Acids
Corn	Lysine, tryptophan, threonine	
Millet	Lysine, threonine	
Oats	Lysine, threonine	
Rice	Lysine, threonine	Methionine
Flour, white	Lysine, threonine	
Legumes		
Beans, mature	Methionine, valine	
Beans, immature	Methionine, isoleucine	
Peas	Methionine, tryptophan	
Oils Seeds and Nuts		
Soybeans	Methionine	Lysine, threonine
Sesame seeds	Lysine	Tryptophan, methionine, cystine, cysteine
Sunflower seeds	Lysine, threonine	Tryptophan, methionine, cystine, cysteine
Peanuts	Lysine, threonine	Tryptophan, methionine
Cottonseed	Lysine	
Coconut	Lysine, threonine	
Vegetables		
Green peas	Methionine, tryptophan	Lysine
Green leafy	Methionine, isoleucine	All others
Gelatin	Methionine, lysine, tryptophan	
Yeast	Phenylalanine	Threonine, tryptophan

potatoes, beans, whole-grain or enriched cereal products, dried fruits, and eggs (if accepted). The iron content of selected plant foods useful for this purpose is given in Table 10-3.

ZINC

Selected food sources of zinc are whole-grain cereals, legumes, oatmeal, dried yeast, and wheat germ. Specific values are shown in Table 10-3. Absorption is decreased by phytates and fiber. Therefore, vegetarians may become deficient in zinc. The phytate in whole wheat is reduced by yeast fermentation. The zinc in leavened bread may therefore be more available than the average of 10 percent availability from plant sources.

CALCIUM

Calcium intake is easily provided for lactovegetarians. Vegans, however, must plan carefully to select plant foods high in calcium, such as dark green, leafy vegetables, broccoli, brussels sprouts, okra, rutabagas,

TABLE 10-2   Complementary Proteins

Grains	+	Legumes	+	Nuts & Seeds	+	Other
Wheat		Legumes				
Corn		Legumes				
Corn		Soy				Milk
Rice		Legumes				
Rice & Wheat		Soy				
Rice						Brewer's Yeast
Rice				Sesame seeds		Milk
Wheat		Soy		Sesame seeds		
Wheat						Milk
Wheat				Peanuts		Milk
Wheat		Beans				
Cornmeal		Beans				
		Beans				Milk
				Peanuts		Milk
Wheat & corn		Soy		Peanuts & sesame		
Wheat & Rice				Peanuts		
				Sesame		
Rice						Brewer's Yeast
Millet or converted rice						Greens

Compiled from: M.T. Goodwin,. *Better Living Through Better Eating*, 2d ed. Montgomery County Health Dept., Maryland, 1974. 19. F.M.Lappe, *Diet for a Small Planet*. New York: Friends of the Earth/Ballantine, 1982.

legumes, dried fruits, and almonds. Specific values are given in Table 10-3. Again, bioavailability is reduced by the oxalic acid and fiber in spinach, chard, and beet greens. Calcium may also be obtained from calcium-fortified soy milk and calcium-precipitated tofu. Calcium supplementation may be needed, in addition to sources, for children and pregnant or lactating women.

RIBOFLAVIN

Milk products are important sources of riboflavin. Those vegetarians who eliminate milk should include in their daily diets two servings of alternative sources—that is, whole or enriched grains, dark green leafy vegetables, asparagus, brussels sprouts, okra, winter squash, mushrooms, nutritional yeast, legumes and nuts, broccoli, or avocado.

VITAMIN B$_{12}$ AND FOLIC ACID

Vitamin B$_{12}$ is not found in plant foods; therefore, it may present a problem in the vegan diet. Vitamin B$_{12}$ deficiency can result in megaloblastic anemia and also causes, over the long term, inadequate synthesis of myelin with resulting neurological damage. Some vegetarians eat a diet containing large amounts of folate, a deficiency of which also contributes to megaloblastic anemia. The intake of large amounts of folate may retard the development of the anemia while the neurological damage progresses unnoticed (11). Therefore, it is important to provide vitamin B$_{12}$ even before anemia is detected.

Vegans must obtain the vitamin by using a supplement or eating vitamin B$_{12}$-fortified foods. Cheerios, Total, Product 19, and Raisin Bran are fortified with vitamin B$_{12}$ but are not acceptable to all vegans. Seaweed and plankton are not reliable sources because their B$_{12}$ content is highly variable. Although adults may take up to 20 years to develop a vitamin B$_{12}$ deficiency, those who develop diseases of malabsorption that interfere with enterohepatic B$_{12}$ absorption, may develop a B$_{12}$ deficiency in less than 3 years (12, 13). Infants of vegan mothers have smaller stores, and a deficiency may develop rapidly (14). Foods, such as spirulina, have been claimed to be high in vitamin B$_{12}$ but contain corrinoids, which lack vitamin activity (14).

TABLE 10-3   Calcium, Iron, and Zinc Contents of Selected Plant Foods

	Serving Size	Calcium (mg)	Iron (mg)	Zinc (mg)
Legumes, cooked				
Blackeyed peas	1 c	43	3.5	6.7
Black beans	1 c		7.9	1.8
Garbanzo beans	1 c		6.9	2.0
Great Northern beans	1 c	90		
Green split peas	1 c		3.4	2.1
Lentils	1 c		4.2	2.0
Lima beans	1 c		4.3	2.0
Navy beans	1 c	95	5.0	
Peanut butter	4 T		1.2	2.0
Peanuts, roasted	1/2 c		2.7	2.2
Pinto beans	1 c		6.4	N/A*
Red kidney beans	1 c		3.6	
Soy beans	1 c		4.9	N/A
Soy milk	1 c	60	1.8	N/A
Tofu	4 oz		2.3	N/A
Cereals and cereal products				
Corn, cooked	1 c		0.7	1.0
Rice, brown, cooked	1 c	7	1.0	1.2
Rice, white, cooked	1 c		1.8	0.8
Oatmeal, cooked	1 c	22	1.7	1.2
Wheat germ, toasted	1/4 c	18	2.0	3.6
Bread, whole-wheat	1 slice	25	0.8	0.5
Bread White	1 slice		0.6	0.2
Nuts (shelled, whole)				
Almonds	1/2 c	166	3.5	1.9
Brazil nuts	4 med			0.76

(continued)

TABLE 10-3 *(continued)*

	Serving Size	Calcium (mg)	Iron (mg)	Zinc (mg)
Cashews	6–8			
Filberts	1/2 c	146		
Pecans	1/2 c		1.2	2.0
Seeds				
Sesame, whole	1/2 c	1160	10.5	
Sesame, hulled	1/2 c	110	2.4	
Soy, mature, cooked	1/2 c	37	1.3	
Soy, milk	1 c	60	1.5	
Sunflower seed kernels	1/2 c	87	4.2	
Vegetables, cooked				
Broccoli	1 c	136–2882	1.6	0.2
Cabbage	1 c			0.6
Carrots	1 c			0.05
Kale	3/4 c	111–206[†]	1.2	N/A
Spinach	1 c	—[*]	4.0	1.3
Greens, beet	1 c	—[‡]		2.8
collard	1 c	220–2522	1.6	
dandelion	1 c	252	3.6	
mustard	1 c	194	2.6	
turnip	1 c	267	1.5	
Peas, green	1/2 c	19	1.5	
Potato, baked with skin	1 med			0.96
Sweet potato	1 small	44	1.0	
Dried fruits				
Apricots, cooked	1/2 c	25	2.0	
Dates, pitted	1/2 c		1.9	0.4
Figs, uncooked	1 large	26	0.6	0.4
Peaches, raw	1		0.5	0.2
Prunes, cooked	1/2 c	28	2.3	0.4
Raisins	1/2 c	48	2.7	0.2
Other fruit and juice				
Banana	1 med			0.3
Mango	1/2 med			0.47
Cranberry-apple juice	8 oz			0.62
Pineapple juice	8 oz			0.38

[*] N/A = information not available
[†] Range of values available from various sources
[‡] Present as soluble calcium oxalate and not available
Compiled from M.T. Fanelli, and R.J. Kuczarski. Food selection for vegetarians. *Dietetic Currents.* 10(1):(1983)1–6; E.R. Williams. Making vegetarian diets nutritious. *Am. J. Nursing.*75:(1975)2168–70.J.A.T. Pennington and H.N. Church. *Food Values of Portions Commonly Used, (15th ed.)* Philadelphia: Lippincott, 1989.

VITAMIN B$_6$

The richest sources of pyridoxine are found in poultry, pork, seafood, organ meats, and eggs. Nevertheless, deficiencies in this vitamin in vegans are not often found. As a precaution, however, the diets should contain rich sources of pyridoxine, such as whole wheat, brown rice, oats, soy, peanuts, and walnuts.

VITAMIN D

Vitamin D may be obtained from fortified cow's milk or fortified soy milk. Sunlight for endogenous synthesis is not always a sufficiently reliable source in many geographical areas. Vitamin D is not present in plant foods. Supplementation should be provided for children and pregnant or lactating women.

MENU PLANNING FOR VEGETARIANS

"Food guides" have been established for ease of planning adequate diets. Given the variations in the degree of diet restriction in vegetarian diets, coupled with the variation in nutrient requirements, several patterns are necessary. The nutrient content of major food groups considered in planning vegetarian diets may be summarized as follows:

> *Meat, poultry, and fish*: protein; kcal; EFA; Fe, Zn; vitamins B$_1$, B$_{12}$, folate
> *Milk*: protein; kcal; Ca; vitamins A, D, B$_{12}$, riboflavin
> *Grains*: protein; kcal; riboflavin, niacin
> *Legumes*: protein; Ca, Fe, Zn
> *Vegetables and fruits*: vitamins A, C; fiber

The following principles can be followed in vegetarian meal planning (1, 5, 15, 16):

1. Reduce high-calorie foods that are not important sources of other nutrients.
2. Use a variety of nutrient-dense foods and plant foods.
3. Replace meat with other animal foods, meat analogs, or complementary proteins from legumes, unrefined cereals, seeds, and nuts.
4. If milk is not accepted, replace with dark green, leafy vegetables, legumes, nuts, seeds, and fortified soy milk.
5. Increase intake of unrefined breads and cereals, legumes, nuts, seeds, and dried fruits as necessary to meet energy needs.
6. Replace fruits that are not accepted; increase vegetables and unrefined grains.
7. Include a food high in ascorbic acid at each meal to improve absorption of nonheme iron.
8. If vegetables are not accepted, increase fruits and unrefined grains.

9. If milk is not used, use a fortified soy milk drink and increase the intake of green, leafy vegetables that are low in oxalate.
10. If goat's milk, low in methionine, is used, recommend intake of a food abundant in methionine at the same meal.
11. For vegans, use nutritional yeast or foods fortified with vitamin B_{12}, or provide a vitamin B_{12} supplement.

A useful guide for lacto-ovo-vegetarian children and adults is given in Table 10-4. The serving sizes appropriate for children of various ages are given in Tables 9-3 and 9-9.

As stated previously, planning an adequate diet becomes more difficult as more groups of foods are excluded from the diet. A suggested food guide for adult vegans is shown in Table 10-5, and guides for use in pregnancy are given in Table 10-6.

Providing nutritionally adequate diets for infants and children of vegans can present special problems. Their diets may be inadequate in energy, calcium, zinc, and vitamins B_{12} and D, as well as, possibly, protein, riboflavin, and iron (17). Some suggestions have been made to overcome these deficiencies (17):

1. To increase energy intake,
   a. Increase intake of legumes, and legume spreads, nuts, and nut butters in favor of vegetables with lower caloric density.
   b Use avocados (remove strings for infants) and dried fruit spreads (puree 1/2 c uncooked dried fruit with 2 t fruit juice).
   c. Do not use honey or corn syrup for infants because of the danger of botulism.
   d. Encourage intake of foods high in complex carbohydrates.
   e. Allow children to eat frequently.
2. Recommend the use of fortified cow milk or fortified soy milk. Commercial soy formulas are Soyalac, Prosobee, Nursoy, and Isomil.
3. Zinc may be provided from legumes, nuts, miso, and tofu.
4. Calcium is contained in soy, navy and pinto beans, tofu, some drinking water, almonds, molasses, and baking powder.
5. Because of their limited capacity, an increase in bulky plant foods of low caloric density is not advisable. In addition, beets, carrots, collard greens, spinach, and turnips are high in nitrates and may need to be limited.
6. Yeast is high in purine content and is not recommended for infants or toddlers.

Suggested diet plans for vegan children to the age of 6 years are given in Table 10-7.

Those who depend on nuts and seeds for a large portion of their protein must remember that these products can become contaminated with aflatoxins. These toxins are produced by the *Aspergillus flavus*

TABLE 10-4   Food Guide for Lacto-ovo-Vegetarian Diets

Food Group	1–3 yr Both sexes	4–6 yr Both sexes	7–9 yr Both sexes	10–12 yr Both sexes	13–17 yr M	13–17 yr F	18–19 yr M	18–19 yr F	20 + yr M	20 + yr F	Standard Serving
I. Cereals, whole grains, breads	3	3–4	4	5	7	5	9	5	8	6	1 slice whole-grain or enriched bread or 3/4 c cooked cereal or 1 oz dry cereal
II. Legumes, meat, analogs, textured vegetable protein (TVP)	1/4	1/4	1/2	1/2	3/4	1/2	1 1/2	1	1	3/4	1 c cooked legume or 2–3 oz meat analog or 20–30 g TVP
Nuts, seeds	1/8	1/4	1/2	3/4	1	3/4	2	1	1	1	1 1/2 oz or 3T
III. Milk, milk products	2–3	2–3	3	4	4	4	2–3	2–3	1 1/2	1 1/2	1 c milk *
Eggs	1	1	1	1 1/2	1 1/2	1 1/2	1 1/2	1 1/2	1 1/2	1 1/2	1 medium egg
IV. Fruits, vegetables	2–3	3–4	4	5	5	5	6	5	6	5	1/2 c juice or 1 medium piece or 1 c raw or 1/2 c cooked
V. Oils	1/3–1	2/3–1	2/3–1	1	1	1	1	1	1	1	1 T

* Common portions of dairy foods and their milk equivalents in calcium: 1-in, cube cheddar-type cheese = 1/2 c milk; 1/2 c yogurt = 1/2 c milk' 1/2 c cottage cheese = 1/4 c milk; 2T cream cheese = 1T milk; 1/2 c ice cream or ice milk = 1/3 c milk.

Reprinted with permission of Ross Laboratories, Columbus, OH 43216

TABLE 10-5 Food Guide for Adult Vegan Diets

Food Group	Minimum Number of Servings Daily[*]	Estimated Protein (g) per Serving[†]
I. Bread	4	2
Whole grains	3–5	4
II. Legumes	2	10
III. Nuts or seeds	1	5
IV. Fruits	1–4	—
Vegetables	4	2
V. Oils	1	—

[*] A serving = 1 slice whole-grain or enriched bread; 1c cooked cereal or whole grains: 1c cooked legumes; 3 T nuts or seeds; 1/2 c fruit juice; 1/2 c cooked or 1 c raw vegetables; and 1 T oil.

[†] Vegan protein balance formula: 60% of protein from grains; 35% of protein from legumes; 5% of protein from leafy, green vegetables (D Calloway, professor of nutrition, University of California, Berkeley).

Reprinted with permission of Ross Laboratories, Columbus, OH 43216.

mold, which grows on nuts or seeds stored at humidities above 70 percent. Aflatoxins are a cause of liver cancer in some countries, but are not usually a problem in the United States. Aflatoxins grow well on peanuts but the level may be reduced by roasting. Vegetarians who use large quantities of nuts and seeds should avoid long-term storage at high humidity. Peanuts should be roasted before eating.

Some vegetarians, particularly those who avoid caffeine, use herb teas. Many of these substances can be hazardous, however. A list of these is given in Table 10-8.

TABLE 10-6 Daily Food Guide for Pregnancy

Food Group	Lacto-Ovo-Vegetarian Pattern	Strict Vegetarian Pattern
Milk and milk products	4	—[*]
Protein foods		
Animal source	1 (2 eggs)	—
Dried beans/peas	2	3
Nuts	1	1
Fruits and vegetables		
Vitamin C-rich	1	1
Dark green/deep yellow	2	2
Other	2	2
Whole-grain or enriched cereal products	6	6
Fats and oils (T)	2	2[†]

[*] 4 c fortified soy milk should be recommended

[†] More fats and oils may be needed for palatability and energy.

TABLE 10-7 Food Guide for Vegan Children

Food Group	Serving size[*]	Minimum Number of Servings Daily[†] 1/2–1 yr	1–3 yr	4–6 yr
Cereal (enriched or whole grains); breads	1–5 T / 1 slice	1	3	4
Protein sources[‡]	1–6	2	3	3
Soy milk (fortified)[§]	1 c	3	3	3
Fruits, citrus	4–8 T	0	2	2
other	2–6 T	3	2	3
Vegetables,				
Green or yellow	4–6 T	1/4	1/2	1
Other	4–6 T	1/2	1	1
Fats	1 t	0	3	4
Brewer's yeast	1 T	0	1	1
Molasses	1 T	0	1	1

[*] Detailed information on serving sizes appropriate for age is contained in Table 9–9.

[†] Foods should be strained or chopped as necessary for age.

[‡] Includes legumes, miso, tofu, seeds, seed butters, nuts, nut butters.

[§] Isomil[R], Nursoy[R], Prosobee[R], or Soyalac[R].

TABLE 10-8 Toxic Effects of Herbal Teas

Effect	Herb
Diuretic, mild patent	Bucker, quack grass, dandelion, green tea Juniper berries, shave grass, horsetail
Cathartic	Buckthorn, senna; dock; aloe
Anticholinergic or psychotogenic	Burdock, catnip, juniper, hydrangea, lobelia, jimsonweed, wormwood, shave grass, horsetail.
Allergenic	Camomile, goldenrod, marigold, yarrow, St. John's wart
Abortifacients	Devil's claw root (South African imported), pennyroyal
Cardiovascular toxicity	St. John's wart
Possible carcinogen	Sassafras oil
Poisons	Mistletoe leaves, stems, berries; Indian tobacco; pokeweed
Gastrointestinal irritant	Juniper, mistletoe, pokeweed
Hormonal effects	Gensing, mandrake, snakeroot

Compiled from J. Dwyer, Vegetarian and other alternative dietary practices. In *Manual of Clinical Nutrition*, Pleasantville, NJ: NPT, 1983,

Anonymous. Toxic reactions to herbal teas. *Nutrition and the M.D.* 5(8):(1983)4.

THERAPEUTIC MODIFICATIONS OF VEGETARIAN DIETS

Most therapeutic diets can be planned as vegetarian diets. The *Diet Manual Including a Vegetarian Meal Plan* (8) is a useful resource for those who plan diets for vegetarian patients or counsel lacto-ovo-vegetarians willing to accept meat analogs in the diet.

TOPICS FOR FURTHER DISCUSSION

1. Do any students in the class use some form of vegetarian diet? What proportion of the class does so? What are their reasons for adopting their type of diet? Ask selected students to describe their meal pattern.
2. How do meat analogs compare in cost to the meat products they resemble?

REFERENCES

1. American Dietetic Association. Position paper of the American Dietetic Association: Vegetarian diets—technical support paper. *J. Am. Dietet. Assoc.* 88:(1988)352.
2. **Vyhmeister, I.B.** Vegetarian diets: issues and concerns. *Nutrition and the M.D.* 10(5):(1984)1–3.
3. **Erhard, D**. The new vegetarians, Parts 1 and 2. *Nutrition Today.* 8(6):(1973)4–12 and 9(1):(1974)20–25.
4. **Ohsawa, G**. *Zen Macrobiotics.* Los Angeles: Ignoramus Press, 1965.
5. **Trahms, C.M.** Vegetarianism as a way of life. *In* B. Worthington-Roberts, ed. *Contemporary Developments in Nutrition,* St. Louis: Mosby, 1981.
6. **Dwyer, J.T., E.M. Andrew, B. Barkey, I. Valadian, and R.B. Reed.** Growth in "new" vegetarian preschool children using the Jenss-Bayley curve-fitting technique. *Am. J. Clin. Nutr.* 37:(1983)815–27.
7. **Pride, C**. *Tempeh Cookery.* Summertown, TN: Book Publishing Company, 1984.
8. *Diet Manual Including a Vegetarian Meal Plan, 7th ed.* Loma Linda, CA: The Seventh-Day Adventist Dietetic Association, 1990.
9. **Dwyer, J.T.** Nutritional consequences of vegetarianism. *Ann. Rev. Nutr.* 11:(1991) 61–81.
10. **Lappe, F.M.** *Diet for a Small Planet (rev. ed.).* New York: Ballantine Books, 1975.
11. **Herbert, V.D., and N. Colman.** Folic acid and vitamin B$_{12}$. *In* M.E. Shils and V.R. Young eds. *Modern Nutrition in Health and Disease,* 7th ed. Philadelphia: Lea & Febiger, 1988.
12. ———. Biology of disease: megaloblastic anemia. *Lab. Invest.* 52:(1985) 3–19.
13. ———, **G. Drivas, C. Manusselis, B. Mackler, J. Eng, and F. Schwartz.** Are colon bacteria a major source of cobalamin analogs in human tissues? 24-hour human stool contains only about 5 micrograms of cobalamin but about 100 micrograms of apparent analog (and about 200 micrograms of folate.). *Trans. Assoc. Am. Phys.* 97:(1984)161–171.
14. **Higgenbottom, M.C., L. Sweetman, and W.L. Nyhan.** A syndrome of methylmalonic acidemia, homocystinuria, megaloblastic anemia, and neurologic abnormalities in a vitamin B$_{12}$-deficient breast-fed infant of a strict vegetarian. *New Eng. J. Med.* 299:(1978)317.
15. American Dietetic Association. Position paper on the vegetarian approach to eating. *J. Am. Dietet. Assoc.* 77:(1980)61–69.
16. ———. Position of the American Dietetic Association: Vegetarian diets. *J. Am. Dietet. Assoc.* 93:(1993) 1317.
17. **Truesdell, D.D. and P.B. Acosta.** Feeding the vegan infant and child. *J. Am. Dietet. Assoc.* 85:(1985) 837–840.

ADDITIONAL SOURCES OF INFORMATION

Acosta, P.B. A view of vegetarianism by a lacto-ovo-vegetarian. *In* J.J.B. Anderson ed *Nutrition and Vegetarianism*, Proceedings of Public Health Nutrition Update, May 1981. Chapel Hill: Health Sciences Consortium, 1981.

Debruyne, L. Vegetarian diets during vulnerable times. *Nutr. Clin.* 4(6):(1989) 1–12.

Dwyer, J. Wonderful world of vegetarianism: Benefits and disadvantages. In J.J.B. Anderson, ed. *Nutrition and Vegetarianism.,*. Proceedings of Public Health Nutrition Update. May 1981. Chapel Hill: Sciences Consortium, 1981.

Fanelli, M.T. and R.J. Kuczmarski. Food selection for vegetarians. *Dietetic Currents* 10(1):(1983) 1–6.

Fanelli, M.T. and R.J. Kuczmarski. Guidelines for lacto-ovo-vegetarian and vegan diets. In J.J.B. Anderson.ed. *Nutrition and Vegetarianism,.* Proceedings of Public Health Nutrition Update. May 1981. Chapel Hill: Health Sciences Consortium, 1981.

Kramer, L.B., D. Osis, J. Coffey, and **H. Spencer**. Mineral and trace-element content of vegetarian diets. *J. Am. Coll. Nutr.* 3:(1984) 3-11.

MacMillian, J.B. and **E.B. Smith**. Development of a food guide for lacto-ovo vegetarians. *J. Canad. Dietetic Assoc.* 36:(1975) 1110.

Mutch, P.B. and **P.I. Johnston**, eds. First International Congress on Vegetarian Nutrition. Proceedings of a congress held in Washington, DC. *Am. J. Clin. Nutr.* 48(Suppl. 3):(1988) 707–919.

Position of the American Dietetic Association: Vegetarian diets. *J. Am. Dietet. Assoc* 88:(1988) 351.

Robertson, L., C. Flinders, and **B. Godfrey**. *Laurel's Kitchen.* New York: Bantam Books, 1978.

Smith, E.B. A guide to good eating the vegetarian way. *J. Nutr. Ed.* 7:(1975) 109–111.

Vyhmeister, I.B., U.D. Register, and **L.B. Sonnenberg**. Safe vegetarian diets for children. *Ped. Clinics N. Am.* 24:(1977) 203–210.

TO TEST YOUR UNDERSTANDING

1. List the nutrients that are provided in important amounts in the following foods:
  a. Fortified soy milk
  b. Tofu
  c. Meat analogs

2. Why might some meat analogs be unacceptable to a vegan? To a lactovegetarian?

3. Why might some cheeses be unacceptable to a lacto- or lacto-ovo-vegetarian?

4. Compare and contrast unsupplemented homemade and commercial soy milk.

5. If a lacto-ovo-vegetarian asked you if he needed injections of vitamin B_{12}, what would you answer? Why? If a vegan asked you the same question, what would you reply?

6. Explain specifically, but succinctly, why the ingredients in each of the following foods complement each other. Use your knowledge of amino acid composition to justify your answer.

7. Examine the following sample menus. Assuming average size servings, explain the following for each menu:
  a. Does it contain a balanced protein (all essential amino acids)?
  b. If so, what foods contribute to the protein?

Menu 1: Greek-style skillet (1 c brown rice, 1/4 c soy grits, eggplant, green beans, seasonings)
Sliced tomato salad
Carrot cake
Tea

Menu 2: Sesame-rice fritters
Citrus salad on romaine lettuce
Oatmeal bread
Cheese cake
Fruit juice

8. The following menu was written for nonvegetarian patients. Modify the menu so that it is acceptable for the diet indicated in the column heading. Be sure to provide for adequacy of all nutrients.

Omnivore menu	*Lacto-ovo-vegetarian*	*Vegan*
Consommé		
Broiled chicken		
Rice pilaf		
Buttered broccoli		
Citrus sections in gelatin on lettuce		
Blueberry crepe		

9. What are sources of ascorbic acid that can be included in a menu to improve iron absorption?

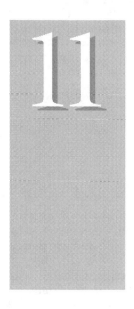

Cultural Factors in Nutritional Care

INTRODUCTION

Culture is passed from generation to generation and consists of the shared beliefs, knowledge, and behaviors of members of a group. In general, a group's culture is derived from the group's nationality, religious beliefs, and race. There also may be cultural differences based on other factors such as economics or geography; for example, cultural differences can be seen between the poor and the middle class. A great deal of overlap of cultural factors may exist among members of a race, a religion, or a nationality. For example, two groups may differ in nationality but share the same religion.

Food is important in cultural identification and has many symbolic meanings related to family traditions, feelings of security, expressions of status, and prestige. Personal habits and preferences may become more pronounced in the elderly and the ill. Consequently, in multicultural nations such as the United States and Canada, competent nutritional care specialists must have a knowledge of the cultures of the various component groups, the effects of these cultures on acceptance of available foods and the response to nutritional counseling and nutritional care.

General principles of patient interviewing and patient counseling are given in Chapters 3 and 7. This chapter will give an overview of modifications to provide more effective nutritional care for patients of cultures other than that of the nutritional care provider. These procedures are referred to as *cross-cultural* or *multicultural*. *Cross cultural* contacts occur when the health care provider and the client are of different cultures, while *multicultural* indicates that several cultural groups are involved. Procedures for cross-cultural and multicultural care have changed greatly in recent years. At one time,

the term *melting pot* referred to the tendency to mix and blend cultures by means of education, intermarriage, and economic factors to establish a new culture. In this process in the United States, Anglo-Saxon norms and values were the usual point of reference. The role of the professional was often to promote *cultural assimilation*, that is, the adoption of mainstream attitudes and behaviors. The procedures were characterized by:

Cultural imposition, the tendency to impose ones's beliefs, practices and values on other cultures in the belief that one's own culture was superior.

Ethnocentrism, the tendency to put one's own culture central in priority and growth, to evaluate other cultures in terms of one's own, and to conclude that other cultures are inferior (1).

A more recent view recognizes that the United States and many other countries are pluralistic as a result of the continuous influx of persons of other cultures and a lack of *structural assimilation* (integration into the social-structure). Given these developments, successful professional attitudes now require:

1. Increased attention and respect for cultural differences.
2. Recognition of the powerful effects of culture on food intake and health-related behaviors.

Additionally, in recent years, demographic changes have affected multicultural nutritional care. The ethnic origins of the minority populations have been changed markedly from those seen in previous generations. For more than a century, the largest increase in the population of the United States resulted from immigration of Caucasian Europeans. In recent years, there has been a shift in the national origin of immigrants and in their racial makeup. Table 11-1 shows the changes since 1980 and the racial distribution in the United States according to the 1990 census.

PREPARATION FOR PROVISION OF MULTICULTURAL NUTRITIONAL CARE

Preparing oneself to provide multicultural nutritional care has become necessary for the competent nutritional care specialist. The process of preparation may be considered to consist of three parts: (1) self-evaluation, (2) development of knowledge of other cultures, and (3) development of cross-cultural interactive skills.

SELF-EVALUATION

People tend to be *culture bound*, that is, to assume that their values, customs, and beliefs are right and admirable and that cultural traits that are different are inferior and undesirable (2). To be a successful counselor, one must be able to recognize cultural differences and avoid making judgments.

A counselor must first become aware of the values of his or her own culture. *Value* in this context is a standard used to assess one's self and others—a belief about what is worthwhile, desirable, and important (2). These values or characteristics of a culture are more subtle than the more overt signs of a culture such as holidays or traditional dress. Table 11-2 lists examples of values that are typically Anglo-American, along with possible corresponding values of other cultures.

Another aspect of self-evaluation is recognition of tendencies to *stereotype*, that is, to categorize individuals in ways that limit their potential. Stereotyping may be demonstrated by statements such as, "All ____ (fill in the blank) are lazy, stupid, emotional, domineering, aggressive, belligerent, etc." In addition to recognizing your own stereotypes, you must consider the stereotypes other groups have about *you*.

Stereotypes are used not only in reference to national and religious groups, but also may include many other identifiable characteristics. Some examples are:

Old vs. young (or teenagers or any other age group)
Rich vs. poor
Male vs. female
Obese vs. normal weight

DEVELOPMENT OF KNOWLEDGE OF OTHER CULTURES

You must understand the interrelationships between food and other aspects of a culture. As you try to learn about these relationships from your patients, you should consider the following variables (3):

TABLE 11-1   Population Distribution by Race in 1990 [*]

Group	% Change in 1980–1990 Decade	% of Population
White	6	80
Black	13	12
Asian or Pacific Islander	108	3
American Indian, Eskimo or Aleut	38	1
Other		4
Hispanic origin (may be any race)	10	
Total	10	100

[*] From 1990 Census data.

1. *The social unit.* What kind of family unit is typical of the culture? What are the roles of various family members? Is there a hierarchy of availability of foods? Is the breadwinner favored, or children, or pregnant women? How permissive is the family in relation to child feeding? Is a child allowed to eat as she or he desires, or is food intake structured?

2. *Social status.* How do food habits and status interrelate? Are specific foods associated with high or low status? What is their nutritional value? Are high-status foods available at reasonable prices? If not, are equally nutritious substitutes available and acceptable? Are these high-status foods an important part of the diet?

3. *Relationship to health.* How is health defined and what importance is put on good health? Is optimal health a valued objective, or is a low level of functioning considered adequate? Does the group use traditional scientific medical services? To what extent does the group adhere to the beliefs and practices of folk medicine? Does the group relate good or poor health to the supernatural or to natural processes? Are there food-related taboos?

4. *Economic factors* Is desired food affordable? Is it available with reasonable convenience? Are preparation methods compatible with employment schedules and time available?

5 *Special events and celebrations* Are celebrations or special observances that involve food an integral part of the culture? What are these events? When and how frequently do they occur? How long do they last? What foods are served? How much? Is there a tradition of fasting? How long and how often? What is the extent of the limitations on food and fluid intake?

Are some foods considered harmful? Conversely, are some foods believed to have special, beneficial properties? Are there certain combinations or groups of foods believed to have special properties? Are herbs and tonics used for special purposes? What items are used, and what are their properties and effects?

Do the food habits characteristic of the culture conflict with the requirements of nutritional care? For

TABLE 11-2 Comparison of Cultural Values

Anglo-American Values	Values of Selected Other Cultures
Change	Tradition
Human equality	Rank, status seeking
Individuality	Group welfare
Competition	Cooperation
Informality	Formality
Directness, openness	Indirectness, "Face"
Materialism	Spiritualism

example, is there a large intake of salt, alcohol, caffeine, or saturated fat?

In order to discuss foods and food habits with patients you will need to be familiar with characteristic foods. Some basic information on various cultural groups is contained later in this chapter. Further information can be obtained from patients and also from visits to ethnic restaurants and travel.

DEVELOPMENT OF CROSS-CULTURAL INTERACTIVE SKILLS

In developing skills in cross-cultural counseling, one must be sensitive to the importance of both verbal and nonverbal communication. These have, in general, been discussed in Chapters 3 and 7; however, some aspects related to a multicultural setting will be addressed here.

Verbal Communication
A language barrier is a frequent problem in counseling persons of other cultures. Clients may not speak English. Unless you speak the client's language, an interpreter will be necessary. In this case, a few guidelines are useful:

> Interpreters may be obtained from bilingual staff, community volunteers, or the client's relatives or friends. Generally, children should not be used, nor should other clients in the waiting room be recruited.
>
> When using an interpreter, seat everyone so your view of the client is not obstructed.
>
> Address the client directly rather than talking to the interpreter.
>
> Avoid slang, lengthy sentences, scientific jargon, complex ideas, and abstractions.

In some cases, clients speak English as a second language. For some of these clients, it is necessary to speak slowly, avoiding technical jargon and avoiding a tendency to increase the volume. Unless the client is hard of hearing, shouting is *not* helpful. The level of reading material must be correlated with reading ability in English.

In other situations, the client speaks English, but cultural differences may still promote misunderstanding. It is therefore important to use a commonly understood terminology. In addition, build opportunities to obtain feedback as described in Chapter 7.

Nonverbal Communication
Nonverbal messages may be communicated by body position, facial expression, distance, eye contact, or silence. The nutritional care specialist must be aware of the effects of these factors on communication. For example, some cultures expect direct eye contact, while others consider this behavior to be rude and aggressive.

Content of Communication
The diet-related cultural practices can be classified as beneficial, neutral, harmful, or unknown. Plans for counseling should then focus on those that are harmful.

In addition, for new immigrants, help may be needed to learn "survival skills." Clients sometimes need assistance in:

> Buying food (i.e., interpreting labels)
>
> Storing food
>
> Preparing unfamiliar foods

Appropriate consideration of these factors may improve compliance with nutritional programs.

FOOD HABITS OF SPECIFIC GROUPS

This section provides some basic information as a starting point for developing an acquaintance with the food habits of other cultures. In addition, there is information on health risks common to these groups. The nutrition counselor should be alert to those risks during the counseling process.

REGIONAL FOOD HABITS IN THE UNITED STATES

The variable climate and geographical features of North America have supported great variety in the food supply. Modern food processing, storage, transportation, and the increasing tendency to "eat out" have, to some extent, moderated the regional differences that once existed. Nevertheless, some of these differences persist. Information on the identity of unfamiliar foods and methods of preparation may be obtained from American recipe books that contain regional recipes. In addition, Southern blacks and Native Americans have been identified with specific foods and food habits. These have been influenced by the history, geographical location, and economic status of these groups.

Southern Black Diet

The typical diet of Southern blacks and poor whites in the Southeast has been known for years, but only recently has it been called "soul food." As the black population has migrated to other parts of the country, it is increasingly likely that you will see some patients who prefer this type of food regardless of your location.

The diet dates back to the days of slavery and originally consisted largely of foods that were available to the slaves. It has evolved since that time, of course. Appendix Table J-1 lists commonly used foods and preparation methods. One must be careful not to assume, however, that every black patient prefers this type of diet.

Health risks

A comparison of the health risks of black populations has shown a reduced life expectancy, increased neonatal and postnatal mortality, and increased incidence of iron-deficiency anemia, lactose intolerance (in 95 percent of the population), obesity, hypertension, stroke, and cancer of the lung, colon, rectum, prostate, and esophagus.

The nutrient intake of the black population has been shown to be low, compared to the RDA, in vitamin B_6, folacin, vitamin E, calcium, magnesium, and zinc in both men and women. Women also have low intake of dietary iron, while men have low vitamin A and riboflavin intakes. The intake of these nutrients should be observed carefully as a preventive public health measure and in nutritional care of black patients with those disorders that occur with increased frequency.

Native American Food Habits

Native Americans, including Alaskan natives as well as American Indians, constitute less than 1 percent of the population. Their diets will vary with the geographic area, residence on reservations or other locations, income, and availability of food. There are over 300 tribes, whose customs vary.

The "traditional" diets of Native Americans consisted of foods available in the geographic area occupied by the tribe. Protein was obtained from wild, large and small game, fish, and eggs. Legumes also served as a protein source, while milk products were not used. Corn was the primary grain, also wild rice in some locations. Fruits and vegetables, nuts and seeds were gathered. Fats were rendered from game and sea creatures. Other items included sugars of honey or tree saps, teas from berries and leaves, and seasonings from plant materials.

Major adaptations have occurred, so that the diet is a blend of traditional and modern processed foods. While there is a high incidence of lactose intolerance in those with a high proportion of Indian heritage, powdered milk and evaporated milk are distributed in the U.S. Commodity program and used in cooking and baking. Among meats, beef, lamb, pork, and luncheon meats are common. Game, of course, is now rare. Apples, bananas, oranges, and many canned fruits are commonly available. Vegetables are less popular. Wheat has replaced corn to some extent. Sweet baked goods, candy, jam, and jelly are popular, as are coffee, tea, and soft drinks. Tortillas and fry bread are common in the Southwest. A summary of these foods is contained in Appendix Table J-2.

Health risks

Alcoholism is prevalent. Heart disease, cancer, cirrhosis, and diabetes are leading causes of death in this population. There is also a high incidence of hypertension, obesity, and dental caries. Nutrition and diet in the treatment of these conditions are discussed in later chapters. Infant death rates are high in comparison to the white population, as is stunted growth in children.

Diets tend to be high in carbohydrate, sugar, sodium, and saturated fat. Sources of calcium may be low but can include the culinary ash from corn dishes and breads to which powdered milk has been added.

Nutritional care specialists working with Native Americans need to acquaint themselves with the specific tribal cultures in their area.

FOOD HABITS OF SELECTED FOREIGN CULTURES

As a nation whose population is primarily composed of immigrants or descendants of immigrants, our food habits are heavily influenced by those of foreign cultures. These cultural influences may be divided into three categories. There are those of such long standing, or universal acceptance, or both, that they have become integrated into the dominant culture. A second category includes those cultural factors characteristic of population groups who have maintained, to some extent, their ethnic identity, despite the fact that they may already be integrated into the dominant culture. Third, there are newly arrived immigrant groups, who are still in the process of adjusting to their new environment. This third group may be in particular need of nutritional counseling.

It is often difficult for the nutritionist to obtain food values of unfamiliar foods for diet evaluation. Some sources of these are given in tables of composition of foreign foods (4–6).

A belief common to many ethnic groups, particularly those from Latin American and Asian cultures, is the classification of foods, beverages, herbs, and drugs as "hot" or "cold." The terms may be *caliente* (hot) or *fresco* or *frio* (cold) in Latin America, or *yang* and *yin* in Eastern cultures. Some foods are considered neutral. The classification is unrelated to the temperature of the food. Although the philosophy of the adherent groups is basically similar, the beliefs vary in detail. Differences between Latin American and Asian forms of these beliefs are discussed later in this chapter. Similar beliefs are found among some vegetarians (see Chapter 10).

Foods and Food Habits of European Ethnic Groups

In various parts of the country are groups who have retained, to varying degrees, their ethnic identity even though they have been in this country for many years. When members of these groups are elderly and ill, ethnic food preferences often become stronger and more important, and it then becomes particularly important for you to understand these food habits (7).

Some established ethnic groups in the United States include the following: Scandinavians in Minnesota and the Dakotas, Finns in upper Michigan, Portuguese in New England and California, Armenians in California, Greeks in Florida, groups of most Central and Eastern European cultures in large cities of the East and Middle West, and some Asian and Mexican American groups in western cities. The food habits of five of the larger European groups are shown in Appendix Table J-3.

Hispanic-American Food Habits and Health Risks

There are many groups with different food habits in the Southwest United States, Mexico, Central and South America, and the Caribbean. They have been referred to by various terms, not all of which are interchangeable, including *Mexican American*; *Chicano* with its political connotations; *Latino*, *Hispanic*, and *Spanish-American*, the original settlers of the Southwest who did not intermarry with the Indians. *Hispanic* and *Latino* have recently become favored all-inclusive terms. Many of the groups from which immigration occurs are Spanish speaking. In the United States, 63 percent of the immigrants are of Mexican origin, 12 percent Puerto Rican, 11 percent Central and South American, 5 percent Cuban, and 9 percent smaller groups. Food habits vary widely but are mostly based on carbohydrate staples such as rice or tortillas made from wheat or corn. Prominent protein sources are vegetable in origin, such as dried beans. Milk and other dairy foods are not emphasized, but corn for tortillas is pretreated and becomes a good source of calcium. Popular vegetables are tomatoes, onions, corn, and sweet potatoes. Many tropical and semitropical fruits are popular.

As the degree of acculturation increases, there is a shift from corn to wheat for tortilla preparation, and an increased use of sugared cereals and sweet baked goods. There is also increased consumption of soft drinks and caffeine-containing beverages.

Overall, Hispanic diets are high in fiber and somewhat lower in proportion of fat. However, they tend also to excess amounts of sodium and energy and often contain less than adequate amounts of calcium, iron, vitamin A, and vitamin C.

Adult Hispanic Americans are at increased risk of obesity and diabetes. They are at lower risk of osteoporosis and associated fractures. The incidence of lactose intolerance is high. In children, there is increased incidence of stunted growth and obesity, particularly in those in low socioeconomic groups. Some information on subgroups of the Hispanic population is useful in selected areas.

Mexican American Foods and Food Habits

Mexican American food habits are a composite of those of the Aztecs, Spanish, French, and Anglo-Americans. The diet of Mexican Americans in the United States has been found to vary somewhat with the number of generations since the family left Mexico. The first generation of immigrants and Mexican nationals are very familiar with the indigenous Mexican diet; second- and third-generation Mexican Americans may be at various stages of acculturation and usually retain some, but not all, of their parents' and grandparents' culture (8). Generally, the speed of acculturation is also proportional to the distance to the United States–Mexico border. Middle- and upper-class Mexican Americans may not differ from Americans of other ethnic origins. When counseling Mexican American patients, therefore, it is important for you to establish the level of acculturation to Anglo-American food habits and the degree to which Mexican food habits are retained.

Many Anglo-Americans are familiar with the dishes served in Mexican restaurants. However, in Mexican American homes, dishes requiring long preparation time, such as tamales and enchiladas, are prepared primarily for Sundays, holidays, and special occasions. Most everyday dishes are easier to prepare and include soups (*caldos*), rice and macaroni dishes (*sopas*), and stews (*guisados*). The staple foods of low-income families are beans and tortillas. Beans are often eaten for more than one meal a day, fried at first and then refried for succeeding meals. Tortillas, made from cornmeal or wheat flour, or purchased ready-made, are used instead of bread. As income improves, meat, eggs, fruits, and vegetables are used in greater quantities (9). A summary table of Mexican American foods is given in Table J-4, in the appendix.

Milk is scarce in Mexico, and refrigeration is a problem. Immigrant families are thus unaccustomed to using milk and often use it in inadequate amounts. Evaporated milk is sometimes used since it does not require refrigeration before opening. Cheese is more commonly used.

Chili, if eaten raw or home cooked, is a good source of ascorbic acid. One-fourth cup of green chili contains about the same amount of ascorbic acid as a serving of cabbage. Commercial red chili sauce is highly variable in vitamin content. Dried chilies and chili powder are poor vitamin sources.

The most common cooking methods are simmering, boiling, frying, and a small amount of baking. Broiling is seldom used in families with the more traditional food habits. This fact may present a compliance problem with some diet modification.

Mexicans in Mexico have four meals a day. As migrants become more acculturated, this pattern, which does not fit well into common work schedules in the United States, tends to vary in the direction of U.S. meal plans. A typical meal pattern in the Los Angeles area, with its high proportion of Mexican Americans, is as follows (10):

Breakfast: Cooked or dry cereal with evaporated milk, coffee, bacon and eggs, if income is not limited, and sweet rolls occasionally.

Lunch: Soup, canned or homemade, sandwich, coffee or soft drink, and fruit.

Dinner: Stew or other dish with meat, fish, or chicken, a rice or macaroni dish, refried beans, bread or tortillas, lettuce and tomato salad, and beverage.

Attention must be called to the belief in the hot-cold (*caliente-frio* in Spanish) system among Mexican Americans and other Latin Americans. The classification varies among individuals, among generations, and from one village of origin to another; therefore, individualized counseling is necessary.

In the *Hippocratic system*, treatment is with opposites, and "hot" diseases require "cold" treatment. In the *homeopathic system*. by contrast, treatment is with like items, so a "hot" disease requires a "hot" treatment.

In general, "cold" foods are most fresh vegetables, tropical fruits, dairy products, and low-prestige meats such as goat, fish, and chicken. "Hot" foods are chili, temperate-zone fruits, cereals, goat milk, cooking oils alcoholic beverages, and high-prestige meats such as mutton and water fowl. "Neutral" foods are beans, legumes, rice, pork, and peaches. Some "hot" or "cold" foods may be neutralized by preparation methods.

Water is considered a strong "cold" food. A problem may arise when a patient with a "hot" disease such as a fever is believed to need only hot food and may be forbidden to drink water.

In Mexico, cold foods are linked with sterility, and the diet is based on "hot" foods. In menstruation, a "hot" condition, homeopathy predominates, and the woman eats only "hot" foods. "Hot" foods are consumed during pregnancy lest the fetus be harmed, and "hot" foods are considered to increase milk production. On the other hand, an excess of "hot" foods is believed to cause *enlechado*, curdling of milk in the stomach of the child. An iron supplement is considered "hot," as is the mother. It may therefore be necessary to dissolve the iron supplement in fruit juice to neutralize it before the mother will take it. This will help ensure that an excess of hot foods is not consumed.

Puerto Rican Foods and Food Habits

The Spanish-speaking population in the East and Midwest is more likely to be from Puerto Rico or other areas of the Caribbean than from Mexico. Food habits in these groups may also vary with the degree of acculturation over the years and are often affected by income limitations.

The food habits may have the Spanish influence in common with Mexican Americans, but the different climate, the island environment, and the absence of Aztec influence result in major differences. For example, while beans are used by both groups, corn is not much used in Puerto Rican foods, nor is chili. Puerto Rican foods are not as highly spiced. Rice and red kidney beans are the Puerto Rican staples.

Beef, chicken, and pork, either fresh, smoked, or in sausage are often used in small pieces in stews and to flavor vegetables. A frequently used seasoning mix is known as *refrito*. Chicken is eaten with red kidney beans or as *arroz con pollo* (rice with chicken). Fish is accepted either fresh or dried and salted and served as a salad with hard-cooked eggs and onions. *Serenata* is a staple dish containing salted cod (*baculao*), avocado, *vianda* (starchy vegetables such as plantain or *platano*, green banana, cassava, *batata*, *name*, *yautia*, *panapin*, *malanga*, and *apio*), onion, and sometimes egg. Other protein sources are the various legumes, lima, navy, pinto, and red beans, and chick peas or garbanzo beans, which are a basic food.

Commonly used cereals are rice, wheat (including white bread), oatmeal as a breakfast cereal, and cornmeal. A common staple, used several times weekly, is a stewed mixture of beans and rice with lard or olive oil, flavored with *refrito*; tomatoes are sometimes added. Spaghetti and noodles are also widely used. A native white cheese, *queso blanco*, is popular but expensive. It is used with pasta. Boiled fresh milk is used when income permits as a beverage for children and in *cafe con leche* (half each coffee and milk) for adults. It is also used in chocolate or cocoa drinks. Vegetables are used in stews or salads of tubers and onions with an oil-and-vinegar dressing. Acceptable vegetables include eggplant (*chayote*), green peppers, beets, tomatoes, green beans, carrots, and okra. In addition, the vegetables known as *viandas* are eaten as such or used in fritters, turnovers, pies, and desserts. *Sofrito*, a tomato sauce, is used with many foods. Popular fruits include plantain, or banana, mashed and mixed with onion, or raw oranges, acerola, mango, guava, papaya, and pineapple.

Common seasonings are garlic, onion, and vinegar and flavorings from lard, ham fat, and olive oil. *Malta* is a common beverage of caramel, malt extract, and sugar. Other beverages are fruit juices and drinks, coffee, beer and rum (10). Some Puerto Ricans believe in the *caliente-frio* system, which must be considered during counseling.

Cuban Foods and Food Habits

Cubans have tended to eat in restaurants and have adapted American eating habits more than have Puerto Ricans (10). At home, however, main staples are rice and beans; black beans, rather than kidney beans, are the most popular. These are cooked in a sauce similar to *sofrito* but with more pork. Beef, lamb, veal, poultry, sausages, all types of fish, and eggs are accepted. The most popular rice dish is *arroz con qui*, rice and black beans. Vegetables in the typical diet include native tubers (*yucca, name, malanga, boniato*—(white yams)—*berenjena*, plantain, and potatoes), tomatoes, and carrots. Accepted cereals include rice, cornmeal, and dry breakfast cereals.

Fresh cow's milk is used for a beverage for children, in coffee for adults, and in sauces and desserts. Native cheese is hard cheese eaten with guava paste.

Lard is popular for cooking. Oil (olive, peanut, or soy) is used on salads and beans. Butter, margarine, and hydrogenated shortenings are also used. Foods are seasoned with vinegar, oregano, garlic, onion, and green peppers.

Desserts are eaten at each meal and as a snack. Ice cream, cake, pie, custard, and pudding are popular. Other sweets are those made from fruit and viandas. Another is *panetelas*, a coconut candylike dish (10). In general, tropical fruits are well liked. Native dessert names are *raspadura, terrejas, boniatillo, bunuelos,* and *cafiroleta.* Coffee, tea, wine, beer, and soft drinks are commonly used beverages.

Asian American and Pacific Islander Food Habits and Health Risks

This is a rapidly growing group with many subcultures. It includes Chinese, Japanese, Koreans, Hawaiians, Filipinos, Samoans, Vietnamese, Cambodians, Laotians, and others. About 7 percent of the total are Pacific Islanders. There is great variation in culture, religion, food habits, health status, and degree of acculturation, but a few generalizations concerning the traditional diet are possible.

Carbohydrate, primarily rice, is the basic source of energy, but rice noodles, tubers, and wheat are also used. Intake of meat and dairy products tends to be low, while diets are high in vegetables, fruits, fish, and shellfish. Sauces from beans, dried fish and pickled vegetables make the diet high in sodium. If tofu, sardines, and leafy vegetables are not used, the diet may be low in calcium. As acculturation occurs, animal protein, fat, simple carbohydrate, and energy intake increases, while sodium and fiber decrease, and there is a tendency to increase the intake of baked goods. Carbonated drinks, butter, margarine, and sweets are increased.

Information on subgroups commonly encountered can be of value.

Chinese Foods and Food Habits

There are five main regions of China, each with a distinctive cuisine. North China, including Peking, was influenced by the Moslems and Manchurians. The resulting Mandarin cuisine contains wheat as the staple grain. The cuisine of Szechwan-Hunan in west and central China, Fukien and coastal China, and eastern China, including Shanghai, are less common. The cuisine of south China and Canton is the type most commonly found in this country since this is the source of most immigrants to North America. However, there are many ethnic Chinese who come most directly from other countries such as Viet Nam.

Raw vegetable consumption is limited, possibly related to the use of human excreta for fertilization in China. Milk products are minimally used, except by immigrants from south China. Tofu is extensively used

and is a good source of protein and iron, and of calcium when the protein is precipitated with calcium salts. The use of sweet or sugar products is limited. Rapidly cooked mixtures of vegetables with fish, pork, and chicken are popular.

A belief in the "hot-cold" system may be encountered, particularly among the elderly. *Chi*, or air, breath, or wind, is believed to be energy, which is broken down when food is metabolized, into categories of yin (cold, female) and yang (hot, male). The elderly believe that yin, or "cold" foods must not be eaten because they contribute to the development of "weak blood" as one ages. Among avoided foods are white turnips, believed to cause indigestion and shortness of breath; seaweed, believed to cause an increase in urination and a decrease in blood pressure; and bean sprouts (11). Many yin foods are also believed to cause cancer. The desire to limit the use of "weak foods" and disease-causing foods must be considered when counseling these elderly patients.

Pregnant and lactating women may also require special consideration. Some patients may believe that foods eaten by the mother will not have an immediate effect on the child, but will, instead, have effects that will become evident years later. Food avoidance includes the following for the reasons given (11):

Food	Belief
Soy sauce	Causes baby to be too dark
Shrimp and shellfish	Causes allergies in adolescence
Watermelon	Causes abortion
Persimmon	Causes "chills"
Deep-fat-fried foods	Causes large birth size
Rice noodles	Causes mother's intestines to twist into the shape of the noodles
Mangoes	Causes severe dermatitis
Mung beans	Causes abortions and glossitis

Dietary intake is reduced during pregnancy, in the belief that the size of the fetus will be reduced and delivery will be easier. Tonics high in iron are used during the last trimester, and ginseng tonic is used to "increase strength for labor." Iron or potassium supplements in capsule form are avoided in order to reduce the "hardening of the bones" of the mother and fetus to allow easier labor (11).

In the postpartum period, the woman is believed to have shifted from yang during labor to yin. Therefore, yin foods are avoided. This has the effects of increasing calories, but decreasing the number of fruits and vegetables eaten. The traditional Chinese belief is that the pores are open following delivery, and cold air enters. Yang foods, such as rice, eggs, vinegar, ginger, peanuts, rice wine, and a soup from chicken and pig knuckles are used during this period.

The meal pattern commonly consists of the following.

Breakfast:	Eggs and fresh milk
Lunch:	Rice, eggs, chicken, ginger
Snack:	Wine
Dinner:	Chicken-pigs' knuckles soup, vinegar, alcohol

Specific rejected foods include the following (12):

During first 30 days of lactation	*Reason/belief*
Turnips and carrots	Cause drying up of mother's milk
Taro root	Prolongs vaginal infection
Ice cream	Causes digestive disorders in infants
Sugar cane	Causes periods of sterility in offspring

After 30 days of lactation	*Reason/belief*
Fresh fish	Causes fever in infants
Melons	Cause diarrhea or measles in infants
Frog legs	Cause leg cramps in infants
Tomatoes	Cause a red face in older infants

Problems resulting from these food habits result in an increased incidence of deficiencies of B vitamins, ascorbic acid, and some minerals. Constipation is also a frequent problem.

Indochinese Foods and Food Habits

A large, somewhat heterogeneous, recent immigrant group consisted of those from Southeast Asia. Many arrived in poor physical, emotional, and financial condition, with educational level ranging from near illiteracy to completion of advanced degrees. Their social customs varied to a great extent from those common in North America. These factors, in addition to language barriers, and the unfamiliar dietary habits of this population, greatly impeded nutritional counseling, as well as the provision of other social services, when the first of these refugees arrived. New immigrants in this group continue to arrive.

The Indochinese comprise distinct subgroups: Vietnamese, Cambodians, and Laotians. The population of Laos is sometimes further classified into three smaller subgroups, based principally on language, but with other cultural differences. One group of these, the *Tai*, which has a number of further divisions, the largest of which are the *Thai-Lao*. There are also minority Tai tribes who lived in mountain valleys, growing rice corn, millet, sweet potatoes, and beans. The second division are the *Mon-Khmer*, or *Lao Theung*, who lived on the hillsides. Third are the *Hmong* and *Yao*, mostly mountain dwellers, who used slash-and-burn agriculture and raised livestock. (They are sometimes called *Meo*, but this is a pejorative term in Chinese and should not be used.) There are some Hmong among the refugees. Their food habits are sufficiently different that they are often considered a separate group.

The Cambodians tend to be the most culturally homogeneous group. Many are highly educated and familiar with urban living. Those Vietnamese and Cambodian refugees who are ethnic Chinese may tend to follow Chinese food habits, rather than those which will be described here.

The Vietnamese. The Vietnamese are the largest of the refugee groups; most now reside in California and Florida, with smaller numbers on the Gulf Coast and elsewhere. Some diet changes have occurred, but most still prefer the typical Vietnamese diet (13, 14).

Rice is the staple food. Long-grain rice is preferred, served with fresh or dried fish or shellfish, or sometimes meat. Accepted meats are pork (most common), including the heart, liver, stomach, intestines, tongue, and coagulated blood, Chinese sausage, chicken and giblets (on special occasions), and some beef. Fish may be fresh, dried, salted, or fermented, but the preferred method of preparation is fried and dipped in fish sauce. A spicy fish sauce, *nuoc mam*, is used extensively for seasoning and is rich in protein and calcium. It is available in Asian grocery stores as "Filipino fish sauce." Other protein foods are soy milk, tofu, peanuts, and legumes in desserts. Milk and dairy products are not typically part of the diet, but small children are sometimes given evaporated milk.

Favorite fruits are banana, mango, melon, orange, pineapple, and papaya. A wide variety of vegetables are acceptable if fresh or frozen, including many vegetables commonly available in North America, plus bamboo shoots, bean sprouts, bok choy, snow peas, bittermelon, dried lily flowers, lotus root, and wintermelon. Bok choy, snow peas, and lotus root are good sources of ascorbic acid. Canned vegetables, which are considered too soft, are not popular.

Among cereal products, besides rice, bean thread and noodles are used. French bread is accepted, a legacy of French colonialism. Other foods in the diet are lard for frying, gluten flour, and seeds. Tea is the main beverage, but coffee, soft drinks, soy milk, sugar cane drink, beer, and wine are accepted. Condensed milk is used in coffee and on bread, and is sometimes given to infants in formula. Soft drink intake has increased markedly in Vietnamese families.

A typical meal pattern is shown in Table J-5. Foods are generally highly spiced with hot chili, ginger root, pepper, onion garlic, herbs, spices, and fish sauce. Most cooked food is boiled, stir-fried, or steamed.

During pregnancy, the Vietnamese woman is expected to eat nourishing food and avoid "unclean" food such as beef. After delivery, preferred foods are salty foods, pork stew, rice, and chicken. All foods must be hot to "keep the stomach warm and avoid heat loss." Cold foods and cold water are not used because they are thought to be bad for the teeth and stomach. Sour foods, which include salads, beef, and all seafood, are forbidden for 6 months (15).

The Laotians. Loatian food habits differ in a few ways from those of the Vietnamese. The meat, fish, fruit, and vegetables they eat are similar. Laotians prefer glutinous rice. Soybean products are eaten by the Hmong, but not by the Lao. A major seasoning is a fermented fish paste called *padek*. Others are chili, fish sauce, coconut milk, tamarind, and curry. Tea, coconut juice, fruit and vegetable juices, a soy bean drink, sugar cane drink, beer, and wine serve as beverages. Diluted condensed milk is used as a beverage for adults and sometimes as an infant formula. Typical meal plans for Laotians and Hmong are shown in Table J-5.

The Cambodians. Cambodian food habits also do not differ markedly from those of the Vietnamese. Fish, fresh, smoked, or dried is common. *Prahoc*, a salted, fermented fish paste is popular. Soybeans are not eaten, except by Chinese Cambodians, but various legumes are made into desserts. Rice may be long- or short-grain, or black, sweet rice, which is used as a dessert. Seasonings include prahoc as well as those used by Laotians and Vietnamese. Beverages are also similar. Sweetened, condensed milk is spread on bread and used for infant formula. The Cambodian meal pattern is also shown in Table J-5.

Health risks
Growth stunting in children is commonly seen in Indochinese refugees, but the relative contributions of genetics and of low economic status are unknown. The adult population may be at risk of hypertension and stroke, but the extent to which diet contributes in the many subgroups is also unknown.

Adaptations that occur on immigration to the United States include increases in consumption of dairy products, meat, milk, and eggs and a decrease in fish consumption. Rice may still be eaten at lunch and dinner but not at breakfast.

RELIGIOUS INFLUENCES IN PATIENT CARE

Religion may also influence a patient's food habits, crossing national and racial influences. It is not only necessary to consider the religion of any individual patient if the religion affects food habits, but it is also important to understand policies based on religious beliefs in church-operated hospitals.

The effects on food habits of beliefs of the world's five major religions—Christianity, Judaism, Islam, Hinduism, and Buddhism—will be discussed. Emphasis is on those religions, followed by larger groups in North America.

In many religions, there are feasts, fasts, and food taboos that may affect nutritional status. Feasts and fasts may be *fixed*, occurring on the same day each year, or *movable*, occurring at different times yearly, often varying with the lunar cycle. Specific foods, seating arrangements, menus, and eating customs may be associated with certain festivals and serve to maintain the traditions.

CHRISTIANITY

In the United States and Canada, Christianity has the most adherents of the five major religions. It may be broadly subdivided into Roman Catholic, Protestant, and Eastern Orthodox.

Roman Catholic Dietary Regulations
The regulations vary somewhat with geographical location; therefore, it is wise to inquire at the office of the local diocese if there is any doubt. The following regulations are typical:*

1. The law of *fast* obliges only on Ash Wednesday and Good Friday. On fast days, one full meal and two other partial meals, which together would not equal a full meal, are allowed. Eating between meals is not permitted, but liquids, including milk and fruit juices, are allowed. *When people are ill or their ability to work would be seriously affected, the laws of fast and abstinence do not oblige.* Fasting is observed by all those between the ages of 21 and 59.
2. The law of *abstinence*, which prescribed the abstention from meat, and soup or gravy made from meat, no longer obliges on Fridays in general. It does, however, oblige on Ash Wednesday, Good Friday, and on all Fridays of Lent besides Good Friday. Abstinence is observed by all those beyond the age of 14 years.

It is important to note the difference between *fast*, in which less food is eaten, and *abstinence*, in which meat and meat products are not eaten. Ash Wednesday and Good Friday are days of both fast and abstinence. Patients may need to be reminded that obligations do *not* apply when they are ill.

Seventh-Day Adventists
The beliefs of Seventh-Day Adventists are discussed in Chapter 10, since many are vegetarians. They usually do not use caffeine-containing beverages—such as coffee, tea, or cola drinks—nor alcoholic beverages. Meat is not served in Seventh-Day Adventist–operated hospitals, except when prescribed by a physician (16).

Mormons
The Church of Jesus Christ of Latter-Day Saints, also known as the Mormon church, disapproves of alcoholic

*These regulations were obtained from the Roman Catholic Diocese of Sacramento, CA.

and caffeine-containing beverages. Although the church is centered in the state of Utah, members are found throughout the United States and Canada, particularly in the West, and also in many foreign countries.

Other Protestant Denominations
The Protestant denominations generally do not emphasize fast days or food taboos. They share some holidays (feast days) and fast days with Roman Catholics, but the degree of observance varies greatly with the denomination and individual choice.

Orthodox Christians
Members of the Eastern Orthodox church were originally the Christians of the Balkan states in Europe, the area northeast of the Mediterranean Sea, Greece, and Russia. Each state church is independent, and is thus called, for example, Greek Orthodox or Russian Orthodox. The head of the state church is the patriarch or archbishop. The patriarch at Istanbul is the spiritual leader.

The Greek Orthodox religion has many fast days: every Wednesday and Friday in the year except two, the 40 days of Lent, and the 40 days of Advent (before Christmas), and two shorter fasts in July and August. The requirements are more severe than in Roman Catholicism. On fast days, no meat—animal products such as dairy products—or fish—with the exception of shellfish—are eaten. The more devout members also abstain from olive oil. A soup of dried beans and lentils is commonly served on fast days.

Easter is the most important event in the Orthodox church calendar. It is preceded by 40 days of Lent. Since the Orthodox calendar is not identical to the Gregorian calendar used by the Roman Catholic and Protestant churches, Easter falls on a different day. Other dates vary in similar fashion.

Lent is preceded by several weeks of preparation. This period includes *Apokreos*, or *Meat-fare Sunday*, 10 days before Ash Wednesday, the first day of Lent. On this day and during the ensuing week, all meat in the house is eaten. A week later is *Cheese-fare Sunday*, the Sunday before Ash Wednesday, when all cheese, eggs, and butter are eaten. As a result, this is a period of feasting.

During Lent, adherents abstain from all animal foods; the only exception is fish, which is allowed on Palm Sunday and on the Day of Annunciation. Lentil soup is eaten on Good Friday. Lamb is traditionally eaten on Easter Sunday.

JUDAISM

Adherents to Judaism constitute the second largest religious group in North America. You will be called on to see Jewish patients in almost every hospital, and their diets may have to be modified to conform to their religious beliefs. In addition, Jewish hospitals in large cities may have broad policies based on Jewish religious beliefs.

The adherence to the "dietary laws" varies among Jews. There are four groups. *Orthodox* Jews observe the laws strictly. They have difficulties in obtaining acceptable food elsewhere, so they eat away from home only in restaurants or homes with kosher kitchens. The *Conservative* Jews generally observe the dietary laws in their own homes, but accept more variations when eating elsewhere. *Reform* Jews may conform to few of the dietary laws, and sometimes none. The last group is the *Reconstructionists*, for whom observance varies from very strict to none at all, based on individual conscience.

In institutions not equipped to prepare kosher meals on the premises, frozen meals may be purchased in many large cities and served on disposable paper plates with disposable eating utensils. When instructing patients for use of diets at home, their beliefs must be kept in mind. The practices of Orthodox Jews will be described in some detail.

The Jewish dietary laws are known as *Kashruth*, or *Kashrus*. They originate in the Torah and were interpreted in the Talmud. They specify the foods that are "fit and proper" (*kosher*, or *kasher*) for Jewish people to eat. The term *glatt kosher* means that the food satisfies even the strictest kosher standards.

The dietary laws divide all foods into three categories (17):

1. Those foods that are inherently kosher, that is, they are "neutral," or *pareve*, and may be eaten in their natural state. Such foods include grains, fruits, vegetables, eggs, tea, coffee, and other foods free of meat, poultry, or dairy products.
2. Foods that require processing in order to be kosher, that is, meat, poultry, and cheese;
3. Foods that are inherently nonkosher, or *trayf*, that is, pork products, fish without scales and fins, and shellfish.

In order to be kosher, meat must come only from "clean" animals, those that chew their cud and have divided (cloven) hooves. Beef cattle, sheep, oxen, goats, and deer are considered clean. Liver, chicken, and turkey are also acceptable, as well as most species of ducks, geese, pigeon, and squab. Pork is not acceptable. Other forbidden foods are winged insects, reptiles, creeping animals, and birds of prey. The latter restrictions are, of course, of little consequence in North America. It is not permissible to eat blood because it is "the life of the animal."

The slaughter of animals must be supervised by a rabbi. The actual slaughter, however, is done by a trained person called a *schochet*, and the animal is killed in such a way as to allow the draining away of a maximum amount of blood. The meat must then be further treated to remove the remaining blood. It is soaked in water for 30 minutes, then salted on all surfaces with a medium-coarse salt, allowed to drain for almost an hour, and then washed three times to remove the salt (16). Iron and B vitamins are probably lost in the process (18). Since the blood cannot be removed from liver by this process, liver must be broiled on a rack designed so that the blood can drip from it as it cooks. Usually, only the forequarter of quadrupeds may be used, so the cuts available in kosher meats are the less tender cuts. Hindquarter cuts are usable only if the hip sinew of the thigh vein is removed.

Many dairy products are not kosher because meat derivatives are used in their manufacture. These include rennin in some cheeses and the gelatin used in making some yogurts, ice creams, and other frozen desserts. Many Orthodox Jews will only eat *cholov yisroel* dairy products or those whose total preparation is supervised by reliable Jewish authorities.

Fish must have fins and scales to be fit to eat. These do not require ritual slaughtering. Shellfish, catfish, frogs, eels, and shark meat are prohibited. The roe of nonkosher fish are also forbidden. Fish may be cooked in or with milk but not with meat. Other taboo foods are animals that died of disease or natural causes, blood, and the internal fat of an animal. Because of this last stricture, soaps made from animal fats are forbidden, and detergents are used instead for dishwashing. For cooking, vegetable fats and oils are permitted.

Another practice important to Orthodox Jews is the prohibition of eating meat and milk in the same meal. In addition, meat and milk cannot be prepared or served with the same dishes and utensils. After meat is eaten, some time must pass before dairy foods may be consumed. The time required may vary with the customs of the national ancestry. Eastern European Jews wait 6 hours; German and West Europeans Jews, 3 hours; and Dutch Jews, 72 minutes (19). On the other hand, milk may be consumed just before eating meat, but not with it (17). Commonly, breakfast and lunch are milk meals, and dinner is a meat meal.

In order to keep meat and milk separate, Orthodox Jewish homes must keep two completely separate sets of cooking utensils, dishes, and silverware. The separation also applies to dishwashing and towel drying. An electric dishwasher can be used for both milk and meat dishes only if it can be properly koshered between washing separate loads of milk and meat dishes.

Meals are therefore meat (*fleischig*) meals or dairy (*milchig*) meals. Allowable fish are eaten with either, as are eggs; however, an egg with a blood spot cannot be used. Pareve foods may be eaten with either type of meal. Some foods are not acceptable on a kosher diet or are considered to be waste products; one of the latter is cream of tartar, made from the sediment remaining after wine is filtered.

Prepared products may be acceptable as kosher if produced within kosher standards, which is indicated by emblems on the *sealed* package. There are many of these emblems (19). The symbol U is used by the Union of Orthodox Jewish Congregations of America, while the symbol K is the emblem of the Organized Kashrus Laboratories. Two emblems are common in Canada: MK from the Montreal Vaad-Harabonim, and COR from the Counsel of Orthodox Rabbis of Toronto.

Food plays an important role in the observance of Jewish festivals and holy days. No food may be cooked on the Sabbath, which extends from sundown Friday to sundown Saturday. Food is cooked in advance on Thursday or Friday, so that the Sabbath can be a day of rest.

The Sabbath dinner on Friday evening is often the most substantial of the week. At that dinner, two loaves of bread (*challah*) are on the table. The two loaves are in remembrance of the double portion of manna provided on Fridays during the 40 years that Jews wandered in the wilderness (20).

Food also has symbolic meanings on other Jewish holy days. The most solemn of these are the 10 days in September or October of each year, which begin with *Rosh Hashanah*, the Day of Judgment and end with *Yom Kippur*, the Day of Atonement. The challah for Rosh Hashanah, which is the Jewish New Year, is commonly made round, to symbolize the desire for a well-rounded year. It may be made with ladders or birds baked on top to symbolize the carrying of family prayers to heaven. The wish for sweetness in the New Year is symbolized by bread and apple slices dipped in honey. Yom Kippur is a day of complete fast for all except children younger than 13 years, people who are ill, and pregnant women (18).

The eight-day *Festival of Pesach*, or *Passover*, occurs in the spring and commemorates the flight of the Israelites from Egypt. This festival requires many preparations in Orthodox Jewish homes. None of the foods in daily use can be used during Passover. Prepared foods that are purchased must be labeled *Kasher L'Pesach* (Kosher for Passover) and certified for use by rabbinical authority. The *Kasher L'Pesach* label alone is insufficient (17).

The home is thoroughly cleaned and all leaven is removed. All leavened products in the home are eaten or disposed of prior to Passover, and no leavened bread or other leavened food can be eaten during Passover. An unleavened wheat crackerlike bread known as *matzo* has been used by Jews for many centuries. It is now prepared commercially under rabbinical supervision.

Flour and grain cannot be used for cooking during Passover since either may become naturally leavened very quickly. The result of this process is called *hametz*. Other *hametz* foods forbidden for use during Passover include coffeelike materials derived from cereals, dry peas, dry beans, and all liquids that contain ingredients or flavors made from grain alcohol. No malt liquors may be used during Passover, including malt vinegar. Matzo, which is finely ground to make *matzo meal*, may be used in food preparation in place of flour. No salt is used in traditional Passover matzo.

If certified for Passover use by rabbinical authority, Passover noodles, candies, cakes, beverages, canned and processed foods, milk, butter, jams, jellies, cheese, relishes, dried fruits, vegetable oils, vegetable gelatin, vinegar, wines, and liquors are acceptable (17). Fresh fruits and vegetables, except peas and beans, are acceptable without certification. Coffee, tea, sugar, salt, and pepper are permitted if the container has not been previously opened (17).

The *Seder* meal is a special feast that occurs the evening of the first day of Passover. In Orthodox homes outside of Israel, the Seder is repeated the second night.

Nearly all Orthodox Jewish homes have separate dishes for use during Passover. An Orthodox Jewish home may thus have four sets of dishes: milk dishes and meat dishes for daily use, and milk dishes and meat dishes for Passover. This may present a financial burden; however, there is a ritual for purifying the everyday dishes for Passover use if the family cannot afford the extra sets. Another alternative is to use disposable table ware during Passover. Passover and other Jewish festivals are listed in Table 11-3.

It is important to realize that foods preferred by individual Jews may be strongly influenced also by their country of origin. More broadly, Jews are often divided into two groups. *Ashkenazie* Jews are those whose background is in Central or Eastern Europe. Foods associated with this group are those most familiar in North America, such as borscht, pickled herring, dark rye bread, gefilte fish, lox, corned beef, and pastrami. On the other hand, the background of *Sephardic* Jews is in North Africa, Spain, and Portugal. Characteristic foods include hummus, tahini, and couscous.

In addition to considerations already described, the following guidelines may be applied where appropriate in planning modified diets for observant Jews:

1. Take a very careful diet history.
2. Many typically Jewish foods are high in salt (e.g., pickled herring, lox, koshered meat). If the diet is sodium-restricted, inquire about these carefully.
3. Many foods are high in fat (e.g., foods cooked with chicken fat; cream cheese). Inquire carefully about these when appropriate.
4. Jewish law accepts that patients may have medical conditions that justify exceptions to dietary observances (e.g., fasting on Yom Kippur). Patients resistant to the exceptions may be advised to consult a rabbi (21).

ISLAM

Adherents to the *Islamic (Muslim or Moslem)* religion reside primarily in the Middle East, North Africa, and across Asia as far as the Philippines. There are also

TABLE 11-3 Summary of Jewish Holidays

Holiday	Approximate Date	Observation	Traditional Foods
Rosh Hashanah (New Year)	September/October	Beginning of Jewish New Year	Carrot tzimmes, honey, honey cakes
Yom Kippur	September/October	Day of Atonement	Fast all day
Sukkoth	October	Harvest festival and Feast of Booths (Booth or shelter in which the Jews lived during flight from Egypt)	Kreplach or holishkes (chopped meat rolled in cabbage leaves): strudel
Hanukkah	December	Festival of Lights: celebrates battle of Maccabees for Jewish independence.	Grated potato latkes and potato kugel
Tu b'Shevat	January	Festival of Trees (Arbor Day); the blossoming time of trees in Palestine	Bokser (St. John's Bread), cakes, raisins, fruits, nuts
Purim	March	Feast of Esther: celebrates fall of Haman and deliverance of Hebrews by influence of Queen Esther on King Xerxes	Hamantaschen (3-cornered cookie), apples, nuts, raisins
Passover	April	Festival of Freedom: celebrates escape of Israelites from slavery in Egypt	Seder meal, matzoth, nuts, wine
Shavuoth	May/June	Feast of Weeks: celebrates Moses receiving the Ten Commandments on Mt. Sinai	Cheese blintzes, cheese kreplach, dairy foods
Tisha b'Av	August	Fast day: commemorates destruction of the First and Second Temples	Meat not eaten on Tisha b'Av or the 9 days preceding it. Blintzes and dairy foods are traditional

Muslims in the Balkan nations of Europe and Russia. Several million Muslims reside in North America, and there are a great many Muslim visitors, such as students. Therefore, although Islam is not a major religion in North America in terms of numbers, it is quite possible that you will encounter Muslim patients in need of nutritional counseling. Detailed information on Muslim customs has been published (22, 23).

Briefly, alcoholic beverages and other intoxicating drugs are prohibited. Pork and pork by-products are also forbidden. Other meats and fowl are acceptable if ritually slaughtered. Kosher foods (see section on Judaism) are considered by most Moslems to fulfill this requirement and are acceptable.

There are a number of ritual fasts. The longest is the fast during *Ramadan*, the ninth month of the Islamic lunar calendar. During this period, a Moslem fasts (no food or drink) from dawn to sunset. Two meals per day are eaten, one before dawn and one just after sunset. Other fasts that may be observed include 6 days in *Shawwal*, the month following Ramadan 3 days each month, preferably on Mondays or Thursdays in other months, and other fasts are less often observed.

Some Moslems are exempt. These include women during menses, pregnancy, and lactation to 40 days after delivery, elderly persons physically unable to fast, mental patients, and those doing hard labor (21).

HINDUISM

Hinduism originated in India and is still the dominant religion in that country. The number of Hindus in North America is quite small, but you may encounter some. It is important to realize that a Hindu's adherence to dietary strictures will depend somewhat on his or her caste. These castes, from high to low, are as follows: the *Brahmins*, currently a large portion of the professional class and those in the universities and the government; the *Ksatriyas*, the soldier class; the *Vaisyas*, the agricultural and commercial class; and the *Sudras*, or Untouchables. Although the caste system, the untouchability in particular, is legally prohibited in India, it is still alive and well in the society. Hindus who come to North America may be imbued with its provisions.

Devout Hindus, particularly of the Brahmin caste, are usually vegetarians. The practice of avoiding meat results from the fundamental tenets of Hinduism regarding reincarnation and reverence for life. Some also do not eat eggs, since eggs are a form of life, but milk and milk products are acceptable. All Hindus regard the cow as sacred and will not eat beef or beef products, such as gelatin. Lower castes may eat other meats, but those who wish to identify themselves with a higher caste are likely to follow the diet of that caste.

Some Hindus, but not all, eat fish. The higher castes are forbidden to eat onions, garlic, turnips, mushrooms, salted pork, and fowl. Even in those lower castes that eat meat, eating of pork and chicken may be eliminated because the animals are regarded as scavengers and therefore unclean. *Ghee* (clarified butter), cow milk, and coconut are sacred foods.

Days of fasting and prayer are called *Vratas*. On these days, the Hindu is expected either to observe a complete fast or to abstain from eating cooked foods (4).

BUDDHISM

Buddhism is the predominant religion in Sri Lanka, Burma, Thailand, Japan, Laos, and Cambodia. Although there are relatively few Buddhists in North America, the number has risen in recent years, partly because the religion has been adopted by many of those involved in the "counterculture" movement. In addition, some of the Indochinese refugees are Buddhists.

The taking of any life is contrary to the tenets of Buddhism. Some Buddhists, however, do eat fish. Intoxicating beverages are forbidden.

SUMMARY

Religion is likely to assume greater importance for patients who are ill. To provide proper nutritional care, it is necessary to plan a diet that is acceptable to the patient's religious beliefs. At the same time, racial and ethnic preferences must be considered, and all must be integrated with the physiological requirements for diet modification. You will have an opportunity in subsequent chapters to modify diets for patients of various ethnic and religious groups.

TOPICS FOR FURTHER DISCUSSION

1. Name some foods, acceptable elsewhere, that are universally considered unacceptable in this country.
2. If there are students in the class from other regions of the country, ask them to describe differences that they have observed in availability of foods and in food habits of the population.
3. Students in the class will have varying ethnic backgrounds. Ask for volunteers to describe how their ethnic background has affected family food habits.
4. Assume that a group of refugees from a culture not previously found in this country begins arriving here in large numbers. The group consists of whole families who are destitute. Few speak English. You are a nutritionist in a public clinic in a large city to which this group has come. List some of the information you will need in order to be able to provide effective nutrition counseling to these refugees. Discuss some of the methods you could use to acquire this information.
5. Class members of various religions can volunteer to describe food habits related to religious observances in their families. How do their religious practices involving food compare to the practices of their grandparents?

REFERENCES

1. **Frankle, R.T., and A.L Owen.** *Nutrition in the Community. The Art of Delivering Services,* 3d ed. (Ch. 5: Working effectively in cross-cultural and multicultural settings.) St. Louis: Mosby, 1993.

2. *Cross-Cultural Counseling, A guide for Nutrition and Health Counselors.* U.S. Dept. of Health and Human Services. FNS-250, Sep., 1986.

3. **Suitor, C.J.W., and M.F. Crawley.** *Nutrition Principles and Application in Health Promotion,* 2d ed.. Philadelphia: Lippincott, 1984.

4. **Hernandez, M., A. Chavez, and H. Bourges.** *Valor Nutritivo de Los Alimentos Mexicanos.* Mexico: Instituto Nacional de la Nutricion, 1977.

5. **Leung, W.-T.W. and M. Flores.** *Food Composition Tables for Use in Latin America.* Bethesda, MD: National Institutes of Health, 1977.

6. **——, R.R. Butrum, and F.H. Chang.** *Food Composition Table for Use in East Asia.* Bethesda, MD: National Institutes of Health, 1973.

7. **Sucher, K.P., P.G. Kittler, and C. Fee.** The greying rainbow: Ethnogeriatric nutrition counseling. *Topics in Clin. Nutr.,* 8(2): (1993) 40.

8. **Romero-Gwynn, E., D. Gwynn, L. Grivetti, R. McDonald, et al.** Dietary acculturation among Latinos of Mexican descent. *Nutr. Today* 28(4):(1993)6

9. **Gladney, V.M.** *Food Practices of the Mexican-American in Los Angeles County.* Los Angeles: Los Angeles County Health Department, 1966.

10. **Yohai, F.** Dietary patterns of Spanish-speaking people living in the Boston area. *J. Am. Dietet. Assoc.* 71:(1977)273–275.

11. **Chang, B.** Some dietary beliefs in Chinese folk culture. *J. Am. Diet. Assoc.* 65:(1974)436–438.

12. **Ling, S., J. King, and V. Lueng.** Diet, growth and cultural food habits in Chinese-American infants. *Am. J. Chinese Med.* 13: (1975)173–80.

13. **Crane, N.T., and N.R. Green.** Food habits and food preferences of Vietnamese refugees living in northern Florida. *J. Am. Dietet. Assoc.* 76:(1980)591–93.

14. *Asian Food Guide for Teachers.* Sacramento, CA: Dairy Council of California, 1980.

15. **Hollinsworth, A.O., L.P. Brown, and D.A. Brooten.** The refugees and childbearing: what to expect. *RN:* Nov. 1980, 45–48.

16. **Hodgkin, G.,** ed. *Diet Manual Utilizing a Vegetarian Diet Plan, 7th ed.* Loma Linda, CA: The Seventh-Day Adventist Dietetic Association, 1990.

17. **Dresner, S.H. and S. Siegel.** *The Jewish Dietary Laws: Their Meaning for Our Time; A Guide to Observance.* New York: Burning Bush Press, 1966.

18. **Kaufman, M.** Adapting therapeutic diets to Jewish food customs. *Am. J. Clin. Nutr.* 5:(1957) 76–82.

19. **Anonymous.** Cultural food practices of elderly observant Jews. *Nutrition and the M.D.* 9(12):(1983) 4.

20. **Lowenberg, M.E., E.N. Todhunter, E.D. Wilson, M.C. Feeney, and J.R. Savage.** *Food and Man.* New York: John Wiley, 1986.

21. *Ethnic and Regional Food Practices* (series). Chicago and Alexandria, VA: American Dietetic Association and American Diabetes Association, 1989.

22. **Sakr, A.H.** Dietary regulations and food habits of Muslims. *J. Am. Dietet. Assoc.* 58:(1971)123–26.

23. **——** Fasting in Islam. *J. Am. Diet. Assoc.* 67:(1975)17–21.

ADDITIONAL SOURCES OF INFORMATION

Debruyne, L.K., F.S. Sizer, and S.R. Rolfes. Ethnic Diets and Health. *Nutrition Clinics* 6:(1991)1–15.

Hoang, G.N. Cultural barriers to effective medical care among Indochinese patients. *Ann. Rev. Med.* 36:(1985)229–39.

Pangborn, R.M. and C.M. Bruhn. Concepts of food habits of "other" ethnic groups. *J. Nutr. Educ.* 2:(1971)106–110.

Ruiz, P. Cultural barriers to effective medical care among Hispanic-American patients. *Ann. Rev. Med.* 36:(1985) 63–71.

Sanjur, F. *Puerto Rican Food Habits: A Sociocultural Approach.* Ithaca, NY: Cornell University, 1970.

Packard, D.P. and M. McWilliams Cultural foods heritage of Middle Eastern immigrants. *Nutr. Today* 28(3):(1993) 612.

Qureshi, B. *Transcultural Medicine,* 2d ed. Boston: Kluwer, 1994.

☑ TO TEST YOUR UNDERSTANDING

1. a Name some locally available foods or categories of foods that are considered specialties of the area in which you live.

b. In what meal(s) are these foods usually used? What place do these foods have in the meal?

c. What are their nutrient contributions?

2. Are there foods that are rare and expensive in your area? If so, name some less expensive substitutes of approximately equal nutritional value.

3. You have a young Chinese patient who is pregnant. During counseling, she tells you that she does not, and will not, drink milk. What alternative high-calcium foods can you suggest?

4. An impoverished Mexican-American family cannot afford citrus fruit, and no one in the family will drink milk. The family consists of two parents, aged 30; a grandmother, 50 years old; and three children, ages 7, 9, and 11. What sources of the following nutrients are available to them in a low-cost, traditional Mexican diet?

> Protein
> Calcium
> Riboflavin
> Ascorbic acid

5. If the family followed a typical Puerto Rican diet, what would be the best sources of these same nutrients?

> Protein
> Calcium
> Riboflavin
> Ascorbic acid

6. A pregnant Mexican-American patient tells you that she will not drink milk, and that she buys ready-made wheat tortillas. What suggestions would you make to her to improve the calcium content of her diet?

7. Visit a retail store that specializes in Mexican or Puerto Rican foods. List the fresh fruits and vegetables that are not sold in most supermarkets. (Ask the grocer their names, if necessary.) List each, describe its use in a typical meal pattern, state its primary nutritional value, and comment on cost.

8. In the same store, scan the shelves of canned goods. List items not commonly seen in most supermarkets, describe the use of each in the meal pattern, state its primary nutritional value, and comment on cost.

9. Consult a table of food values and compare the food value of evaporated and condensed milk. If an Indochinese mother told you she was using condensed milk to feed her infant, what would you recommend? Why?

10. In the following table, mark an X in the column in which the food would be included by an Orthodox Jew:

Food	Pareve	Fleischig	Milchig	During Passover	Trayf
Orange Juice					
Oatmeal					
Poached egg					
Whole-wheat toast					
Cereal					
coffee					
Cream					
Oxtail soup (from kosher-killed beef, with vegetables)					
Salmon salad					
Sliced tomato					
Breaded shrimp					
Roast lamb					
Carrots					
Harvard beets					
Molded fruit salad					
Fried liver and onions					
Angel food cake					

(continued)

TO TEST YOUR UNDERSTANDING *(continued)*

11. An elderly Conservative Jew has been admitted to your hospital. He is willing to make some adjustments for the fact that you do not have a kosher kitchen. You plan to order some commercial frozen kosher meals for him and serve them with disposable tableware. It will take 2 days to get delivery. In the meantime, how would you adjust the following hospital menus to satisfy as many of his expectations as possible? Write the menu as you would modify it in the space below.

Breakfast

1/2 grapefruit
Cornflakes/milk/sugar
Soft-cooked egg
Salt and pepper
White toast/butter/jam
Coffee/cream/sugar

Dinner:

Lamb chops, broiled
Mint jelly
Baked potato/butter
Buttered peas
Fruit salad (melon, strawberries, banana, grapes)
Maple-nut ice cream

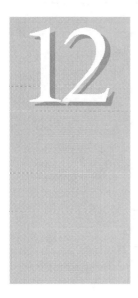

Routine and Transitional Diets

Patients' voluntary food intake may vary in quantity from large amounts to little or none. Some patients have voracious appetites; at the other extreme are those who are unable or unwilling to take any food. The nutrient needs of patients may also vary greatly. Some patients need to have their intakes of one or more nutrients reduced, while others have increased needs.

For patients who are willing and able to make the necessary alterations in their diets, the function of the nutritional care specialist involves providing the necessary foods when they are hospitalized and providing the necessary education when they are to be discharged or when they are outpatients. For the patient who is having difficulty complying with the diet or is unable to do so, however, nutritional care becomes more challenging.

In providing nutritional care, consideration must be given not only to the nutrient content of the diet, but also to the methods of feeding. Patients may obtain food in the usual manner, eating at meals from trays or at the table. For some patients, however, the usual manner of eating does not meet their needs, and they must be given formula feedings directly into the gastrointestinal tract via *tube feedings*. Still others do not have functional digestive systems and take nutrients directly into the circulatory system via parenteral feeding.

These methods are introduced in this and the next two chapters without reference to specific diagnoses. This chapter will discuss some procedures for feeding patients by conventional methods of oral feeding and several of the more common methods for increasing intake. As you proceed, you may wish to refer to background material in your text.

ROUTINE HOSPITAL DIETS

The diets classified as "routine" include the house diet and modification in consistency, usually called *soft* and *liquid* diets; these may differ slightly among institutions, but they are generally similar. A table of routine diets typical of those used in many general hospitals is reproduced in Table 12–1.

The *house*, or *general*, diet is intended for adult patients who do not require diet modifications. Many hospitals provide a restaurant–like "selective" menu from which the patient makes choices. In other institutions, a single, set menu is planned. It is important that the menu be planned so that it is nutritionally adequate or so that the patient is able to select a nutritionally adequate diet. The menu should also be planned to provide foods most patients are willing to eat. It may be used, in addition, to teach principles of good nutrition by example.

In some institutions, other diets are used as the general house diet. In a hospital in which most patients are vegetarians, for example, the house diet might be a vegetarian diet.

The *soft* diet serves as a transition diet between the liquid diet and the house diet. It varies from one institution to another in minor ways. Many institutions have several soft diets which vary in consistency. The *soft diet* or *whole soft diet* generally contains tender cuts of meats and whole, cooked vegetables and fruits, usually without skin or seeds. The *pureed diet* commonly include pureed–consistency foods. The *soft* and *pureed* diets given in Table 12–1 are typical examples. They should be planned to be nutritionally adequate.

TABLE 12-1 Summary of Routine Hospital Diets

Food Group	Clear Liquid *	Full Liquid	Pureed†	Soft	House
Soup	Broth, bouillon (fat-free)	Broth, bouillon (fat-free), and strained cream soups	Broth, bouillon (fat-free), and strained cream soups	Broth, bouillon (fat-free), and strained cream soups	All
Cereal	None	Refined or strained in gruels	Refined or strained	Refined , cooked; cornflakes, rice, pasta products	All
Bread	None	None	White or refined wheat; seedless rye; toast	Foods from preceding column; rolls, crackers	All
Meat and substitutes	None	Pasteurized or dried eggs in milk drinks, eggs in custards; strained meat or poultry in soup	Eggs; ground, or blenderized meats or poultry, white fish (not fried); no pork, small-curd cottage cheese;other cheeses in sauces	Eggs, milk, cheese, tender whole or ground beef, lamb, veal, bacon, poultry (not fried)	All
Vegetables	Tomato juice (in some institutions)	In strained cream soups only; vegetable juices	Potatoes (not fried); strained or pureed bland cooked vegetables	Potatoes (not fried); whole tender or chopped bland cooked vegetables; tomato	All
Fruits	Clear juice (e.g. apple, cranberry, grape), str. lemonade, Hawaiian punch, powdered beverage mixes	All juices	Strained or pureed; juice	Cooked or canned; raw banana; citrus sections without membrane; melon, juice, leaf lettuce	All
Desserts	Gelatin, fruit ice, popsicle	As in previous column, sherbet, ice cream, custard, pudding	As in previous column	As in previous column; cakes & cookies without nuts or coconut	All
Beverages	Tea, coffee, cereal beverages; carbonated drinks	As in previous column	All	All	All
Milk	None	Milk and milk beverages; cocoa; yogurt, plain or without particulate additions	As in previous column	As in previous column	All
Miscellaneous	Sugar, honey; hard candy; salt	Foods from preceding column; butter, margarine, oil, cream in cream soups; honey, syrup;cocoa, chocolate syrup; mild spices. Mocha Mix, mild seasonings as tolerated	Foods from preceding column; plus pepper; jelly; and jam without seeds; well-cooked, pasta, rice	Foods from preceding columns; mayonnaise or similar dressing; gravy; crisp bacon; avocado	All

* Adust to patient's capacity. Meal size is usually small. If patient is nauseated, it may be helpful to avoid fruit and tomato juice. Avoid any food not listed.
† Avoid fried foods, any foods containing nuts, seeds, pickles and pickle relish, whole meats, fruits and vegetables.

These diets may be the basis for other modifications. In many institutions, the soft diet is also used when a "bland" diet or low–residue diet is ordered, since the soft diet is "bland" according to most definitions and is also reasonably low in residue. Therefore, they do not usually contain highly spiced foods, fried foods, or "strong–flavored" or "gas–forming" vegetables. The latter terms usually refer to cabbage–family, or *cruciferous,* vegetables (cabbage, cauliflower, broccoli and Brussels sprouts) and onion–family vegetables (onions, leeks). Vegetables are not served raw, and those with large amounts of indigestible material, such as corn, are eliminated (1–4).

Some patients require adjustments between the pureed and whole soft diets. Many institutions provide these as *mechanical soft* or *surgical* soft diets (1–4). Patients with immobilized jaws, surgery of the head or neck or radiation treatment in that area are among those that need this type of diet. In some cases it may be necessary to ensure that the diet can be taken through a straw.

The liquid diets include the full liquid and clear liquid diets, similar to those shown in Table 12–1. The clear liquid diet, as usually served, contain 600 to 900 kcal per day. It comprises mostly carbohydrate, with some protein, largely of low biological value, and little fat. Obviously, it is nutritionally inadequate and should be used only for a short period. In some institutions, use of the clear liquid diet for more than 3 days is considered to place the patient at nutritional risk and indicates the need for nutritional support.

The full liquid diet is more adequate, but is often inadequate in niacin, folacin, and iron. With its high water content, however, its caloric density is low. Patients are often given between–meal snacks to increase their intake. Vitamin and mineral supplements should be ordered if the diet is used for more than a few days. This diet may be further modified for special purposes. The milk or fruit juices are sometimes eliminated to adjust to patients' tolerances. These diets may be given special titles, such as the *surgical liquid diet.*

Another variation is the "cold semiliquid", or "T and A" (*t*onsils and *a*denoids), diet, which is used following throat surgery. Foods on this diet are soft, smooth, and either cold or lukewarm. Acid juices and very hot soups and beverages must be used carefully. Chocolate products are not used because they interfere with the detection of hemoptysis (blood in sputum). The cold semiliquid diet is inadequate in ascorbic acid, thiamin, niacin, folacin, and iron.

Some patients require a liquid diet containing higher levels of nutrients. These are variously referred to as "high–calorie, high–protein," "fortified," and "wired–jaw" diets. The latter title refers to the fact that the wiring the jaws is often required following broken–jaw injuries.

INCREASING NUTRIENT INTAKE

Persons who are ill often have depressed appetites, and many simultaneously have increased nutrient needs. Under these circumstances, the nutritional care specialist may use some of the following techniques for increasing nutrient intake.

ENCOURAGE EATING AT MEAL TIME

When the patient does not eat sufficient food in three regular meals, it is sometimes sufficient to undertake the following adjustments:

Use a selective menu if this is not in routine use, and cater to the patient's preferences.

Ensure an environment conducive to eating, including absence of offensive odors, provision of comfortable temperature, and acceptable light and ventilation.

Provide assistance as necessary for self–feeding, or arrange for the patient to be fed.

Schedule meals adequately so that appetite can return.

Relieve pain.

Review drug intake as a source of food intake problems.

Many of these interventions require the cooperation of the attending physician and the nursing staff.

INCREASE NUMBER AND SIZE OF SERVINGS

If a patient has an increased appetite as well as increased requirements, it is occasionally sufficient to increase the sizes of servings. For example, patients may be given larger glasses of juice and milk, extra bread and rolls, two pork chops instead of one, or two eggs at breakfast instead of one.

In addition, foods may be added to the menu. Here are some examples:

Add appetizers and salads to menus on which they do not already appear.

Give both fruit and juice at breakfast.

Provide both jelly and honey for bread and rolls at all meals.

Add mayonnaise to sandwiches, and mayonnaise or other salad dressings to salads.

Use sour cream or yogurt as a topping on vegetables and fruit, and whipped cream on desserts and hot chocolate.

Add ice cream to milk drinks.

Add peanut butter to crackers and fruit.

INCREASE NUTRIENT DENSITY

A patient may be limited in the total volume of food which can be tolerated. If nutrient needs cannot be met within that volume, the total nutrient density can sometimes be successfully increased. These steps are specifically intended to increase intake of protein and energy, since vitamins and minerals will accompany properly chosen protein– and energy–containing foods or can be given as supplements.

The energy content of the diet can be increased by taking some of the following steps (5, 6):

Stir butter or margarine into hot cereals, soups, rice, mashed potatoes, gravies, and casseroles.

Fry foods rather than baking, broiling, or boiling.

Substitute half and half for milk in cooking

Add dried fruits to baked goods.

Add less water when reconstituting beverages.

The following steps will increase the protein content of the diet:

Stir skim–milk powder into milk beverages and milk used in cooked dishes, such as cereals, scrambled eggs, mashed potatoes, casserole dishes, meat balls, patties, or loaf, soups, gravies, and baked goods.

Substitute milk or half and half for water in recipes for cereals, soups, puddings, and canned soups.

Add ground or diced meats to soups and casseroles.

Sprinkle grated cheese on vegetables and salads.

Substitute instant breakfast mix for milk beverages.

As well as these additions of familiar foods, some special concentrated sources are available that can be added to foods:

Protein sources: Maxipro HBV, Pro–Mix, ProMod, Propac.

(See Table K–2 for specific content.) These can be added to other foods.

Lipid sources: Calogen, High Fat Supplement, Liquigen, Lipomul, Microlipid, MCT Oil. (See Table K–2) For rationale for use of these products, see Chapters 13 and 16.

Carbohydrate sources: CalPower, Hy–Cal, Maxijul, Moducal, Polycose, Sumacal.

In addition, there are protein–energy supplements, such as those seen in Table K–1 in beverages and puddings.

The clear–liquid diet presents a special problem in increasing nutrient intake. If the patient cannot be advanced to a more adequate diet, the following procedures may be useful:

Add Polycose powder (6 oz. contains 170 g carbohydrate and 680 kcal). (See Table K–2)

Add 6 oz Citrotein (Table K–2) as a drink t.i.d. in standard dilution (provides 65.5 g carbohydrate, 21.5 g protein, and 1 g fat, for a total of 354 kcal).

Combining the two procedures just listed will provide 235.5 g carbohydrate, 21.5 g protein, 1 g fat, and 1.034 kcal.

Substitute Ross SLD (see Table K–2) for the clear–liquid diet, or add the product to the clear–liquid diet.

INCREASE FREQUENCY OF FEEDINGS

Some patients must be fed at more frequent intervals. If this procedure is not carried out carefully, however, it may be self-defeating. It is a common practice for patients to be given additional feedings in the mid––morning (10:00 or 10:30 AM), midafternoon (2:00 or 3:00 PM), and evening ("HS feeding"), usually at about 8:00 PM. The midmorning and midafternoon snacks, in particular, may reduce the appetite for the next meal.

Some patients are given the usual diet divided into six meals instead of three. A typical diet order might read "small, frequent feedings," with hot foods served at the regular meal times and cold foods, such as salad and desserts, served with a beverage at the between meal feedings. This procedure reduces the volume of individual feedings, promoting intake in the patient with limited capacity.

An increase in nutrient intake may be provided by adding between meal snacks *in addition to* the full meals on the menu served at the usual time. There are two broad categories of between–meal snacks. Some consist of the usual types of foods and beverages served at other meals, such as fruit, juice, milk beverages, sandwiches, and dessert items. Other useful foods are nuts, dried fruits, candy, popcorn, cheese, crackers, and granola.

Commercially available liquid formula products are alternatives for adding energy and protein to the patient's intake. Many of these are listed in Table K–1. It is important to note that these formulas may not be nutritionally complete. Other formulas for oral supplementation are included in Table K–3 with the notation that they can be used for either oral or tube feeding. Most of these formulas are nutritionally complete.

Several questions must be kept in mind when choosing a supplement:

1. Is the patient lactose intolerant, so that a lactose–free formula must be chosen?
2. Is the patient capable of digesting and absorbing fat?
3. Does the patient need a supplement low in residue, protein, sodium, or potassium, separately or in combination?
4. Does the supplement have an acceptable taste, odor, and consistency?

TOPICS FOR FURTHER DISCUSSION

1. Assume you have a patient who is 6 feet, 3 inches tall and of normal body weight. His digestive system is intact, but he will require a liquid diet for several weeks because his jaws are wired. Enough space has been left between his teeth to admit a large–caliber straw. How could you modify the routine full–liquid diet to make it higher in protein and calories to more nearly meet his needs? How could you provide greater variety in his diet?

2. Some institutions list routine diets other than those shown in Table 12–1. Survey other diet manuals to which you have access and list the routine diets they contain. Explain the purpose of each one that differs from those in Table 12–1.

3. Some diet manuals list soft, bland, and low–residue diets. If your diet manual is one of these, compare and contrast the content of these diets.

REFERENCES

1. Clinical Dietetic Section, Hospital Department of Nutrition. *Manual of Clinical Dietetics*. Los Angeles: University of California, 1986.
2. American Dietetic Association. *Manual of Clinical Dietetics*, Chicago: American Dietetic Association, 1988.
3. *Mayo Clinical Diet Manual*, 6th ed. Toronto: B.C. Decker, 1988.
4. *Diet Manual Including a Vegetarian Meal Plan*, 7th ed. Loma Linda, CA: The Seventh Day Adventist Dietetic Association, 1990.
5. **Escott–Stump, S.** *Nutrition and Diagnosis–Related Care*. Philadelphia: Lea & Febiger, 1985.
6. **Walker, W.A. and K.M. Hendricks.** *Manual of Pediatric Nutrition*. Philadelphia:W. B. Saunders, 1985.

TO TEST YOUR UNDERSTANDING

1. A sample house diet menu is given below. Assume that this is a menu for the general hospital in which you are a clinical nutritionist and that it is your responsibility to modify this menu to plan the remaining routine diets. Your modifications should be based on the diets listed in your diet manual or on those given in Table 12–1. Your instructor will specify which to use. If your diet manual has diets with titles other than those given on the menu, you will need to change the titles at the top of the columns. When planning this menu, be sure to abide by the following policies:

a. Use as many items from the house diet as possible, and limit the number of separate items that must be prepared by using the same item if possible. For example, if

the house diet said "fried chicken," you could write baked chicken in the soft–diet column. Be sure to make a choice of one only when there are two usable items on the house menu. In other words, do not make a "selective menu" for the soft, pureed, and liquid diets.

b. Make all menus as nutritionally adequate as possible.

c. Take care to apply the usual principles of menu planning so that diets are acceptable to patients. Try, for example, to provide for a variety of colors and flavors, and follow a commonly accepted meal plan.

Menu Plan				
General	Soft	Pureed	Full Liquid	Clear Liquid
Breakfast Orange juice Stewed prunes Farina Bran flakes Fried egg Bacon Waffles				

Lunch
Beef-vegetable soup
Saltines
Lamb patty
Tuna salad (w./onions, celery,
    pickles) on bed of lettuce
Potato chips
Buttered peas
Spiced canned peach half
Sliced tomato salad with French
    dressing
Blueberry muffins
Baked caramel custard				

Dinner
Tomato juice/lemon wedge
Breaded shrimp
Roast beef/gravy
Mashed potatoes
Buttered broccoli
Buttered carrots
Fresh fruit salad (Orange sections,
    sliced banana, diced pineapple) on
    lettuce leaf
Maple-nut ice cream
Sugar cookies				

(continued)

TO TEST YOUR UNDERSTANDING *(continued)*

2. Standard accompaniments are not usually written on the menu plan. Instead, institutional policies state which items are to be automatically included in the patient's meal. The items listed on the form below are those which are usually available for inclusion with the diets you have just planned. Put an X in each column for each item that would be acceptable on the diet specified in the column heading.

Standard Menu Accompaniments					
Food	House	Soft	Pureed	Full Liquid	Clear Liquid
Bread, white					
wheat					
rye					
Butter					
Margarine					
Jelly					
Milk, whole					
skim					
Coffee					
Sugar					
Tea					
Lemon					
Salt					
Pepper					

3. You have a patient who is capable of eating any food, but who needs an increased protein and calorie intake. The patient has a large appetite. Modify the menu provided by your instructor to provide an intake of about 3,500 kcal in three meals plus an evening snack.

4. You have a patient who requires three between-meal formula feedings to supplement his regular meals. The patient is unable to digest lactose.
   a. How are your choices of formula limited for this patient?
   b. Name some formula products you might choose to give this patient?

5. You are planning to mix a protein supplement into the food of a protein– depleted, anorexic patient. The patient is lactose intolerant and has shown some evidence of mild fat malabsorption.
   a. What protein source would you use and why?
   b. What other dietary component is it important to supplement?

6. A patient is receiving, in addition to her three meals, 240 ml of Sustacal Liquid at midmorning, 240 ml of Meritene Liquid in mid–afternoon, and 240 ml of Delmark Milkshake at bedtime. How much protein and energy are added to the patient's daily intake by providing each of these supplements? (The information necessary for your calculations is given in Appendix K.)

13 Tube Feeding

Some patients are unable to eat enough food in familiar forms to maintain or restore good nutritional status, even though they have a functioning gastrointestinal (GI) tract. Under these circumstances, the patient may be fed through a tube into the gastrointestinal tract with a formula mixture used either as a supplement to other food intake or as the sole source of nutrition. For the patient without a functioning gastrointestinal tract, the patient may be fed a formula mixture directly into a vein, avoiding the GI tract. This is commonly called *parenteral nutrition*. Parenteral nutrition will be discussed in Chapter 14.

This chapter will explain, without reference to specific diagnoses, the characteristics of formulas used for, and the procedures involved in administering, tube feedings. Before proceeding, you should review the information on tube feeding in your text and the material on fluid and electrolyte balance in Chapter 4.

CHARACTERISTICS OF TUBE-FEEDING FORMULAS

A familiarity with the nutritional and physical characteristics of tube-feeding formulas is essential in planning for tube feeding. The formula composition and concentration, physical properties, rate of feeding, and delivery systems must be carefully integrated.

NUTRIENT CONTENT OF FORMULAS

An understanding of the nutritional composition of tube-feeding formulas is needed in order to evaluate different formulas.

Caloric Density

Caloric density is defined as the amount of energy per unit volume of food. For tube feedings, it is usually expressed in kcal/mL. Most tube feedings contain 1 kcal/mL, but some are more concentrated—1.5 to 2 kcal/mL—and others may be more dilute—0.5 kcal/mL. Patients whose caloric need are high, whose appetites are depressed, or whose tolerance to volume is limited are candidates for feeding with more calorically dense formulas. The patient must, however, be able to tolerate the higher osmolality of such formulas and must also receive adequate fluid for excretion of the high renal solute load. Another consideration is that greater density delays gastric emptying. In particular, a high-fat content has a significant effect (1). On the other hand, patients whose gastrointestinal mucosa has been damaged or unused and atrophied from disease may have improved tolerance to a more dilute formula. This more conservative approach allows time to restore the integrity of the tissue and to replete enzyme concentrations (2).

Protein

Various methods are used to express protein quality. *Protein efficiency ratio* (PER) is obtained by measuring the growth of laboratory rats in relation to protein intake:

$$PER = \frac{\text{weight gain in g}}{\text{protein intake in g}} \quad \text{(13-1)}$$

Casein, the reference protein, has a PER of 2.5. Low–quality proteins have a lower PER. When PER is 2.5 or more, 45 g of the material will provide the adult RDA of protein.

Biological value (BV) indicates the amino acid ratio of the protein. Specifically, it measures the retention of absorbed nitrogen (3).

$$BV = \frac{N \text{ retained}}{N \text{ absorbed}} \times 100 \qquad (13\text{-}2)$$

Whole egg has a biological value of 100. Values for other materials commonly used in tube feedings are (4):

Cow milk	90
Lactalbumin	84
Soybean	75
Casein	72

In general, lower biological value requires a greater amount of protein to reach equilibrium.

An *amino acid profile* consists of a list of the specific amino acids and their amounts. The list is usually available from the manufacturer of the product. The amino acid content must be examined critically in relation to the patient's normal body needs, needs as affected by the illness, and information on possible essentiality of amino acids such as glutamine.

Patients must receive sufficient total protein to meet their normal needs as well as to meet the increased needs resulting from illness. The protein must also be of high biological value in order to provide the required amino acids. On the other hand, excessive amounts of protein in the diet will markedly increase the renal solute load. The amount of fluid necessary for excretion of the load must be provided in the formula or as added free water. It is generally recommended that the protein portion of formulas provide no more than 15 percent of the calories.

Calorie–to–Nitrogen Ratio

The composition of the formula must be such that sufficient energy from nonprotein sources is available so that protein is not used for energy. A useful technique for evaluating a tube–feeding formula is the calculation of the *calorie-to-nitrogen* (C:N) ratio. The nitrogen content is calculated from the protein content, on the assumption that nitrogen is 16 percent of the protein. The C:N ratio is then calculated by using the following equation:

$$C:N \text{ ratio} = \frac{\text{kcal per day}}{\text{g N per day}} \qquad (13\text{-}3)$$

The kcal/day may represent total energy intake or may indicate energy from carbohydrate and fat, but not protein, that is, nonprotein kcal (nonpro kcal). An acceptable ratio of kcal per g of N in a normal adult male may be 300 if *nonprotein* kilocalories are used as the basis for calculation:

$$\text{Nonprotein kcal/g N} = \frac{\text{total kcal} - \text{kcal from protein}}{\text{g N}}$$

$$(13\text{-}4)$$

For the critically ill patient, the nonpro kcal:N ratio often needs to be in the range of 100 to 200, providing a greater proportion of protein. Ratios greater than 200 may be inadequate in protein, while those less than 100 usually provide a formula that requires the use of protein as a source of energy. Recommended C:N ratios to provide for anabolism in a patient are based on total kcal, within the same range. It appears, therefore, that a ratio of 150 is a useful guideline.

Carbohydrate

Carbohydrates commonly provide about 55 percent of the energy in tube–feeding formulas. Some formulas contain milk and thus contain lactose, but many patients are deficient in lactase (a problem discussed in more detail later). These patients, if tube fed, need a formula that is lactose–free.

Fat

Fat provides a concentrated energy source in tube feedings, serves as a carrier for fat-soluble vitamins, and, in many formulas, is a source of essential fatty acids. It improves the flavor and palability of the formula, but does not contribute to the osmolality.

Fiber

The term *fiber* encompasses plant polysaccharides and lignin that are resistant to hydrolysis by digestive enzymes. It is a heterogenous mixture that has a water-holding capacity, viscosity, and ion-exchange capacity.

At one time most tube-feeding formulas were low in residue. More recently, fiber-containing formulas have become available. The fiber most often used in these formulas is soy polysaccharide in amounts of 5 to 14 g per liter of formula. It provides 2 kcal per gram. Fiber is discussed in more detail in Chapter 18.

Water

Most enteral formulas contain between 690 mL (2.0 kcal/mL) to 860 mL (1.0 kcal/mL) of water per liter of formula.

Vitamins and Minerals

The majority of ready-to-use tube-feeding formulas are nutritionally complete. They provide the NRC recommended dietary allowance of vitamins and minerals when caloric requirements are satisfied. Three precautions must be observed, however:

1. Some patients have disorders that increase the need for one or more vitamins or minerals. As the specialist in nutritional care, it is your responsibility to monitor these requirements and recommend supplements.when indicated.
2. Some formulas that are otherwise complete do not contain vitamin K. A weekly supplement has been recommended as a precaution (6). Such a supplement may be particularly important for patients with fat malabsorption.

3. A current recommendation states that therapeutic doses of vitamins should not exceed 10 times the RDA level. For fat–soluble vitamins, however, this dose may be excessive (7).

PHYSICAL PROPERTIES OF FORMULAS

Physical properties must also be considered in choosing a tube-feeding formula for an individual patient.

Osmolality

Osmolality has an important effect on the patient's tolerance of the formula. Gastric emptying is delayed by hypertonic solutions and may result in gastric retention, nausea, and vomiting. In the duodenum, solutions in the lumen are adjusted to isotonicity by adding or removing water. If a solution is very hypertonic and is delivered into the duodenum, a large fluid shift into the lumen of the gut will follow, since the membranes of the enterocytes are semipermeable. Severe diarrhea and dehydration can result.

It is important, therefore, to be aware of the osmolality of feeding formulas that you recommend for patients. Information on osmolality of unflavored formulas and the effects of the use of the flavor packets is provided by the manufacturers. Flavoring materials may be particularly high in osmotic effect.

Renal Solute Load

Renal solute load (RSL) is a major consideration in pediatric feeding. Recall that, for any patient, if the solute load is excessive, a larger quantity of water will be required to excrete it. If sufficient water is not given, the patient may become dehydrated, *hypernatremic* (having a high serum Na), and *azotemic* (having a high serum N), with weight loss, oliguria, fever, cyanosis, and irritability.

Convulsions, brain damage, and coma may ensue. At the same time, the ill tube-fed patient, adult or child, may have other conditions that add to the fluid requirement. These include impaired urine-concentrating ability and excessive water losses from fever, diarrhea, vomiting, or burns. Protein catabolism will also add to the load.

In summary, in choosing a formula, you must carefully consider the osmolality and renal solute load in relation to the patient's disease, renal-concentrating ability, and ability to ingest liquids. A frequent problem occurs as a consequence of the administration of a high-protein formula with a volume of fluid insufficient to excrete the resulting high RSL. Under these conditions, the patient may develop a dehydration, known as *tube-feeding syndrome,* which can be life–threatening if not corrected (8, 9).

Viscosity

The viscosity of the formula is determined by its composition. In general, larger molecules increase viscosity; more calorically dense formulas are also more viscous. Viscosity, in turn, will determine the size of the feeding tube that must be used. Less viscous formulas may be administered in a smaller tube, which is more comfortable for the patient.

FORMULA INGREDIENTS

In order to use tube feedings, you must have a thorough knowledge of the content of the formula and be able to relate that content to the patient's digestive ability to tolerate the feeding. A major consideration is the molecular size of the substrates, which relates to osmolality, and the patient's ability to digest the substrates. Digestive ability varies with the area of the gastrointestinal tract that lies below the end of the feeding tube. For example, if the tip of the tube lies in the jejunum below the site of action of pancreatic enzymes, the content of the tube feeding cannot consist of materials that require pancreatic enzymes for digestion.

Carbohydrates

Carbohydrates used in tube feedings are listed in Table 13–1. They may vary considerably in molecular size. The larger molecules are less sweet and exert less osmotic pressure. They also require more digestion, but most patients have sufficient amylase to digest starch. Starch may consist of 400 to several thousand glucose units and thus contributes very little to formula osmolality. It has limited use because it is relatively insoluble.

Starch molecules can be made smaller by hydrolysis to molecules of shorter lengths. *Glucose polysaccharides* have more than 10 saccharide units and require pancreatic amylase for digestion. Smaller units, called *oligosaccharides*, are soluble glucose polymers with 2 to 10 units and do not require amylase for digestion. Further hydrolysis of cornstarch results in *maltodextrins, maltose*, and, eventually, *glucose*. As the molecular size decreases, osmotic activity increases.

Glucose may be used in formulas but will markedly increase osmolality and is very sweet. It does not require any digestion, however. In clinical situations, glucose is commonly called *dextrose*.

Sucrose and lactose are sometimes used in formulas, but their use also increases the formula's osmolality. Sucrose, lactose, and maltose require specific disaccharidases for digestion and are therefore not tolerated by patients with deficiencies of these enzymes.

A list of the carbohydrates contained in a formula is called a *saccharide profile*. It may contain the exact sugar, such as glucose or sucrose. Alternatively, it may list categories, such as mono-, di-, and polysaccharides.

Protein

Four major categories of protein are used in tube–feeding formulas (see Table 13–1). They differ in the amount of digestion that is required prior to absorption.

Intact Proteins. Intact proteins are in their original, natural form and require complete digestion. Examples include milk, eggs, and pureed meat. Some intact proteins have been separated from the original food. These are sometimes called *isolates*, such as "soy protein isolate." Lactalbumin and casein are isolates from milk with removal of lactose, and albumin may be isolated from egg white. Some are used in combinations. Caseinate, which is expensive, may be combined with the cheaper soy isolate. This reduces cost while still providing high–quality protein. All intact proteins require normal amounts of pancreatic enzymes for digestion. Intact proteins promote stimulation of growth factor and gut hormone release. Since they are large molecules, they do not appreciably affect formula osmolality.

Partially Hydrolyzed Proteins. These products may be made from some of the same proteins or from fish, whey, or meat, and then hydrolyzed with enzymes. The enzyme hydrolysis results in a mixture of peptides of various sizes. Some formulas have added free amino acids to improve the protein quality of the formula. These formulas are useful for patients with problems of reduced absorptive surface or exocrine pancreas insufficiency. They also promote stimulation of growth factor and gut hormone release, but to a lesser degree than does intact protein.

Dipeptides and Tripeptides. These are a subcategory of partially hydrolyzed proteins that are further hydrolyzed from the same basic protein. They are categorized separately because they are absorbed by passive diffusion. Absorption may be improved in patients with compromised gastrointestinal function or hypoalbuminemia. Nitrogen balance, growth, and hepatic function may also be improved.

Pure Crystalline Amino Acids. Amino acids require no digestion but require active transport for absorption. These products are indicated for patients with reduced absorption, pancreatic insufficiency, and amino acid transport disorders. The amino acids markedly add to the osmotic load. It is particularly important to examine the amino acid composition of these products, since not all provide the necessary amino acids within the amount of protein provided in the feeding (10). For anabolism, it is suggested that essential amino acids comprise at least 40 percent of the total. These formulas tend to be very unpalatable.

Fat

Most tube–feeding formulas contain lipid from a vegetable source such as soy, corn, safflower, or sunflower seed, or, in the case of milk-based formulas, from butterfat. The fatty-acid chains in these products are long—14 carbons or more—and the lipid is called *long–chain triglyceride* (LCT).

The amount of essential fatty acids (EFA)—that is, linoleic and linolenic acids—required has not been specifically determined, and recommendations vary. About 3 to 6 percent of total kcal intake is recommended by the NRC for adults (11). LCT sources provide generous quantities of linoleic acid (13), as shown in Table 13–2.

For patients who are unable to digest and absorb LCT, feedings that contain medium-chain triglycerides (MCT) may be formulated. MCT is prepared by fractionating coconut oil and isolating fatty acids with 6 to 12 carbon atoms. The triglyceride prepared from these fatty acids provide 8.3 kcal/g. Each 15-mL tablespoon of oil weighs 14 g and thus contains about 115 kcal. Since the product is rapidly hydrolyzed in the intestinal lumen, it adds to the osmolality of a tube-feeding formula. MCT does not provide essential fatty acid, an important consideration if MCT is the only lipid. Other problems arise from the side effects sometimes produced. Nausea, vomiting, diarrhea, and abdominal distension occur. MCT is oxidized to ketone bodies and carbon dioxide in the liver and may result in excess ketogenesis. It should be added to formulas gradually to avoid the side effects.

TABLE 13-1 Sources of Ingredients in Commercial Formulas

Carbohydrates

Polysaccharides: Hydrolyzed cereal solids, pureed vegetables, modified food starch, tapioca starch; soy polysaccharides

Glucose polymers: Glucose polysaccharides (>10 glucose units), glucose oligosaccharides (2–10 glucose units), glucose polymers (partial hydrolysis of cornstarch), maltodextrins, corn syrup, corn syrup solids

Disaccharides: Lactose (from milk), sucrose, maltose (by-product of oligosaccharide or starch digestion)

Monosaccharides: Glucose (dextrose), fructose

Protein

Intact: pureed beef, egg white solids, soy protein isolates, casein, lactalbumin, dry milk, caseinate of sodium or calcium, whey

Partially hydrolyzed to shorter chains such as oligopeptides: from casein—whey, soy, meat protein, lactalbumin, collagen

Dipeptides and tripeptides: protein hydrolyzed as above into di- and tripeptide fragments

Crystalline amino acids: L-amino acids

Fat

Long-chain triglycerides: butterfat, corn oil, safflower oil, soy oil, sunflower oil

Medium-chain triglycerides: MCT (manufactured from coconut oil)

Lecithin

Diglyceride

Monoglycerides

TABLE 13-2 Linoleic Acid Content of Vegetable Oils

Source of oil	Linoleic acid (%)
Corn	58
Safflower	74
Sesame	74
Soy (not hydrogenated)	51
(hydrogenated)	39
Sunflower	66

Many ready-to-use formulas contain both LCT and MCT. The LCT provides essential fatty acids, while MCT improves the overall digestion and absorption of the formula. MCT adds appreciably to the cost of a formula.

A third form of fat found in enteral formulas is known as *structural lipid*. These are triglycerides that are modified, as described for MCT, using both polyunsaturated fatty acids (PUFA) from vegetable oils, including EFA, and with medium-chain acids for ease of digestibility.

TYPES OF COMMERCIAL FORMULAS

There are now a wide variety of commercial tube-feeding formulas available from a number of manufacturers. One of the functions of the nutritional care specialist is to recommend the products that will meet the needs of particular patients. For this reason, it is useful to be able to classify formulas according to their content, digestibility, purpose, and other properties relevant to the patient's needs.

Two broad categories of commercial tube-feeding formulas are available: fixed-ratio formulas and modular formulas.

Fixed–Ratio Formulas

Fixed–ratio formulas are those that contain protein, fat, and carbohydrate in "ready–to–use" form. The ratio of the ingredients relative to each other is thus fixed, except if they are altered by further addition of ingredients. Some require the addition of water.

Fixed-ratio formulas can be categorized in a variety of ways. For example, they often are classified on the basis of the form of protein, whether blenderized, isolates, or hydrolyzed.

Blenderized formulas are based on intact protein, starch, and long-chain triglycerides. This type of formula is available commercially and can also be made in the hospital from common ingredients such as pureed meat, strained fruits and vegetables, nonfat dry milk, and added carbohydrate, oil, vitamins, and minerals. They are moderate in osmolality, high in viscosity, and low in cost. They usually contain 25 to 35 g lactose per liter. The most common caloric density is 1 kcal per mL. These feedings require intact digestion and absorption; therefore, patients need a normal, functioning gastrointestinal tract. Blenderized formulas are used for patients who have difficulty ingesting food. These include those who have esophageal disease, head or neck surgery, or sequelae of a cerebrovascular accident. They are placed via the feeding tube into the patient's stomach.

Milk-based formulas are the most palatable types of tube-feeding preparations and may also be used as an oral supplement. They should be used with caution when administered by tube, because they have a high protein content and, thus, a high renal solute load. Osmolality is usually 500 to 700 mOsm per kg. They are best used in tubes into the stomach, but are contraindicated in lactose intolerance.

Formulas with intact nonmilk protein are usually lactose-free formulas composed of protein isolates, oligosaccharides, oil, vitamins, and minerals. Some contain medium-chain triglycerides. Many are low in osmolality (300 to 400 mOsm per kg) compared to milk-based formulas. They are less viscous than blenderized or milk-based formulas and can thus be used with a smaller-diameter tube. Most commercial formulas yield 1 kcal per mL. A few are especially formulated to yield 2 kcal per mL for patients with high-energy requirements but low volume tolerance.

Hydrolyzed protein–based chemically defined feedings are composed of amino acids or small peptides or both as a source of protein, plus glucose, or glucose oligosaccharides, as a source of carbohydrate, and minimal amounts of triglycerides. They are used for patients with problems of malabsorption. They are hyperosmolar and must be used with caution. These same formulas are sometimes classified on the basis of

Calories: usually 1 kcal/mL vs. increased (1.5 or 2.0 kcal/mL) or reduced (0.5 kcal/mL)

Protein concentration: usually about 15% of kilocalories

Lactose content: lactose–containing or lactose-free

Osmolality

Fiber content: fiber–free or fiber added

Fat content: concentration, relative amounts of LCT and MCT

An additional category consists of disease-specific formulas available for patients with renal failure, hepatic failure, pulmonary disease, glucose intolerance, fat malabsorption, trauma, sepsis, or severe metabolic stress. Table K–3 gives the properties of many of the tube feedings categorized above. The disease-specific formulas will be discussed in later chapters describing nutritional care in those diseases.

Modular Formulas

There are some patients whose needs are not met by any fixed-ratio formula and who may benefit from an individualized modular formula. A *module* is a single nutrient, or combination of a few nutrients, that can be used to prepare an individualized formula suited to a patient's unique needs. Modules may be used to prepare the whole feeding or can be added to a fixed-ratio formula.

Several modules are available, providing various forms of carbohydrate, fat, and protein. These are listed in Table K–2. Vitamin and mineral modules are under development.

Alternatively, a module-style tube feeding can be made by blenderizing regular foods. This is a simple and economical method of preparing a tube feeding, but it has definite disadvantages. The risk of contamination is high, and the mixture is viscous, necessitating a large-bore tube. Therefore, tube feedings are seldom formulated in this fashion. The planning of modular feeding requires greater expertise than that needed for the use of fixed-ratio feedings.

SELECTING A FORMULA

When you are asked to recommend a tube feeding for a patient, major considerations are the capacity of the patient for digestion and absorption, as well as the patient's fluid needs and renal function. Polymeric formulas must be administered only to patients who are physiologically capable of digestion and absorption of their ingredients.

Monomeric formulas are chosen for patients who need a feeding that is residue-free or fat-free, or for which no digestion is required. In general, they can be absorbed if the patient has 100 cm of functioning jejunum, an ileocecal valve, and 150 cm of ileum.

Here are some pointers to keep in mind in special circumstances:

1. A patient who was taking nothing by mouth (NPO) for a few days or who has gastroenteritis may best tolerate a low–osmolality, lactose–free formula.
2. It is commonly recommended that a patient who is in transition from total parenteral nutrition to tube feeding be given a low-residue formula. Most tube-feeding formulas are low in residue.
3. Special guidelines may apply to children:
   a. Premature infants requiring tube feeding because of immature suck, swallow, or gag reflexes will often benefit from breast milk.
   b. If an infant is less than 6 months of age and has normal bowel function, an infant formula or breast milk may be given by tube.
   c. An older child with normal bowel function who needs a tube feeding can often be given the nutritionally complete formula for adults. However, care must be taken that the formula has an appropriate C:N ratio, that sufficient vitamins and minerals are provided, and that renal solute load does not exceed renal capacity.

FORMULA DELIVERY

In designing a tube-feeding regimen, the choice of a formula must be integrated with both a delivery system and a protocol for administering the tube feeding. Other important considerations are anticipated duration of tube feeding and anticipated risk of aspiration of the formula into the lungs.

TUBE PLACEMENT

It is essential that you know the location of the tube in the patient who is being tube fed. Some tubes can be placed without surgery, but surgical procedures are required for others. The tip of the tube lies either in the stomach or in the duodenum or jejunum of the small intestine.

Nonsurgical Tube Placement

In hospitalized patients, tubes are usually placed by nurses or physicians. Nutritional care specialists in outpatient settings, however, sometimes work with tube-fed patients and will insert tubes. They may also instruct patients, or parents of child patients, on tube insertion. If you are expected to do this, it is essential that you ask for detailed coaching on techniques. The procedure will not be described in detail here.

In any setting, tubes should not be inserted until 3 hours after the patient's last intake of food or fluid. This precaution is observed because of the danger of vomiting and aspiration when the tube is inserted. Tubes are usually inserted via the nasal passages into the stomach (*nasogastric*, or *NG*, tube), into the duodenum (*nasoduodenal*) or into the jejunum (*nasojejunal* or *nasoenteric*). (See Fig. 13–1).

Vomiting and aspiration are hazards in ventilator-dependent patients, those who have depressed levels of consciousness or depressed gag reflexes, or those who are restrained. Feeding for such patients should be administered using a nasoduodenal tube with a weighted tip. The nasal routes are used in tube placement if possible. Tubes are relatively easy to insert, but there is a hazard of tube insertion into the trachea. Tubes are withdrawn if the patient is coughing.

Rarely, an orogastric tube is placed in an adult. The tube is inserted through the mouth instead of the nasal passages and is usually removed after each feeding. In premature infants, orogastric tube placement is used because the infants are obligate nose breathers. In addition, the nasal passages may be too small to accommodate the tube.

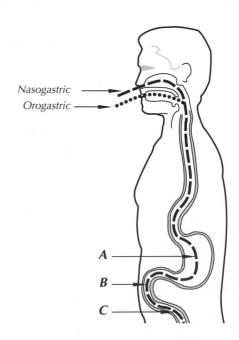

FIGURE 13-1   Location of nonsurgically placed feeding tubes. Nasal and oral access sites are shown. A) end of nasogastric tube; B) end of nasoduodenal tube; C) end of nasojejunal tube.

In an adult, the normal distance from the mouth to the cardia of the stomach is about 45 cm, and from the cardia to the duodenum, 15 cm. Excessive length of tube insertion may indicate that the tube is coiled in the stomach. If the tip is pointed toward the head, vomiting and aspiration may result. Tube placement should preferably be confirmed radiologically. Many brands of tube are radiopaque to make them visible on X–ray.

Tubes are well tolerated if the appropriate type is chosen. On the other hand, the nasogastric tube, in particular, is easily removed by a patient who is uncooperative or disoriented.

Surgically Placed Tubes

Surgical placement is necessary if an obstruction through the nasal passages or esophagus exists. It is also useful if very long-term tube feeding is anticipated, since the opening for the tube (an *ostomy)* is not usually visible when the patient is clothed. Ostomies may be placed into the esophagus at the level of the cervical spine (*cervical esophagostomy*) or into the stomach (*gastrostomy*). (See Fig. 13-2). These are placed by the surgeon under anesthesia. A *percutaneous endoscopic gastrostomy* (PEG) is less costly and placed under local anesthesia. A tube may also be placed into the jejunum (*jejunostomy*), also shown in Fig. 13-2. A *needle-catheter jejunostomy* tube is a small polyethylene catheter introduced into the jejunum through a large–bore needle (trocar). This procedure is done during the patient's surgery. A *percutaneous endoscopic jejunostomy* (PEJ) is place by a method analogous to the PEG.

Gastrostomy and jejunostomy placement reduces the likelihood of aspiration, and patients are less self-conscious about appearance. Duodenostomy is seldom used because the duodenum swings toward the back and is not easily available via the anterior abdominal wall. Also, there is danger of leakage into the abdominal cavity.

EQUIPMENT

Three types of equipment are required for tube feeding: feeding tubes, the container for the feeding, and, sometimes, a pump. This equipment is shown assembled for use in Figure 13–3.

Types of Feeding Tubes

For the comfort of the patient, the tube (1) should have the smallest diameter through which the formula will flow and (2) must be as pliable as possible. The diameter of feeding tubes is measured in *french* (F) units. 1 F unit = 0.33 mm.

Modern feeding tubes tend to be quite small in diameter, commonly 8 F or 9.6 F. They usually are made of polyurethane, silicone rubber (silastic), or a combination of these, and tend to remain relatively pliable for long periods, even if left in place. Tubes may be radiopaque and weighted with tungsten, stainless steel, or silicon for ease of insertion and ease of determining location. Some brands contain a wire stylet in the lumen to stiffen it for easier insertion. When the tube is in place, the stylet is withdrawn. Some tubes are treated with a substance to provide lubrication when wet. Recommended tube sizes are given in Table 13–3, and some commercially available sizes are described in Table 13–4. Polyvinyl chloride (PVC) and polyethylene (PE) tend to become stiff and uncomfortable, and increase the danger of perforation. It is usually recommended that they not be used in tubes.

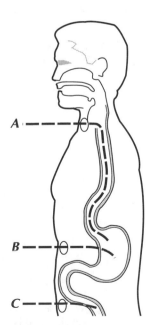

FIGURE 13-2 Location of surgically placed feeding tubes. A) cervical esophagostomy; B) gastrostomy; C) jejunostomy.

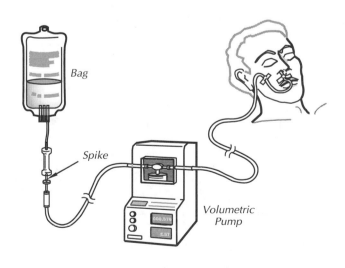

FIGURE 13-3 Combined setup for nasoduodenal feeding. A volumetric or peristaltic pump may be used. Correct taping of the tube will reduce pressure on the nares for greater patient comfort.

TABLE 13-3 Feeding Tube Sizes and Preferred Uses

Formula type	Size* Gravity	Pump	Preferred use
Blenderized	10.0–18.0	8.0–9.6	Gastric feeding
Milk-based†	8.0 9.6	7.3	Gastric feeding
Lactose-free†	7.3–9.6	7.3–9.6	Gastric and duodenal feeding
Defined formula	5.0–6.0	5.0–6.0	Duodenal and jejunal feeding

*french units.
†Protein isolates.

Feeding Containers

A number of feeding containers and feeding sets are available. Many are available from the manufacturers of the formulas. You need to be knowledgeable about the advantages and limitations of each. Some of the factors for consideration include the following:

1. Container size must be considered. Volumes as large as 1 L are available. They are convenient for the nursing staff, but the formula they contain must be used within a limited time to control bacterial contamination. Sets that can attach to the manufacturer's bottle of formula can reduce contamination.
2. Some sets are designed to be used with pumps.
3. Accurate flow rates are essential.

Pumps

A pump is often needed to obtain more accurate control of the tube-feeding rate. Pumps are essential if the feeding is to go directly into the small intestine. They are also needed for the more viscous formulas. They make it possible to reduce the tube size and thus improve patient comfort. Two types of pumps are available: peristaltic and volumetric. Generally, peristaltic pumps are used for tube feedings since they are less expensive then the volumetric pumps.

PROTOCOLS FOR FEEDING

Protocols for administering a tube feeding must take into consideration the frequency, volume, and concentration of formula to be infused.

Frequency and Amount of Feeding

One protocol for delivery involves administration of a large volume (*bolus*) of formula at widely spaced intervals. For example, a patient receiving 2,400 mL per day might be given 400 mL of feeding every 4 hours. The

TABLE 13-4 Characteristics of Selected Small-Caliber Tubes for Forced Enteral Feeding

Tube	Composition	Length (in)	External Caliber (French)*	Tip	Comment
Dobbhoff (Biosearch)	Polyurethane	43 55	8, 12 8	7 g tungsten Bolus weight	Stylet radiopaque
Duo-Tube (Argyle-Quest)	Silicone elastomer	40	5, 6, 8 6, 8	1 g silicone 5 g tungsten	Radiopaque, no stylet required; outer PVC tube for insertion
Entriflex (Biosearch)	Polyurethane	36, 43 43 36, 43	8 10 12	3-g tungsten- filled up	Lubricant
Flexi-flo (Ross Laboratories)	Polyurethane	36 36 45 45	12 14 8, 10 8 8,10,12	No 3 g tungsten 3 g tungsten	No stylet Radiopaque Stylet radiopaque Y-access port
Keofeed II (IVAC)	Polyurethane	30 36 43	6 8 8, 12	Tungsten-filled tip 0.75g 3 g 3 g, 5 g	Radiopaque stylet Stylet
Vivonex Tungsten Tip (Norwich-Eaton)	Polyurethane	45	8	Flexible tungsten bolus weight (8 F)	Avoids any disposal of mercury-weighted tubes.

* 1 F = 0.33 mm outside diameter.

entire feeding is given from a large syringe within a few minutes. This method is often poorly tolerated, leading to nausea, vomiting, diarrhea, distention, cramps, or aspiration. The advantages of this system are that it requires the least equipment and nursing time, and it does not limit the movement of an ambulatory patient. Bolus feeding is given into the stomach, not into the intestine.

An alternative to bolus feeding is the administration of the formula by *intermittent gravity drip* over a 20-to 30- or 60-to-90 minute period. Although tolerance may also be poor by this method, it is usually better than that produced by bolus feeding. This method can be quite successful if the patient is allowed to gradually adapt to it. It also does not confine the ambulatory patient.

Another alternative is the *continuous feeding*, whereby the formula is administered over 16 or 24 hours. A closed, sterile administration system can be used. This method should be chosen if hypertonic solutions are to be fed directly into the small intestine. It is the best tolerated of the three methods, but it requires a pump and is thus more expensive. The patient receiving 2,400 mL per day in 16 hours would receive 150 mL per hour, a volume more likely to be tolerated than are the more rapidly administered feedings.

Volume and Rate

The most recent policy for gastric feeding is to administer isotonic or hypertonic formulas at full strength, but to control the rate carefully. For nasoduodenal or nasojejunal, the feeding is often first given at half-strength to avoid osmotic diarrhea.

Nasogastric Feedings. In general, the most common recommendations are to begin with slow administration of 20 to 50 mL/hr. The amount is progressed at 10 to 25 mL/hr every 8 to 24 hours followed by an increase in concentration, until the desired concentration and total volume are reached. This may take several days.

In intermittent feeding, the procedure may begin with 120 mL of an isotonic formula given at the rate of 30 mL/minute or less every 4 hours. This schedule is advanced with an additional 60 mL every 8 or 12 hours if tolerated.

The feeding remaining in the stomach (*gastric residual*) should be measured every 4 to 6 hours if a pump is used, or before each feeding in intermittent gravity drip. This procedure consists of using a syringe to gently withdraw the stomach contents through the tube. Patients should not receive additional feeding if the residual exceeds 100 to 150 mL. Nasoduodenal feeding may be necessary if gastric residuals are greater than 100 mL 2 hours after the last feeding. Feeding must be stopped if the patient vomits.

The measurement of gastric residuals is usually a nursing responsibility. The resistance of very small-bore tubes makes them unpopular with nurses. More important, the residual volumes are unreliable when the small-bore tubes are used.

Nasoduodenal or Nasojejunal Feedings. Osmolality is a particularly important consideration in this feeding location. A common protocol is to begin feeding at 50 mL/hour and increase 25 to 50 mL/hr each day, or per 8-hour shift, as tolerated, until the desired volume is reached, provided there is no diarrhea, glycosuria, or intestinal obstruction. A pump for continuous administration is usually necessary. With postpyloric feeding sites, there will usually be little or no residual.

Other Considerations

To guard against dehydration or overhydration ("water intoxication"), particularly in the patient unable to communicate, the patient's total fluid requirements must be calculated, and actual fluid intake must be determined. Fluid intake includes the water content of the tube feeding and of any food or liquid taken orally, the fluid used to flush the tube, and any fluid taken with oral medication. Free water in the tube feeding is estimated by subtracting the protein, fat, and carbohydrate content from the total volume. The difference between intake and need must be provided as free water in order to prevent dehydration.

The temperature at which tube feedings are given is believed to affect formula tolerance. Although there is some disagreement on the question (12), cold formulas are generally believed to cause cramping and diarrhea. Therefore, tube feedings are usually given at room temperature.

The patient's head should be elevated during feeding and for 30 minutes after an intermittent feeding to reduce the risk of aspiration (see next section). A sample tube feeding order form is shown in Table 13–5.

COMPLICATIONS OF TUBE FEEDING

The avoidance of complications demands that great care be taken in the process of tube feeding. In general, the complications may be categorized as those related to (1) the mechanical process, (2) the patient's gastrointestinal function, (3) the patient's metabolism, (4) infectious processes, and (5) psychological factors.

MECHANICAL COMPLICATIONS

Mechanical complications include nasopharyngeal discomfort such as erosions and abscesses, excessive gagging, esophageal and laryngeal ulceration or rupture of varices, and inability to withdraw the tube. These complications are usually related to the pliability and size of the feeding tube. Since small-lumen, tungsten-weighted, polyurethane and silicon rubber tubes have been available, the incidence of complications of this type has decreased markedly. Irritation from large-bore tubes can frequently be relieved by using small-bore (<10 F) tubes. The viscosity of the formula, size of the tube, and other equipment must be carefully integrated, as described earlier in this chapter, to avoid complications.

TABLE 13-5 Tube Feeding Order Form

University Medical Center Enteral Feeding Orders

(Check boxes, circle items, fill in blanks as needed.)

1. Formula _____

2. Vitamins _____

3. Insert _____ feeding tube.

   Location _____

   _____ Stomach

   Begin feeding when tube is in place, confirmed by aspiration of gastrtic contents.

   _____ Continue to advance tube 1–2 cm/hr to duodenum.

   _____ Leave on right side 2 hrs. Leave 15–21 cm showing ABO, X-ray in 24 hrs. to confirm placement.

   _____ Do not begin feeding until placement in duodenum is confirmed.

4. Head of patient elevated 30° during feeding + 30 min.

5. Fill container with feeding for _____ hrs. + 1/2 t blue food coloring

6. No formula to hang more than _____ hrs.

7. Change feeding container and tubing q 24 hrs.

8. Start formula at _____ mL/hr, _____ strength

9. Increase rate to _____ mL/hr in _____ hrs if there is no N&V, abdominal distension, or gastric residuals more than _____ mL.

   Then:

_____ mL/hr	_____ strength	_____ time	_____ date
_____	_____	_____	_____
_____	_____	_____	_____
_____	_____	_____	_____

10. If diarrhea occurs, administer _____ after checking for impaction.

11. Check gastric residuals every _____ hrs and record. If more than _____ mL, hold feeding.
    Flush tube with water.
    Recheck residual in 2 hrs.
    Restart feeding when residual less than _____ mL.

12. Flush tube with _____ mL water or cranberry juice q _____ hrs, following delivery of crushed medication and when tube is disconnected

13. Urine sugars q _____ hrs × _____ hrs, then _____ .
    Notify physician if > or = to 1%.

14. Record I & Os. Chart volume of feedings separately from water or other oral intake for each shift.

15. Measure weight.

16. Weigh pt. now and Q.O.D. Chart on graph.

17. Blood sugars and lytes, now and q M,W,F.

18. Calorie count daily for _____ days and then _____ .

19. SMA-12,[*] CBC, TIBC, serum Fe, mg weekly.

20. SMA-6[†] every Mon and Thurs.

21. 24-hr. urine collections for urea to start 8:00 AM on _____ in conjunction with calorie count for nitrogen balance calculation.

[*] total protein, albumin, Ca, PO_4, cholestorol, creatinine, bilirubin, alkaline phosphatase, CPK, LDH, SGOT, and uric acid
[†] Na, K, Cl, HCO_3, glucose, BUN.

Use of a small-bore more pliable tube may also be helpful for patients at risk of developing acute sinusitis or otitis media.

High gastric residuals are included among the mechanical complications. The patient with a gastrostomy tube with continuous feeding should have residuals checked immediately prior to the tube feeding and every 4 hours thereafter. If the residual cannot be checked, monitoring of abdominal girth may be substituted. Abdominal girth is measured by the distance between the anterior superior iliac crests. An abdominal girth more than 8 to 10 cm greater than the patient's baseline girth suggests gastric retention.

Approaches to the prevention or therapy of gastric retention include:

Maintain head of bed 30 degrees above the horizontal for 30 minutes for bolus–fed or intermittent–fed patients to use gravity for gastric emptying.

Switch from bolus or intermittent feeding to continuous feeding.

Ambulate the patient if possible.

Position end of tube in lower duodenum or jejunum rather than gastric tube.

Use medications that stimulate gastric mobility, but not secretion, e.g., metoclopramide.

Dislodgement of the feeding tube is an additional mechanical complication. Tubes may be dislodged upward because of coughing or vomiting. On the other hand, peristalsis may move the tube downward. In either case, the tube must be carefully anchored while still avoiding irritation.

Lastly, a recurring problem is *obstruction of the lumen of the tube* from (1) inadequate irrigation of the tube, (2) attempts to put insufficiently crushed medication through the tube, (3) precipitation of tube feeding with fruit juice or carbonated beverage, or (4) inadequate mixing of the feeding prior to administration.

The incidence of tube obstruction may be reduced by thorough mixing or blenderizing before use, straining the formula and flushing tubes before and after each use for bolus or intermittent feeding, every 4 hours for continuous feeding. For this purpose, 20 to 30 mL of water is used. To unclog an obstructed tube, sometimes water in a syringe can be used to force through the material. If the tube remains clogged, a papain and bicarbonate solution (meat tenderizer) may be effective.

GASTROINTESTINAL COMPLICATIONS

The most common gastrointestinal complications are nausea, vomiting, and diarrhea; on the other hand, some patients become constipated. Table 13-6 lists the problems, causes, prevention, and therapy of these conditions in tube-fed patients. This table shows that many of the causes are within the responsibilities of the nutritional care specialist; therefore, you should study the table carefully.

A number of pathogenic mechanisms unrelated to tube feeding can cause diarrhea; however, diarrhea can be produced in a tube–fed patient who does not have a diarrheal disease. An important etiologic factor is hyperosmolality of the feeding solution, particularly if the feeding is delivered directly into the small bowel. The hyperosmolar solution may delay the passive diffusion of water from the intestinal lumen, or it may even cause a net secretion of water into the lumen to correct the high osmolality. In the case of extremely hyperosmolar solutions delivered very rapidly, the movement of fluid from the vascular system into the intestinal lumen may be rapid enough to cause vascular collapse. As indicated in Table 13–6, hyperosmolar tube feedings may be diluted at first so that they are approximately isoosmotic, and they are given slowly. If the tube feeding is isoosmotic at full strength, further dilution is unlikely to be necessary, and the feeding is simply initated at a slower rate.

If reduction of volume and osmolality do not help resolve the problem, an antidiarrheal agent—such as tincture of opium (paregoric), in a dose of 6 to 10 drops every 6 to 12 hours, kaolin, pectin, 30 mg codeine sulfate every 6 hours, diphenoxylate HCl (Lomotil), or loperamide (Imodium)—is sometimes ordered by the physician and added to the feeding. The intestinal flora of a patient who has been receiving antibiotics may be restored with buttermilk or Lactobacillus tablets.

Some tube–fed patients complain of constipation. The causes, therapy, and prevention are also shown in Table 13-6. Of those therapeutic and preventive measures listed in the table, your responsibility will center on observing the patient's intake and output and providing additional free water as necessary. For some patients, it may be helpful to use a feeding with added fiber. You should keep in mind that patients on lactose–free feedings will have a markedly diminished stool volume, which is not constipation.

METABOLIC COMPLICATIONS

The metabolic complications common in tube-fed patients are overhydration, dehydration, and nutrient imbalances. These are usually avoidable if the patient is carefully monitored. The causes, therapy, and prevention of these complications are listed in Table 13–7, which should be studied carefully. Dehydration is a particular hazard for tube–fed patients, especially infants and patients who cannot express thirst, such as those who are confused or unconscious.

INFECTIOUS COMPLICATIONS

The most common infectious complications are the result of aspiration or contamination of formula.

TABLE 13-6 Gastrointestinal Complications

Problem	Causes	Prevention or Treatment
Abdominal distention, cramping	Gastric retention	Decrease flow rate.
	Rapid infusion	Decrease flow rate.
	Cold feedings	Warm to room temperature; reduce flow rate.
	Hyperosmolar formula	Change to isotonic formula.
	Lactose intolerance	Use lactose-free formula.
	Intestinal atrophy	Reduce volume, start at 1/2 strength, isotonic formula.
	Medication	Evaluate side effects; suggest antispasmodics?
Nausea and vomiting	Incorrect patient position	Elevate head 30–45 degrees; turn to right side.
	Rapid infusion	Slow rate to previous tolerated level; advance more slowly.
	Incorrect tube	Check placement; aspirate contents.
	Hyperosmolar formula	Dilute formula or change to isotonic; advance slowly.
	Gastric retention	Stop feeding 2 hr and check residuals; ambulate if possible.
	Lactose intolerance	Use lactose-free formula.
	Excess fat	Use lower fat formula.
	Unpleasant odor	Add flavoring (be careful of osmolal changes).
Diarrhea	Rapid infusion	Decrease rate.
		Change bolus to continuous feeding.
	Volume overload	Decrease amount; advance more slowly
	Hyperosmolar formula	Change to isotonic; start with diluted formula; reduce rate; advance slowly every 12–24 hours.
	Lactose intolerance	Use lactose-free formula.
	Fat malabsorption	Use lower fat formula; Evaluate for pancreatic insufficiency; supplement pancreatic enzymes?
	Cold feedings	Warm feedings; reduce rate.
	Impaction	Provide adequate water; medication?
	Contaminated formula	See Table 13-7.
	Medications	Evaluate side effects; suggest antidiarrhea drug?
	Decrease bulk	Change formula.
Constipation	Dehydration	Monitor I and O. Add water so I > 0 by 500–1,000mL.
	Inactivity	Ambulate if possible.
	Medications	Evaluate side effects, suggest stool softeners, bulk formers?
	Obstruction	Stop feeding.
	Impaction	Add water..

Compiled from D.B.A. Silk and J.J. Payne-James. Complications of enteral nutrition. In J.L. Rombeau and M.D. Caldwell. *Clinical Nutrition: Enteral and Tube Feeding, 2d ed.* Philadelphia: Saunders, 1990; K.T. Ideno. Enteral nutrition: In: Gottschlich, L.E. Matarese, and E.P. Shronts. eds. *Nutrition Support Dietetics Core Curriculum, 2d ed.* Silver Spring, MD:ASPEN, 1993; M. Bernard, and L. Forlaw. Complications and their prevention. In: J.L. Rombeau, and M.D. Caldwell. *Enteral and Tube Feeding.* Philadelphia: Saunders, 1984: and American Dietetic Association. Handbook of Clinical Dietetics, 2d ed. New Haven: Yale University Press 1992.

Aspiration Pneumonia

Pneumonia can develop as a result of vomiting or regurgitation and aspiration of stomach contents. A major preventive measure is to keep the patient's head elevated 30 degrees at all times during continuous feeding and for 2 hours following intermittent feeding. Aspiration is more likely to occur in patients with decreased mental ability or with decreased ability to close the glottis. These include those with a tracheostomy, for example, patients after radical neck surgery, or those with an endotracheal tube, such as patients on respirators. Other patients at high risk are those with head or neck surgery or respiratory problems and those who have trouble swallowing their own saliva. It is helpful in those patients to use nasoduodenal, in preference to nasogastric, feeding and to elevate the patient's head 30 degrees if possible. The volume of gastric contents should be minimized. Since high osmolality retards gastric emptying, you will need to dilute hypertonic fluids and build up to concentrated forms slowly. High-fat formulas also retard gastric emptying, and reducing fat content may be helpful. Table 13-8 summarizes methods for prevention.

Contaminated Formulas and Equipment

Commercially prepared formulas are generally preferred over those prepared in the hospital because they reduce

TABLE 13-7   Metabolic Complications

Problem	Possible Causes	Prevention or Treatment
Dehydration / hypernatremia	Inadequate fluid intake	Monitor fluid I and O.
		Monitor body weight daily.
	Excess fluid loss	Monitor serum electrolytes, SUN, serum creatinine,, urine specific gravity daily.
	Hypertonic, high-protein feeding	Replace fluid loss and give maintenance fluids daily.
		Dilute or change formula if necessary. Reduce flow rate.
Overhydration / hyponatremia	Refeeding; PCM; some cardiac, renal, or hepatic disease	Decrease volume; Restrict fluids,
		Use concentrated feeding,,
		Diuretic therapy.
Hyperglycemia	Refeeding	Stop feeding or slow rate.
	Metabolic stress	Give insulin?
	Diabetes?	Monitor blood glucose.
		Increase fat, decrease carbohydrate.
Hypoglycemia	Fluid overload	Monitor blood glucose daily;
	Sudden stop in feeding of patient receiving hypoglycemic agents	Taper feeding gradually
Hyperkalemia	High-K-feeding	Monitor serum K daily.
	Renal insufficiency	Change formula; reduce K
	Metabolic acidosis	Suggest insulin, glucose.
Hypokalemia	Refeeding	Monitor serum K daily.
	Diuretics	Supplement K and Cl..
	Excess loss	
	Metabolic acidosis	
	Insulin therapy	
Hyperphosphatemia	Renal insufficiency	Change formula to lower phosphate
		Give phosphate binders.
Hypophosphatemia	Malnutrition	IV phosphate or supplement phosphate enterally.
Essential fatty acid deficiency	EFA deficiency in formula	Add 5 ml safflower oil daily, change formula..
Abnormal liver function	Unknown	Stop or change formula? (Reverts to normal when feeding is stopped).
Excess CO_2	Overfeeding carbohydrate	Increase fat to 30–50 % of total kcal; decrease carbohydrate in formula.

Compiled from D.B.A. Silk, and J.J. Payne-James. Complications of enteral nutrition. In: J.L.Rombeau, and M.D. Caldwell. *Clinical Nutrition: Enteral and Tube Feeding,* 2d ed. Philadelphia: Saunders, 1990; K.T. Ideno, Enteral nutrition. In: M.M. Gottschlich, L.E. Matarese, and E.P. Shronts. eds. *Nutrition Support Dietetics Core Curriculum,* 2d ed. Silver Spring, MD: ASPEN, 1993; M. Bernard, and L. Forlaw. Complications and their prevention. In: J.L. Rombeau, and M.D. Caldwell. *Enteral and Tube Feeding.* Philadelphia: Saunders, 1984; and American Dietetic Association. *Handbook of Clinical Dietetics,* 2d ed. New Haven: Yale University Press, 1992.

the risk of contamination. Many formulas are now available in a sterile, prefilled, closed system. Hospital-prepared formulas are prepared in the pharmacy in some institutions and by the Department of Dietetics in others. In any case, clean technique should be used during preparation. You may need to be familiar with this technique in order to instruct employees in formula preparation.

Policies regarding the length of time a formula can be left hanging vary among institutions. In some hospitals, it is believed that enteral formulas can be hung for 8 to 12 hours at room temperature without clinically significant contamination. Feeding equipment, except for the tube, should be changed every 24 hours. Formula preparation should be limited to the amount used in 24 hours. See Table 13–8 for prevention of infection.

PSYCHOSENSORY COMPLICATIONS

You may be able to assist the patient with the psychosensory deprivation that accompanies tube feeding. Some patients are distressed by the lack of taste of food.

If they are cooperative, they may be allowed to chew, and then spit out, food. Other patients have considerable discomfort from dryness of the mouth and nasal passages. Depending on the specific condition, the patient might be given additional water, ice, chewing gum, or hard candy. Some patients are particularly in need of reassurance.

MONITORING THE TUBE-FED PATIENT

All patients receiving tube feeding must be carefully monitored by the Nutrition Support Service. Usually, the nursing staff will monitor gastric residuals, flow rate, and vital signs and will record the intake and output of fluid and formula. A nutritionist should monitor patients for indicators in three areas: tolerance to the formula, state of hydration, and nutritional response. It is important to use these indicators, as well as routine nutritional assessment methods (see Chapter 5) to establish baseline data; thereafter, repeated measurements are made to monitor progress. The laboratory test panels commonly used in monitoring the tube–fed patient are those listed as Preliminary Screening and Broad Spectrum Screening in Table E-5. You should be familiar with normal values (see Tables E-3 to E-4) and the significance of abnormal values in the tube-fed patient.

TABLE 13-8 Infectious Complications

Causes	Prevention
Contamination in "homemade" formula	Use sterile, commercial formulas. Sanitize equipment.
Contamination of reservoir	Use larger containers to reduce handling
Contaminated equipment	Sanitize equipment. Use "clean technique" in handling. Use sterile commercial formulas.
Poor personal hygiene	Careful handwashing by caretakers.
Improper storage	Store covered, refrigeration temperature. Limit storage time to 24 hours Limit hang time per institution policy (8 hours?)
Aspiration of formula	Verify tube placement every 4-8 hours Monitor gastric residuals. Raise head of bed. Reduce caliber of tube to <10.F. Change to post-pyloric tube location?

Compiled from D.B.A. Silk, and J.J. Payne-James. Complications of enteral nutrition. In J.L. Rombeau, and M.D. Caldwell. *Clinical Nutrition: Enteral and Tube Feeding,* 2d ed. Philadelphia: Saunders, 1990: K.T. Ideno, Enteral nutrition. *In:* M.M.Gottschlich, L.E. Matarese, and E. P Shronts. eds. *Nutrition Support Dietetics Core Curriculum,* 2d ed. Silver Spring, MD: ASPEN, 1993; M. Bernard, and J.L. Forlaw. Complications and their prevention. *In* J.L. Rombeau, J.L. and M.D. Caldwell. *Enteral and Tube Feeding.* Philadelphia: Saunders, 1984: and American Dietetic Association. *Handbook of Clinical Dietetics,* 2d ed. New Haven: Yale University Press, 1992

INDICATORS OF FORMULA TOLERANCE

Stool frequency and consistency will be noted in the medical record by the nursing staff, who will also note any vomiting that occurs. The patient can be questioned concerning untoward symptoms such as abdominal distention and bloating. When these occur, it may be necessary to stop the feedings until symptoms subside and then restart them on a more conservative schedule.

Blood glucose is an indication of carbohydrate tolerance. It should be tested daily until the patient is stable and goal flow rate of formula has been reached. It may then be monitored 2 to 3 times/week in the nondiabetic patient, but continued daily if the patient is diabetic. For stable long–term tube–fed patients, recommended intervals are every 6 months for nondiabetics, and daily if the patient is diabetic (11).

If the diabetic, septic, or severely stressed patient cannot metabolize the carbohydrate, insulin is sometimes given, rather than reducing the carbohydrate content, and thus the energy level, of the formula. The use of a continuous feeding to replace intermittent feeding is also helpful.

INDICATORS OF HYDRATION STATUS

The patient should be weighed initially and at frequent intervals thereafter. Some protocols require daily weighing, while others require weights 3 times per week. Daily measurements of input and output of formula and of water, recorded separately, are essential. This is generally a nursing responsibility. If the patient suddenly gains or loses weight, a disturbance in hydration status should be investigated. Indicators of dehydration will include hypernatremia and azotemia, hyperchloridemia, hyperglycemia, and elevated hematocrit. In addition, the dehydrated patient will show evidence of dry mucous membrane, poor turgor, decreased blood volume with low blood pressure, and increased levels of serum protein, hematocrit, and blood cells. Overhydration may be indicated by weight gain, elevated blood pressure, edema, and jugular vein distention.

In a typical protocol, laboratory values available in the patient's chart are BUN, serum glucose, serum sodium, serum potassium, serum chloride, serum albumin (done twice a week), Broad–Spectrum Screening (done weekly), and a CBC with red–cell indices (done weekly). (See Table E-3 and Chapter 4).

EVALUATION OF NUTRITIONAL RESPONSE

Nutritional assessment of the tube-fed patient must be more detailed than is the case for many orally fed patients. Body weights and the selected laboratory values just described are useful. In addition, the following have been recommended for evaluation of nutritional response:

1. Calorie count daily for 5 to 7 days, and then weekly. Monitor the amount actually administered compared to the amount ordered.
2. Urinary urea nitrogen and urine creatinine for original nutritional assessment and weekly thereafter for assessment and calculation of nitrogen balance.
3. Determination of nitrogen intake to calculate nitrogen balance.
4. Estimation of energy expenditure initially and repeated any time a change is likely to have occurred.
5. Serum albumin until the patient is stable, then monthly; twice yearly in long-term patients.
6. Serum iron and transferrin or TIBC weekly until the patient is stable and twice monthly thereafter.
7. Serum magnesium biweekly in the severely malnourished patient.
8. Phosphorus and liver function twice weekly; twice yearly in long-term patients (12)

DOCUMENTATION OF THE TUBE FEEDING

The medical record is an essential tool in communicating information on the tube feeding to other members of the health care team. The information documented by the nutritionist varies with the division of responsibility. You may be expected to include the following:

1. Recommendations on the type of feeding tube, if not surgically placed.
2. Recommended formula
3. Recommended method and rate of delivery
4. Actual formula intake, with kcal and protein content
5. Patient's tolerance to tube feeding; complications
6. Recommended corrective action
7. Education about tube feeding provided to the patient

In most institutions, your recommendations for items 1 through 3 and 6 must be countersigned by the attending physician.

TOPICS FOR FURTHER DISCUSSION

1. New tube–feeding products are frequently developed, and changes are continually being made in existing formulation. What methods and sources of information could you use to keep up to date in this area?
2. Discuss the content and purpose of new products not listed in Appendix K.

3. Why are most tube–feeding formulas not recommended for use in newborn infants?

REFERENCES

1. **Davenport, H.W.** *Physiology of the Digestive Tract, 4th ed.* Chicago: Yearbook Medical Publishers, 1977.
2. American Dietetic Association. *Handbook of Clinical Dietetics, 2d ed.* New Haven: Yale University Press, 1992.
3. **Mitchell, H.H.** A method of determining the biological values of protein. *J. Biol. Chem.* 58:(1924)873.
4. **Aser, B.L.** Method for ingesting essential amino acid content in the nutritional evaluation of protein. *J. Am. Dietet. Assoc.* 27:(1951)396.
5. **Kinney, J.M.** Energy requirements of the surgical patient. In W.F. Ballinger, J.A. Collins, W.R. Drucker, S.J. Dudrick, and R. Zeppa. eds. *Manual of Surgical Nutrition,* Philadelphia: Saunders, 1975.
6. **Shils, M.E.**, et al *Liquid Formulas for Oral Feedings.* New York: Memorial Sloan-Kettering Cancer Institute, 1979.
7. Council on Scientific Affairs. Vitamin preparations as dietary supplements and as therapeutic agents. *J.A.M.A.* 257:(1987) 1929–36,.
8. **Engel, F.L., and C. Jaeger**, Dehydration with hypernatremia, hyperchloremia, and azotemia complicating nasogastric tube feeding. *Am. J. Med.* 17:(1954)196.
9. **Gault, M.H., and M.E. Dixon**, Hypernatremia, azotemia, and dehydration due to high protein tube feeding. *Ann. Int. Med.* 68:(1968)778.
10. **Marable, N.L., M.L. Hinners, N.W. Hardison, and N.L. Kehrberg**. Protein quality of supplements and meal replacements. *J. Am. Dietet. Assoc.* 77:(1980) 270–276.
11. **Ideno, K.T.** Enteral nutrition. *In* M.M. Gottschlich, L.E. Matarese, and E.P. Shronts, eds. *Nutrition Support Dietetics. Core Curriculum, 2d ed.* Silver Spring, MD: American Society for Parenteral and Enteral Nutrition, 1993.
12. **Kagawa–Busby, K.S., M.M. Heitkemper, B.C. Hansen R.L. Hanson, and V.V. Vanderburg.** Effects of diet temperature on tolerance of enteral feedings. *Nurs. Res.* 29:(1980)276–280.

ADDITIONAL SOURCES OF INFORMATION

Smith, J.L. and S.B. Heymsfield. Enteral nutrition support: Formula preparation from modular ingredients. *JPEN* 7:(1983) 280– 288.

Rombeau, J.L. and M.D. Caldwell, *Clinical Nutrition: Enteral and Tube Feeding, 2d ed.*, Philadelphia: Saunders, 1990.

✓ TO TEST YOUR UNDERSTANDING

1. How many grams of protein would be contained in 2,000 ml of a formula with a caloric density of 1kcal/mL, 15% of which are from protein?

  a. What is the nonpro kcal:N ratio?

2. A patient is receiving a tube feeding that contains the following: 1,000 mL, 2 kcal/mL, 20% of energy from crystalline amino acids, 5.0 mEq Na$^+$/100 mL, 2.5 mEq K$^+$/100 mL, and 7.8 mEq Cl$^-$/100 mL.

  a. What is his renal solute load? (Show your calculations.)

  b. If the patient had a renal disease in which his maximum renal concentrating ability were 200 mOsm/L, what would be the consequences of giving this formula? Why?

  c. What would you recommend for this patient?

3. Your instructor will provide some samples of supplementary feedings and tube feedings. On the form on the next page, evaluate these formulas. Fill in the form after examining and tasting the products.

4. Suggest some characteristics of tube feeding you might recommend for the following patients. Explain your answers.

  a. A patient who has been NPO for 4 days

  b. An adult patient with severely decreased gastrointestinal function

  c. A patient in transition from total parenteral nutrition (TPN) to tube feeding

  d. A patient who complains of constipation

5. A patient who had a traumatic injury to his head and neck, followed by major plastic surgery, has a feeding gastrostomy created by the surgeon. The end of the feeding tube lies immediately distal to the pyloric sphincter. The patient is underweight and is losing more weight. He is known to be lactose intolerant.

  a. What category of tube feeding would you recommend the patient be given?

  b. What diameter tube would be required?

6. A comatose patient is receiving 2,000 mL of a tube–feeding formula which provides 1 kcal/mL. Composition is as follows: carbohydrate 54.5% of kcal, protein 14% of kcal, and fat 31.5% of kcal. It is given in eight bolus feedings of 250 mL each. The tube is rinsed with 20 mL of water as previously described. How much free water does the patient receive in 24 hours? Show your calculations.

7. Describe the type of complication you might expect in the following situations and describe preventive measures.

  a. A blenderized feeding given through an 8F tube into the stomach

  b. 2,000 mL of formula, 900 mOsm/kg, containing 30% intact protein

8. A patient in a coma is being fed by tube a lactose–free formula containing soy protein isolate. The protocol includes 100 mL of water to follow each feeding. What purpose(s) does this water serve?

9. What change in a tube–feeding protocol might be indicated by the following developments?

  a. Elevated temperature (fever) in the patient

  b. Large amount of exudate from a wound

  c. Warm environment

  d. Loss of ability to concentrate urine

10. List possible actions that might be taken to correct the following in the tube–fed patient.

  a. Dehydration

  b. Constipation

  c. Hyperglycemia

(continued)

Evaluation of Special Feeding Products

	Appearance (Check One)				Viscosity (Check One)			Taste & Acceptability (Check all that apply)			
PRODUCT	Clear	Cloudy	Opaque	Color	Watery	Syrupy	Semiliquid	Very acceptable	Marginally acceptable	Distasteful	Repulsive

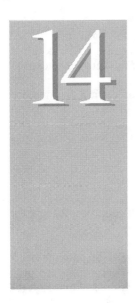

14 Parenteral Nutrition

Parenteral feeding includes any method of feeding that bypasses the digestive tract. The term *parenteral nutrition* (PN) includes the provision of partial or total nutritional requirements by the intravenous route. Parenteral nutrition can be used in addition to enteral feedings or as a sole source of nutrients. When it fills all the nutrient requirements, it is commonly referred to as *total parenteral nutrition* or TPN. Dudrick and his colleagues (1) first developed the technique of TPN in the mid-1960s, and it is now a widely used, often life-saving technique for the provision of nutritional support.

Many institutions have *nutrition support teams* that assist in the management of the nutritional care of patients who require specialized enteral-parenteral feeding systems. The nutrition support team comprises a physician, who is often a surgeon, a pharmacist, a nurse, and a nutritional care specialist. Other specialists who may advise the team, especially if home parenteral nutrition is being considered, include a social worker, psychiatrist or psychologist, and an expert in reimbursement issues.

The role of the nutrition care specialist in the care of patients receiving PN has many aspects that may include: evaluating nutritional status through nutrition assessment (Chapter 5); taking medical and dietary histories (Chapter 6); calculating nutrient requirements; recommending parenteral prescriptions; assessing the adequacy of intake and tolerance to parenteral formulations; monitoring laboratory data, clinical status, and outcome of therapy; and educating the patient (Chapter 7) (2). A knowledge of the composition of solutions used in PN and the protocols for administering TPN are essential for the nutrition care specialist. In addition, recording of nutrient intake and parameters reflecting nutritional status in the medical record may serve as the basis for decisions concerning the discontinuation of parenteral feeding. Once the transition to enteral tube feeding or oral feeding is started, monitoring nutrient intake is especially important.

This chapter will explain, without reference to specific diagnoses, the composition of PN solutions, the assessment of parenteral nutrient needs, protocols for administering TPN, and transitional feeding from parenteral to enteral nutrition. After completing this chapter and the "To Test Your Understanding" questions, you should be able to design a parenteral feeding regimen. Considerations in pediatric PN are discussed briefly at the end of this chapter.

TERMINOLOGY

Parenteral feedings can be administered peripherally, usually into the veins of the arm, or centrally. *Central parenteral nutrition* (CPN) usually involves infusion into the superior vena cava, which is reached via the internal jugular or subclavian vein (Fig. 14-1). *Peripheral parenteral nutrition* (PPN) involves infusion into small veins, usually in the arm (Fig. 14-2). Parenteral feedings, either PPN or CPN, may be given concurrently with enteral feeding. In this chapter we will use CPN to denote central administration and PPN to denote peripheral administration of PN, whether or not enteral feeding is also used.

Total nutrient admixture (TNA) refers to the increasingly common practice of adding all of the components of TPN— i.e. dextrose, amino acids, lipid emulsion, electrolytes, vitamins, trace elements, and other additives— into a single container for infusion into the patient. The preparation of PN solutions is done in the

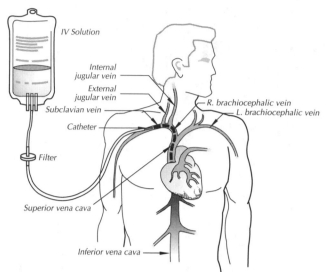

FIGURE 14-1   Central parenteral nutrition (CPN) is administered into large veins such as the superior vena cava, which is reached via the internal jugular or subclavian vein.

pharmacy, and if TNA solutions are prepared, an automated compounding device that is interfaced with a computer is usually used to provide rapid and accurate mixing of the parenteral solutions.

INDICATIONS AND CONTRAINDICATIONS

The primary indication for the use of parenteral feeding is that sufficient calories cannot be ingested or absorbed enterally. Parenteral nutrition is used to feed patients who either are already malnourished or have the potential for developing malnutrition.

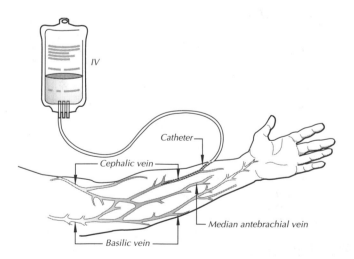

FIGURE 14-2   Peripheral parenteral nutrition (PPN) is administered into small veins, usually in the arm.

Clinical presentations that may indicate the need for parenteral feeding include:

1. Intestinal dysfunction/failure including inflammatory bowel diseases such as Crohn's disease, and ulcerative colitis, short-bowel syndrome, and chronic intestinal pseudo-obstruction
2. Excessive nutritional needs that cannot be met by enteral feeding, and accompanying hypermetabolic states, such as burns, multiple trauma, or sepsis
3. Organ failure including liver, kidney, pancreas, or respiratory failure
4. Cancer including AIDS and bone marrow transplantation (3)
5. Neurologic impairment
6. Severe malnutrition or refusal to eat, as in anorexia nervosa

Specific guidelines for the use of PN in patients with these and other specific diseases and conditions are provided by the American Society for Parenteral and Enteral Nutrition, or ASPEN (4).

There are two major contraindications to TPN. The first is the presence of a functioning gastrointestinal tract. A useful guideline is the adage "If the gut works, use it!" The second contraindication is the existence of a terminal condition for which aggressive medical therapy is not provided. Advanced inoperable cancer is an example.

COMPONENTS OF PARENTERAL NUTRITION SOLUTIONS

The nutrient needs of a patient fed parenterally are similar to the requirements of a patient fed enterally. As always, the six major categories of nutrients—carbohydrate, protein, fat, vitamins, minerals, and fluid—must be considered, as must adequate energy intake. However, the form of many nutrients must be specialized for direct infusion into the blood without prior digestion.

CARBOHYDRATE

Carbohydrate is given as *dextrose* or glucose monohydrate. This yields 3.4 kcal per g, rather than the general 4 kcal per g, because of the attached noncaloric water molecule. Commercial dextrose preparations are available in concentrations from 2.5 to 70 percent, although the 70-percent solutions are most commonly used for TNA.

PROTEIN

Protein is supplied as solutions of crystalline amino acids, which are available in various concentrations. The 10- and 15-percent concentrations are often stocked in hospital pharmacies because they can be easily diluted to the desired final concentration. Several types of amino acid solutions are available. These include not only conventional amino acid solutions for patients with normal organ function but also some special-purpose formulations, such as those containing a high proportion of branched-chain amino acids for trauma and liver failure, essential amino acid formulations for renal failure, or specialized formulations for rapidly growing neonates. The special-purpose amino acid solutions are more expensive than standard amino acid solutions and should be used only when indicated.

The amino acid compositions of several different types of parenteral solutions are summarized in Table 14-1. Standard commercial amino acid solutions usually contain 40 to 50 percent essential amino acids and 50 to 60 percent nonessential amino acids. The amino acid profile of standard adult solutions differs in a number of ways from the amino acid profile of enteral formulas. These differences include the absence or reduced levels of glutamic and aspartic acids, low levels of cysteine and tyrosine, which are relatively insoluble, and higher levels of arginine, alanine, and glycine. Amino acid solutions provide an equivalent amount of protein, on the basis of a gram of amino acid per gram of protein, and are calculated to provide 4.0 kcal/g when oxidized for energy.

TABLE 14-1 Intravenous Amino Acid Solutions

Composition	Conventional Aminosyn 10% (Abbott)	Conventional Novamine 15% (Clintec)	NephrAmine[*] 5.4 % (McGaw)	Aminosyn-HBC[†] 7 % (Abbott)	Heptamine[‡] 8% (McGaw)
Amino Acid concentration (g/100mL)	10	15	5.4	7	8
Nitrogen (g/100mL)	1.57	2.37	0.65	1.12	1.2
Essential amino acids (mg/100mL)					
Isoleucine[§]	720	749	560	789	900
Leucine[§]	940	1,040	880	1,576	1,100
Lysine	720	1,180	640	265	610
Methionine	400	749	880	206	100
Phenylalanine	440	1,040	880	228	100
Threonine	520	749	400	272	450
Tryptophan	160	250	200	88	66
Valine[§]	800	960	640	789	840
Nonesential amino acids (mg/100mL)					
Alanine	1,280	2,170	—	660	770
Arginine	980	1,470	—	507	600
Aspartic acid	—	434	—	—	—
Cysteine	—	—	< 20	—	< 20
Glutamic acid	—	749	—	—	—
Glycine	1,280	1,040	—	660	900
Histidine	300	894	250	154	240
Proline	860	894	—	448	800
Serine	420	592	—	221	500
Tyrosine	44	39	—	33	—
Electrolytes (mEq/100mL)					
Acetate	14.8	15.1	4.4	7.2	6.2
Chloride	—	—	< 0.3	—	0.3
Phosphate (mmol/L)	—	—	—	—	1.0
Potassium	0.54	—	—	—	—
Sodium	—	—	0.5	0.7	1.0
Osmolarity (mOsm/L)	1,000	1,388	435	665	785

[*] Renal failure formula
[†] Branched-chain amino acid–enriched stress formulation.
[‡] Hepatic failure formula.
[§] Branched-chain amino acids.

FAT

Fat is needed during PN as an energy source and to provide the essential fatty acids (EFA) linoleic and linolenic. At present, 10- and 20-percent fat emulsions are available in a variety of volumes. The basic ingredients in the fat emulsion include 10 or 20 percent fat from soy or a blend of safflower plus soy oil, 1.2 percent egg yolk phospholipid for use as an emulsifying agent, and 2.2 to 2.5 percent glycerin to make the emulsion isotonic. The 10-percent fat emulsions provide 1.1 kcal per mL, while 20-percent fat emulsions provide 2.0 kcal per mL. Both 10- and 20-percent fat emulsions are isotonic to blood. The emulsions composed of a blend of safflower and soybean oil supply approximately 66 percent of fatty acid content as the EFA linoleate, while the emulsions containing soy oil supply 50 percent of fatty acids as linoleate. The composition of representative fat emulsions is summarized in Table 14-2. EFA requirements can be met by providing 500 mL of a 10 percent fat emulsion 2 to 3 times a week, or 200 mL daily.

ASSESSING PARENTERAL NUTRIENT NEEDS

An assessment of parenteral energy and protein needs is the first step in planning a parenteral-feeding regimen. In general, the techniques for calculating parenteral energy and protein needs are similar to those discussed for enteral feeding in Chapter 5. However during TPN, frequent reevaluations of body weight, nitrogen balance, serum albumin level, any dietary intake, and other parameters of nutritional status are necessary to monitor the adequacy of the parenteral feeding regimen. For example, a critically ill patient may undergo several stressful periods during the course of the illness, such as surgery, septic complications, and development or resolution of a fistula, and nutrient needs would be likely to change throughout these periods.

ENERGY

If possible energy needs should be determined by measurement of gas exchange through indirect calorimetry. However, this technique may not be available in all settings and may be inaccurate in patients maintained with ventilators. Thus, energy needs can be calculated using the Harris and Benedict equation, followed by multiplication by an activity and injury factor: Eq. (5-19) to (5-21). In practice, only a few conditions require use of an injury factor greater than 1, e.g., burns, head injury, or multiple trauma. Thus, the calculation of total parenteral energy needs is often simplified to BEE multiplied by an activity factor, where an AF of 1.2 is used for patients confined to bed, 1.3 for patients who are ambulatory, and 1.5 for normally active people, as may occur for someone on home TPN.

Another approach to the estimation of calorie needs is based on requirements expressed on the basis of kcal per kg of body weight per day, as shown in Table 14-3. These recommendations also consider the severity of injury and a direct relationship between nitrogen excretion and caloric expenditure (6). *As a general rule, a range of calories from 30 to 35 kcal per kg body weight per day*

TABLE 14-2 Composition of Intravenous Fat Emulsions

Product[*]	Osmolarity (mOsm/L)	Glycerin (%)	Fatty Acid Content (%)		
			Linoleic	Linolenic	Other[†]
Soybean oil based					
Intralipid 10% or 20%	260	2.25	50	9	41
Liposyn III 10% or 20%	292	2.5	54.5	8.3	37.2
Nutrilipid 10%	280	2.21	49–60	6–9	31–45
Nutrilipid 20%	315	2.21	49–60	6–9	31–45
Soyacal 10%	280	2.21	49–60	6–9	31–45
Soyacal 20%	315	2.21	49–60	6–9	31–45
Safflower and soybean oil–based (50%/50%)					
Liposyn II 10%	276	2.5	65.8	4.2	30
Liposyn II 20%	258	2.5	65.8	4.2	30

[*] Intralipid is manufactured by Kabi-Vitrum, Liposyn by Abbott, Nutrilipid by McGaw, and Soyacal by Alpha Therapeutic. All products with 10% lipid provide 1.1 kcal/mL those with 20% lipid provide 2.0 kcal/mL. All products contain 1.2% egg yolk phospholipid, which provides 15 mmol of phosphorus per liter.
[†] Other fatty acids: oleic, palmitic, and stearic.

TABLE 14-3 Considerations in Parenteral Carbohydrate, Protein, and Fat Infusion

Caloric Density	Availability	Requirements / Tolerance
Carbohydrate: dextrose monohydrate		
3.4 kcal / g	5%, 10%, 20%, 30%, 40%, 50%, 60%, and 70% in a wide range of volumes.	Maximum tolerance of 0.36 g dextrose / kg / hr (range of 4–6 mg / kg / min); may provide up to 70% energy. Peripheral venous infusion is tolerated if the final dextrose concentration is less than 7%.
Protein: crystalline amino acid		
4.0 kcal / g amino acid or protein	4–15% in a wide range of volumes. Special formulations are available for renal or hepatic disease or for neonates.	1.2–1.5 g pro/kg for mild–moderate stress. kcal: N ratio of 100–150: 1 for anabolism.
Fat: emulsion of soybean or safflower oil		
1.1 kcal / cc (10%), 2.0 kcal / cc (20%)	10% and 20% solutions in units of 50, 100, 200, 250, and 500 mL.	2%–4% kcal as fat to prevent EFA deficiency; 8% kcal to correct EFA deficiency. Maximum level of 60% kcal as fat or 0.5–2.5 g / fat / kg /day. Fat emulsions usually supply 10–40% of energy. Larger amounts of fat are given if decreased CO_2 production is desired or fluid must be restricted.

or 1.5 times BEE is sufficient for maintenance in most patients with mild to moderate stress. For the obese patient, calculation of BEE using actual weight may yield excessive calories, and BEE may have to be decreased by 20 to 30 percent based on actual weight. An alternative is to calculate calorie needs for the obese patient using ideal body weight.

Parenteral infusion of calories in excess of 40 kcal per kg body weight should be avoided unless clearly indicated for maintenance of body weight in conditions such as burns or severe trauma. The provision of excess calories by the parenteral route may lead to such complications as hepatomegaly, liver dysfunction, pulmonary distress, increased energy expenditure, and hyperglycemia-induced osmotic diuresis. In providing nutritional support to the catabolic patient, the initial goal is usually to *preserve* lean body mass and then, later, when the patient is more stable, actually to *replenish* nutrient reserves.

The nutritional support of the depleted patient must be carried out gradually. Depleted patients incorporate nitrogen more efficiently and at lower caloric levels than do normal patients, so it is easy to overestimate their caloric needs. Overzealous nutritional support of the depleted patient can lead to a "refeeding syndrome," that is characterized by hypophosphatemia, hypokalemia, hyperglycemia, fluid retention, and cardiac arrest (7).

PROTEIN

According to the Recommended Dietary Allowance (RDA), a healthy adult needs 0.8 g pro per kg ideal body weight. *For the majority of patients with mild to moderate stress, 1.2 to 1.5 g protein per kg ideal body weight is indicated to promote anabolism.* Needs may increase up to 2.5 g protein per kg, with conditions accompanied by increased nitrogen excretion, such as burns, severe trauma, or presence of a fistula (Table 14-4). Protein restriction may be indicated in hepatic encephalopathy, or in renal failure where dialysis is contraindicated.

The calorie to nitrogen ratio (kcal:N) must be considered in determining protein needs, as an adequate

TABLE 14-4 Energy and Protein Requirements of Hospitalized Patients

Patient Condition	Energy Requirements (kcal / kg / day)	Nitrogen Excretion (g / day)	Protein Requirements (g / kg / day)
Normal	25–30	5–10	0.8–1.0
Elective surgery	28–30	8–10	1.0–1.5
Severe Injury	30–35	10–15	1.5–2.0
Severe trauma / burns	45–55	>15	2.0–2.5

Adapted from C.L. Long, and W.S. Blakemore, Energy and protein requirements in the hospitalized patient. *JPEN* 3:(1979)69–71.

energy intake is necessary to support use of protein for anabolism. *A kcal:N ratio of 200 to 300 kcal:1 g N is adequate for normal body maintenance. In stressful conditions, a kcal:N ratio of 100 to 150 kcal:1 g N is indicated to promote anabolism.* Some clinicians calculate only nonprotein calories when evaluating PN prescriptions because, in theory, amino acids are being provided for protein synthesis and repair (2). Thus, the *nonprotein kcal:N ratio* is sometimes used. The adequacy of protein intake can be assessed by determination of nitrogen balance Eqs. (5-22) and (5-23). If possible, adequate protein should be given to maintain a positive nitrogen balance of 2 to 4 g N per day.

CARBOHYDRATE

There is a limit to the quantity of parenteral dextrose that can be oxidized for energy without serving as a substrate for lipogenesis. Many of the earlier problems noted with TPN, such as fatty liver and liver dysfunction, are thought to have been the result of infusion of excess dextrose calories. Postoperative surgical patients have been shown to oxidize a maximum of 4 to 6 mg per kg per minute, or 0.24 to 0.36 g per kg per hour, of intravenous dextrose (8, 9). In designing a parenteral-feeding regimen, the quantity of dextrose calories will be determined in large part by deciding the percentage of calories to provide as fat. *However, dextrose should not be given at a rate greater than 0.36 g per kg body weight per hour.*

LIPID

The provision of fat in parenteral nutrition reduces the calories required from dextrose and more closely approximates an enteral diet. However, liver dysfunction and impaired lipid clearance and immune function have been associated with the parenteral infusion of excess lipid calories. The prevention of EFA deficiency requires administration of 2 to 4 percent of calories as linoleic acid, or approximately 10 percent of calories from soy or safflower oil emulsions. Most patients receive 10 to 40 percent of daily energy needs from intravenous fat emulsions, or 0.5 to 1.0 g fat per kg. An upper limit of 60 percent of calories as fat or no greater than 2.5 g fat per kg in adults is usually set. Absolute contraindications to the administration of intravenous fat emulsions include pathologic hyperlipidemia, lipoid nephrosis, severe egg allergy, and acute pancreatitis associated with hyperlipidemia (10). Administration of 30 to 50 percent of calories from fat may benefit patients with compromised respiratory function who often develop respiratory acidosis due to increased carbon dioxide production when excessive dextrose is given. The oxidation of fat produces less carbon dioxide compared to the oxidation of dextrose.

Although rare, acute adverse reactions may occur with parenteral infusion of fat emulsions. The reactions usually occur immediately after initiation and include, fear, chills, oily taste, and respiratory difficulties (2). The reactions may be related to the dose of fat emulsion and the rate of infusion. A test dose of 1 mg lipid per minute for 30 minutes can be used to evaluate the possibility of side effects. Lipid tolerance should be assessed during hospitalization by monitoring serum triglyceride levels before and 6 hours after lipid infusion. If an individual is unable to tolerate intravenously administered fat emulsions, recommendations for supplementation with EFA include cycling the PN therapy to allow endogenous release of EFA from fat stores or daily oral intake of fat (2).

The provision of fat as a continuous infusion or as part of a TNA is preferred because less fluctuation in serum triglyceride concentrations and improved fat oxidation occur when fat emulsions are given continuously in moderate doses. Parenteral-feeding solutions composed of higher proportions of fat are often used in PPN, as fat has the advantage of providing a high caloric density with low osmolarity.

A summary of various considerations affecting the provision of parenteral carbohydrate, protein and fat is shown in Table 14-3.

FLUID

The fluid requirements of a patient will determine the percentage of dextrose needed in designing a parenteral-feeding regimen. Methods for estimating fluid requirements are outlined in Table 4-2. Adults generally need 30 to 40 ml fluid per kg body weight to maintain hydration. Fluid requirements are increased with increased renal, gastrointestinal, dermal, or respiratory losses. Fluid requirements are decreased with cardiac or renal insufficiency.

ELECTROLYTES

Electrolytes in maintenance or therapeutic doses need to be added daily to the parenteral nutrition solution to maintain electrolyte homeostasis. Electrolyte requirements in parenteral nutrition vary, but representative levels are shown in Table 14-5.

The need for electrolytes is decreased in conditions where normal losses of electrolyte are reduced, such as

TABLE 14-5 Representative Electrolyte Levels

Electrolyte	Amount / Day (mmol)
Sodium	60–150
Potassium	60–150
Chloride	60–150
Phosphorus[*]	20–40
Calcium[†]	10–20
Magnesium[†]	8–24

[*] Potassium phosphate provides 0.68 mmol P / mmol K; sodium phosphate provides 0.75 mmol P / mmol Na.
[†] Calcium gluconate and magnesium sulfate are the preferreed salts for parenteral use.

congestive heart failure or renal failure. Alternatively, the need for electrolytes is greater when losses increase due to diarrhea, ostomies, vomiting, fistulas, or nasogastric suctioning, as often occurs in gastrointestinal diseases. Malnutrition usually results in the loss of muscle tissue, with a subsequent decrease in intracellular fluid and an increase in extracellular fluid. With refeeding and the synthesis of new lean tissue, requirements for the major intracellular electrolytes (potassium, phosphorus, and magnesium) may be quite elevated. Thus, frequent monitoring of these electrolytes is needed during refeeding of malnourished patients. Weight loss may also be observed with refeeding due to increased urine output that accompanies the decrease in extracellular fluid.

Electrolytes may be added to parenteral nutrition solutions using single- or multiple-entity products or as part of amino acid solutions that contain added electrolytes. In addition, most amino acid products contain substantial amounts of chloride and acetate salts. Sodium and potassium are routinely provided as salts of acetate or chloride. Chloride and acetate are often administered as a ratio of 2 chloride to 1 acetate, but this may vary with acid-base status. Acetate salts metabolize to yield net bicarbonate ions and are often used in greater proportion in metabolic acidosis.

The combination of calcium and phosphorus salts in parenteral nutrition solutions may result in crystalline precipitates, depending on the volume and pH of the solution and mixing procedures. A maximal combined dose of 45 mmol of calcium and phosphorus is sometimes recommended (10). Fat emulsions provide 15 mmol phosphorus per liter because of the egg yolk phospholipid.

VITAMINS

Multivitamin formulations containing both fat soluble and water soluble vitamins are available for incorporation into parenteral nutrition solutions. These products have been formulated according to guidelines developed by the American Medical Association and the American Academy of Pediatrics (11, 12). Most institutions use a multiple-entity product (MVC 9 + 3, LyphoMed, Deerfield, IL) that contains 12 (adults) or 13 (pediatrics) vitamins, as outlined in Table 14-6. The adult formulations do not contain vitamin K because it antagonizes the effects of coumadin in patients receiving this drug. In adults, vitamin K can be administered by adding 1 to 2 mg per day to the parenteral nutrition solution or by giving 5 to 10 mg per week intramuscularly or subcutaneously (10). Many of the vitamins are marketed in single-entity parenteral formulations including: vitamin A, D, E, K, thiamine, riboflavin, niacin, pyridoxine, folic acid, vitamin B12 ,and vitamin C. For optimal retention the daily dose of vitamins should be diluted with the entire daily volume of PN solution. Vitamins are usually added to the PN solutions just prior to administration because of problems with degradation.

TABLE 14-6 Recommended Daily Intake for Parenteral Vitamins

Vitamin	Units of Measurement	Infants and Children <11 years	Adults
Fat soluble			
A	RE* (IU)†	690 (2,300)	990 (3,300)
D	μg‡ (IU)	10 (400)	5 (200)
E	mg§ (IU)	4.7 (7)	6.7 (10)
K	μg	200	—
Water soluble			
Ascorbic acid (C)	mg	80	100
Biotin	μg	20	60
Cyanocobalamin (B$_{12}$)	μg	1.0	5.0
Folic acid	μg	140	400
Niacin	mg	17	40
Pantothenic acid	mg	5.0	15.0
Pyridoxine (B$_6$)	mg	1.0	4.0
Riboflavin (B$_2$)	mg	1.4	3.6
Thiamine (B$_1$)	mg	1.2	3.0

* RE = retinol equivalents.
† IU = International units.
‡ As cholecalciferol
§ As dl-α-tocopherol.
Adapted from JPEN.3:(1979)258–262, and Am. J. Clin. Nutr.48:(1988)1324–42.

TRACE ELEMENTS

Trace elements are usually added to parenteral nutrition solutions daily. Guidelines are available for parenteral supplementation with four trace elements: zinc, copper, chromium, and manganese (13). In addition, recent evidence suggests that selenium stores are depleted in patients on long-term TPN or in those with burns, AIDS, or liver failure, so many clinicians now routinely add selenium to TPN solutions (14). Current recommendations for supplementation with these trace elements are provided in Table 14-7. In addition, commercial solutions of molybdenum and iodine are available, although parenteral guidelines for these trace elements have not been established. Iron is not routinely added to parenteral solutions because of instability.

Toxicity of trace elements during TPN is a potential problem for patients with cholestatic liver disease, because some trace elements are excreted though the biliary tract. For example, manganese and copper are excreted in the bile, and toxicity of manganese has been reported during TPN (14, 15). Zinc, chromium, and selenium are excreted renally and generally do not accumulate during TPN. Zinc requirements are the

TABLE 14-7 Recommended Daily Intakes for Parenteral Trace Elements

Trace Elements	Adults	Children	Neonates
Chromium	10–15 µg/day	0.14–0.2 µg/kg/day	0.14–0.2 µg/kg/day
Copper	0.5–1.5 mg/day	20 µg/kg/day	20 µg/kg/day
Manganese	150–800 µg/day	2–10 µg/kg/day	2–10 µg/kg/day
Selenium	40–80 µg/day	23 µg/kg/day	2–3 µg/kg/day
Zinc	2.5– 4 mg/day	100 µg/kg/day	300 µg/kg/day

Adapted from *JPEN* 3:(1979)263–267.

largest of all the trace elements. They increase dramatically in patients with gastrointestinal diseases who show significant ostomy or diarrheal losses. An additional 12.2 mg of zinc is needed for each liter of small bowel fluid lost, and an additional 17.1 mg of zinc is needed per kg of stool or ileostomy output (13). Zinc requirements are also increased in metabolic stress secondary to increased urine output. An additional 2.0 mg of zinc per day is suggested for an adult in an acute catabolic state (13, 14).

The effectiveness of parenteral trace element and vitamin formulations is the subject of continued research. Little is known about the parenteral requirements of vitamins and minerals during acute and chronic disease. Ongoing assessment and monitoring of biochemical and clinical markers of these nutrients, especially trace elements, is needed during TPN (14).

DESIGNING A PARENTERAL FEEDING REGIMEN

The preparation of TPN solutions is done in the pharmacy. However, a familiarity with preparation and administration techniques is helpful when designing a parenteral feeding regimen.

All component parenteral solutions must be sterile, and solutions are mixed aseptically. Random samples of TPN solution are routinely cultured to monitor for bacterial contamination, and assay of electrolyte content is also routinely done.

The use of TNA, or the combination of carbohydrate, protein, and fat into one container for PN, has simplified the preparation and administration of TPN solutions. However, TNA provides a better growth medium for bacteria than does a conventional PN infusion system. In a conventional PN infusion system, intravenous fat emulsions are usually not mixed with the dextrose-amino-acid- base solution but are instead infused from a separate sterile bottle. The fat is administered "piggyback" via a Y connector into the same line through which the dextrose-amino acid base is infused. An in-line filter (0.22 micron) is usually placed in the dextrose-amino acid line to ensure sterility of the solution being delivered. Fat is infused into the line past the filter, as the fat particles are too large (0.45 micron) and would be impeded by the filter. With a TNA system an in-line filter cannot be used. A diagram of a conventional PN infusion systems is shown in Figure 14-3.

An order for CPN using a conventional infusion systems might read as follows:

Daily infusion of 2L/day TPN solution composed of 25% dextrose, 4% amino acids with standard electrolytes, vitamins, and minerals supplemented with 500 ml 10% fat emulsion. Run dextrose-amino acid solution at 83 mL / hr, and piggy-back fat emulsion over 10 hr at 50 mL / hr.

PERIPHERAL VERSUS CENTRAL PARENTERAL NUTRITION

The decision to recommend CPN versus PPN is based on the number of calories needed, the expected duration of parenteral feeding, the need to restrict total fluids, and other metabolic considerations relevant to the medical history. Hypertonic nutrient solutions with a high osmolarity due to high dextrose concentrations cannot be infused into peripheral veins. The low blood flow in these veins can lead to inflammation followed by thrombosis when hypertonic solutions are infused. In practice, parenteral nutrition solutions with an osmolarity of 250 to 600 mOsm/L can be infused peripherally.

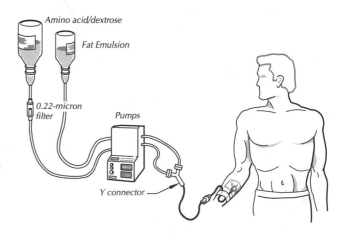

FIGURE 14-3 Coinfusion of fat emulsion in peripheral parenteral nutrition (PPN). If a total nutrient admixture is used, all of the components of TPN are mixed into a single container for infusion into the patient.

However, these limitations do not allow enough protein and energy to be given to meet the needs of some patients. If the solution has a higher osmolarity, it must be given centrally. The high blood flow in central veins results in quick dilution of hypertonic solutions.

In general, CPN is used to provide nutrients at greater concentrations and smaller fluid volumes than is possible with PPN. CPN is usually indicated when calorie needs exceed 2,000 kcal per day and parenteral feeding is needed for more than 10 days.

PPN is typically used for patients for whom parenteral feeding is needed for less than 10 to 14 days (16). PPN is not the optimal choice for feeding patients with significant malnutrition, severe metabolic stress, or large nutrient or electrolyte needs, especially potassium, a strong vascular irritant. The primary advantage of PPN is that it avoids many of the mechanical and septic complications associated with placement and maintenance of central catheters (16).

Osmolarity

The osmolarity of a parenteral solution is an important factor in determining whether the solution will be infused via the peripheral or central route. Note that for parenteral solutions we calculate tonicity as *osmolarity* instead of *osmolality,* which is used for enteral formulas (Chapter 13). Osmolarity is used because parenteral solutions are prepared using a defined number of grams of solute diluted to a final solution volume (Chapter 4). Thus, percent concentration of a parenteral solution indicates the number of grams of solute present in 100 mL of solution.

The osmolarity of a solution of known dextrose concentration can be readily calculated. For example, a 5-percent dextrose solution has 50 g dextrose per L divided by the atomic weight of dextrose monohydrate, 198.2 g per mole (50 g/L ÷ 198.2 g/mole), which gives 252.3 mOsm per L. A short method for calculating the osmolarity of a dextrose solution is to multiply the percentage of solution by 50. For example, the osmolarity of $D_{20}W$ would be 1,000 mOsm per L. The osmolarity of amino acid solutions can also be calculated by a quick method that multiplies the percent amino acid concentration by 100. Using this method, a 2.5-percent amino acid solution would have an osmolarity of approximately 250 mOsm per L. Intravenous fat has an osmolarity of approximately 300 m Osm /L. The addition of electrolytes, vitamins, and minerals also increases the osmolarity of PN solutions by approximately 300 to 400 mOsm per L.

In calculating the osmolarity of a PN solution, the component osmolarities are added together. Here is an example:

If 500 ml $D_{50}W$ (50% × 50= 2,500 mOsm/L × 0.5 L = 1,250 mOsm) and 500 mL 8.5% amino acids (8.5% × 100 = 850 mOsm/L × 0.5 L = 425 mOsm) are mixed to make 1L of solution, the final osmolarity would equal 1,250 + 425 = 1,675.

CENTRAL PARENTERAL NUTRITION

As an example, we will calculate a CPN regimen for Mr. Smith, a mildly depleted 60-year old who is experiencing an exacerbation of ulcerative colitis. Mr. Smith weighs 140 pounds (63.6 kg) and measures 5 foot 10 inches in height (178 cm).

First we establish his daily nutrient needs as follows:

35 kcal / kg × 63.6 kg = 2,230 kcal
1.5 g pro / kg × 63.6 kg = 95 g pro or 15.3 g N
30 mL fluid / kg × 63.6 kg = 1910 mL

We will assume that Mr. Smith will receive 2 L of TPN solution per day, which will be prepared as a TNA. His macronutrient needs are calculated assuming a final volume of 2 L of TPN solution. The volume needed for supplementing each liter of TPN solution with additives, including electrolytes, vitamins, and trace elements, will be disregarded as the total volume for additives is generally less than 10 percent of the final volume of TPN solution. Many pharmacies allow a 10 to 20 percent overfill in their calculation of TPN solutions (10).

In calculating the TNA we assume that the following parenteral solutions are available for mixing: 20 percent lipid emulsion, 70 percent dextrose, and 10 percent amino acid solutions. We assume that 25 percent of daily energy will be provided by the lipid emulsion.

Next we calculate the volume of lipid, amino acids and dextrose needed for each liter of Mr. Smith's CPN formulation.

Lipid:

2230 kcal × 25% = 560 lipid kcal
560 lipid kcal × 1 mL / 2kcal 20% lipid emulsion =
    280 mL 20% lipid emulsion /day or *140 mL / L CPN*

Amino Acids:

95 g protein / day × 100 mL / 10 g amino acids=
    950 mL 10% amino acids/day or *475 mL / L CPN*

Dextrose:

Assume that the energy from protein is not calculated as part of daily energy needs. Thus, if fat provides 25 percent energy, then dextrose provides 75 percent of energy.

2,230 kcal × 75% = 1675 dextrose kcal
1,675 dextrose kcal × 1 g dextrose/3.4 kcal = 495 g
    dextrose/day
495 g dextrose × 100 mL / 70 g dextrose=
710 mL 70% dextrose / day or *355 mL / L CPN*

Thus, each L of CPN would contain:
140 mL 20% lipid emulsion
475 mL 10% amino acids
355 mL 70% dextrose
Total: 970 mL plus 30 to 70 mL additives

The final concentrations of nutrients would be:

Lipid:

$$140 \text{ mL / L} \times 20 \text{ g lipid / 100 mL} \times 1 \text{ L/1000 mL} =$$
$$0.028 \text{ g lipid / mL} \times 100 \text{ mL} = 2.8\% \text{ lipid}$$

Amino Acids:

$$475 \text{ mL / L} \times 10 \text{ g amino acids/100 mL} \times 1 \text{ L/1000 mL}$$
$$= 0.0475 \text{ g amino acids/mL} \times 100 = 4.75\% \text{ amino acids}$$

Dextrose:

$$355 \text{ mL / L} \times 70 \text{ g dextrose / 100 mL} \times 1 \text{ L / 1,000 mL} =$$
$$0.2485 \text{ g dextrose / mL} \times 100 = 24.85\% \text{ dextrose}$$

The intake of lipid and dextrose per kg of body weight is calculated as follows:

Lipid:

$$2,000 \text{ mL / day} \times 2.8 \text{ g lipid / 100 mL} = 56 \text{ g lipid}$$
$$56 \text{ g lipid / 63.6 kg} = 0.88 \text{ g lipid / kg / day}$$

This easily provides for EFA requirements.

Dextrose:

$$2,000 \text{ mL / day} \times 24.85 \text{ g dextrose / 100 mL} =$$
$$497 \text{ g detrose}$$
$$497 \text{ g dextrose / 63.6 kg} = 7.8 \text{ g dextrose / kg / day}$$
$$7.8 \text{ g dextrose / kg / 24 hr} = 0.325 \text{ g dextrose / kg / hr}$$

The amount of dextrose in this CPN regimen is within the range of tolerance for a patient with normal respiratory function.

The kcal to N ratio is calculated as follows:

$$560 \text{ lipid kcal} + 1675 \text{ dextrose kcal} + (95\text{g amino acids}$$
$$\times 4 \text{ kcal / g}) = 2,615 \text{ total kcal / day}$$
$$2,615 \text{ kcal / 15.3 g N} = 170 \text{ kcal: g N}$$

The nonprotein kcal to N ratio is calculated as follows:

$$560 \text{ lipid kcal} + 1,675 \text{ dextrose kcal} = 2,235 \text{ nonprotein}$$
$$\text{kcal / day}$$
$$2,235 \text{ kcal / 15.3 g N} = 146 \text{ nonprotein kcal: g N}$$

These ratios are appropriate to support anabolism in this mildly depleted patient.

Summary of CPN:

Total volume = 2,000 mL over 25 hr; 83 mL / hr
Nonprotein Energy = 2,235 kcal (25% lipid and 75% dextrose)
Protein = 95 g
Total kcal to N ratio = 170:1

A sample TPN order for administration of the previously described CPN regimen might read as follows:

2L / day of 25% dextrose, 2.8% lipid and 4.75% amino acids solution with standard additives to run at 83 mL / hr.

PERIPHERAL PARENTERAL NUTRITION

Now we can consider how to formulate a parenteral feeding regimen for delivery into a peripheral vein for Mr. Smith. Because the high osmolarity of dextrose-amino acid solutions dictates that a greater percentage of calories be provided by fat in PPN, we will calculate Mr. Smith's PPN formulation with 50 percent of energy from the 20 percent lipid emulsion and 50 percent from carbohydrate. Thus, we will need 1,115 kcal (2,230 kcal × .50) or approximately 560 ml 20 percent lipid emulsion per day. This means that 1,115 kcal would be provided by dextrose or approximately 330 g of dextrose per day (1,115 kcal dextrose × 1 g dextrose/3.4 kcal = 330 g dextrose).

Because a 10% dextrose solution is the most concentrated solution tolerated in PPN, the final daily volume of TPN will exceed 3 L per day in order to meet energy needs. This volume of fluid may not be tolerated by Mr. Smith. Alternatively, the total volume could be reduced somewhat if 60 percent of energy was provided by fat. Thus, considerations regarding fluid needs and tolerance to intravenous lipid emulsions, as well as the expected duration of parenteral nutrition, affect the decision to use PPN versus CPN.

A typical order for PPN using a TNA might read as follows:

3.5 L/day of 10% dextrose, 2.85% lipid, 3% amino acid solution with standard additives to run at 145 mL / hr.

PROTOCOLS FOR PARENTERAL NUTRITION

COMPLICATIONS ASSOCIATED WITH PARENTERAL NUTRITION

In general, complications associated with PPN have tended to be fewer and less serious than those resulting from CPN (16). A common complication with PPN is infiltration at the catheter site, necessitating placement in a new peripheral venous site.

Complications arising from CPN fall into three major categories: catheter-related problems, metabolic abnormalities, and gastrointestinal complications (17). One of the most common catheter-related problems is *catheter sepsis*, a blood stream infection that originates from a contaminated catheter or catheter site, contaminated PN solution, or both. Other catheter-related problems that may arise during central vein cannulation include pneumothorax, air embolus, catheter malposition, and arterial puncture or subclavian laceration, which may lead to hemothorax or hematoma.

Metabolic problems associated with PN include both hyper- and hypoglycemia, glycosuria, compromised respiratory function, mineral and electrolyte abnormalities, and elevation of hepatic enzymes. Gastrointestinal complications associated with PN include fatty liver, which can be prevented by using balanced amounts of fat and dextrose and avoiding overfeeding, and cholestasis and gastrointestinal atrophy, which can be prevented by introduction of enteral feeding when possible. Table 14-8 outlines the symptoms, etiology, and treatment of specific metabolic complications associated with PN.

MONITORING GUIDELINES

Ongoing monitoring of both metabolic and nutritional status are important in order to detect and prevent complications due to PN. The following guidelines are often used:

1. Measure electrolytes and blood urea nitrogen (BUN) daily for the first week of parenteral feeding to monitor adequacy of hydration, renal function, and electrolyte balance. Serum calcium, phosphorus, and magnesium should be measured until blood levels stabilize.
2. Measure blood glucose levels daily, and spot-check urine for glucose and acetone. The detection of 2 + or 3 + glycosuria should prompt blood glucose determination and possible insulin supplementation of the parenteral-feeding solution.
3. Monitor liver enzymes—serum glutamic oxaloacetic transaminase (SGOT) or serum glutamic pyruvic transaminase (SGPT), lactic hydrogenase (LDH), and alkaline phosphate-and serum bilirubin weekly to detect hepatic dysfunction related to the TPN.
4. Monitor weight daily for fluid overload. Weight gain of 1.5 kg per week or less is expected from intensive PN therapy. Weight gain above this amount probably indicates fluid and sodium retention.

Once the PN is stable, weekly monitoring is usually adequate. Nutritional monitoring should include recording of patient weight 2 or 3 times per week, documentation of total calories and protein received from parenteral and enteral nutrition, and evaluation of nitrogen balance to assess the adequacy of protein intake. Other indices of nutritional status as discussed in Chapter 5 may also be used.

TRANSITIONAL FEEDING

Transitional feeding refers to the gradual progression from one mode of feeding to another, while maintaining nutrient requirements. For example, transitional feeding is used when a patient is gradually switched from TPN to enteral tube feeding or oral feeding, or when a tube-fed patient begins oral feeding. Enteral feedings should be initiated as soon as it is safe to use the gut, because significant atrophy of the gastrointestinal tract accompanies PN and contributes, in part, to many of the long-term complications associated with TPN. Frequently, the patient is the best judge of when oral feedings will be tolerated; however, patients on TPN are generally not hungry. Some of the benefits of early enteral feeding

during PN include maintenance of the gut barrier, which contributes to improved immune function, maintenance of digestive and absorptive functions, and promotion of gut trophic hormones. The use of even occasional enteral feedings during PN is likely to reduce the length of time needed for transitional feeding (17).

The nutrition care specialist plays an important role in the decision to initiate transitional feedings and the assessment of nutrient intake during transitional feeding. It is essential to maintain nutrient intake during transitional feedings to prevent a decline in the patient's nutritional status. This is accomplished by careful monitoring of nutritional status and documentation of total calorie and protein intake from both parenteral and enteral feedings. Excess nutrient intake may occur during transitional feeding, resulting in complications of overfeeding such as hyperglycemia, fluid retention, hypokalemia, respiratory insufficiency, and hepatic dysfunction. Careful monitoring of nutritional status and total nutrient intake throughout the transitional feeding period will prevent problems due to both under- and overnutrition.

The approach to transitional feeding is largely empirical; that is, little scientific evidence exists to support the current methods of transitional feeding (18). Factors to consider in designing a transitional feeding regimen include the following:

1. Feeding should be introduced slowly with gradual increases in volume;
2. Selection of a tube feeding or an oral diet must consider the patient's digestive capacity;
3. Monitoring is essential to prevent complications such as aspiration pneumonia, gut dysfunction, overfeeding, or a decline in nutritional status due to inadequate nutrient intake;
4. At least one-third to one-half of nutrient needs must be provided by tube feeding or oral feeding before a decrease or "weaning" from the original feeding method is begun (17).

The average time needed to achieve full nutrient intake from tube feeding or oral feeding after intestinal surgery is approximately 4 to 10 days (19). However, patients given PN for prolonged periods, such as in home TPN, require much longer periods of transitional feeding.

This section includes a discussion of how to assess the status of the gastrointestinal tract and a summary of methods of transitional feeding for progression from PN to either enteral tube feeding or oral feeding. Procedures and formulas used for tube feeding are discussed in Chapter 13.

ASSESSING THE GASTROINTESTINAL TRACT

An assessment of the state of the gut and its functional capacity must be considered before initiation of a transitional feeding regimen. The decision to initiate

TABLE 14-8 Possible Metabolic Complications of TPN and Their Management

Complications	Characterized By	Usual Cause	Treatment
Hyperglycemia	Blood glucose >200mg / dL Metabolic acidosis Polyuria, polydipsia	Too rapid an initiation of TPN Sepsis, postoperative stress or diabetes Use of steroids Chromium deficiency	Slow initiation and advancement of TPN Reduce dextrose concentration Search for infection Consider insulin
Hyperosmolar nonketotic dehydration	Hyperglycemia Dehydration Increase in serum osmolarlity and serum sodium Somnolence Seizures Coma	Failure to recognize initial hyperglycemia and increased glucose in urine.	Give insulin to correct hyperglycemia Give 5% dextrose and hypotonic saline (1/4 to 1/2 strength), rather than TPN, to correct free-water deficit. Continue to monitor serum glucose, osmolality, sodium, and potassium.
Hypoglycemia	Hypothermia Somnolence or lethargy Peripheral vasoconstriction Shallow respiration	Abrupt discontinuation of TPN. Insulin overdose	Immediatelly begin dextrose infusion Monitor serum glucose and potassium
Hypokalemia	Muscle weakness Cardiac arrhythmias Altered digitalis sensitivity Nausea	Excessive gastrointestinal or urinary potassium losses Inadequate potassium in TPN	Increase potassium in TPN 3 mmol of potassium per g of nitrogen needed with anabolism
Hypomagnesemia	Cardiac arrhythmias Muscle weakness Convulsive seizures with or without tetany	Inadequate magnesium in TPN Medications: diuretics or cyclosporin Excessive gastrointestinal or renal losses	Increase magnesium in TPN In an emergency, give $MgSO_4$ solution immediately
Hyponatremia	Lethargy Confusion Hypotension	Excessive gastrointestinal or urinary sodium losses Excessive fluid administration	Increase sodium in TPN Restrict fluid intake
Prerenal azotemia	Lassitude Elevated serum BUN	Dehydration Excess protein intake Inadequate nonprotein calorie intake	Increase fluid intake Decrease protein intake Increase nonprotein calories
Hypertriglyceridemia	Serum triglyceride level 300–350 mg / dL, 6 hr post lipid initiation Elevated level in previously stable patient, i.e., sepsis	Excess lipid infusion Medications such as cyclosporin Sepsis, multisystem organ failure, pathologic hyperlipidemia	Decrease lipid volume Use continuous lipid infusion Avoid lipid infusion >2.5 g / kg / d or >60% of total calories.
Hyperchloremic metabolic acidosis	Decrease in blood pH Decrease in serum [HCO_3^-] Decrease in blood base excess Increase in serum [Cl^-] Increase in serum [Na^+]	Excessive renal or gastrointestinal losses of base Infusion of preformed hydrogen ion Cationic amino acids greater than the concentrations of anionic amino acids in TPN solution Excessive chloride in TPN	Decrease chloride excess in TPN solution by exchanging chloride ion with acetate ion.

transitional feeding is the physicians' responsibility; however, to function as a part of the medical team, the nutrition care specialist needs to understand the clinical factors affecting the state of the gut and its functional capacity. In general, safe usage of the gut is characterized by the absence of nausea, vomiting and abdominal distention (18).

State of Gut

The state of the gut is assessed by considering three types of information. First, the presence of factors that are overt contraindications to enteral feeding, such as peritonitis, gut perforation, or ileus due to mechanical obstruction. Ileus is defined as intestinal obstruction associated with failure of peristalsis resulting in abdominal pain, distention, vomiting, and constipation. The treatment for ileus is constant suction, often nasogastric suction, to remove gastric fluids that would otherwise accumulate and result in aspiration. The second consideration in assessing the state of the gut is the length of time that the gut has been subjected to starvation. This reflects the degree of atrophy and, thus, the total length of time needed for transitional feeding. Third, the degree of gut damage and dysfunction due to the patient's diagnosis and clinical course must be considered. Examples of clinical factors that affect the gut include: sepsis; shock resulting in ischemia and hypomotility of the bowel; physical trauma to the gastrointestinal tract, for example, a gunshot wound; malignancy and treatment with chemotherapy or radiation, resulting in diarrhea and enteritis; inflammatory bowel disease, such as Crohn's disease or ulcerative colitis; surgical alteration of the anatomy of the gut; and temporary, postoperative ileus.

Functional Capacity

The functional capacity of the gut is usually assessed by considering the presence of bowel sounds, abdominal distention, and the passage of flatus or stool. These factors must be assessed individually and in relation to other pertinent clinical symptoms.

Bowel Sounds. Bowel sounds must be present for several days before initiation of enteral feeding. Hypoactive bowel sounds suggest that gut function is starting to return, but initiation of feeding should wait until bowel sounds are heard consistently. Hyperactive bowel sounds suggest that diarrhea may occur with feeding.

Abdominal Distention. In general, the abdomen should be soft before the initiation of enteral feeding. A hard, distended abdomen may indicate ileus. If ascites is present, a firm abdomen is often noted, although, in many cases, enteral feeding can still be given.

Passage of Flatus or Stool. The passage of flatus or stool is usually a positive indicator that gut function is adequate for enteral feeding. However, in cases of partial bowel obstruction the patient may still pass stool even though the gut is not ready for enteral feeding.

Other Considerations. The use of medications must also be considered when initiating enteral feeding. Medications that may cause diarrhea, such as antibiotics, or alter gut motility, such as morphine or smooth muscle depressants, may affect the methods of transitional feeding.

In some cases tube feeding may be possible when intermittent nasogastric suctioning is still needed. If the aspirate is less than 300 cc per day and the patient tolerates clamping of the nasogastric suction tube without nausea or vomiting, a gradual initiation of tube feeding may begin. If nasogastric aspirates total 1,000 cc per day or greater, it is probably too early to begin tube feeding, although progressive clamping of the nasogastric suction tube and assessment of tolerance can be used to monitor the return of gut function.

Lastly, it is possible in some cases to utilize a functional part of the gastrointestinal tract for feeding even though portions of the gut proximal or distal to the healthy section are dysfunctional. Feeding an elemental diet through a needle catheter jejunostomy is one example of how this might be accomplished.

TRANSITION FROM PARENTERAL NUTRITION TO TUBE FEEDING

Information about the state and functional capacity of the gastrointestinal tract and the expected duration of tube feeding will determine placement of the feeding tube and the type of enteral formula used. Jejunal feeding is preferred instead of gastric feeding in patients at risk for aspiration. If the duration of tube feeding is expected to be longer than 6 weeks, jejunostomy, gastrostomy, percutaneous endoscopic gastrostomy, or percutaneous endoscopic jejunostomy are recommended (17). Polymeric formulas are used for patients with adequate digestion and absorption, whereas hydrolyzed or elemental formulas are used if impaired digestion and absorption exists (Chapter 13). In either case, infusion at 25 to 50 mL per hour at isotonic concentrations are used initially. If the patient tolerates the formula and rate of administration, as evidenced by the absence of nausea, diarrhea, and cramps, the tube feeding may be advanced in increments of 20 to 25 mL per hour every 12 to 24 hours (17). When the patient is receiving one-third to one-half of calorie needs from tube feeding, the CPN may be decreased or the PPN may be discontinued to reduce the fluid load. When the patient is receiving two-thirds to three-fourths of calorie needs from the tube feeding, CPN may be discontinued by reducing the flow rate over several hours.

TRANSITION FROM PARENTERAL NUTRITION TO ORAL FEEDING

In order to begin the transition from PN to oral feeding, the patient must clearly indicate the desire to eat by mouth and not be at risk for aspiration. On the first day of feeding, low-fat clear liquids are offered, which the patient is instructed to sip slowly at frequent intervals. Full liquids are offered on the second day of feeding, with monitoring for lactose intolerance. If the patient tolerates the full liquid diet, solid foods are offered on the next day. In cases where there is evidence of impaired digestion or absorption, low-fat, lactose-free solids may be used initially. When the oral intake is at least 500 calories per day, the volume of CPN may be reduced and the CPN may be discontinued when the patient is consuming two-thirds to three-fourths of nutrient requirements (17). PPN is often discontinued when the patient begins solid foods to reduce fluid intake. Between-meal supplements may be used, and cyclic PN at night may help to encourage return of appetite and an increase in oral intake during the day.

PEDIATRIC PARENTERAL NUTRITION

Parenteral feeding is widely used in pediatrics, particularly in neonatology. More than 1 percent of all births in the United States include infants weighing less than, 1,500 g, i.e., very low birth weight. These infants require PN for the first several weeks of life because of immaturity of the gastrointestinal tract. Parenteral feeding results in delayed maturation or atrophy of the gastrointestinal tract. Thus, it is desirable to initiate enteral feedings in the premature infants or children as soon as possible. Enteral feedings stimulate enzymatic development and activity, promote bile acid flow, and increase small intestinal villous growth. A detailed discussion of PN for the pediatric population is beyond the scope of this text but can be found in other references (20). The information in this section will review the assessment of parenteral nutrient needs for the pediatric population, with particular emphasis on premature or LBW infants. The method of calculating parenteral feeding regimens are generally similar for adults and children, as previously discussed.

Representative compositions of central and peripheral PN solutions appropriate for a premature infant are given in Table 14-9.

ASSESSING NUTRIENT NEEDS

Energy

Parenteral energy requirements for premature infants differ from enteral energy requirements, as digestive losses do not occur. Infants require 50 to 60 kcal / kg / day for maintenance and 70 to 120 kcal / kg / day for growth. For children older than 1 year of age, BEE (kcal / kg / day) can be estimated as: 1 to 8 years, 70 to 100; 8 to 12 years, 60 to 75; and 12 to 18 years, 45 to 60. Total daily energy needs can be calculated as BEE times 1.25 (mild stress), 1.50 (nutritional depletion), or 2.00 (high stress) for children (21).

Protein

Protein requirements range from 1.5 to 4.0 g / kg / day with approximately 2.5 to 4 g / kg / day required in infants weighing less than 1,500 g, 2.0 to 2.5 g / kg / day from 0 to 12

TABLE 14-9 Composition of Nutrient Infusates Suitable for Central Vein and Peripheral Vein Infusion in Preterm Infants.*

Component	Central Vein (Amount / kg / day)[†]	Peripheral Vein (Amount / kg / day)[†]
Amino Acids	3–4 g	2.5–3.0 g
Glucose	15–25 g (83–139 mmol)	10–15 g (56–83 mmol)
Lipid emulsion	0.5–3.0 g	0.5–3.0 g
Sodium	2–3 mEq (46–69 mg)	2–3 mEq (46–69 mg)
Potassium[‡]	2–4 mEq (78–156 mg)	2–4 mEq (78–106 mg)
Calcium	80–100 mg (4–5 mEq)	40–80 mg (2–4 mEq)
Magnesium	3–6 mg (0.125–0.25 mmol)	3–6 mg (0.125–0.25 mmol)
Chloride	2–3 mEq (71–107 mg)	2–3 mEq (71–107 mg)
Phosphorus [‡]	43–62 mg (1.4–2.0 mmol)	43–62 mg (1.4–2.0 mmol)
Zinc[§]	200–400 µg (3–6 µmol)	200–400 µg (3–6 µmol)
Copper [§]	20 µg (0.3 µmol)	20 µg (0.3 µmol)
Iron[§]		
Vitamins (M.V.I. Pediatric) [‖]		
Total volume	120–130 mL	150 mL

* In general, the peripheral vein regimen is appropriate for the transitional period and as a supplement to tolerated enteral feedings; the central vein regimen is appropriate for the stable growing infant dependent upon parenteral nutrition.

[†] For all nutrients, the amount / kg / day is expressed in the most commonly used unit; these amounts expressed in alternative units are shown in parentheses.

[‡] With a lower calcium intake (40–60 mg / kg / day or 1–1.5 mmol / kg / day), a phosphorus intake in excess of 1.4 mmol / kg / day, or 43 mg /kg / day. the amount given with a daily potassium intake of 2 mEq/kg/day or 78 mg/kg/day as a mixture of KH_2PO_4 and K_2HPO_4, frequently results in hyperphosphatemia. Although this may not be true with the calcium intakes suggested here, a potassium intake of more than 2 mEq / kg / day should be given initially as KC1, and the infant should be monitored carefully to assess the adequacy of phosphorus intake.

[§] Iron Dextran (Imferon, Fisons Corp., Bedford, MA) can be added to the infusate of patients requiring parenteral nutrition but the dose should be limited to 0.1 mg/kg/day. Alternatively, the indicated intramuscular dose can be used intermittently, either as the sole source of iron or as an additional dose.

[‖] M.V.I. Pediatric (distributed by Astra Phamaceufical Products, Inc., Westborough, MA; manufactured by Armour Pharmaceutical Co., Kankakee, IL) is a lypholized product. When reconstituted as directed, 2 mL. added to the daily infusate provides 280 µg vitamin A, 2.8 mg vitamin E, 80 µg vitamin K, 4 µg (64 IU) vitamin D, 32 mg ascorbic acid, 520 µg thiamine, 560 µg riboflavin, 400 µg pyridoxine, 6.8 mg niacin, 2 mg pantothenic acid, 8 µg biotin, 56 µg folic acid, and 0.4 µg vitamin B_{12} . See Table 14-6.

Reproduced with permission from W.C. Heird, and M.R. Gomez, Parenteral nutrition. *In*: R.C. Tsang, A. Lucas, R. Uauy, and S. Zlotkin, eds. *Nutritional Needs of the Preterm Infant,* Baltimore:Williams and Wilkins, 1993(Table 15.1)p. 227.

months in the normal-weight infant, 1.5 to 2.0 g / kg / day from 1 to 8 years, and 1.0 to 1.5 g / kg / day from 8 to 15 years. Specialized amino acid solutions should be used for rapidly growing neonates. Compared to adult solutions, these solutions contain a greater proportion of essential amino acids with increased amounts of tyrosine and taurine.

Fluid and Electrolytes
Fluid requirements for children can be calculated using the guidelines in Table 4-2. Fluid requirements for LBW infants range from 125 to 150 mL / kg / day. The electrolytes sodium, potassium and chloride are provided in amounts ranging from 2 to 4 mmol / kg / day for LBW infants with normal organ function.

Carbohydrate
Dextrose is the principal calorie source, as it is for adults. Preterm infants may demonstrate glucose intolerance secondary to immaturity and metabolic instability that may include both hypo- and hyperglycemia. Preterm infants often begin with an initial rate of glucose infusion of 4 to 6 mg / kg / minute, and term infants may begin with a rate of 8 to 9 mg / kg / minute.

Fat
Provision of EFA is especially important for rapidly growing neonates who have minimal fat stores. Provision of 0.5 to 1.0 g lipid/kg/day is needed to prevent EFA deficiency. Total parenteral fat intakes should not exceed 2 to 3 g/kg/day.

Vitamins and Trace Elements
Vitamin and trace element requirements are not well established for premature infants but are generally similar to those of term infants. Guidelines for parenteral supplementation of vitamins and trace elements are found in Tables 14-6 and 14-7, respectively.

REFERENCES

1. **Dudrick, S.J., D.W. Wilmore, H.M. Vars,** and **J.E. Rhoads**. Long-term total parenteral nutrition with growth, development and positive nitrogen balance. *Surgery* 64:(1960)134–42.
2. **McCrae, J.D., R. O'Shea,** and **L.M. Udine**. Parenteral nutrition: hospital to home. *J. Am. Dietet. Assoc.* 93:(1993)664–70..
3. **Ziegler, T.R., L.S. Young, K. Benfell, M. Scheltinga, K. Hortos, R. Bye, F.D. Morrow, D.O. Jacobs, R.J. Smith, J.H. Antin,** and **D.W. Wilmore**. Clinical and metabolic efficacy of glutamine-supplemented parenteral nutrition after bone marrow transplantation. *Ann. Int. Med.* 116:(1992)821–28.
4. A.S.P.E.N. Board of Directors. Guidelines for the use of parenteral and enteral nutrition in adult and pediatric patients. *JPEN* 17(4): supplement, 1993.
5. **Long, C.L.,** and **W.S. Blakemore**. Energy and protein requirements in the hospitalized patient. *JPEN* 3:(1979)69–71.
6. ——— , **N. Schaffel,** and **J.W. Geiger**. Metabolic response to injury and illness: estimation of energy and protein needs from indirect calorimetry and nitrogen balance. *JPEN* 3:(1979)452–56..
7. **Weinsier, R.L.,** and **C.L. Krumdieck**. Death resulting from overzealous total parenteral nutrition: the refeeding syndrome revisited. Am. *J. Clin. Nutr.* 34:(1980)393–99.
8. **Wolfe, R.R., T.F. O'Donnell, M.D. Stone, D.A. Richmond,** and **J.F. Burke**. Investigation of factors determining the optimal glucose infusion rate in total parenteral nutrition. *Metabolism* 29:(1980)892–900.
9. **Goodenough, R.O,.** and **R.R. Wolfe**. Effect of total parenteral nutrition on free fatty acid metabolism in burned patients. *JPEN* 8:(1984)357–60.
10. **Dickerson, R.N., R. O. Brown,** and **K.G. White**. Parenteral nutrition solutions. *In* J.L. Rombeau, and M.D. Caldwell, eds. *Parenteral Nutrition*, 2d edition. Philadelphia: Saunders, (1993)310–33.
11. American Medical Association, Department of Foods and Nutrition. Multivitamin preparations for parenteral use. *JPEN* 3:(1979)258–62.
12. **Green, H.L., K.M. Hambidge, R. Schanler, et al**. Guidelines for the use of vitamins, trace elements, calcium, magnesium, and phosphorus in infants and children receiving total parenteral nutrition. Report of the Subcommittee on Pediatric Parenteral Nutrient Requirements from the Committee on Clinical Practice Issues of the American Society for Clinical Nutrition. *Am. J. Clin. Nutr.* 48:(1988)1324–342.
13. American Medical Association, Department of Foods and Nutrition. Guidelines for essential trace element preparations for parenteral use. *JPEN* 2:(1979)263–67.
14. **Fleming, C.R**. Trace element metabolism in adult patients requiring total parenteral nutrition. *Am. J. Clin Nutr.* 49:(1989)573–79.
15. **Malecki, E.A., H.-C. Lo, H. Yang, C.D. Davis, D.M. Ney,** and **J.L. Greger**. Tissue manganese concentrations and antioxidant enzyme activities in rats given total parenteral nutrition with and without supplemental manganese. *JPEN* 19:(1995) 222-226.
16. **Payne-James, J.J.,** and **H.T. Khawaja**. First choice for total parenteral nutrition: the peripheral route. *JPEN* 17:(1993)468–78.
17. **Gottschlich, M.M., L.E. Matarese,** and **E.P. Shronts**, eds. *Nutritional Support Dietetics Core Curriculum*, 2d ed. Silver Spring, MD:American Society of Parenteral and Enteral Nutrition 1993
18. **Guenter, P., S. Jones, D.O. Jacobs,** and **J.L. Rombeau**. Administration and delivery of enteral nutrition. *In:* J.L. Rombeau, and M.D.Caldwell eds. *Enteral and Tube Feeding*, 2d edition. Philadelphia: Saunders, 1990, pp 192–203.
19. **Biasco, G., C. Callegari, F. Lami et al**. Intestinal morphological changes during oral feeding in a patient previously treated with total parenteral nutrition for small bowel resection. *Am. J. Gastroent.* 79:(1984)585–88.
20. **Heird, W.C.** and **M.R. Gomez**. Parenteral nutrition. *In* R.C. Tsang, A. Lucas, R. Uauy, and S. Zlotkin, eds., *Nutritional Needs of the Preterm Infant*. Baltimore: Williams and Wilkins, 1993, 225–42.
21. **Khalidi, N., A.G. Coran,** and **J.R. Wesley**. Guidelines for parenteral nutrition in children. *Nutritional Support Services* 4:(1984)27–8.

☑ TO TEST YOUR UNDERSTANDING

1. Calculate the osmolarity and the caloric content of one liter of a 20% dextrose solution. Show your calculations.

2. Calculate the grams of protein and nitrogen, and the caloric content of 1 liter of a 8.5% amino acid solution. Show your calculations.

3. a. What is the caloric content (kcal / mL) of a solution composed of 225 mL of a 10% amino acid solution and 350 mL of a 50% dextrose solution? Show your calculations.

b. If the solution just described were infused at 20 mL/ hr, and a 10% fat emulsion was simultaneously infused at 10 mL/ hr, what would the hourly caloric infusion rate (kcal / hr) be?

4. a. What concentration (% or g / 100 mL) of a 1-L dextrose solution would it take to equal the calories in 500 mL of a 20% fat emulsion?

b. Could this dextrose solution be infused in a peripheral vein? Explain.

5. Calculate the calorie and protein needs of Mr. C.W., a 45-year old who is 6 ft tall and weights 80 kg. He is confined to bed while recovering from elective gastrointestinal surgery. Use an allowance of 1.5 g pro/kg, and calculate calorie needs by BEE × activity × injury, BEE × 1.5, and 30 kcal / kg. How do these calorie levels differ? Use the intermediate calorie level to calculate the kcal:N ratio.

a. _____ g protein
_____ kcal (BEE × AF × IF)
_____ kcal (BEE × 1.5)
_____ kcal (30 kcal / kg)
_____ kcal:N

b. Using a factor of 35 mL/kg body weight to estimate Mr. C.W.'s initial fluid requirements, what would be his daily total fluid needs in mL/ day? Rounding this to the nearest 500 mL gives _____L/ day.

6. Assume that Mr. C.W. receives a total volume of 3 L/day of a TNA parenteral nutrition solution administered as CPN and that 30% of total energy is provided as fat.

a. Calculate the number of kcal from dextrose that Mr. C.W. will need in his parenteral feeding solution in order to receive 2,655 kcal/ day. How many g of dextrose would this be per day? Show your calculations.

_____ dextrose kcal / day
_____ g dextrose / day

b. Would this amount of dextrose be tolerated by Mr. C.W. as part of a CPN formulation? Explain your answer, i.e. in g dextrose/kg/hr.

c. What final concentrations of dextrose, amino acids and lipids would be needed in each liter of TNA parenteral nutrition solution.

_____ % dextrose
_____ % amino acids
_____ % lipids

7. How do CPN and PPN differ in regard to the following factors?
Duration of PN support needed
Calorie needs
Fluid status

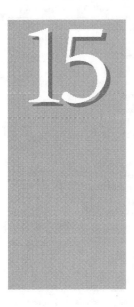

Nutritional Care of Allergic Patients

There are a number of conditions included in the broad category of *adverse reactions* or *food sensitivities. Food intolerance* is "any abnormal physiological response to an ingested food" (1). The mechanism is unknown but may be metabolic, emotional, toxic, or pharmacologic. *Food toxicity* or *food poisoning* is caused by a toxin in the food. The toxin may be produced by bacteria or an innate part of the food, such as the toxin in some fish. An *allergy*, whether to food or another substance, involves the immune system. Food allergy is also sometimes called *food hypersensitivity*. Food allergy must be distinguished from *food idiosyncrasy* in which the reaction resembles an allergic response but is not immunologic. It may involve a genetic predisposition. Lastly, some patients develop *food aversions*, a psychologic intolerance and avoidance of certain foods (1, 2, 3). This chapter will emphasize particularly the allergic response to food.

Food allergies are usually diagnosed and treated on an outpatient basis. The function of the nutritional care specialist is to interview and counsel the patient. This counseling often includes a considerable amount of instruction on food composition and preparation, so the nutritionist must be knowledgeable about these matters. Skills in patient interviewing and counseling, which are covered in Chapters 3 and 7, are extremely important.

Occasionally, an allergy patient is hospitalized. Those with respiratory manifestations are particularly sensitive to infections. In addition, any hospital patient with any diagnosis may have food allergies.

Nutritional care of allergic conditions may be directed toward prevention of sensitization, toward diagnosis, including identification of specific antigens, or toward management. It is the nutritional care specialist's responsibility to ensure that all patients who have food allergies are served an appropriate diet in which all conditions are considered.

Prior to proceeding with this chapter, you should review the anatomy and physiology of the immune system and the discussion of hypersensitivity in your text.

PREVENTION OF SENSITIZATION

Preventive actions are primarily directed toward genetically vulnerable infants—that is, those whose parents or siblings have a history of allergy. There is some evidence that infants can be sensitized in utero during pregnancy or via breast feeding postnatally (4). Foods in the mother's diet which have been implicated in the development of allergy in infants in utero are milk, eggs, wheat, soybean, and peanuts, but the occurrence of in utero sensitization is believed to be rare (4).

Some studies of breast feeding and allergy suggest that breast feeding prevents or delays allergy, while others indicate that it does not. Nevertheless, some exclusively breast-fed infants do develop allergies. It has been suggested that the infant may be sensitive to human milk protein (rare) or to antigens transmitted to human milk from the mother's diet. Food antigens previously shown to be transmitted in human milk include cow's milk and cheese, egg, citrus, wheat, and chocolate (4).

Despite these uncertainties, certain diet recommendations are commonly given for prevention of allergies in atopic women and infants at risk:

During pregnancy:
Omit all foods to which you are allergic (6).

Omit all foods to which members of the immediate family are allergic (6).

If allergic to cow milk, substitute meat or soy; supplement calcium (6).

Take calcium and phosphorus supplements (5, 6, 7).

Take one multivitamin and iron tablet per day (7).

During lactation:
Omit eggs, cow milk and cheese, and peanut butter (5, 8).

Limit milk to one pint of boiled milk per day (5).

Take calcium supplements.

Use reduced amounts of wheat, soy, citrus, and fish (8).

Avoid excess consumption of allergenic foods (5).

Avoid synthetic coloring agents (5).

For the infant:
No cow milk first month; promote breast feeding if necessary; use soy milk (5, 9).

Breast feed for 6 months; no soy or cow milk; may add Nutramigen (8).

Add nonallergenic solids at 6 months (8).

Add cow milk at 12 months (8).

Add egg around 24 months (8).

Add wheat cereal at 13 to 18 months (8).

Add legumes, corn, and citrus during 13 to 18 months, but after wheat (8).

As you can see, researchers do not agree on the recommendations. In addition, other publications state that no significant differences were found between groups who restricted diets prenatally and those who did not (10, 11). As a consequence, one cannot ensure that the above dietary manipulations will be effective in all patients, but they may be useful for some.

As a precaution, patients at risk can be advised to avoid a preponderance of any particular food during pregnancy. Instead, a mixed diet without emphasis on a limited number of foods is recommended. This advice should apply particularly to those foods that are known to be especially allergenic. Common food allergies are listed in Table 15-1.

At the age of 4 to 6 months, the baby may be given cereal, fruit, vegetables, and meat in the amounts and consistency described in Chapter 9. The introduction of the foods within these groups that are common allergens may be delayed further. For example, the introduction of cereal may begin with rice, since it is less often allergenic than are other cereals commonly fed to infants. Following the introduction of rice, other cereals are added at intervals, with wheat, a common allergen, added last. Cereals should also be added one at a time so that the offending allergen may be identified if allergic symptoms arise. Consequently, the use of mixed cereals for infants at risk should be discouraged. Similarly, when fruits and vegetables are given, apple sauce, pears,

TABLE 15-1 Common Food Allergens

Children 2 years +	Older Children and Adults
Cow milk	Cow milk
Chocolate / cola	Chocolate/cola
Wheat	Corn
Corn	Legumes
	Egg (whites)
	Citrus
	Tomato
	Wheat
	Pork
	Cinnamon
	Fish; crustacea; mollusks
	Nuts
	Peanuts
	Soybeans
	Green peas
	Potato
	Peach
	Papaya
	Rice
	Buckwheat

Compiled from: J.C. Breneman,. *Basics of Food Allergy.* Sprinfield, IL: Charles C. Thomas. 1978: G.J. Lawlor Jr., and T.J. Fisher. *Manual of Allergy and Immunology.* Boston: Little Brown. 1981; Speer. F. *Food Allergy* (2nd ed.). Boston: John Wright. PSG Inc., 1984, and S.L.Taylor, Chemistry and detection of Food Allergens. *Food Tech.* May 1992;146.

carrots, and squash may be given early, with others added later. Mixtures should not be used until it is established that the infant is not sensitive to any of the individual components. Lamb is commonly used as the first meat. Vitamins for infants at risk should be uncolored (2); the reason for this will become clear later in this chapter. Eggs and citrus juices are often avoided until the infant is a year old.

Several problems can arise in connection with the protocol just described. There is evidence that infants may be sensitized to allergens in breast milk (3). Some allergic reactions have been reported to occur after the mother ate oranges, eggs, chocolate, cow milk, strawberries, tomatoes, apples, bananas, coffee, or tea (4). When such reactions occur, the lactating mother must be counseled on avoiding the allergen. If many foods are restricted, she must also be given advice on planning a diet for herself which is adequate for lactation. (See Chapter 8).

A special formula is required if the infant is allergic to cow milk and if the mother is unable to breast feed. An artificial formula that is tolerated by the infant must be used. Among these are:

1. *Casein hydrolysate-based formulas* have low allergenicity. Some are also lactose-free. Specific examples are given in Appendix H, Table 2.
2. *Soy protein-based formulas* may be useful, but must be chosen from those that are supplemented with calcium and vitamins (see Appendix H, Table 1). In addition, some infants develop a sensitivity to soy (12).

3. *Goat milk* is sometimes useful, but it has several limitations. It has an excessively high solute load for infants and must be supplemented with vitamins A, D, C, B_{12}, and folate. If it is purchased fresh, it must be boiled for 2 minutes to render it bacteriologically safe and to reduce allergenicity. However, it is also available canned or dried in some areas. In any form, goat milk contains lactose, a problem for some infants with gastrointestinal allergy or other accompanying disorder.

DIAGNOSIS

The signs and symptoms of food allergy include many that are nonspecific, including vomiting and diarrhea as well as rashes, itching, coughing, irritability, and anemia. It is therefore necessary for the physician to differentiate food allergy from a number of other conditions. Once the condition is diagnosed as an allergy, it is necessary to determine whether the patient is sensitive to food or to pollens, drugs, or other materials. Last, the specific food antigen must be identified. The nutritional care specialist can have an important role first in confirming or disproving the existence of suspected food allergy. The specific antigen within a food is not usually known. Most are proteins, but in shrimp, a nonprotein antigen, transfer ribonucleic acid, has been identified (13).

Diagnostic approaches include a thorough physical examination, some laboratory tests, and a detailed clinical history, of which the diet history is an important component (14). If these methods are inconclusive, diagnostic diets may be used.

PHYSICAL EXAMINATION

The physical examination includes careful observation for signs characteristic of allergy. It may be helpful in differential diagnosis to rule out other conditions, but is not generally useful in identifying specific food antigens. The physical examination also identifies malnutrition and other effects secondary to allergy.

LABORATORY TESTS

The *enzyme-linked immunosorbent assay* (ELISA) measures the level of IgE or other immunoglobulins, but a positive test must be confirmed by dietary challenge tests, which will be described later. A variety of other tests of immune function are less useful (14, 15, 16).

CLINICAL HISTORY

The clinical history is often the most useful diagnostic procedure. Information is obtained, usually by the physician, about the following:

Nature and severity of symptoms
Age of onset
Possible precipitating factors
Time relationship between exposure to any suspected antigen and onset of symptoms
Other allergic phenomena

DIET HISTORY

The diet history may be useful both in ruling out or confirming food allergy and in identifying the allergen. To accomplish these objectives, it is necessary for the nutritional care specialist to interview the patient thoroughly and to have a detailed knowledge of foods.

The diet history interview must include a number of questions requiring detailed answers. In allergy clinics, a questionnaire form is used as a guide. Table 15-2 lists information often needed and can give you an idea of the amount of detail required.

THE FOOD DIARY

If the identity of the food allergen is not obvious to the patient and cannot be established by analysis of the diet history, the patient may be asked to keep a *food diary*. The number of days for which the diary should be kept will depend on the frequency of the symptoms. There must be enough days on which symptoms occur to make it possible to establish the relationship to intake of specific foods.

Unless the nutritional care specialist provides detailed directions to the patient, the procedure will be useless. The information required is similar to that listed in Table 15-2. The time of intake of each food or other ingestant must also be noted, along with the time of onset and a description of symptoms. This procedure should be undertaken only if the diet history is not helpful since interpretation is time-consuming and difficult.

DIAGNOSTIC DIETS

A number of diets have been used for diagnosis of food hypersensitivity. In general, they can be classified as *food challenges* or *elimination diets*. These may be necessary if other methods are uninformative or inconclusive.

Food Challenge Test
When an allergy to a specific food is suspected based on a diet history or food diary, the diagnosis may be tested by a food challenge. It is helpful if a diet free of all suspect foods can be followed first with the objective of having all symptoms subside. Preferably, the challenge test is a "double blind" test, in which neither the patient nor the physician knows what has been given. In an ideal situation, used when the patient is an older child or an adult, a third person places either dextrose or a dehydrated form of the suspected allergen in nonallergenic capsules. The patient is then given one or the other type of capsule and is observed for signs of allergic reaction.

Since neither the patient nor the physician knows if the patient has received the allergen, the observation can be quite objective. If this method is not possible, a "single blind" test can be conducted, in which the patient, but not the physician, is unaware of the material given. For small children, the suspected offending food can be hidden in another nonoffending food. In any case, all medications, especially antihistamines and corticosteroids, should be discontinued 1 week before the test. Patients with anaphylactic responses should not be challenged.

The challenge test may be repeated with gradually increasing doses up to 8 g. If this is tolerated, the food is given openly in large amounts conventionally prepared to evaluate the effects of preparation procedures. It may also be repeated at intervals to see if the child has "outgrown" the allergy.

Elimination Diets

Elimination diets may eliminate a few or many foods from the diet. The simplest type is *elimination of a single suspected food*. This is a useful procedure when only one food is suspected. In a child, for example, the parents may suspect a sensitivity to milk, wheat, or eggs, all common antigens in children. Since these foods are often hidden within processed foods, you will need to counsel

TABLE 15-2 Areas of Inquiry in the Diet History for Suspected Food Allergy

Food-related questions

1. List foods eaten, with frequency and amount
2. For each food, was it home prepared? If so, describe ingredients.
3. If foods were eaten away from home, where were they obtained? Give brands and specific ingredients.
4. Was each food eaten cooked or raw?
5. Were artificial colors or flavors used in food preparation?
6. Describe the meal pattern; include the time, amount, and frequency of food intake.
7. Are any foods eaten in especially large quantities?
8. Do other family members have allergies? To foods? Which foods? Does the patient eat these foods?
9. Do symptoms develop from smelling or handling certain foods?

Other Related Questions

1. List symptoms and time of onset.
2. Do symptoms develop only in certain locations or during certain activities?
3. Does the patient chew gum? When? How often? Brand?
4. What cleaning compounds are used, including soaps, detergents, and scouring powders for dishwashing?
5. List all drugs, cosmetics, and personal hygiene products and give brand names, and time and frequency of use. Include information on toothpaste, mouthwash, lipstick, throat lozenges, prescription drugs, laxatives, and other over-the-counter drugs.
6. Is the patient under constant or recurrent emotional stress?

the patient or the patient's parents on procedures for total elimination of the foods from the diet. Further information on specific foods to eliminate is given later in this chapter in the section on treatment.

When a single food has not been identified as the culprit and the antigens have not been identified, a diet might be formulated to eliminate those foods which, by previous experience, are known to have a high probability of allergenicity. The diet, sometimes called a *probability multiple-elimination diet*, eliminates common offenders for 2 to 3 weeks. If there is improvement in the symptoms, the foods eliminated are reintroduced one at a time as a challenge to identify the antigenic foods.

A difficulty may arise in deciding which foods to eliminate. Opinions differ about which foods are common offenders. There is general agreement, however, that milk is an important one, particularly in children. The list of common offenders (Table 15-1) should be coupled with the clinical and diet histories and the food diary in deciding which foods to eliminate.

If this procedure does not identify the allergen, a more stringent elimination diet may be required. A number of variations of this type of diet have been published. The principle common to all is that each consists of a limited number of foods chosen primarily from those which have been shown by past experience to be allergenic only rarely. At the same time, a sufficient number of foods must be included to make possible a diet adequate in protein and calories and provide a little variety for acceptability. Since the number of foods allowed are quite limited, however, compliance is improved if you provide some guidance on methods of preparation and meal planning. The patient is also likely to need supplementation of vitamins and minerals in a hypoallergenic form.

Some suggested combinations of allowable foods that have been used as elimination diets are shown in Table 15-3. Those given are well known as *Rowe elimination diets*, named after their originator. Since all foods are potentially allergenic, there is no guarantee that all symptoms will subside in all patients. If symptoms do not subside with one diet, another composed of a different combination of foods may be tried.

For infants, elimination diets may consist of the following foods:

Less than 3 months—milk substitute

3–6 months—milk substitute & rice cereal

6–24 months—milk substitute, rice cereal, applesauce, pears, carrots, squash, and lamb.

If the diet results in improvement of symptoms, foods can be added one at a time at intervals of 4 to 5 days, regardless of the patient's age. Any food that causes the patient's previous symptoms to reappear should be eliminated from the diet. The response might be tested again in 6 to 12 months.

TABLE 15-3   Examples of Foods Allowed with Typical Elimination Diets

Rowe Elimination Diet # 1	Rowe Elimination Diet # 2	Rowe Elimination Diet # 3	Rowe Elimination Diet # 4
Cereals			
Rice	Corn	Tapioca	
Puffed Rice	Rye	Bread of any combination of soy,	
Rice Flakes	Corn pone	lima bean, potato starch and	
Rice Krispies	Corn-rye muffin	tapioca flours	
Tapioca	Ry-Krisp		
Rice biscuit			
Rice bread			
Vegetables			
Lettuce	Beets	White potato	
Chard	Squash	Tomato	
Spinach	Asparagus	Carrot	
Carrot	Artichoke	Lima beans	
Sweet Potato		String beans	
Yam		Peas	
Fruit or Juice			
Lemon	Pineapple	Apricot	
Grapefruit	Peach	Grapefruit	
Pear	Apricot	Peach	
	Prune		
Meat			
Lamb	Capon (no hens)	Beef	
	Bacon	Bacon	
Other			
Cane sugar	Cane or beet sugar	Cane sugar	Cane sugar
Maple sugar	Karo corn syrup	Maple sugar	Milk
Cane sugar syrup flavored with	Sesame oil	Cane sugar syrup flavored	Cream
maple	Mazola oil	with maple	Plain cottage cheese
Sesame oil	Gelatin, plain or flavored with	Sesame oil	Tapioca
Olive oil	pineapple	Soybean oil	
Gelatin, plain or flavored with	Salt	Gelatin, plain or flavored with	
lime or lemon	Baking powder	lime or lemon	
Salt	Baking soda	Salt	
Baking powder	Cream of tartar	Baking powder	
Baking soda	Vanilla extract	Baking soda	
Cream of tartar	White vinegar	Cream of tartar	
Vanilla extract		Vanilla extract	
Required Supplements			
1. multivitamin supplement	multivitamin supplement	multivitamin supplement	multivitamin supplement
2. 1 tbsp bid Calcium-Sandoz	1 tbsp bid Calcium-Sandoz	1 tbsp bid Calcium-Sandoz	
Syrup	Syrup	Syrup	

OTHER CONSIDERATIONS IN IDENTIFYING ALLERGENS

Biological Classification

According to some beliefs, a patient who is hypersensitive to a food may also be hypersensitive to other foods in the same *biological classification*. Some believe this phenomena is rare, while others are of the opinion that this cross-reactivity is common and that patients should be tested and counseled accordingly (16, 17). Groups of biologically related foods are shown in Table 15-4.

Intolerances to Food Additives and Other Foods

It has been suggested that patients may have an allergy or other form of intolerance to additives used in food processing. Some of these additives include monosodium

TABLE 15-4   Biological Classification of Foods

Family	Members
	Plants
Apple	Apple (cider, vinegar, apple pectin), pear, quince, loquat
Arrowroot	Arrowroot
Arum	Poi, taro
Banana	Banana, plantain
Beech	Chestnut, beechnut
Birch	Filbert, hazelnut, oil of birch (wintergreen)
Buckwheat	Buckwheat, rhubarb
Cactus	Tequila
Carob	Gum acacia
Cashew	Cashew, mango, pistachio
Citrus Fruits	Angostura, citron, grapefruit, kumquat, lemon, lime, orange, tangelo, tangerine
Cola nut, cacao	Coffee, chocolate, cola, cola drinks, tea
Cocheospurnum	Guiac gum, guar gum
Composite	Artichoke, chicory, dandelion, endive, escarole, head lettuce, leaf lettuce, oyster plant, sunflower, sesame, safflower, vermouth
Ebony	Persimmon
Fungi	Mushroom, yeast, antibiotics
Ginger	Cardamom, ginger, turmeric
Gooseberry	Currant, gooseberry
Goosefoot	Beet, beet sugar, spinach, Swiss chard
Gourd	Cantaloupe, casaba, cucumber, honeydew, muskmelon, Persian melon, pumpkin, squash, watermelon, citron, vegetable marrow.
Grains (Grass)	Barley, malt, cane (cane sugar, molasses, corn oil, glucose), corn (cornstarch), oats, rice, rye, sorghum, wheat (bran, gluten flour, graham flour, wheat germ), wild rice
Grape	Grape, cream of tartar, raisin
Heath	Blueberry, cranberry, huckleberry, loganberry
Honeysuckle	Elderberry
Iris	Saffron
Laurel	Avocado, bay leaves, cinnamon
Lycethis	Brazil nut
Legumes	Acacia, black-eyed peas, kidney bean, lentil, licorice, lima bean, navy bean, pea, peanut, peanut oil, senna, soybean, soybean oil, stringbean, gum tragacanth
Lily	Aloes, asparagus, chive, garlic, leek, onion, sarsaparilla
Mallow	Cottonseed, okra (gumbo)
Maple	Maple syrup (maple sugar)
Mint	Basil, marjoram, mint, oregano, peppermint, sage, savory, spearmint, thyme
Morning glory	Sweet potato, yam
Mulberry	Breadfruit, fig, hop, mulberry
Mustard	Broccoli, Brussels sprouts, cabbage, cauliflower, celery cabbage, collard, cress, horseradish, kale, kohlrabi, mustard, radish, rutabaga, turnip, watercress
Myrtle	Allspice
Nutmeg	Nutmeg, mace
Olive	Green olive, ripe olive, olive oil
Orchard	Vanilla
Palm	Coconut, date, sago, palm oil

(continued)

TABLE 15-4   *(continued)*

Family	Members
Papaw	Papaya, papain, papaw
Parsley	Angelica, anise, caraway, carrots, Celeriac celery, coriander, cumin, dill, fennel, parsley, parsnip
Pea	Bean, lentil, pea, peanut, soy, alfalfa, clover, licorice, tamarind
Pedalium	Sesame, sesame oil
Pepper	Black pepper, white pepper
Pineapple	Pineapple
Plum	Almond, apricot, cherry, nectarine, peach, persimmon, plum, (prune), sloe (gin)
Pomegranate	Pomegranate
Poppy	Poppy seed
Potato (nightshade)	Chili, eggplant, green pepper, paprika, pimiento, potato, cavenne pepper, red pepper, tomato
Rose	Apple, blackberry, dewberry, loganberry, loquat, quince, raspberry, strawberry, youngberry
Seaweed	Agar, longan
Spurge	Tapioca, cassava
Sterculia	Cacao (chocolate), kola bean, gum karaya
Sunflower	Jerusalem artichoke, sunflower seed oil, cardoon, chicory, endive, tarragon
Walnut	Black walnut, butternut, English walnut, hickory nut, pecan
Miscellaneous	Honey
	Animals
Crustaceans	Crab, crayfish, lobster, prawn, shrimp, squid
Fish (with fins)	Anchovy, barracuda, bass, bluefish, buffalo fish bullhead, butterfish, carp, catfish, caviar, chub, codfish, croaker, cusk, corvina, drum, eel, flounder, haddock, hake, halibut, harvestfish, herring,, mackerel, millet, muskellunge, perch, pickerel, pike, pollock, pompano, porgy, rosefish, salmon, sardine, scrod, scup, shad, smelt, snapper, sole, sturgeon, sucker, sunfish, swordfish, trout, tuna, weakfish, whitefish
Fowl	Chicken (chicken eggs), duck (duck eggs), goose (goose eggs), grouse, guinea hen, partridge, pheasant, squab, turkey
Mammals	Beef (butter, cheese, cow milk, gelatin, veal), goat (cheese, goat milk), horsemeat, mutton (lamb), squirrel, venison
Mollusks	Abalone, clam, cockle, mussel, oyster, scallop
Reptiles	Turtle

Compiled from C. Collins-Williams, and L.D. Levy, Allergy to foods other than milk, in *Food Intolerance.* R.K. Chandra, ed., New York: Elsevier. 1983. M.K. Farrell, Food allergy, *In* G.J. Lawlor Jr. and T.J. Fischer, eds., *Manual of Allergy and Immunology.* Boston: Little Brown, 1981; J.M. Sheldon, R.G. Louell, and K.P. Matthews, Food and gastrointestinal allergy *In A Manual of Clinical Allergy* Philadelphia: Saunders, 1967 and J. Monro, Food allergy and migraine, *Clin. Immun. Allergy*, 2:(1982) 137–164.

glutamate, metabisulfites, and sodium nitrate, but attention has tended to focus particularly on the artificial coloring agent tartrazine, or FD&C yellow No. 5, which is used in many processed foods, and on salicylate, a structurally related compound that occurs naturally in some foods and in aspirin. Although the subject is controversial, some allergists use tartrazine-free and "salicylate-free" diets for diagnosis and treatment.

This chapter considers allergies to foods. However, other patients may have *intolerances* to some of these same foods. Lactose intolerance, for example, is discussed in Chapter 17.

TREATMENT

Once the offending foods have been identified, the diet is modified to avoid the foods in question. This type of diet is called by the general term *avoidance diet*. It is thus distinguished from an elimination diet used for diagnosis.

AVOIDANCE DIETS

Planning a diet to avoid only one or a few foods is not difficult, provided the foods to be avoided are usually eaten singly. If a person is allergic to shrimp and papaya, for example, avoiding these foods is easily arranged. On the other hand, if the patient is allergic to many foods or if the offending foods are those in common use within many mixtures, there may be great difficulty. In particular, management of sensitivities to wheat, milk, eggs, soy, or corn is difficult.

Before we describe techniques for specific avoidances, some general principles may be established:

1. The diet should be planned initially for total avoidance of all forms of the offending foods. For some individuals, the diet can be modified later to include certain tolerated forms of the offending foods. Some milk-sensitive patients, for example, can tolerate milk if it is boiled. Some patients can tolerate a food if it is eaten in small quantities or at intervals at least 4 days apart, or both.
2. Nutritional adequacy must be carefully planned. When foods are omitted from the diet, alternative sources of nutrients may need to be included. If a milk-free diet is used, adequate dietary protein, energy, calcium, riboflavin, and vitamin D must be planned for. Foods or supplements suggested for replacement must be nonallergenic.
3. Specific guidance on diet management must be given to the patient. Patients must be helped to identify sources of the allergens. This is particularly true when there are many hidden forms of the allergen. Instructions on reading labels and identifying forms of the offending foods are important. Many patients also need helpful food preparation suggestions in the form of recipes.
4. It may be necessary for the patient to inquire of the manufacturer concerning the ingredients in a product. If you counsel allergy patients frequently, you will need to keep up-to-date lists of manufactured food products free of wheat, corn, milk, egg, soy, and, possibly, tartrazine and salicylates.

In addition to these general principles, each food sensitivity has its unique aspects. Consult your diet manual or diet therapy text (18) for general guidelines for diets free of cow milk, egg, corn, soy, and wheat. Each of these foods are present in many foods, often in hidden form, and present problems in avoidance. The avoidance of wheat is particularly troublesome since there is no completely adequate substitute for wheat flour in baked goods. Table 15-5 lists substitutes for use in recipes and gives suggestions for their use. In addition, many wheat-flour products contain yeast, which is also known to be an allergen in its own right.

As previously mentioned, there is a growing belief that allergies may be developed to chemicals in foods, certain food additives, and food contaminants such as

TABLE 15–5 Alternative Ingredients in Cooking for the Allergy Patient.

Milk	Fruit juice (in cooking)
Corn Cornstarch	Equal amounts arrowroot starch or potato starch Double the amount of whole wheat, soy, or barley flour
Baking Powder containing cornstarch (1 t)	1/4 t baking soda + 1/2 t cream of tartar
Egg as emulsifier	Egg substitutes (some brands contain egg white) 2 T whole-wheat flour, 1/2 t oil, 1/2 t baking powder & 2 T milk, fruit juice, or water
Cocoa Chocolate (1 sq)	Equal amounts of carob powder 3 T carob powder + 2 T milk, butter, margarine, or water
Butter	Willow Run Margarine and Parv are kosher, milk-free butter substitutes
Wheat 1 c*	1 1/3 c ground rolled oats 1 1/4 c rye flour 1 c corn flour, fine cornmeal, rye meal 3/8 c rice flour 3/4 c coarse cornmeal or coarse oatmeal 3/8 c potato flour 1/2 c barley flour 1/2 c rye flour + 1/2 c potato flour 2/3 c rye flour + 1/3 c potato flour 3/8 c (10 T) rice flour and 1/3 c rye flour 1c soy flour + 3/4 c potato starch
Wheat flour as thickener, 1 T	1/2 T cornstarch, potato starch, arrowroot starch, rice flour

Compiled from M.A. Ohlson,. Experimental and Therapeutic Dietetics, (2d ed.) Minneapolis: Burgess, 1972, 142–3; and G.J. Lawlor and T.J. Fischer, ed,. *Manual of Allerrgy and Immunology*, Boston: Little Brown, 1981, 467.
* To improve product quality in baking.
1. Always use soy flour in combination with another flour.
2. For smoother texture, mix rice flour or cornmeal with the liquid in the recipe, bring to boil, and cool.
3. In baking, use lower temperature and longer time. Increase leavening to 2 1/2 t baking powder/c of any coarse meals or flour.
4. Bake muffins and biscuits in small sizes. Yeast breads are not satisfactory without wheat flour.
5. Apply frosting or store in closed containers to preserve moisture.

molds and yeasts. Many believe that hypersensitivity to salicylates and tartrazine causes hyperactivity and other abnormal responses, especially in children. The salicylate-free, tartrazine-free diet, often called the *Feingold diet*, is frequently used despite weak evidence of its effectiveness. This diet and the mold-free and yeast-free diets are found in more detailed diet manuals (19).

INDIVIDUAL FOODS AND FOOD INGREDIENTS

Nutritional care specialists must be knowledgeable about sources of foods and manufacturing procedures. This section will provide you with information useful both in identifying allergens and in counseling patients with allergies and some other types of food intolerance (20, 21).

Food Additives
Sugar, salt, smoke, vinegar, and wine have been used for centuries as additives to preserve foods and improve color and flavor. A wide variety of other substances are now used in food processing as acids, antioxidants, colors, emulsifiers, flavoring agents, mold inhibitors, preservatives, sequestrants, stabilizers, and thickeners. Many additives are listed as "generally recognized as safe" (GRAS) by the FDA. Items are sometimes removed from the GRAS list, however, when information casts doubt on their safety. An item is more commonly removed from the list because it has become a suspected carcinogen than because it causes allergies. Nevertheless, many patients believe that additives in foods are the source of their allergies and will ask you about them. It is important for you to be able to answer their questions.

Acid Additives. The organic *acids—acetic, benzoic, citric, fumaric, malic, oxalic, quinic, succinic,* and *tartaric*—are found in many fruits and some vegetables. They are often used in food processing and may be listed on labels as "fruit acids". *Phosphoric acid*, an inorganic acid, is also sometimes used. Acids are usually added to give tartness and flavor, to prevent discoloration of vegetables during processing, and to provide sufficient acid in making jams and jellies.

Antioxidants. Agents used to prevent oxidation or unwanted browning of fruits and vegetables and rancidity of fats and oils are ascorbic acid, vitamin E, erythorbic acids, sodium sulfite, sulfur dioxide, butylated hydroxyanisole (BHA), butylated hydroxytoluene (BHT), and propyl gallate. BHA and BHT have been reported to cause rhinitis, wheezing, headache, and somnolence.

Coloring Agents. Coloring agents, which may be natural or synthetic, are added to foods to improve consumer acceptance. The naturally occurring colors include beet juice, fruit juice, grape skin extract, paprika, saffron, turmeric, and caramel, all of which are plant products. Products that require an oil-soluble coloring agent, such as butter, oil, cheese, and salad dressings, are colored with carotenoids or annatto. Annatto, from the seeds of the annatto tree, is used infrequently. Of these substances, only turmeric has been reported to act as an allergen.

The question of safety of synthetic dyes has led to a great deal of confusion. Decisions about approval for use have been based on political pressure generated by those who fear that they are "poisons" or "cause cancer." The following colors have been implicated in adverse reactions: (22)

Tartrazine (FD&C Yellow #5)
Brilliant blue (FD&C Blue #1)
Citrus Red #3 (to color orange skins)
Erythrosin (FD&C Red #3)
Ponceau (FD&C Red #4 to color maraschino cherries)
Sunset Yellow (FD&C Yellow #6)
Indigotine (FD&C Blue #2)

As an example of the confusion, amaranth (formerly FD&C Red #2) has been banned in the United States, while allure red is approved. In Canada, on the other hand, allure red is banned and amaranth is approved. At present, 90 percent of the manufacture of colorants consists of allure red, tartrazine, and sunset yellow.

There is some evidence of sensitivity to synthetic coloring agents. Although interest has focused on tartrazine, intolerance to other dyes may be more common. The mechanism of the adverse reaction is unknown and may be intolerance rather than allergy. Because of the attention given to tartrazine, manufacturers must list it on labels. For others, consumers must judge for themselves whether a particular dye is present, based on the color of the product.

Common FD&C dyes used in carbonated beverages, for example, are the following:

Orange	Yellow #6, or 96% Yellow #6 + 4% Red #40
Cherry	99.5% Red #40 + 0.5% Blue #1
Grape	80% Red #40 + 20% Blue #1
Strawberry	Red #40
Lime	95% Yellow + 5% Blue #1
Lemon	Yellow #5

Emulsifying Agents. Emulsifiers serve to disperse one liquid in another. Oil-in-water emulsions are prepared in shortenings, margarine, salad dressings, ice creams, ices, sherbets, some soft drinks and baked goods. The agents used are generally mono- and diglycerides. Soy lecithin and sorbitan monostearate are used in many foods.

Flavoring Agents. Synthetic flavoring agents are used in a wide variety of foods. Common artificial flavors include the following:

Allyl caproate (pineapple)

Allyl disulfide (onion or garlic)

Anisic alcohol (peach)

Benzaldehyde (cherry)

Ethyl acetate (strawberry)

Ethyl vanillin (vanilla)

Methyl anthranilate (orange)

Methyl salicylate (wintergreen)

Mold Inhibitors. Mold inhibitors, mostly sodium diacetate and calcium or sodium propionate, are widely used in baked products. These products are presumed to be helpful to those with allergy to molds.

Preservatives. Many have questioned the safety of nitrites used in prepared fish and meat products. Nitrites also occur naturally in some vegetables, including spinach and beets. They react with amino acids to form nitrosamines, which have been suspected of being carcinogens. Allergic reactions have not been reported.

Sequestrants. Sequestrants are chelating agents used to deactivate undesirable metals in foods that otherwise catalyze lipid oxidation and cause clouding of soft drinks, and off-tastes and deterioration of foods such as canned shrimp and beans, potato salad, sandwich spreads, and other mayonnaise-containing foods.

Stabilizers and Thickeners. These materials are used to prevent separation of the contents of peanut butter, ice creams, cheese spreads, pie fillings, and salad dressings. The most common items in this category are gelatin, carboxymethyl cellulose, various vegetable gums, and cornstarch.

Useful Facts about Some Specific Foods

To advise the allergic patient, the counselor must be very familiar with foods, including their use in a menu and their appearance, preparation, availability, and nutritional value. This section contains information on specific food items that may be of use in identifying offending foods and in planning avoidance diets.

Baking powder: Ingredients are sodium bicarbonate (baking soda), cream of tartar (potassium acid tartrate), tartaric acid, and either monocalcium phosphate or sodium aluminum sulfate. These are not allergenic; however, some contain wheat flour, cornstarch, or powdered egg white, which may cause an allergic response.

Beef: Beef does not cross-react with cow milk allergy. Rare beef may be more allergenic than well-done beef in some sensitive individuals.

Beer: Ingredients are yeast, hops, corn, malt, usually made from barley, and sometimes other grains. The yeast may cause difficulty for the mold-sensitive patient, and some patients are sensitive to one or more of the grains.

Buckwheat: Buckwheat is in a different botanical family from wheat, and can thus be used as a substitute for other grains, but it can be an allergen itself. Buckwheat is available as a flour and as a groat, called kasha.

Chewing gum: Chicle and a variety of other materials, including natural or artificial rubber and various waxes, preservatives, flavors, and colors, are used in gum manufacture. Allergies to one or more ingredients have been reported (20).

Chicken: Chicken and chicken-egg allergies do not cross-react.

Chocolate: Chocolate is prepared from the cacao nut. The defatted product is cocoa. Milk chocolate contains 20 percent milk. Chocolate is a common allergen. It cross-reacts closely with cola, and patients allergic to one are often sensitive to the other. Both contain caffeine.

Cinnamon: Cinnamon may be prepared from "true cinnamon" (*Cinnamomum zeylanicum*) or from cassia (*Cinnamomum cassia*). Either may be an antigen.

Cola (Kola): This nut is a native African plant material closely related to the South American chocolate. It is contained in cola soft drinks.

Flaxseed (Linseed): Flaxseed is contained in some whole-grain cereal. Otherwise, patients are not usually exposed to this material, and sensitivities are rare.

Honey: The hexoses (glucose and fructose) in honey are nonallergenic, but honey contains about 2 percent protein specific to the flower from which the honey is made. Some patients who are allergic to honey may also be sensitive to legumes and licorice if the source of the honey was a leguminous plant such as alfalfa. Honey allergy does not cross-react with bee venom allergy.

Licorice: Licorice is prepared from the rootstock of a legume. There is sometimes cross-reactivity between licorice and other legumes.

Milk: Allergy to milk can be a hypersensitivity to lactalbumin or casein. Albumin is species-specific and heat sensitive. A patient who is allergic to cow milk lactalbumin may be able to tolerate goat milk or boiled milk. The film that forms on the top of boiled milk should be removed. Casein is neither species-specific nor heat sensitive.

Nuts: English walnuts, black walnuts, pecans, and butternuts frequently cross-react. Useful substitutes are Brazil nuts, hazelnuts, almonds, and macadamia nuts. The oil in peanut butter may be corn oil.

Onion: Onion or related vegetables may be contained in items with "flavoring agents" listed on the label.

Sulfites: Sulfating agents include sulfur dioxide and potassium and sodium salts of bisulfite or metabisulfite. They are used to prevent darkening of potatoes on standing. Sulfites may cause asthmatic reactions in individuals allergic to sulfite compounds.

Surimi: Surimi is a fish paste prepared by mincing fish flesh and adding natural or artificial flavors. Sorbitol, sugar, and salt are also usually added. Surimi is used to prepare various foods which simulate shellfish, such as crab, scallop, shrimp, and lobster-like products. It may be in the form of flakes, chunks, prebreaded portions or morsels, tails, sticks, or legs. It is often prepared from Alaskan pollock and may have a percentage of meat from the shellfish being simulated.

DRUGS

Drugs are sometimes used in management of allergies. Cromolyn sodium is thought to block mast cell degranulation in the digestive tract and thereby reduce symptoms, allowing the patient to eat restricted amounts of the offending food. Because it is poorly absorbed from the digestive tract and is used in the treatment of asthma, it is usually administered as an inhalant. Oral cromolyn sodium has been used in the treatment of food allergies. The major justification for its use is for the patient whose nutritional status could not be adequately maintained otherwise. Antihistamines and theophylline are given for symptomatic treatment, as are corticosteroids if reactions are severe. Table 15-6 lists the side effects of drugs used in the management of allergic symptoms.

TOPICS FOR FURTHER DISCUSSION

1. Do you think a child's hypersensitivity could have been inherited from his atopic parents if the child is allergic to different foods and shows different allergic manifestations?
2. Do any members of the class have food allergies? Describe problems and management.
3. Groups of students may visit a nearby supermarket and examine the items in the frozen food-case, canned food sections, dairy case, or baked good sections. What items would be usable by a person with an allergy to wheat? Corn? Soy? Cow milk? Egg? All five? Evaluate these products in terms of nutrient composition, indications for use, cost, and palatability. Discuss some techniques for counseling these patients about the use of convenience foods.
4. Compile a bibliography of recipe books for allergy patients.

REFERENCES

1. **Hamburger, R.N**. Introduction: A brief history of food allergy, with definitions of terminology in food intolerance. *In:* R.N. Hamburger, ed. *Food Intolerance in Infancy: Allergology, Immunology and Gastroenterology,* New York: Raven Press, 1989.
2. **Anderson, J.A.** Food allergy or sensitivity terminology, physiologic bases, and scope of the clinical problem, In: J.E. Perkin, ed. *Food Allergies and Adverse Reactions,* Gaithersburg, MD, Aspen Publishers, 1990.
3. **Krey, S.H. and R.L. Murray,** Modular and transitional feedings. *In:* J.L. Rombeau and M.D. Caldwell , eds. *Clinical Nutrition. Enteral and Tube Feeding,* 2d ed., Philadelphia: Saunders, 1990.
4. **Perkin, J.E**. Maternal influences on the development of food allergy in the infant. *In* J..E. Perkin., ed. *Food Allergies and Adverse Reactions,* Gaithersburg, MD: Aspen Publishers, 1990.
5. **Lawrence, R.A**. Prenatal dietary prophylaxis of atopic disease *In* R.A. Lawrence, *Breastfeeding: A Guide for the Medical Profession.* St. Louis: Mosby, 1985.
6. **Glaser, J. and D.E.Johnstone,** Prophylaxis of allergic diseases in the newborn. *J.A.M.A.* (1953)153–620
7. **Chandra, R.K., S. Puri, C. Suraiya, C. and P.S. Cheema,** Influence of maternal food antigen avoidance during pregnancy and lactation on incidence of atopic eczema in infants. *Clin. Allergy* 16:(1986)563.
8. **Hamburger, R.N., S. Heller, S.H. Mellon , R.D. O'Connor, and R.S. Zeiger,** Current status of the clinical and immunologic consequences of a prototype allergic disease prevention. *Am. J. Allergy* 51:(1983)281.
9. **Stentzing, G, and R. Zetterstrom,** Cow's milk allergy incidence and pathogenetic role of early exposure to cow's milk formula. *Acta Paediatr. Scand.* 68:(1979)383.
10. **Zeiger, R.S.** Prevention of food allergy. *In* A.T. Schneider, and F. Lifshitz, eds. *Food Allergy: A Practical Approach to Diagnosis and Management,* New York: Marcel Dekker, 1988.
11. **Lilia, G. A. Danaeus, K. Falth-Magnusson. et al.** Immune response of the atopic woman and foetus: effects of high- and low-dose food allergen intake during late pregnancy. *Clin. Allergy* 18:(1988)131.
12. **Kibort, P.M. and M.E. Ament.** Cow's milk and soy protein intolerance in childhood. *Ped. Ann.* 11:(1982)1, 119–123.
13. **Taylor, S.L.** Chemistry and detection of food allergens. *Food Tech.* May 1992, 146.
14. **Farrell, M.K.** Food allergy. *In* G.J. Lawlor Jr., and T.J. Fischer, eds., *Manual of Allergy and Immunology,* Boston: Little, Brown, 1981.
15. **Chandra, R.K. and S. Jeevanandam.** Diagnostic approach. *In* R.K. Chandra, ed. *Food Intolerance,* New York: Elsevier, 1983.
16. **Anderson, J.A. and J.E. Perkin.** *In:* J.E. Perkin, ed. *Food Allergies and Adverse Reactions,* Gaithersburg, MD: Aspen Publishers, 1990.
17. **Perkin, J.E**. Major food allergies and principles of dietary management. *In:* J.E. Perkin, ed. *Food Allergies and Adverse Reactions,* Gaithersburg, MD: Aspen Publishers, 1990.
18. **Zeman, F.J.** *Clinical Nutrition and Dietetics,* 2d ed. New York: Macmillan, 1991.
19. **C.M. Pemberton and C.F. Gastineau, eds.** *Mayo Clinic Diet Manual,* 5th ed., Philadelphia: Saunders, 1981.
20. **Speer, F.** *Food Allergy,* 2d ed. Boston: John Wright, PSG Inc., 1983.
21. **Breneman, J.C.** *Basics of Food Allergy,* 2d ed. Springfield, IL: Charles C Thomas, 1984.
22. **Perkin, J.E.** Adverse reactions to food additives and other food constituents. *In* J.E. Perkin, ed. *Food Allergies and Adverse Reactions,* Gaithersburg, MD: Aspen Publishers, 1990.

TABLE 15-6 Nutrition-Related Side Effects of Drugs Used in Management of Allergies

Generic Name	Nutrition-Related Effects
Antihistamines	Gastrointestinal complaints common: take with meals Dry mouth is common Weight gain: do not use in newborn or premature infants.
Corticosteroids	Weight gain, gastrointestinal disturbances, emotional disturbances, growth retardation in children, negative nitrogen balance, hyperglycemia, hyperlipidemia, negative calcium balance, interference with vitamin D metabolism, gastrointestinal bleeding, pancreatitis, fatty liver, peptic ulceration.
Theophylline	Nausea: plasma clearance is decreased by high-carbohydrate diet or dietary methylxanthines; decrease in low-carbohydrate, high-protein diet, charcoal-broiled meats

ADDITIONAL SOURCES OF INFORMATION

Brostoff, J., and S.J. Challacombe, eds. *Food Allergy and Intolerance*. London:Braillier Tindal, 1987.

Chandra, R.K. ed. *Food Intolerance*. New York: Elsevier, 1984.

Dong, F.M. *All About Food Allergy*. Philadelphia: Stickley, 1984.

Dwyer, J. Commercial additives. *In* E.F.P. Jelliffe and D.B. Jelliffe, eds. *Adverse Effects of Foods*, New York: Plenum, 1982.

Metcalfe, D.D., H.A. Sampson, and R.A. Simon, eds. *Foods and Food Additives. Adverse Reactions to Foods and Food Additives*. Boston: Blackwell Scientific, 1991.

Metcalfe, D.D. The nature and mechanisms of food allergens and related diseases. *Food Tech*. May 1992, 136.

National Advisory Committee on Hyperkinesis and Food Additives, *Final Report to the Nutritional Foundation*. New York: Nutrition Foundation, 1980.

Stevenson, D.D., and R.A. Simon. Sensitivity to ingestion of metabisulfites in asthmatic subjects. *J. Allergy Clin. Immunol*. 68:(1981)26–32.

 ## TO TEST YOUR UNDERSTANDING

1. You are counseling a pregnant patient who has been sent to you by an obstetrician for information on normal, adequate diet. The patient, Mrs. H., is 25 years old, 5 feet, 4 inches tall, and weighs 110 pounds. She is 2 1/2 months pregnant.

Mrs. H. is a teacher in a nursery school with 50 children and must be quite active. She also tells you that she has suffered from hay fever for 10 years. Her husband develops hives when he eats shellfish and strawberries. Neither has any other abnormal condition.

A 24-hour recall gives you the following meal pattern, which the patient states is typical of her week days. On the weekends and holidays, she does not eat the snacks.

Breakfast:
4 oz orange juice
Scrambled eggs (2)
Sweet roll
8 oz milk
Coffee/sugar

Snack (with children at school):
8 oz carton of milk
2 graham crackers

Lunch (eaten with children at school):
3/4 c cream of tomato soup
1 1/2 egg salad sandwich on whole-wheat bread
Baked custard
8 oz milk

Snack (with children at school):
8 oz carton of milk
2 oatmeal cookies

Dinner:
4 oz meat loaf
1/2 c broccoli with 1/4 c Hollandaise sauce
Sliced tomato salad/Thousand Island dressing
1/6 lemon meringue pie

a. State the basic principle(s) on which your nutritional counseling will be based.

b. The patient is required to eat lunch with the children at the nursery school. She cannot change the menu, but it is posted a week in advance so that she knows what the meals will consist of. Indicate at the right of the menu in part how you would suggest she modify her breakfast and dinner. Suggest two alternative box lunches for days that the school menu does not offer appropriate choices.

c. Mrs. H. is later referred to you by a pediatrician. She now has a baby boy who is 6 weeks old. Although she has been breast feeding him, she says this is too limiting on her freedom and wants to stop. What would you suggest to her and why?

2. Write a menu for a Rowe Elimination diet #1.

3. A patient tells you he carries his lunch, but he needs a Rowe elimination diet #2. Write a list of foods that he could pack for lunch.

4. When a commonly used food or a food category is removed from a diet, the intake of certain nutrients may become inadequate. Name the nutrients that might be deficient in the diet of a patient who is allergic to the following foods, and suggest alternative sources.
a. Milk, wheat, and egg (adult patient)
b. Citrus fruits and tomatoes (adult patient)
c. Chocolate, cola, and nuts (teenage patient)

5. A patient's food diary indicates that she developed hives after eating the following items: Sunday—Roast lamb: Monday—Pepperoni pizza; Thursday—Roast turkey and bread stuffing.
What allergy would you suspect?
What questions would you ask the patient?

6. A patient asks you if the mold inhibitor put into bread can cause cancer or asthma. What would you reply?

Nutritional Care in Food Allergy

Part I: Presentation

Present illness Barbara R. is a 22 y.o. commercial artist referred to Allergy Clinic by her family-practice physician. The patient C/O sporadic abdominal distention, cramping, and diarrhea 1–2 hr following some meals, with a 13# weight loss in 2 mo. She denies other symptoms. Referral states tests had ruled out infection, chronic inflammation, abnormality of anatomy or motility of intestinal mucosa, pancreatic insufficiency, abnormality of enterophepatic circulation, and endocrine disease or malignancy; treatment for irritable bowel syndrome was not successful.

Past medical history: Rubella and chickenpox in childhood, milk allergy as an infant, hayfever in spring for past 10 yr.

Family history: Father has sensitivity to insect venom. Mother has asthma. No history of GI disease in immediate family.

Social history: Single, recent college graduate in first job. Shares apartment with female friends. Pt describes her employment as "very stressful,"

Review of systems: Pt has no complaints except those related to abdomen and recent weight loss.

Physical Exam:
General: White female. Ht 5 ft., 5 in, wt 112#, medium frame. Abdomen distended, diffusely but minimally tender. No rebound. Bowel sounds normal. No hepatosplenomegaly. Remainder of exam WNL.

Laboratory: RBC 4.0×10^{12}/L, Hct 0.42, Hgb 12.2 g/L, plasma fasting glucose 5.6 mmol/L, serum albumin 38 g/L, WBC 5.0×10^9/L, lymphs 1.35, eos 0.06.

Impression: Moderate GI distress 2° to possible hypersensitivity to unknown antigens in 22 y.o slightly underweight female with positive family history of allergy.

Plan: Nutrition Clinic referral for detailed diet history for identification of possible antigen and nutritional counseling. Primary physician to continue symptomatic treatment of GI symptoms.

QUESTIONS

1. Discuss the significance of the family history and employment history.

2. Compare this patient's laboratory values with normal values:

		Normal	Patient	Interpretation
A.	Hct	_____	_____	
B.	Hgb	_____	_____	_____
C.	Blood glucose	_____	_____	_____
D.	Plasma albumin	_____	_____	_____
E.	Leukocytes	_____	_____	_____

Part II: Nutrition Consult

Barbara R. is first evaluated in the nutrition clinic by a dietetic technician (DT), who obtains a preliminary diet history and nutritional assessment. The DT reports a TSF of 14.0 mm and a MAC of 25.7 cm, and a 24-hr recall:

Breakfast
    4 oz orange juice
    3/4 c ready-to-eat corn cereal/ 4 oz whole milk
    3 Ry-Krisp wafers
    Coffee/1 t sugar

Lunch
    Cold plate
    4 oz sliced ham
    3 oz potato chips (1 oz = P-2; F-8; C-37 g)
    1/2 c sliced tomato/lettuce
    "A few" celery sticks
    Watermelon slice, 1 serv
    Iced tea/sugar, 1 tsp

Snack
    12 oz cola drink (C-37 g)

Dinner
    4 oz baked salmon/lemon
    1/2 c buttered peas
    1/2 c fresh fruit salad
    2 chocolate brownies (P-2; F-8; C-26 g)
    Coffee/1 t sugar

QUESTIONS

3. Complete Forms C and D as shown in Appendix M for this patient. Does the diet appear to be deficient in any of the vitamins and minerals listed?

4. List additional questions related to the 24-hr recall that you would ask this patient when you interview her after studying the available data.

5. Your questioning reveals that her symptoms worsen when she eats chocolate. Summarize your observations, assessment, and plan in a SOAP note.

Part III: Diagnostic Diet

Three weeks after your initial consultation, the patient returns to the nutrition clinic. She states that she has followed your advice, but that her symptoms have not totally subsided, although they occur less frequently. Her physician has requested that she be instructed on the use of a Rowe elimination diet #3, which she is to follow for 2 weeks.

QUESTIONS

6. Explain the rationale for diet.

7. Modify the diet provided by your instructor to conform to the prescribed diet.

8. If the patient refuses to eat the meats on the Rowe #3 diet, what would you do?

9. List the essential points of your diet instructions. (Review Chapter 7 if necessary.)

10. Two weeks later, the patient reports that all her symptoms have disappeared. The physician now authorizes additions to the basic diet. Describe how you would advise the patient to proceed.

    a. At what intervals would you recommend each new addition?

    b. How often should the newly added food be eaten during that interval?

11. If your first addition is wheat, what wheat-containing food would you recommend the patient use? Why?

Part IV: Avoidance Diet

The above procedure suggested that Barbara R. was also sensitive to wheat, milk, and eggs. You instruct her on a diet that is free of these foods and her previous avoidances.

QUESTIONS

12. For each of the following items, decide whether you would advise the patient to avoid the food. If you advise avoidance, state your reason.

    a. Sliced bologna
    b. Rye bread
    c. French bread
    d. French toast
    e. Buckwheat pancake and waffle mix
    f. Consomme (canned)
    g. Chicken-noodle soup
    h. Kosher frozen dinner with beef
    i. Root beer
    j. Cola drink

13. Name the nutrients that are likely to be marginal in this patient's diet. Name two acceptable sources of each for use in her diet.

14. Using the sample menu provided by your instructor, indicate the modifications necessary to make a diet allergen-free for Barbara R.

Part V: Drugs in the Treatment of Allergy

Two years later, Barbara R. tells you she is engaged to John H. who is also a patient at the clinic. John was seen first in the ER a year ago. He was wheezing and pale. Closer physical examination revealed urticaria across the abdomen.

John stated at that time that he was allergic to peas, beans, and soy, and the symptoms were similar to previous reactions from these foods. He was not aware of having eaten any of these items, but had been to a potluck supper held by his athletic club.

John was given epinephrine 0.4 ml sc to relieve the respiratory symptoms, and oxygen was administered. Since he responded rapidly to these measures, it was felt he did not need theophylline or corticosteroids. He was released from the ER on an antihistamine, diphenhydramine HCI (Benadryl), 50 mg t.i.d.

QUESTIONS

15. Describe some "hidden" sources of soy John might have eaten at the potluck supper that caused his condition.

16. Since John is allergic to peas, beans, and soy, what other foods should be investigated for allergenic effects in this patient?

17. List the main points you would make in your nutritional counseling with John.

18. Using the menu provided by your instructor, modify the menu as you would instruct John to do.

Part VI: Prevention of Allergy

After Barbara and John had been married for a year, Barbara reappears at the Nutrition Clinic. She tells you she is two months pregnant and asks if there is any advice you can give her about diet during pregnancy to prevent allergies in her baby.

QUESTIONS

19. Summarize briefly the main points of your advice.

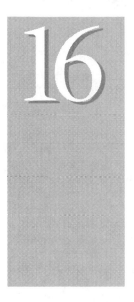

Nutritional Care of Patients with Diseases of the Upper Digestive System

Digestive system discomfort is a common experience often arising from unwise eating and drinking. Most such disorders are mild, brief in duration, and do not require professional nutritional care. However, a few conditions become sufficiently severe or chronic that nutritional care is indicated. Before proceeding, you should review, if necessary, the material in your text on diseases of the upper digestive tract.

In some circumstances, interference with food intake may be an integral part of a disorder of the gastrointestinal (GI) tract. The nutritional care specialist will thus have use for the various procedures that help improve nutrient intake. These procedures, described in Chapter 12 through 14, will not be described again here. However, they may need to be integrated with the nutritional care procedures described in this and subsequent chapters. In addition, most patients will have preconceived ideas that certain foods cause distressing symptoms or, alternatively, provide unusual benefits. These beliefs, whether or not they are justified, must be considered in planning nutritional care.

Symptoms related to the gastrointestinal tract, such as loss of appetite, taste changes, and dry mouth, may be caused by disorders unrelated to the GI tract. In this chapter, we will describe nutritional care in these conditions, as well as in selected diseases of the esophagus and stomach.

APPROACHES TO COMMON SYMPTOMS IN THE DIGESTIVE SYSTEM

During the onset and course of many disorders, the patient may seek advice concerning symptoms relating to the digestive system. The nutritional care specialist may be very helpful to patients by providing suggestions on approaches to alleviate the discomfort. Some of these are as follows:

LOSS OF APPETITE

Appetite loss may be rather benign in short-term mild illness, but in other illnesses it may be very severe and long-lasting (e.g. cancer) and may lead to severe tissue loss, malnutrition and dehydration. Some of the following suggestions may be helpful in promoting food and fluid intake:

Have a relaxing walk or other relaxation before meals.

Use a glass of wine or beer before meals to stimulate the appetite (subject to physician approval).

Make meal times relaxed and pleasurable.

If appetite loss is sporadic, eat larger meals at times when appetite is best (e.g., large breakfast or lunch with smaller dinner).

Get plenty of rest.

If food preparation is stressful, use ready-to-eat and easily prepared foods and use time-saving appliances.

Eat slowly and take breaks during meals.

If you cannot maintain acceptable weight: Try to eat regularly, even if in small quantities. Keep nutritious snack foods on hand. Try high-caloric liquids or supplements (See Table K-1)

Consult physician if weight loss persists.

ABNORMAL SENSE OF TASTE

Abnormal taste sensations can develop in patients with malignancies, those receiving chemotherapy, for some neurological disorders or infections in the mouth, including the teeth or in the pharynx and sinuses. Unpleasant tastes may contribute to the loss of appetite described above. Depending on the specific problem, some of the following may be helpful:

A metallic taste may be reduced with tart foods such as citrus juice, cranberry juice, and pickles.

Use plastic, instead of metal, utensils.

Add sugar to reduce salty flavor; add salt to decrease excess sweetness.

Unpleasant flavors can sometimes be masked by marinating foods in strong-flavored sauces or by adding strong seasonings such as hot peppers or curries.

If meat has an unusual taste, substitute chicken, fish, dairy products, or eggs (in place of lamb, beef, or pork, for example).

Use cold foods such as fish or egg salads, cold cuts, cold drinks.

Freshen taste in mouth with fruits, chewing gum, sugarfree candy, or 1 teaspoon baking soda in 2 cups warm water.

An unpleasant aroma of some liquids may be reduced by using a straw in *very* cold liquid.

NAUSEA AND VOMITING

Nausea may occur with or without vomiting. Severe, prolonged vomiting can result in electrolyte imbalance and dehydration in addition to malnutrition and weight loss. If the condition is severe, the following may be suggested:

Loose clothing and fresh air are helpful.

Remain upright at least 2 hours after eating.

Eat frequent, small, dry meals; eat slowly; chew food well.

Have 8 or more cups of fluid daily *between* meals.

Eat cold foods without a strong aroma, e.g., cold cereals, crackers, dilute juices, frozen desserts, gelatin, potatoes.

Avoid fried, high-fat, or very spicy foods.

Put ice bag on back of neck..

DRY MOUTH

A dry mouth can occur as a result of disorders that affect salivary secretions. It can also be a side effect of some drugs. The patient can alleviate this condition with some of the following:

Sip on fluids at frequent intervals.

Use gravies, sauces, and salad dressings to moisten food.

Dunk or soak foods in liquids.

Suck on ice chips or hard candies.

Chew gum.

In extreme cases, use "artificial saliva."

NUTRITIONAL ASSESSMENT

Many disorders of the mouth, pharynx, esophagus, and stomach can severely affect nutritional status by altering intake. Therefore, detailed nutritional assessment is important in the care of patients with disease in these tissues. These patients should be routinely considered at nutritional risk and should receive an in-depth nutritional assessment (see Chapter 5). You may need to inquire about specific problems described in the following sections.

MOUTH

Are teeth carious, missing, absent?

Are dentures well fitted? Ill fitted?

Is there periodontal disease? Ulceration of mouth or gums?

Are teeth or mouth sensitive to heat? Cold?

Is mouth abnormally dry?

ESOPHAGUS

If the patient complains of *dysphagia* (impairment or loss of ability to chew or swallow), ask about its frequency. Related to liquids? Solids? Both? Greater with cold liquids or warm? If the patient complains of *odynophagia* (pain on swallowing) ask if the pain is precipitated by cold liquids? Spicy foods? Acid foods? Fatty foods? Does pain occur immediately on swallowing? After meals?

STOMACH

Is distress caused by food intake? Which foods or groups of food?

Is pain relieved by food intake?

GENERAL

Life-style: Smoking? Alcohol intake? Rest? Stress? Activity, including in relation to meals? Medications?

Diet history: Does the diet include fiber? What is the average meal size and frequency? Obtain information about specific offenders. Ask about caffeine intake and liquid intake.

ESOPHAGEAL DISORDERS

There are many esophageal disorders that have important effects on nutrition because they interfere with food intake. Some of these are primary diseases of the esophagus, such as strictures or tumors in or adjacent to the esophagus, reducing lumen size. Others involve neurological or muscular diseases or other conditions. Table 16-1 lists these disorders.

DYSPHAGIA

The nutritional care specialist can be a valuable part of the care team that treats *dysphagia* (swallowing disorders) in cooperation with speech and language pathologists, physicians, nurses, occupational and physical therapists, radiologists, and others. If you are to participate in a dysphagia team, you must understand the normal process.

Normal Swallowing

There are four stages in normal swallowing:

1. In the voluntary *oral preparatory* or *anticipatory phase*, food or liquid is taken into the mouth and prepared to be swallowed. The teeth, tongue, and cheeks move the food around the mouth, including between the teeth as necessary. The food is gathered in a ball (bolus), which the tongue holds against the hard palate.
2. In the *oral phase*, also voluntary, the tongue presses against the palate, and the food or liquid is moved to the back of the throat. When the bolus passes the faucial arches of the soft palate, the swallowing reflex occurs. This should take about 1 second.
3. In the *pharyngeal phase,* the soft palate rises to close off the nasopharynx: Vocal chords close, larynx elevates, and epiglottis drops. This closes off the airway so that food does not enter the trachea. It also creates a negative pressure to pull food to the esophagus. Peristalsis carries the bolus of material into the esophagus. Total time normally is 1 second.
4. In the *esophageal phase*, the muscular movements plus gravity carry the material down the esophagus into the stomach. Total time is 8 to 20 seconds.

Common Problems in Swallowing

Problems in swallowing can be divided among the phases of the normal swallow (1–3). Common problems are:

1. Oral preparatory phase:

   Drooling
   Poor lip closure or poor lip control or both
   Difficulty in moving the food around or to the back of the mouth
   Pocketing food between the cheek and gums, under tongue, against hard palate.

2. Oral phase:

   Food collects in cheeks
   Patient cannot feel where food is located
   Problem triggering pharyngeal stage of swallowing (delayed swallow)
   Food sticks in throat

3. Pharyngeal phase:

   Food caught in valleculae
   Copious secretions
   "Gurgly" voice; poor vocal chord elevation or closure
   Coughing; choking
   Cricopharyngeal inadequate function
   Aspiration
   Delayed swallow

TABLE 16-1 Conditions That Frequently Lead to Swallowing Problems

Neurologic Disorders	*Mechanical Disorders*	*Other Disorders*
Cerebral vascular accident	Stricture of pharynx or esophagus	Inflammation of pharynx or esophagus
Closed head trauma	Tumor or other obstruction of pharynx or esophagus	Complications of AIDS (e.g., thrush)
Cerebral palsy	Surgery of the head or neck	History of aspiration
Poliomyelitis		History of pneumonia
Parkinson's disease		Reflux esophagitis
Amytrophic lateral sclerosis		Encephalitis
Multiple sclerosis		
Muscular dystrophy		
Myotonic dystrophy		
Myasthenia gravis		
Dystonia		
Huntington's chorea		
Alzheimer's disease		
Anoxia		
Spinal cord injury		

4. Esophageal phase:

> Food "stuck in throat"
>
> Reflux of food when lying down
>
> Solid foods cause difficulty, but pureed foods are handled well
>
> Impaired contraction or motility
>
> Constriction or fistulas

Some patients will have more than one of these problems.

The patient's reflexes must be evaluated. The ability to cough in order to clear the airway is especially important. On the other hand, the existence of rooting and suckling reflexes are normal in infants. Their existence in brain-damaged adults indicates the level of cognitive function of the patient.

Assessment in Dysphagia

The assessment of swallowing disorders is frequently done by the speech and language pathologist (SLP). The nutritional care specialist may suspect a swallowing problem and refer the patient for evaluation.

Patients with conditions listed in Table 16-1 should be observed carefully for evidence of dysphagia. If dysphagia is suspected, the nutritional care specialist should observe the patient at mealtime within 48 hours. (1) A videofluoroscope is used in cases hard to diagnose. This instrument makes a video tape of the function of the internal structures when swallowing.

If dysphagia is diagnosed, the patient's nutritional status should be re-evaluated and monitored regularly. Nutritional requirements should be estimated. The dysphagic patient is in danger of *malnutrition* because of problems in chewing and swallowing. In addition, dysphagic patients can easily become *dehydrated* because they may have difficulty in swallowing liquids. For the patient who aspirates food or liquid, the danger of *aspiration pneumonia* increases. These patients must be monitored in the same manner as would any patients with these same conditions from other causes.

Dysphagia patients are sometimes fed with TPN or gastrostomy (PEG) feedings. These patients should be monitored as described in Chapters 13 and 14. Indications for nonoral feedings are aspiration, especially of more than 10 percent of a bolus, absent or delayed pharyngeal swallow (more than 10 seconds), or severe oral motility impairment(4).

The Dysphagia Diet

There is no one dysphagia diet. Instead, the diet is individualized to provide food the patient can manage, and then is progressed to allow the patient to improve. In general, solid foods are easier to manage and are fed first.

Variations in Consistency

Solid foods. When severely dysphagic patients are first orally fed, ice chips are introduced for evaluation and training. Ice is less hazardous if aspirated than many other ingested materials, and the low temperature makes its presence easy to sense.

The patient may then progress to a strained and then to a pureed diet. A typical starting point is apple sauce or mashed banana. Other appropriate foods are pureed fruits and vegetables, mashed potatoes, custards, puddings, stiff gelatin cubes, yogurt, and ice cream. None of these should include solid bits. A suggested sequence in consistencies is shown in Table 16-2.

Foods with the following characteristics should be chosen:

> Approximate consistency of apple sauce
>
> Cold or very warm
>
> Uniform texture
>
> Cohesiveness to form a single bolus.

Foods that often need to be avoided include peanut butter or white butter, which are sticky, bread, cake, tough meat, hard fruit, and spicy, fibrous, and greasy foods. Also, foods of variable consistency (e.g., soup with pieces of vegetables or meat) should be avoided, as well as foods such as rice, and plain ground meats or thin hot cereals, which tend to disintegrate in the mouth.

After the patient learns to manage the pureed diet, foods that require chewing can be added. These can include soft, cooked, cut-up fruits and vegetables, scrambled eggs, minced or ground poultry, and soft fish.

Further steps in the progression include cut, rather than ground, meats, larger pieces of fruits and vegetables, and foods with more than one texture. The patient progresses to a routine mechanical soft diet and eventually to a regular house diet. Some institutions have established multistage "dysphagia diets"; others have only a few. In every case the diet must be individualized to as many stages as necessary for the patient. Raw fruits and vegetables are not added until the patient can manage a regular diet.

TABLE 16-2 Suggested Consistency Levels in Diets for Dysphagia Patients

Solid Foods

Stiff gelled (add unflavored gelatin to strained foods)
Gelled (puddings and dessert gelatins)
Strained
Pureed
Soft diet (with ground meats)
Soft diet (meat not ground)
Regular house diet

Liquid Foods

Thick liquids only ("spoon thick" may be made with thickening agent)
Medium-thick liquids (some include thickening agents)
Cold thin liquids
Hot thin liquids

Adapted from J. Schmitz, Dysphagia. *In* D.J. Gines, ed. *Nutrition Management in Rehabilitation.* Rockville, MD: Aspen, 1990.

The ultimate goal is to return the patient to the regular diet, although the pureed diet is the limit for some patients. In either case, while the patient is progressing through the pureed diet, every effort should be made to provide a diet whose flavor, aroma, and appearance are attractive. Several lines of commercial pureed products that hold their shape are available and are helpful for acceptability and safety.

Liquid foods. Liquids are more difficult for the patient to handle and are often introduced later than solid foods. The ability to swallow liquids is unrelated to the ability to swallow solid foods. When giving liquids, it is useful to start and finish with a few ice chips to cleanse the area.

Training in swallowing liquids begins with such thick liquids as frozen milkshakes, any liquid thickened with gelatin, slushes, nectars, tomato juice, buttermilk, and thickened cream soups. Ice cream and sherbets are included. These are often referred to as "spoon-thick" liquids.

The patient may progress from thick to "medium-thick" (milk shakes, nectars, tomato juice, eggnog) and then thin liquids (see Table 16-2). Foods commonly classified as thin include water, broth, carbonated drinks, such fruit juices as apple and cranberry juice, coffee, and tea.

Liquids are classified according to the speed with which their presence in the mouth can be sensed and how rapidly and completely they pass through the mouth and pharynx. Thin liquids are harder to sense, are harder to control, and pass through quickly. Thicker liquids can be sensed more quickly, but they may accumulate in the pharynx and be aspirated.

Thickening agents

Various materials are used to adjust the thickness of liquids to the needs of patients. Some of these are commonly available food items such as baby rice cereal, baby apple flakes, apple sauce, canned and instant puddings, bread crumbs, graham cracker crumbs, yogurt, and tofu. The characteristics of these items vary in many criteria that might be used for selection. Baby rice cereal can thicken all liquid bases at least cost and is effective at all viscosity levels. It also adds the least volume (5).

Therefore, it is frequently recommended for home use.

There are also commercial thickening agents that are moderate in cost, can be used to produce varying viscosities, and do not add flavors to the base liquid. They are less easily available and must be ordered from the manufacturer or distributor. The available products and their characteristics are listed in Table 16-3. Directions for use are on the package but must be adjusted for the needs of the patient.

Milk

Another food item that requires consideration is milk. It is sometimes stated that milk intake thickens mucus to form "phlegm" (6 7); however, there is little or no scientific evidence to that effect. It has been suggested that milk may adhere to mucus and increase its volume.

Planning the diet

The specific disorder causing dysphagia is highly variable; therefore, the recommended diets also are varied. Common to all dysphagia patients is the need to position the patient appropriately, upright if possible (7). Adaptive equipment should be provided if needed (8).

Consistency levels and positioning must be chosen for specific disorders. Some of these are given in Table 16-4. If a patient has combinations of these problems, the diet may need to be adjusted further.

In case of long-term dysphagia, it is likely that the patient will need TPN or tube feeding or each in succession. The nutritional care specialist must monitor the patient's food intake and progress in relearning to swallow, and make recommendations for advancing the patient from TPN to tube feeding and to oral intake (see Chapters 13 and 14).

ACHALASIA AND ESOPHAGEAL REFLUX

Nutritional care of esophageal disorders frequently requires measures to ensure adequate nutrient intake in general (see Chapters 12 and 14). In addition, there are considerations specific to certain disorders. Nutritional care procedures are given in Table 16-5 for achalasia and Table 16-6 for esophageal reflux.

TABLE 16-3 Thickening Agents

Product	Manufacturer	Characteristic
Nutra-Thick	Menu Magic	Vitamin and mineral fortified; grainy; starchy taste; based on modified food starch
Puree Plus	Diamond Crystal	No taste change; has 5 forms for red meat, white meat, vegetables, dessert/beverage, and multipurpose
Thicken Right	Menu Magic	Dissolves quickly; mixes without lumping
Thick-it	Milani Foods	Smooth; little flavor change; based on modified cornstarch
Thick 'N Easy	American Institutional Products	Modified constarch-based; no cooking required
Thick-N-Quick	Associated Systems	No flavor change; no cooking required; vegetable gum-based; contains ascorbic acid
Thick-Set	Bernard Fine Foods	Lumpy; changes flavor
Thixx	Bernard Industries	Grainy; thickens further on standing

TABLE 16-4   Dietary Treatment in Dysphagia

Swallowing Disorder	Recommended Diet Consistency and Position
Mechanical disorders:	
Surgical Removal of:	
Part of tongue	Semisolid foods that can maintain cohesive bolus Moist foods, add sauces and gravies as necessary
Base of tongue	Semisolid in cohesive bolus Use caution with thin liquids
All of tongue	Very individual May require nonoral feeding
Floor of mouth	Consistency that forms a cohesive bolus May be semisolid or soft
Palate	Very individual May need foods not requiring chewing: liquid or semisolids
Supraglottic laryngectomy	
Total	Use caution with thin liquids Use foods that form a cohesive bolus May try supraglottic swallow (Hold breath; put in mouth; tilt head back, swallow; cough)
Partial	Tip head forward during swallow (usually temporary) if resection is unilateral vertically For more extensive resections, patient may never be able to take liquids p o
Neuromuscular disorders:	
Slow, weak, or uncoordinated swallow	Increase stimulus to swallow with highly seasoned foods and extremes of temperature Use foods that form a cohesive bolus and that require mastication Avoid sticky or bulky foods and thin liquids; use tube feeding for liquid feeding Small frequent meals Chin down on chest

Reduced oral sensation	Maximize sensation with:
	  Highly seasoned foods
	  Colder temperatures
	  Single texture in a food
	  Feeding into most sensitive area

Reduced tongue movement	Use thick liquids Swallow with chin up
Cricopharyngeal dysfunction	Use liquid to pureed diet Turn head to side to swallow (turn to weaker side if any)
Laryngeal elevation decreased	Use medium-thick liquids or soft solids Avoid sticky or bulky foods Use foods that form a cohesive bolus Chin down; turn head to damaged side (if any)

Compiled from Consultant Dietitians in Healthcare Facilities. *Dining Skills: Practical interventions for the Caregivers of the Eating Disabled Older Adult.* Pensacola, FL: Retirement Research Foundation, 1993, *Manual of Clinical Dietetics.* Chicago: American Dietetic Association, 1988, American Dietetic Association Chap. 6: Controlled consistency, modified fluid (dysphagia) diet. In: *Handbook of Clinical Dietetics,* 2d ed. New Haven: Yale University Press, 1992, B. Sperling,. Feeding the patient with impaired swallowing. *In:* A. Skipper, ed. Dietitian's *Handbook of Entereal and Parental Nutrition,* Rockville, MD: Aspen, 1989.

OTHER TREATMENT

Medical management of reflux esophagitis is usually effective. It may consist of antacid therapy given 1 hour and 3 hours after food intake, and 300 mg of cimetidine at bedtime and with onset of symptoms for 2 to 4 weeks. Mechanical measures to reduce reflux include elevating the head of the bed on blocks (*not* propping the head on pillows), avoiding heavy exercise that increases intra-abdominal pressure, not smoking, and wearing loose clothing. The patient should be advised not to lie down within 2 hours after eating and to avoid stooping over.

When these measures are insufficient, other medication can be added. These include bethanechol chloride, 25 mg q.i.d., to increase muscle tone of the lower esophageal sphincter (LES), or metoclopramide hydrochloride, 10 mg q.i.d., to increase esophageal clearance and LES tone. If weight loss continues, a stricture forms, or there is intractable pain, surgery may be undertaken.

TABLE 16-5 Nutritional Care in Achalasia

Give semisolid or liquid foods as tolerated.
Provide small, frequent meals as tolerated.
Reduce protein and carbohydrate and increase fat in the diet to promote reduced gastric secretion and a decrease in lower esophageal sphincter pressure.
Avoid temperature extremes in foods.
Avoid foods such as citrus juices and highly spiced foods, which can injure the esophageal mucosa if retained
Use a low-fiber diet if the patient finds it easier to swallow.
Encourage the patient to eat slowly.

From Frances J. Zeman, *Clinical Nutrition and Dietetics* 2e New York: Macmillan. 1991, 199. Used by permission of the publisher

In mild cases of LES, teaching the patient to avoid precipitating foods and other factors may be sufficient. Pain may be relieved with 0.3 mg sublingual (SL) nitroglycerin or 5 mg SL isosorbide dinitrate. The LES is sometimes dilated with a pneumatic bag. Surgery (myotomy) is the treatment for severe cases.

Achalasia is usually treated mechanically. Surgery is undertaken if mechanical treatment is ineffective.

PEPTIC ULCER DISEASE

Drugs are the mainstays of treatment. Surgery may be undertaken for those patients who do not respond adequately to drugs, however. In drug treatment, *antacids* are often prescribed for use after each meal and at bedtime. Cimetidine (Tagamet A), ranitidine (Zantac), or famotidine may be used to reduce acid secretion. Any of these may cause diarrhea as a side effect. Cimetidine may precipitate pancreatitis. Famotidine may cause nausea, vomiting, and constipation. Cessation of smoking and alcohol intake are often recommended.

Years ago, diets for patients with peptic ulcer disease (PUD) were highly restricted. The diet consisted initially of large quantities of milk and cream and progressed through additions of soft, "bland," or white foods such as soft cooked eggs, baked custard, and cottage cheese. In recent years, less restrictive diets have been used since the rationale for the previously used diets could not be scientifically supported. It has, in fact, been demonstrated that milk can actually increase, rather than decrease, acid production.

Modern treatment of PUD centered on the use of antacids and cimetidine. Diet restrictions have not been shown to increase the healing of ulcers (9). Caffeine does not stimulate acid secretion (10). It has been suggested that a high-fiber diet (11) or a diet high in essential fatty acids may be beneficial, but these diets have not been tested. Recommendations vary somewhat, depending on whether the patient is symptomatic or asymptomatic, as follows:

1. *Avoid alcohol intake.* Alcohol is believed to cause back diffusion of hydrogen ion from the lumen into intercellular sites, resulting in injury to the gastric mucosa. There is some evidence, however, that beverages with an ethanol content below 12 percent do not have this effect. For the asymptomatic patient who does not comply with a more severe restriction, it may therefore be acceptable to suggest moderate beer or wine intake (<12 percent alcohol), with avoidance of higher-proof beverages. When the patient is symptomatic, total abstinence is recommended.

2. *Avoid ground peppers.* Peppers may be irritating to the gastrointestinal tract. The patient may thus be more comfortable when avoiding their use. There is no evidence that pepper causes an ulcer or increases gastric acid secretion.

3. *Avoid fruit juices or foods with very low pH if they are irritating to the patient.*

4. *Avoid any food the patient routinely finds irritating.* You should monitor the patient's diet to ensure that it does not become so restricted that it is nutritionally inadequate.

5. *Avoid food intake before bedtime to avoid nocturnal hypersecretion.*

Some institutions list the "bland" diet in their diet manuals, despite a lack of scientifically based rationale

TABLE 16-6 Nutritional Care in Gastroesophageal Reflux

Increase lower esophageal sphincter pressure
Increase protein in diet
Decrease fat in diet to < 45 g/day
Avoid alcohol, peppermint, spearmint
Avoid coffee, strong tea, and chocolate if not well tolerated
Use skim milk

Decrease irritation in the esophagus
Avoid irritants: citrus juices, tomato, coffee, spicy foods, carbonated beverages
Avoid any other foods that regularly cause heartburn (may include rich pastry and frosted cakes)

Improve clearing of the esophagus
Do not recline for > 2 hr after eating
Elevate head of bed

Decrease frequency and volume of reflux
Elevate head of bed
Do not recline for > 2 hr after eating
Eat small meals, more frequent meals if necessary
Reduce weight if overweight
Sip only small amounts of fluids with meals
Drink most fluids between meals
Include enough fiber to avoid constipation (straining increases intraabdominal pressure)

Nutritional and other considerations
Monitor effect of citrus and tomato avoidance on ascorbic acid status; supplement as necessary
Monitor effect of antacids on iron status; supplement if necessary
Avoid chewing gum (causes air swallowing)
Avoid smoking immediately following meals

From Frances J. Zeman. *Clinical Nutrition and Dietetics*, 2e. New York: Macmillan 1991.201. Used by permission of the publisher.

for its use. It is sometimes prescribed because patients associate symptom exacerbation with diet indiscretions and expect to be given a restricted diet. You should therefore be familiar with the diet, but cautious in recommending its use.

Recently, there is evidence that peptic ulcers may be associated with the organism *Helicobacter pylori*. The treatment of the condition with antibiotics such as amoxicillin is still being evaluated. Some questions that might be asked include:

Is the organism the *cause* of the ulcer?

If the cause, can it be treated with antibiotics alone or with accompanying other treatment?

Will diet modification still be necessary, even if only-to improve patient comfort?

FEEDING THE GASTRIC SURGERY PATIENT

For those patients in whom conservative medical treatment is insufficient, surgery may be undertaken. The problems of nutritional needs in major surgery are discussed in Chapter 22. For the present, it is important for you to understand the procedures that precede and follow surgery in which general anesthesia is used.

All foods and fluids are usually withheld for at least 8 hours prior to surgery. This procedure helps to ensure that the stomach is empty, thus avoiding regurgitation and aspiration during, or immediately following, anesthesia and recovery.

In the immediate postoperative period, there may be a lack of peristalsis, known as *ileus*, in the GI tract. Ileus usually occurs following surgery on the GI tract. The patient cannot be given fluid or food orally until peristalsis returns. In the meantime, fluid and electrolyte balance is maintained by intravenous infusion.

The return of peristalsis is detected with the use of a stethoscope. The patient is lying down, and the stethoscope is placed on the abdomen. If peristalsis has returned, bubbling or gurgling noises, called *bowel sounds*, can be heard every 5 to 15 seconds. The patient is also asked whether he has passed any gas, because flatulence is another sign of the return of bowel activity. Last, the patient's abdomen should be soft and flat. (Tenderness may be present for several days after abdominal surgery and, of itself, is not a reason to delay oral feeding.)

DUMPING SYNDROME

Of the various potential complications following ulcer surgery, *dumping syndrome* most clearly involves nutritional care. The treatment of dumping syndrome is largely dietary and provides an opportunity for you to perform a valuable service to the patient. General guidelines for a diet for dumping syndrome are given in most hospital diet manuals, but the condition is highly variable. It is

TABLE 16-7 Nutritional Management of Dumping Syndrome

Individualize the diet to the patient's tolerance. Consult the patient frequently concerning his or her response to individual food items and to portion sizes. The following items are general guidelines.

Reduce intake of carbohydrates to 100–200 g/day. Avoid simple sugars to prevent rapid movement of food into the jejunum with formation of a hyperosmolar solution. Use *unsweetened* fruits.

Increase fat content to 30%–40% of calories to retard stomach emptying and to provide calories for weight gain.

Increase protein to 20% of calories for tissue formation and to supply energy. Include some protein in each meal.

Meals should be low in bulk, dry, and frequent: Six or more per day is common. Increase portion sizes as the patient's tolerance increases.

Provide low-carbohydrate fluids between meals, at least 1/2–1 hr after a meal, to retard gastric emptying. Avoid high-carbohydrate fluids.

All food and drink should be moderate in temperature. Cold drinks, especially, cause increased gastric motility.

Encourage the patient to eat slowly and then lie down for 20–30 min.

Encourage the patient to eat a variety of foods to provide an adequate diet and achievement of ideal body weight. It may be necessary to urge him or her to try foods that were being avoided preoperatively.

The possibility of lactose intolerance exists. Milk should be avoided until it is established that the patient tolerates milk.

To progress toward a more normal intake, add moderate amounts of carbohydrate with caution if the patient shows no symptoms of dumping in the first several days. Use sugar in the form of sweetened fruits and fruit juice and desserts such as sponge cake and cookies. If these are well tolerated, add more concentrated carbohydrates and food at temperature extremes. Fresh fruits and vegetables may be added in 2–3 wk. They should be chewed thoroughly. The diet may be progressed rapidly in some patients and may be lifelong in others.

From Frances J. Zeman, Clinical Nutrition and Dietetics, 2d ed., New York: Macmillan, 1991,212.

important to *recognize*, first, that development of the syndrome can be prevented by judicious postoperative feeding. Second, some patients have only the early symptoms of dumping, while others have only late symptoms, and still others have both. Some patients have more severe symptoms only temporarily, while others may have permanent symptoms. Thus, you must individualize the diet.

Although your diet manual will list specific foods to be used or restricted, the characteristics of the diet can be summarized as follows:

Early dumping:

Avoid concentrated sources of carbohydrate.

Restrict amounts of carbohydrate-containing foods such as fruits, cereals, and some vegetables.

Eliminate alcohol.

Use small, frequent feedings.

Do not use liquids until at least 1/2 to 1 hour following meals. Note that some fruit juices (grape and apple, for example) and carbonated beverages are very hyperosmolar and are thus inappropriate.

Increase protein and fat intake as indicated to achieve and maintain normal weight.

Late dumping:

Avoid concentrated sources of carbohydrate.

Restrict amounts of carbohydrate containing foods, such as fruits, cereals, and some vegetables.

In addition, patients are sometimes advised to eat in a reclining position to retard stomach emptying. Milk must be eliminated from the diet of patients who do not tolerate it. The recommended diet and related factors are summarized in Table 16-7.

In time, many patients adapt, and the diet can be liberalized. Additions to the diet should be made slowly, in small quantities, until it is established that the patient can tolerate them.

REFERENCES

1. **Schmitz, J.** Dysphagia.*In:* D.J. Gines, ed. *Nutrition Management in Rehabilitation.*. Rockville, MD: Aspen, 1990.

2. American Dietetic Association. Controlled-consistency, modfied-fluid (dysphagia) diet. In *Handbook of Clinical Dietetics,* 2d ed., New Haven: Yale University Press, 1992.

3. Chicago Dietetic Association. *Manual of Clinical Dietetics.* Chicago: American Dietetic Association, 1988.

4. **Melazzo, L.S., J. Buchard,** and **D.A. Lund**. The swallowing process; effects of aging and stroke. *In* R.V. Erickson, ed. *Medical Management of the Elderly Stroke Patient. Phys. Med. Rehab* 3:(1989)489.

5. **Stanek, K., C. Hensley,** and **C. Van Riper**. Factors affecting use of food and commercial agents to thicken liquids for individuals with swallowing disorders. *J. Am. Dietet. Assoc.* 92:(1992)486.

6. **Hester, D**. Neurologic impairment. *In* M.M. Gottschlich, L.E. Matarese, and E.P. Shronts, eds. *Nutrition Support Dietetics: Core Curriculum,* 2d ed. Silver Spring, MD: American Society for Parenteral and Enteral Nutrition, 1992.

7. **Krey, S.** and **R.L. Murray.** Chap. 7: Modular and transitional feeding. *In* J.L. Rombeau and M.D. Caldwell, eds. *Clinical Nutrition: Enteral and Tube Feeding,* 2d ed. Philadelphia: Saunders, 1990

8. **O'Sullivan, N.** *Dysphagia Care Team Approach with Acute Long-Term Patients.* Los Angeles, CA. Cottage Square, 1990.

9. **Sleisenger, M.H.,** and **J.S. Fordtran,** eds. *Gastrointestinal Disease, Pathophysiology, Diagnosis, Management,* 5th ed. Philadelphia: Saunders, 1993.

10. **Macarthur, K.E., D.L. Hogan,** and **J.I. Isenberg**, Relative stimulating effects of commonly ingested beverages on gastric acid secretion in humans. *Gastroenterology* 83:(1982) 199.

11. **Rydning, A., A. Berstad, E. Wadlud,** and **B. Adegaard.** Prophylactic effect of dietary fibre in diuodenal ulcer disease. *Lancet* 2:(1982)736.

Additional Sources of Information

Consultant Dietitians in Health Care Facilities. *Dining Skills: Practical Interventions for the Caregivers of the Eating-Disabled Older Adult.* Pensacola, FL: Retirement Research Foundation, 1993

Pardoe, E.M. Development of a multistage diet for dysphagia. *J.Am. Dietet. Assoc.* 93:(1993)568.

Williams, M. Dysphagia: The New Frontier. *Nutrition Today* 27(3):(1992)26.

Yankelson, S., J.E. Handkins and **C.M. Medford**. Dysphagia: a unique interdisciplinary treatment approach. *Topics Clin. Nutr.* 4(1):(1989)43.

TO TEST YOUR UNDERSTANDING

M.H. is a 22 y.o. male with a head injury resulting from a motorcycle accident. The nutritional care specialist reported a possible swallowing problem. Therefore, a radiologist and a speech/language therapist were called. After videofluoroscopy, they reported evidence of a slow and uncoordinated swallow.

1. What position would you recommend for this patient at meal time?

2. Mark an X next to each food you would restrict for this patient until he has had some swallowing therapy.

____ Cornflakes	____ White bread
____ Orange juice	____ Fresh apple
____ Boiled rice	____ Broth
____ Peanut butter sandwich	____ Vegetable soup

3. Explain briefly the theories concerning the mechanisms by which the manifestations of dumping syndrome are produced.

4. Using the diabetic exchange lists, list the exchanges that would need to be limited in a diet for dumping syndrome.

5. List categories of foods in the diabetic exchange lists that would need to be limited or possibly omitted from a diet for dumping syndrome.

6. You have a dumping syndrome patient who is 5 pounds below ideal weight. What nutrients and categories of foods would you increase in the diet to ensure that no more body weight will be lost?

7. What advice would you give this patient concerning the form of fruit in his diet?

8. Mrs. R. is a 47 y.o,. postpartial gastrectomy patient (Billroth I) who has developed early dumping syndrome. Using a hospital menu provided by your instructor, modify the diet for Mrs. R. Assume she is 8 days postop. Use your diet manual as a guide.

9. Using the same menu, modify the menu for this patient, assuming she has developed late dumping syndrome.

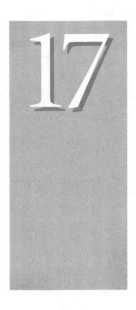

Nutritional Care of the Malabsorbing Patient

The intestine plays an essential role in digestion and nutrient absorption. Therefore, most diseases of the intestinal tract have a detrimental effect on nutritional status. The resulting nutrient deficiencies may, in turn, exacerbate the intestinal disease.

A number of disorders of the small intestine have malabsorption, diarrhea, and other symptoms in common and also have common nutritional consequences. In general, malabsorption can be the result of a deficiency of pancreatic enzymes, deficiency of bile, or impairment of intestinal absorptive capacity. These will be the primary focus of this chapter.

It is important that you understand the general nutritional care procedures indicated by malabsorption and diarrhea regardless of their origin. Since the mechanisms by which diarrhea and malabsorption are produced vary, however, you will also need a command of the nutritional care procedures mandated by some of the more commonly occurring specific disease processes. Thus, this chapter will discuss the use of lactose-restricted, fat-restricted, and gluten-restricted diets. Before proceeding, you should review the related material in your textbook.

DIAGNOSIS

The diagnostic tests for malabsorption are usually used in combination, because individual tests do not establish a specific diagnosis. Those tests that must be preceded by intake of specific foods are described here.

Quantitative fecal fat tests require a diet containing 50 to 150 g (usually 100 g) long-chain triglycerides for 2 days prior to and during the test. Stool is collected for 72 hours. The normal stool contains 1 to 3 g of fat per day

if the patient has been on a usual diet; a value greater than 6 g per day is abnormal. The test establishes the existence of fat malabsorption but does not determine whether the lesion is due to pancreatic insufficiency, bile salt depletion, or ileal dysfunction.

D-xylose absorption tests may help localize the lesion. D-xylose is a 5-carbon sugar that is absorbed without pancreatic digestion and is excreted in the urine. The patient is fasted overnight, because xylose absorption is delayed by food. The patient then ingests 25 g D-xylose, and serum and urine are collected for 5 hours while the patient is on bed rest and without food. For adults, normal serum xylose in 1 to 2 hours is greater than 30 mg per 100 ml; normal urine value in 5 hours is greater than 4.5 g (3.5 if the patient is over age 65). Impaired absorption indicates disease of the intestinal mucosa.

The *lactose tolerance test* measures the rise in blood glucose following intake of a lactose load of 50 g in adults or 50 g per M^2 of surface area in children. An increase of less than 20 mg per dL is considered positive for lactose intolerance.

The *hydrogen breath test* measures the amount of hydrogen produced by the action of colon bacteria on carbohydrate. This test is most frequently used in the diagnosis of lactose intolerance. An adult is given 1.75 g lactose per kg of body weight. Excess hydrogen production (more than 20 ppm) 90 minutes after carbohydrate ingestion indicates malabsorption of carbohydrate. The test may also be used in the diagnosis of bacterial overgrowth.

Some specialized tests include *assays for serum levels of gastrointestinal hormones*, and a test for *urinary 5-hydroxyindoleacetic acid* (5-HIAA), the metabolic breakdown product of serotonin, which is increased in carcinoid intestinal tumors. The 5-HIAA test diet requires the avoidance of bananas, tomatoes, red plums, avocado, eggplant, walnuts, papaya, and pineapple juice.

NUTRITIONAL ASSESSMENT IN GASTROINTESTINAL DISORDERS

Gastrointestinal disorders may have a profound effect on the patient's nutritional status. Nutritional assessment is therefore of great importance. In addition to the standard procedures of nutritional assessment described in Chapter 5, some additional questions that may be useful are listed below. Not all are appropriate for every patient, so you will need to choose. In addition, some questions will be answered in the patient's medical record, while others are appropriate for an interview.

In general:

Weight loss? When? How much?
Anorexia?
Nausea and vomiting? How often? When (in relation to meals)?
Clinical evidence of vitamin and mineral deficiencies? Which nutrients?
Anemia? Type?

Specific to the gastrointestinal tract:

Drainage? How much? Composition?
Absorption site affected by past surgeries? Indicated by diagnostic procedures?
Constipation?
Diarrhea? Duration? Nature of onset? Frequency?

Social history:

Drug exposure? (Antibiotics? Laxatives?)
Alcohol consumption?
Food intolerance? Allergies?
Prior dietary restrictions? Compliance? Duration?
Illnesses (diabetes, inflammatory bowel disease) in self or family?

Medications:

What drugs are being given?
Are any likely to cause problems, e.g., gluten or lactose content?
Do they contain large amounts of sodium? alcohol?
Do any of the drugs cause nutrient loss? Which drugs? Which nutrients?

The following screening tests are often recommended in suspected malabsorption: calcium, phosphate, carotene, vitamin A, alkaline phosphatase, cholesterol, triglyceride, folate, vitamin B_{12}, magnesium, iron, TIBC, zinc, and prothrombin time.

APPROACHES TO NUTRITIONAL CARE IN MALABSORPTION SYNDROMES

Nutritional care in malabsorption can be divided into two categories: supportive and specific.

SUPPORTIVE THERAPY

Some intestinal diseases leave the patient without sufficient digestive or absorptive capacity to maintain good nutrition, and it is necessary to feed the patient parenterally. In other circumstances, the patient must be fed by tube. (The procedures used are those described in Chapters 13 and 14.) Regardless of the method of feeding, fluid and electrolyte balance are important considerations.

Electrolyte and Fluid Balance

The volume of GI secretions in the adult may total 8 to 9 L. Normally, these are reabsorbed, and only about 150 mL of water are excreted daily in the feces. When the amount of fluid in the intestine is compared to a plasma volume of about 3,500 mL, it is obvious that severe fluid imbalances may result if fluid losses from the digestive tract are abnormally high. Abnormal fluid imbalance can be the consequence not only of malabsorption syndromes and diarrhea but also of conditions such as intestinal obstructions and fistulas. You may, therefore, apply this information to the care of patients with a variety of gastrointestinal disorders.

A number of abnormal routes of fluid exchange are common in GI diseases. The patient may receive additional fluid via gastric or duodenal gavage or in an enema. Some routes of abnormal loss are shown in Table 17-1. Loss of gastric juice may reach as much as 6,000 mL in some conditions. Gastric suction or prolonged vomiting are common routes of loss. Losses from "third spacing" can also occur, for example, in intestinal obstruction.

The loss of electrolytes depends not only on the volume of fluid lost but also on its composition. The site of loss is a major determinant of composition. Gastric juice contains H^+ and Cl^- plus some Na^+ and K^+, and its loss can lead to fluid deficit, metabolic alkalosis (as a consequence of H^+ and Cl^- loss), and Na^+ and K^+ deficits.

The contribution of Cl^- loss to alkalosis may require some explanation. Cl^- combines with cations in competition with bicarbonate (HCO_3^-). When Cl^- is decreased, HCO_3^- is increased to compensate because the numbers of anions and cations must equal. Therefore, when Cl^- is lost, HCO_3^- is retained, producing *hypochloremic metabolic alkalosis.*

When a patient's gastric contents are being suctioned, water or ice should not be given by mouth. The water increases the loss of electrolytes, which are suctioned off, leaving the patient in severe alkalosis. Instead, ice chips can be made from an electrolyte solution. Commercial oral electrolyte solutions are useful (see Table K-2).

Intestinal fluid may be lost from diarrhea, intestinal suction, or fistulas. In addition to fluid deficit, loss of intestinal juice can result in metabolic acidosis (HCO_3^- loss) and Na^+ and K^+ deficits. Bile can be lost from fistulas or from drainage following gallbladder surgery and results in Na^+ deficit and acidosis (HCO_3^- loss).

TABLE 17-1 Examples of Fluid and Electrolyte Losses by Abnormal Routes

Route	Fluid Volume mL/24 hr	Na$^+$	Electrolytes K$^+$	(mEq/L) Cl$^-$	HCO$_3^-$
Vomiting	100–6,000	140	4.5	100	24
Saliva drainage	1,500–2.000	20–80	10–20	20–40	20–60
Suction drainage, intubation losses Gastric juice					
with HCl*	2,500	20–100	5–10	120–160	0
achlorhvdric		8–120	1–30	100	20
Bile	700–1,000	134–156	3.9–6.3	83–110	38
Pancreatic juice	>1,000	113–153	2.6–7.4	54–95	110
Small intestine juice (Miller-Abbott suction)	3,000	72–120	3.5–6.8	69–127	30
Ileostomy, new	100–4,000	112–142	4.5–14.0	93–122	30
adapted	100–500	50	3	20	15–30
Cecostomy	100–3,000	48–116	11.1–28.3	37–70	15
Transudates	Variable	130–145	2.5–5.0	90–110	
Diarrhea. secretory	500–17,000	50–60	30–50	40–45	45

* Plus approximately 90 mEq H$^+$/ L; K$^+$ losses may be higher due to increased urinary excretion of K$^+$ in alkalosis.
Compiled from E.A. Goldberger, *Primer of Water, Electrolyte and Acid-Base Syndromes* (5th ed.). Philadelphia: Lea & Febiger. 1986: Stroot. V.R., C.A.B. Lee, and C. A. Barrett. *Fluids and Electrolytes: A Practical Approach*, 3d ed. Philadelphia: Davis, 1984.

Pancreatic juice loss depletes Na$^+$, HCO$_3^-$, and Cl$^-$, resulting in metabolic acidosis and deficits of fluid, sodium, and calcium.

The losses from osmotic and secretory diarrhea are dissimilar, and these differences must be taken into account when fluid and electrolyte balances are calculated. A comparison is given in Table 17-2. In secretory diarrheas, such as bile salt enteropathy, diarrhea from islet cell tumors, and Escherichia coli enteritis, sodium and potassium and their cations provide a stool osmolality about equal to serum osmolality. In osmotic diarrhea, such as that found in the use of magnesium-containing cathartics and in lactase deficiency or other carbohydrate malabsorptive states, less sodium and potassium are lost. The solute gap represents contributions of osmotically active solutes other than sodium, potassium, and their anions, including magnesium and organic ions. As Table 17-2 shows, loss of these materials is particularly severe in osmotic diarrhea. The patient tends to become hypernatremic because the intestine conserves sodium and chloride more effectively than it conserves water

Minor fluid and electrolyte deficits can be corrected by dietary alterations alone. Intravenous feedings are usually ordered to correct more substantial deficits. In either case, you must be aware of the effects of fluid and electrolyte deficiencies on indicators of nutritional status. Serum albumin and hematocrit values, for example, will be elevated in the dehydrated patient (see Ch. 4).

Continuing fluid and electrolyte losses must also be considered when making recommendations for the volume and composition of tube-feeding and parenteral-feeding formulas. You will also be asked to cooperate in measuring fluid intake.

General Nutritional Support

Vitamins and Minerals. Patients with malabsorption disorders usually need vitamin and mineral supplements. The recommended dosages for long-term oral

TABLE 17-2 Comparison of Clinical Features of Osmotic and Secretory Diarrhea

Clinical Feature	Osmotic Diarrhea	Secretory Diarrhea
Daily stool volume, L	<1	>1
Stool osmolality, mOsm/kg	400	290
Stool electrolytes, mEq/L		
Na$^+$	50	100
K$^+$	35	40
Response to fasting	subsides	continues

Compiled from J.D. Gardner, Pathogenesis of secretory diarrhea. *In* M. Field, ed. *Secretory Diarrhea*, American Physiological Society, 1980, 154: G.J.Krejs, G.J. Diagnostic and pathophysiologic studies in patients with chronic diarrhea. *In* M. Field, ed. *Secretory Diarrhea*. American Physiological Society, 1980, p.142.

supplementation are given in Table 17-3. In some cases, parenteral administration may be necessary. These supplements are usually administered as drugs. As the specialist in nutritional care, however, you should be alert to evidence of existing or potential nutrient deficiency and recommend supplementation when it is appropriate.

The nutrients at risk will vary with the location of intestinal involvement. Here is a general summary:

1. Proximal bowel (duodenum and upper jejunum) involvement, seen in Billroth II reconstruction, jejunal resection, nontropical sprue, and afferent loop syndrome:

    Iron, calcium, fat-soluble vitamins
    Fat, carbohydrates, amino acids

2. Midbowel (middle and lower jejunum) involvement, seen in extensive intestinal resection:

    Magnesium
    Amino acids, carbohydrates

3. Distal bowel (ileum) involvement, seen in ileal disease, ileal resection, regional enteritis, nontropical sprue, and lymphoma:

    Vitamin B_{12}, bile salts

Protein and Energy. Many patients need replacement of calories and protein, with consideration of needs for essential fatty acids and amino acids (Procedures for increasing oral intake are discussed in Chapter 12). If the diet assessment indicates insufficient protein and energy intake, some patients may be assisted with the use of a high-protein, high-calorie liquid supplement. The patient unable to ingest enough food by these means may be given supplemental tube feedings. (Procedures are described in Chapter 13). The feeding formula chosen must be appropriate to the patient's disorder, as discussed in the next section. If GI function is inadequate to maintain normal nutritional status by these methods. TPN may be used (see Chapter 14).

SPECIFIC NUTRITIONAL THERAPY

Three diet modifications are most often useful in nutritional care of specific types of malabsorption: *fat restriction, lactose restriction,* and *gluten restriction.* They may be used separately or in combination, depending on the patient's needs.

The Fat-Restricted Diet

Malabsorption can affect many nutrients, but malabsorption of fat is the most common. The resulting steatorrhea may occur in the presence of bile salt deficiency, pancreatic insufficiency, or defects in the absorptive capability of the intestinal mucosa itself.

Most of these conditions require a low-fat intake as part of their treatment. In these diets, the term *fat* refers to triglycerides and does not consider other lipids, such as cholesterol. The diet does not reverse the abnormal physiology; instead, it helps control the symptoms. As a

TABLE 17-3   Guidelines for Nutrient Doses for Patients with Malabsorption Syndromes

1. **Calcium:** 500 mg elemental Ca as carbonate or gluconate, 500 mg t.i.d. or q.i.d., p.o.
2. **Magnesium:** *Oral:* 150 mg elemental Mg as glucoheptonate or gluconate q.i.d.
    Intramuscular: 290 mg Mg as sulfate 1–3/wk IM or IV
3. **Iron:** $FeSO_4$ liquid, 60 mg elemental Fe as Fe SO_4 liquid, po.
4. **Zinc:** Zinc gluconate, 25 mg elemental Zn or gluconate q.i.d., po.
5. **Fat-Soluble Vitamins:**
    a. Vitamin A: 10,000 to 50,000 I.U./day po.
    b. Vitamin D: 1,600 I.U./day po., 0.25–0.50 ug/day po.
    c. Vitamin E: 30 units/day
    d. Vitamin K: 5 mg/day
6. **Folic Acid:** 5 to 10 mg daily
7. **Vitamin B_{12}:** 200 µg./month, IM
8. **Vitamin B Complex:** Any multivitamin preparation that contains daily requirements (thiamine 1.6 mg, riboflavin 1.8 mg, and niacin 20 mg). Use 2 or 3 tablets daily. Intramuscular preparations are available for severe deficiencies.

Adapted from S. Klein, and K.N. Jeejeebhoy. Long-term nutritional managemen of patients with maldigestion and malabsorption. *In* M.H. Sleisinger and J.S. Fordtran eds. *Gastrointestinal Disease: Pathophysiology/Diagnosis/Management,* 5th ed Philadelphia: Saunders, 1993.

consequence, the level of restriction must vary with the degree of malabsorption.

The diet manuals of many institutions list several levels of fat restriction from which to choose as a baseline for planning. These diet levels may be based on a percentage of total energy, such as a mild (30 to 35 percent of total kcal), moderate (25 percent), or severe (10 to 15 percent) restriction. Alternatively, diets may be planned for a specified number of grams of fat, such as 30, 50, 70, or 40, 60, 75 (1–3). A commonly used low fat-diet contains 50 g fat for an adult. It could contain about six lean meat exchanges and 3 to 5 g fat exchanges per day. A more severe restriction with 25 g of fat can be achieved with 5-oz lean-meat exchanges with no fat exchanges (3). In any case, the diet should be adjusted to the needs of the individual patient.

For patients with minimal impairment, avoidance of high-fat meats and fried foods may be a sufficient modification. The exchange lists shown in Appendix C may be used to calculate the basic diet plan and to estimate fat content for more restricted diets. Fat exchanges should be planned so that the fat intake is evenly distributed among meals.

Examples from a more detailed list of foods and their fat content, given as "fat portion exchanges," are listed in Table B-3 (4). These values are based on the same concept as the exchange lists in Appendix C. Each item and quantity listed provides one "fat exchange" containing 5 g fat. Using this system, a patient who requires a 50 g fat diet could be advised to make up the day's diet to include ten fat portion exchanges.

Although exchange lists are useful while you are learning to plan these diets, they are seldom used for this purpose by experienced nutritional care specialists in clinical situations. Some guidelines for planning specific menus are given in Table 17-4.

When fat is restricted, the diet becomes high in carbohydrate and in osmolality. If the carbohydrate is in small molecules, a carbohydrate-induced diarrhea may develop (see Chapter 4).

When fat is severely restricted, protein intake may be limited, since most protein foods also contain fat. If the diet does not then meet the patient's needs, it may be necessary to add a supplement to provide additional protein. At the same time, the supplement must be low in fat.

A fat-restricted diet may not meet the patient's energy needs, because many calorie-dense foods are removed. Medium-chain triglycerides are useful to increase the energy intake of the patient who cannot digest and absorb sufficient sources of energy.

Medium-chain triglycerides are derived from coconut oil. The oil is fractionated to separate the fatty acids that are 8 (octanoic) and 10 (decanoic) carbon atoms in length, as compared with most dietary fats, which have 16 and 18 carbon atoms in the fatty acids. When the isolated medium-chain fatty acids are reesterified, a thin, clear oil is produced. It is available as MCT Oil (Mead Johnson, Evansville, IN) and as a component in selected tube-feeding and infant formulas.

The caloric yield of MCT Oil is described in Chapter 13 and should be reviewed if necessary. It is important to note that MCT Oil contains no essential fatty acids.

MCT Oil should be added to the diet gradually. Most patients can tolerate 20 to 60 g, but side effects may develop if larger amounts are fed or if intake is suddenly increased. The limit on caloric yield is thus about 400

kcal. Side effects include nausea, vomiting, diarrhea, and abdominal pain and distension. MCT Oil is sometimes given as a medication; if it is used as a food, information must be provided to the patients on its use in foods and food preparation. Some suggestions are contained in Table 17-5. Recipes are available from the manufacturer (5) and elsewhere (6, 7).

MCT Oil is also available as an ingredient in Portagen Powder. Its fat content is 86 percent MCT, with the remainder as corn oil, and it is supplemented with vitamins and minerals (see Appendix H). The powder is reconstituted with water to make a milklike drink. Since Portagen provides a high osmotic load, it should be given cautiously, 1 to 2 glasses per day, sipped slowly to start. Because of the high osmotic load, it is also important to maintain fluid intake.

The Lactose-Restricted Diet

Lactose intolerance may be present as the patient's sole complaint or may be secondary to other conditions. It may occur with, and aggravate, the symptoms of gluten-sensitive enteropathy and regional enteritis, for example, or it may become aggravated by these conditions. Patients who are deficient in lactase will benefit from a reduction in the lactose content of their diets, but "lactose-intolerant" individuals vary widely in their ability to digest lactose. Many patients can tolerate 12 g lactose per day, the amount in 8 oz of milk, while some patients may tolerate as little as 3 g. Total lactose avoidance is not usually necessary except in galactosemia, which is described in Chapter 23 and in the congenital disorders Holzel and Durand syndromes.

The goals of the diet for the lactose-intolerant patient are (1) to reduce lactose intake to a level that will not cause intestinal symptoms, and (2) to provide for adequate nutrient intake.

TABLE 17-4 General Guidelines for Planning Fat-Restricted Diets

1. Use skim milk in severe restriction; for higher fat levels, 2% milk may be useful.
2. Avoid cream cheese, hard cheeses: choose low-fat (1%) cottage cheese, sapsago cheese, other skim milk cheeses.
3. Avoid high-fat meats. Use low-fat or medium-fat meats as calculated into the diet. Meat exchanges should be broiled, baked, or boiled, not fried. Remove skin from chicken and turkey.
4. Avoid most baked desserts, such as cakes, cookies, pies, and pastries. Exception: angel food cake.
5. Avoid cream sauces and gravies.
6. Avoid bread and cereal products made with fat. Examples: doughnuts, fritters, muffins.
7. Avoid candies made with chocolate, nuts, or any fat.
8. Use plainly prepared vegetables, not creamed, fried, or with sauces containing fat. Avoid olives.
9. Use fruit as desired. Exception: avocado.
10. Use fat exchanges only as calculated into the diet plan.
11. Use fat-free desserts; avoid dessert containing fat, chocolate, or nuts unless included in fat allowance.
12. Use spices and herbs as desired.
13. Limit alcohol.
14. Plan for nutritional adequacy.

TABLE 17-5 Procedures for the Use of Medium-Chain Triglycerides in the Diet

1. Combine MCT Oil with beverages:
   a. Combine 1–2 T MCT Oil with fruit juice, tomato juice, or carbonated beverages.
   b. Combine 1–2 T MCT Oil with 1/2 c skim milk.
   c. Combine 2–4 t MCT Oil with 1/3 c nonfat dry milk powder and 2/3 c water. Mix in a blender. Sugar and nonfat flavorings may be added.
2. Substitute MCT Oil for vegetable oils in mayonnaise, salad dressings and sauces.
3. Use MCT Oil to stir-fry vegetables.
4. Use MCT Oil in grilling meats; use low heat because MCT Oil has a low smoke point.
5. Use MCT Oil in baking in place of regular oil, such as pancakes, waffles, muffins, and chiffon cakes. Use egg whites in place of whole eggs and skim milk in place of whole milk in such recipes.

Compiled from C.M. Pemberton and C.F. Gastineau, eds. *Mayo Clinic Diet Manual* (5th ed.), Philadelphia: Saunders, 1981.

Diet Planning. Institutional diet manuals may contain a "lactose-free" diet for those who need complete lactose restriction, or they may present diets varying in lactose levels. In either case, the diet should be adjusted to the individual patient's tolerance. Making such adjustments is difficult, however, since information on the lactose content of foods is limited. As a result, a trial and error process may be required. Table 17-6 lists some values that may be helpful in initial planning, Table 17-7 offers general guidelines for a completely lactose-restricted diet and for modifications for less severe restrictions.

Lactose tolerance may be improved if milk is taken as whole milk or along with other food to delay gastric emptying. Milk tolerance may also be improved if milk intake is divided into small, more frequent servings.

You may want to offer your nutritional-counseling patients some references for milk-free recipes. You can also give directions for use of acidophilus milk and Lact-Aid, which will be described in the next section. These may help the patient maintain an adequate calorie intake when other nutrients, such as fat or gluten, are also restricted.

TABLE 17-6 Lactose Content of Selected Foods

Food	Amount	Lactose (g)
Milk, whole or skim	1 c	11
2% fat	1 c	9–13
buttermilk	1 c	10.3–12.0
skim	1 c	11–14
powdered skim	30 g	15.5
chocolate	1 c	10–12
condensed sweetened	1 c	35
goats'	1 c	8.1
Cream, light	1 T	0.6
half and half	1 T	0.6
whipped topping	1 T	0.4
sour	4 oz	4–5
Ice cream, regular	1 c	9
sherbet	1 c	4
ice milk	1 c	10
Butter	2 t	0.1
Cheese, Parmesan, Gouda, blue	1 oz	0.6–0.8
American, Cheddar	1 oz	0.50.
Processed cheese	1 oz	2–3
Camembert, Limberger	1 oz	0.1–0.2
Cream	1 oz	0.8
Cottage, regular	1 c	5–6
low fat	1 c	7–8
Yogurt	1 c	11–15
Milk Chocolate	100 g	8.1

Compiled from Alpers, D.H., R.E. Clouse, and W.F. Stenson, *Manual of Nutritional Therapeutics*, Boston: Little Brown, 1983; C.R. Gallagher, A.L. Molleson, and J.H. Caldwell, Lactose intolerance and fermented dairy products. *J. Am. Dietet. Assoc.* 65:(1974)418-419; T.T. Jensen, J.E. Staggers, and M. Johnston, eds. *Handbook of Clinical Dietetics*, Salt Lake City: Utah Dietetic Association, 1977; Haringe, M.H. et al. Carbohydrates in foods. J. Am. Dietet. Asoc. 46:(1965)197–204: Walser, M., A.L. Imbembo, S. Margolis, and G.A. Elfert. *Nutritional Management*. Philadelphia: Saunders, 1984

TABLE 17-7 General Guidelines for Planning Lactose Restricted Diets

In General

1. Avoid or restrict as necessary milk in liquid, canned, or powdered form.
2. Labels should be read carefully for the content of milk, milk products, milk solids, skim milk, skim milk powder, skim milk solids, milk sugar, and lactose. Restrict foods containing these items as necessary to the tolerance of the patient.
3. Small amounts of cheese and butter may be tolerated.
4. Avoid use of large quantities of milk or cream in cooking.
5. Plan for nutritional adequacy. Supplementation may be necessary.

For diets with 3 g or less lactose per day:

1. Omit all milk and milk products, yogurt, ice cream, sherbet, ice milk, prepared puddings, milk drinks, malted milk products. Use soybased milks, whipped toppings, nondairy creamers.
2. Limit cheese to 1 oz/day or less.
3. Read labels carefully. Avoid products containing "lactose," "dry milk solids," or "milk sugar." "Lactic acid," "lactate," "lactalbumin," and "lactylate" are tolerated.
4. Avoid creamed or breaded meats, vegetables; avoid vegetables with lactose added in processing. (Read labels.)
5. Avoid meat products that contain lactose. (Read labels.)
6. Avoid fruits with lactose added in processing. (Read labels.)
7. Avoid prepared mixes, dry cereals with added lactose (Total, Special K, Fortified Oat Flakes, Cocoa Krispies, Instant Cream of Wheat), bread and rolls containing milk products, commercial cakes, cookies, pastries with cream fillings, or lactose-sweetened fillings.
8. Avoid any products containing chocolate.
9. Avoid instant coffee, powdered soft drinks with lactose, Kool-Aid, many candies, monosodium glutamate, soy sauce.

For patients with a greater tolerance:

1. Some patients who tolerate 10–25 g lactose may have 1–2 c milk or ice cream/day; 1/2 c milk or ice cream will provide 5–6 g lactose.
2. Patients tolerate lactose better if milk is taken with other foods and in small amounts throughout the day.
3. Some patients have a greater tolerance for warmed milk, buttermilk, or yogurt.
4. Consider the use of Lact-Aid to increase milk intake. Advise patients on procedures for its use.

Special Products. Special products are available for the lactose-intolerant patient and may be helpful in menu planning. Some have the nutrient content of milk and are useful in providing for nutritionally adequate diets.

Sweet acidophilus milk is a low-fat (2 percent) milk to which a Lactobacillus acidophilus culture has been added. The culture causes the hydrolysis of lactose to glucose and galactose, resulting in increased sweetness. The taste is otherwise similar to that of low-fat milk. Since the product contains reduced lactose (80 to 90 percent less), it is often tolerated by lactose-intolerant patients.

Lact-Aid (Sugar Low Company, Atlantic City, NJ) consists of packets of lactase enzyme, each of which is sufficient to treat 1 quart of milk. If the contents are added to 1 quart of fresh milk, mixed well, and allowed to stand in the refrigerator for 24 hours, at least 70 percent of the lactose present will be converted to simple sugars. There is 90-percent conversion in 2 to 3 days. Severely lactose-intolerant patients can convert the milk sugar to a greater degree by adding more packets to the fresh milk. Three packets per quart, for example, will convert 98 percent of the lactose present in 24 hours. The single-packet treatment is balanced to provide lactose conversion sufficient to permit 80 percent of lactose-deficient patients to enjoy treated milk.

The milk used for treatment can be fresh fluid, skim, or reconstituted from dried milk; cultured milks and dairy products other than milk cannot be treated this way. Once treated, lactose-modified milk can also be used in cooking, for preparing yogurt or buttermilk, or in any other application for which milk would be used.

Lact-Aid incorporates lactase derived from *Kluveromyces lactis*, a common food yeast, diluted with dextrose. The application of heat must be carefully controlled because the enzyme is inactivated at temperatures above 105° F. The enzyme is also pH sensitive in the acid ranges, so use of poor-quality milk interferes with the lactase action.

Enzyme replacement may also be effective. *Lactrase* (Kremes, Urban, Co., Milwaukee, WI) is beta galactosidase in a capsule. it has been shown to reduce symptoms if taken just before or after lactose intake (8, 9).

Products such as Mocha Mix, Coffee Rich, and Vita-Rich may also be useful in the lactose-restricted diet. These are milk-free, cholesterol-free dairy supplements that can be used as milk substitutes. Sugar content and osmolarity are high, and the taste may not be entirely acceptable. Various soy-based and lactose-free supplementary feedings and tube feedings are listed in Appendix K, Tables 1 and 3.

The Gluten-Restricted Diet

The gluten-restricted diet eliminates gluten from the diet. More specifically, the toxic material is believed to be *gliadin*, the alcohol-soluble fraction of gluten, or one of its parts. The diet is thus sometimes called *gliadin-free*. Glutens are contained in wheat, rye, oat, barley, and triticale protein, or in any derivatives from these cereals. Rice and corn contain different glutens that are not toxic and need not be eliminated. Other cereals that must be tested before they can be recommended include amaranth, buckwheat, millet, quinoa, spelt, and teff (3). Until this is done, these materials are not used in the diet.

General guidelines for nutritional care of the gluten-intolerant patient are listed in Table 17-8. Lists of foods allowed and not allowed, stated in general terms, are contained in most diet manuals. Such lists give information on avoiding obvious forms of wheat, rye, barley, and oats, but they often provide less information on hidden forms of gluten. In order to provide adequate care, the

TABLE 17-8   General Guidelines for Nutritional Care in Gluten Tolerance

1. Omit toxic gluten from the diet.
   a. Omit wheat, rye, barley, oats, and triticale.
   b. Substitute corn, rice, potato flour, soy bean flour tapioca, sago, arrowroot.
   c. Avoid foods containing flours or cereal products of unspecified origin, graham flour, bran, bulgur, groats, starches of unspecified origin, emulsifiers, stabilizers, hydrolyzed vegetable protein, hydrolyzed plant protein, malt, malt flavoring, malt syrup, malt vinegar, malted milk, modified starch, modified food starch, mono- and diglycerides using a wheat-starch carrier, monosodium glutamate of unspecified origin, oat germ, oatmeal, "flavoring" of unspecified origin, soy sauce or soy sauce solids, vegetable gum, wheat germ, wheat gluten, wheat starch.
   d. Read labels carefully.
   e. Use fresh meats, fish, eggs, milk, fruits, and vegetables.
   f. Unless certain that specific brands are gluten-free, be cautious about:
      Cereal-based beverages (Ovaltine, Postum, beer, ale, instant coffee, root beer
      Commercial ice cream, cakes, cookies and similar baked goods
      Salad dressings
      Canned or processed meats
      Canned soups, cream soups
      Candy bars
      Mustard, catsup
      Breaded, creamed, or scalloped products
      Chocolate milk
      Frozen foods with sauces
      Processed cheese

2. Plan the diet to ensure adequate intake of all nutrients, since the diet is long-term. Supplement with vitamins and minerals if necessary.

3. Instruct patient carefully on
   Foods to use
   Foods to avoid
   Hidden sources of gluten
   Label reading
   Diet planning for nutritional adequacy
   Preparation of gluten-free products

4. Instruct patient on the following, if appropariate:
   Choosing a diet in a restaurant
   Additional restrictions of other nutrients (e.g. lactose, fat)

nutritional care specialist must know these sources and instruct the patient on label reading to detect their presence. A list of food materials of which the patient must be aware is also contained in Table 17-8.

It is also helpful to the patient to have a list of commercially prepared foods that are usable on a gluten-restricted diet. You should prepare a list of those that are available in your area and update it when ingredients and manufacturing procedures change. Exacerbations of the disease are often the consequence of diet errors.

The primary foods eliminated are cereals and cereal products. This obviously limits the use of many foods of which the patient may be fond, such as baked desserts.

Therefore, you may want to provide suggestions and directions for substitutes. These ready-made products are expensive, however.

As an alternative to ready-made products, patients can be given directions on food preparation with acceptable alternative cereal products. Some general directions are given in Table 17-9. These are useful for the patient or caregiver who can use initiative and imagination in food preparation. Most patients will also find recipes helpful. Such information is likely to increase diet compliance, encourage greater variety in food intake, and improve the likelihood that the diet will be nutritionally adequate.

Another substance that may be useful is xanthan gum, a polysaccharide obtained from the *xanthomonas campestris* organism. Xanthan gum, obtainable as a powder, may be used to provide smooth texture to salad dressing, gravy, sauces and ice cream. It also acts as a stabilizer and improves the texture when used in baked goods such as cakes, breads, and pizza crust (3).

SOME CONSIDERATIONS IN NUTRITIONAL SUPPORT

The methods for nutritional support described in Chapters 13 and 14 are generally applicable to patients with diseases of the digestive system, but some special considerations in choice of feeding formulas are appropriate. Unless enteral feeding is impossible, it is preferable to parenteral feeding, since nutrients in the intestinal lumen help to maintain structural and functional integrity of the digestive system. Their absence leads to atrophy of the pancreas and the intestinal mucosa. In addition, there are "gut specific" fuels available in tube-feeding formulas, but not found in parenteral formulations.

GLUTAMINE

Glutamine is apparently useful for patients with inflammatory bowel disease and short-bowel syndrome, and in sepsis and stress. It seems to have a role in maintaining structure and function of the intestinal tract (11). It plays a role in preventing mucosal injury and bacterial translocation. A recently developed formula, AlitraQ, (see Table K-3) contains 15.5 g glutamine per 1,000 kcal. (11).

SHORT CHAIN FATTY ACIDS

The short-chain fatty acids—acetate, butyrate, and propionate—are the end products of fermentation of undigested carbohydrate in the colon. They have trophic effects throughout the intestinal tract. Formulas containing fiber are available for patients with inflammatory bowel disease, short-bowel syndrome, enterocolitis, or intestinal atrophy secondary to parenteral nutrition (11). Fiber-containing formulas are listed in Table K-3.

TOPICS FOR FURTHER DISCUSSION

1. What conditions of organs other than the GI tract indicate a need for a low-fat diet?
2. What conditions other than lactose intolerance indicate a need to reduce milk intake? Compare the degree of restriction required for each.
3. Taste-test some of the special products described in this chapter.
4. Discuss modification of fat-, lactose-, and gluten-restricted diets for patients with ethnic origins common to your area.
5. Discuss nutritional support in inflammatory bowel disease; short bowel syndrome.
6. Discuss other tests for pancreatic and intestinal malfunction. What are normal values? Explain rationale for each.

TABLE 17-9   Substitutes for Wheat Flour

Substitutes for 1 c wheat flour
In baking

1 c	cornflour
3/4 c	coarse oatmeal
1 c (scant)	fine oatmeal
5/8 c	potato flour
7/8 c	rice flour
1 1/4 c	rye flour
1 c	rye meal

As a thickener:

1 T wheat flour = 1/2 T cornstarch, potato starch, arrowroot starch, rice flour, or 2 t quick-cooking tapioca

Cooking and baking tips

Bake more slowly and for a longer period.
   Use soy flour in combination with other flours.
When cooking with rice flour or cornmeal, mix with the liquid in the recipe, bring to boil, cool before adding to the other ingredients.
Increase leavening to 2 1/2 t/c when using coarse forms of wheat substitutes
Bake items in small sizes.
Cakes made with wheat-flour substitutes tend to be dry. Store in closed containers. Add frosting.

Compiled from G.J. Lawler, Jr., and T.J. Fischer, eds. *Manual of Allergy and Immunology* Boston: Little Brown, 1981 p.467; M.A. Ohlson, eds *Experimental and Therapeutic Dietetics*, 2d ed. Minneapolis: Burgess. 1972. pp. 142–143.

REFERENCES

1. American Dietetic Association. *Handbook of Clinical Dietetics,* 2d ed. New Haven: Yale University Press, 1992.
2. **C.M. Pemberton and C.F. Gastineau,** eds *Mayo Clinic Diet Manual,* 6th ed. Toronto: Decker, 1981.
3. Chicago Dietetic Association, *Manual of Clinical Dietetics,* Chicago: American Dietetic Association, 1988.
4. **Boyar, A.P. and J.R. Loughridge.** The fat portion exchange list: a tool for teaching and evaluating low-fat diets, *J. Am. Dietet. Assoc.* 85:(1985)589–94.

5. *Recipes Using MCT Oil and Portagen,* Evansville, IN.: Mead Johnson and Co., 1977

6. **Schizas, A.A., J.A. Cremen, E. Larson, and R. O'Brien.** Medium-chain triglycerides: use in food preparation. *J. Am. Dietet. Assoc.* 51:(1964)228–32.

7. **J.R. Senior**, ed. *Medium-Chain Triglycerides*, Philadelphia: University of Pennsylvania Press, 1968.

8. **Moskovitz, M., C. Curtis, and J. Gavaler.** Does oral enzyme replacement therapy reverse intestinal lactose malabsorption? *Am. J. Gastroenterol.* 82:(1987)632.

9. **Di Palma, J.A,. and M.S. Collins,** Enzyme replacement for lactose malabsorption using a beta-D-galactosidase. *J. Clin. Gastroenterol. Nutr.* 11:(1989)290.

10. **Klein, S.**, and **C.R. Fleming**. Enteral and parenteral nutrition. *In* M.H. Sleisenger, and J.S. Fordtran, eds. *Gastrointestinal Disease. Pathophysiology/Diagnosis/Management.* Philadelphia: Saunders, 1993.

11. **Babst, R., H. Horig, P. Stehle, et al.** Glutamine peptide supplemental long-term-total parenteral nutrition: Effects on intracellular and extracellular amino acid patterns, nitrogen economy, and tissue morphology in growing rats, *JPEN* 17:(1993)566.

ADDITIONAL SOURCES OF INFORMATION

C.C. Booth and G. Neale., eds. *Disorders of Small Intestine*, Boston: Blackwell, 1985.

Sleisenger, M.H. and J.S. Fordtran *Gastrointestinal Disease. Pathophysiology/Diagnosis/Management* 5th ed. Philadelphia: Saunders 1993.

✓ TO TEST YOUR UNDERSTANDING

1. Name some specific disorders in which steatorrhea is the result of the following (consult your text):
  a. Pancreatic enzyme deficiency
  b. Bile deficiency
  c. Impaired intestinal absorptive capacity.

2. List the diagnostic tests that require diet manipulation as part of the test procedure and give the diet requirements.

3 Your institution lists three levels of fat-restricted diets in its diet manual. The moderate restriction is set at 25% of total calories. You estimate that your patient needs 2,400 kcal per day.
  a. How many grams of fat would you give a patient requiring a moderate fat restriction?
  b. How many "fat portion exchanges" would you give?
  c. How many grams of fat would you give at each of three meals?

4. You have a patient who requires a diet containing 45 g of fat. Make a list of the exchanges from Appendix C, and note the numbers of servings of each that should be included in the diet to provide this amount of fat.

5. Why is a patient receiving MCT always given some sources of long-chain triglycerides?

6. List oral or supplemental formulas containing medium-chain triglycerides in the following categories:
  a. Hydrolyzed protein
  b. Non-milk-based feeding
  c. Milk-based with intact protein
  d. Blenderized feeding

7. How many kcals can be obtained from 1/4 c of MCT oil? Show your calculations.

8. What formula would be most useful for a 3-month-old-infant with severe fat malabsorption?

9. You have a patient who needs a 1,600 kcal diet with 30 g fat. Using a menu provided by your instructor, plan 1 day's diet for this patient.

10. a. List the nutrients that are most likely to be deficient if a patient's diet must be milk-free. For each, give alternative food sources and commonly used supplements.
  b. Discuss the ease or difficulty of obtaining sufficient amounts of these nutrients in a milk-free diet.

11. Your patient says that she can manage 12 oz of milk per day if she does not drink more than 4 oz in 4 hours. In order to provide her with greater flexibility in menu planning, you give her a list of alternative foods that have about the same amount of lactose as 4 oz of milk. What serving sizes would you suggest for each item?

a.	Ice cream	___ c
b.	Yogurt	___ c
c.	Cottage cheese	___ c
d.	Cream soup	___ c

12. You have a patient who requires a lactose-free diet. Using a menu provided by your instructor, write a day's diet for your patient.

13. What nutrients must be considered if cereals are removed from the diet?

14. Mr. R. is suffering from an exacerbation of his gluten intolerance. He gives you the following 24-hour recall. Circle those items that might account for his current symptoms and about which you should inquire in further detail.

Breakfast:
Orange juice
Cornmeal/milk/sugar
Poached eggs
Rice crackers (no wheat)
Instant coffee

Lunch:
Ham sandwich with gluten-free bread/lettuce/catsup
Malted milk

Snack:
Chocolate-nut bar

Dinner:
Roast beef
Baked potato
Creamed peas
Head lettuce/Thousand Island dressing
Fresh-fruit cup

15. Using a menu provided by your instructor, write 1 day's diet for Mr. R.

16. Using a menu provided by your instructor, write 1 day's diet for a gluten-intolerant patient who has also developed fat malabsorption and a lactase deficiency. He can tolerate 40 g fat and 8 oz milk per day.

Malabsorption

Part I: Presentation

Present illness: Jocelyn W. is a 20 y.o. nursing student referred for evaluation of chronic diarrhea. She denies presence of blood or mucus in her stools. She C/O weight loss, fatigue, weakness, and diarrhea of 1 month's duration with production of 4–5 bulky, semiformed, foul-smelling stools per day. The symptoms had occurred previously but were more severe and prolonged this time. She denies recent travel to a foreign country. No one else in her residence has similar Sx, and she has no fever or joint pains. She has had no contact with any patient with diarrhea in her work as a student nurse.

Past medical history: She had measles in childhood and a broken leg about 10 years ago. There is a history of exacerbations and remissions of diarrhea since childhood.

Family history: An older sister died in infancy of undiagnosed diarrhea.

Social history: Single. Lives in dormitory for students and eats in student cafeteria. Very active: runs, swims.

Review of systems: Patient has no complaints except for excess flatulence and diarrhea.

Physical exam: Black female, 5 ft 6 in, 113#, medium frame. Abdomen is protruberant, with a doughy consistency on palpation. No tenderness. Oral mucosa slightly dry. There is a slight tachycardia with mild postural change. Stool is hemenegative. Remainder of exam is WNL.

Laboratory:		*Normal*
Serum albumin, g/L	30	_____
Total lymphocytes x 10^9/L	1.2	_____
RBC x 10^{12}/L	4.0	_____
Hgb, g/L	120	_____
Hct, vol, fraction	0.38	_____
Serum Na, mmol/L	135	_____
Serum K, mmol/L	3.5	_____
Serum Cl, mmol/L	95	_____
Serum HCO_3, mmol/L	20	_____
Serum P, inorganic, mmol/L	0.7	_____
SUN, mmol/L	70	_____
Serum creatinine, mmol/L	1.2	_____
Urine specific gravy	1.040	_____
TSF, mm	12.2	_____
MAMC, cm	18.1	_____

Impression: Chronic diarrhea and dehydration in a 20 y.o., slightly underweight black female with a positive history of sporadic, chronic diarrhea.

Plan: R/O gluten-sensitive enteropathy, diffuse intestinal lymphoma, Zollinger-Ellison syndrome, early collagenous sprue.

QUESTIONS

1. Fill in the normal values in the spaces provided above.

2. Briefly evaluate the patient's nutritional and hydration status. Indicate the data that support your evaluation.

Part II: Diagnosis
Further laboratory studies produced the following:

		Normal
Fecal fat, g/day	10	_____
Plasma cholesterol, mmol/L	3.4	_____
D-xylose absorption/5-hr urine, vol. fraction	0.15	_____
Serum amylase, µkat/L	2.0	_____
Serum lipase, µkat/L	0.015	_____
Serum carotene, µmol/L	0.8	_____
Serum vitamin A, µmol/L	0.25	_____
Fecal occult blood	Negative	_____
Prothrombin time, sec	14.8	_____
Stool O&P	None seen	_____

Roentgenogram of the small intestine following a barium meal showed dilation of the small intestine with obliteration of the mucosal folds. The barium meal was fragmented and flocculent in the upper and middle portions of the jejunum. Ileal mucosa appeared normal.

Endoscopic biopsy, following treatment with vitamin K given IM, revealed a flat mucosal surface with no intestinal villi. Intestinal crypts were elongated. The cells on the epithelial surface were cuboidal, with a markedly reduced brush border. Crypt cells were markedly increased, with an increased number of mitoses.

QUESTIONS

3. In the spaces provided above, give the normal values for each lab test.

4. a. Which laboratory test are indicators of pancreatic function?
   b. Based on these results, what would you conclude about this patient's pancreatic function?

5. List the signs, symptoms, and laboratory results in the case study that indicate or are compatible with the following:
   a. Acidosis
   b. Electrolyte depletion
   c. Malabsorption

6 Why is a prothrombin time value obtained prior to intestinal biopsy?

(continued)

7. List evidence from the case study that suggests that the patient might be malabsorbing the following nutrients:
   a. Protein
   b. Fat
   c. Carbohydrate
   d. Vitamin (specify which)
   e. Minerals (specify which)

Part III. Continued Treatment

The patient's fluid and electrolyte balances were corrected with IV feeding, after which the following laboratory results were obtained.:

Hgb, g/L	112
Hct, vol. fraction	0.36
RBC x 10^{12}/L	3.8
SUN mmol/L	6.1
Serum creatinine, μmol L	100

The medical record now lists the following problems:
   1. Gluten-sensitive enteropathy.
   2. Fat malabsorption
   3. Anemia, 2° to Problem 1
   4. Malnutrition, 2° to Problem 1
Plan: R/O lactose intolerance

QUESTIONS

8. List the basis on which anemia was included as a problem.

9. Explain why this evidence of anemia did not appear when the pt was first admitted.

Part IV: Nutritional Care

Interview of the patient elicited the following information:

Intake of large quantities of milk recently made symptoms worse. Patient had restricted milk intake to no more than 8 oz/day. Patient stated she "might be allergic" to milk, but denied other allergies.

An attempt to obtain a 24-hr recall revealed that the patient had eaten little for 3 days PTA. Her intake the previous day totaled 800 kcal and 20 g protein. Further interview elicited the following as a sample typical menu when she was feeling well:

Breakfast:
   1/4 cantaloupe
   3/4 c Rice Krispies, 1/4 c milk
   1 egg
   1 Danish pastry
   Coffee, 1 t sugar

Lunch:
   3 oz hamburger (high fat) on sesame seed roll, catsup
   3 oz potato chips
   1/2 c ice cream
   12 oz soft drink

Dinner:
   5 oz roast pork
   1/2 c sweet potato
   1/2 c buttered frozen peas
   Tossed salad with Thousand Island dressing
   Apple pie with 1/2 oz sliced cheese garnish
   Tea, lemon

QUESTIONS

10. The attending gastroenterologist has corrected the fluid and electrolyte imbalances and has ordered a "gluten-free, low-fat diet; low-lactose diet as tolerated." Write the SOAP note you would place in this patient's medical record at this point.

11. Describe the mechanisms by which fat malabsorption and lactose intolerance were produced.

12. Using a menu provided by your instructor, plan a diet for one day for this patient.

13. a. What changes would you make in the diet recommended in question 10 for this patient to use when discharged from the hospital?

   b. Prior to the present illness (PI), the patient had maintained normal weight. What difficulties would you expect her to have on the presently prescribed diet? What suggestions would you give her?

18 Nutritional Care in Diseases of the Large Intestine

Disorders of the intestine vary from simple discomfort, such as benign flatulence, at one extreme, to life-threatening conditions, such as toxic megacolon, at the other. Nutritional care may be provided for any of these disorders; however, the procedures used are generally not specific to individual conditions. Like the fat-restricted diet, they are of use in a variety of circumstances. In this chapter, you will be introduced to the use of fiber-modified diets and to nutritional care of the ostomy patient. Before proceeding, you should review, if necessary, the relevant chapter in your text.

MODIFICATIONS OF FIBER

Although fiber is not classified as a nutrient, it has been recognized as having important health-promoting effects. Diets with *increased* fiber are reported to be protective against constipation, diverticulosis, hemorrhoids, and colon cancer. They are also sometimes recommended for patients with diabetes and with atherosclerosis. Diets with *decreased* fiber content are useful in preparation for barium enema or surgery of the intestine, and in acute diarrheal diseases, intestinal fistulas, short-bowel syndrome, diverticulitis, and bleeding lesions.

TERMINOLOGY

The term *fiber* refers to relative indigestible materials usually associated with plant products. The term includes lignin, cellulose, hemicellulose, and other materials such as pectins, gums, mucilages, and algal polysaccharides (1). They may be divided into water-soluble and insoluble fractions that have been noted to have different physiological effects. For example, foods with high concentrations of insoluble fiber, such as whole-grain cereals or bran, are useful for constipation, whereas foods with high concentrations of soluble pectins and gums, such as fruits and vegetables, are useful for patients with diabetes or hypercholesterolemia.

Some tables give values for *crude fiber*—the residue remaining after the sample has been treated with solvents and boiling acid and alkali. In contrast, the fiber that cannot be digested and absorbed, a much milder process, is known as *dietary fiber*. Dietary fiber has been defined physiologically as the sum of polysaccharides and lignin not digested by the endogenous secretions of the human gastrointestinal tract (2).

Fiber-Modified Diets

Diets with altered fiber content may bear a variety of titles. The alternative terms *roughage* and *bulk* have sometimes been used to refer to fiber. These terms are not synonymous, although they are often used as if they were. The term *dietary fiber* has become the more commonly used term and the term we will use in this book.

Residue refers to the material left in the large intestine after digestion and absorption have been completed. It includes indigestible fibers, plus some fat, minerals, undigested starch, and intestine, even if nothing has been eaten. In addition, it is important to note that all food will leave some residue. Therefore, no diet is "residue-free."

Diets that have increased and reduced fiber content are often called *high-fiber* and *low-fiber* diets, respectively. The terms *minimal fiber* and *minimal residue* are used in some institutions to indicate the lowest level that can be achieved. Because accurate information is not readily available, fiber-modified diets are not usually precisely defined. It has been estimated that the Western-type diet contains 10 to 20 g of dietary fiber each day (1). The National Cancer Institute has recommended that Americans consume 25 to 35 g dietary fiber daily, which represents a doubling of current dietary fiber intake (1).

In general, low-fiber diets will contain up to 3 or 4 g per day, and minimal fiber or minimal residue diets contain 1 g or less of fiber per day. For patients who are tube fed and need fiber restrictions, chemically defined formulas and those based on milk or hydrolyzed protein (see Table K-3) are classified as *low residue* or *low fiber*. In contrast, blenderized formulas contain moderate amounts of fiber.

Values for the crude fiber content of foods are available, but unfortunately they have no consistent relationship to the dietary fiber values for human foods. Dietary fiber values usually are 3 to 5 times higher than crude fiber values (1). Correction factors cannot be used to calculate dietary fiber from crude fiber values because the relationship between the two values is too variable. Values for dietary fiber should be used for diet planning, although accurate information about the dietary fiber content of food and, in particular, the individual types of fiber in foods are limited. A table providing updated values for the dietary fiber content of foods selected to be representative and frequently consumed fiber sources is given in Table B-2 (3).

High-fiber diets, on the other hand, are often defined relative to the patient's previous intake. In a patient whose usual dietary fiber intake is 3 to 4 g, an increase to a level of 12 to 14 g might be considered to be high in fiber. A high-fiber diet is more often defined as containing greater than 30 g of fiber per day. Available research suggests that only vegetarians consume 30 to 50 g of dietary fiber per day (1). Thus, a diet history is essential in defining increased fiber for a specific patient. For formula-fed patients needing increased fiber, high-fiber formulas such as Enrich (Ross Laboratories) are available and can still be administered through a small-lumen tube.

THE HIGH-FIBER DIET

Diet Planning
A normal diet can be modified to increase fiber content by increasing the intake of fruits, vegetables, legumes, whole-grain cereal, and nuts. A diet plan might contain, for example, four servings of whole grain-cereals, one serving of legumes, four servings of fruit, and four servings of vegetables. Depending on specific choices, these foods could provide 25 to 35 g of fiber. Table 18-1 offers some general guidelines for planning the high-fiber diet and for patient counseling.

High-fiber diets often recommend raw fruits and vegetables, but the effect of cooking is controversial. However, it seems clear that if fruits and vegetables are peeled before cooking or canning, the total fiber content is reduced compared to the unpeeled item.

TABLE 18-1   Planning a High-Fiber Diet

1. Increase the amount of vegetables, fruits, legumes, and nuts in the diet.
2. Emphasize unpeeled fruits and vegetables when possible.
3. Use whole-grain bread and cereal in place of refined products.
4. Reduce the use of low-fiber, high-energy foods as necessary to maintain normal body weight.
5. Bran (1/4–1 c) may be added to cereal, breads, and casseroles if constipation is a problem.
6. The addition of bran and other high-fiber foods should be made gradually and in divided doses throughout the day.
7. Increase fluid intake.

Side Effects
Large amounts of fiber in the diet may bind minerals. It has been reported that small children and malnourished adults may develop mineral deficiencies if given a high-fiber diet (>30 g). Zinc is most likely to be bound to fiber and excreted in the stool, as are iron, copper, and calcium. As a consequence, high-fiber diets are not often recommended for these two categories of patients. Alternatively, mineral supplements may be given.

Some components of fiber, particularly soluble polysaccharides such as pectin and guar gum, can be fermented by colonic bacteria, producing excess gases such as hydrogen, carbon dioxide, and methane. Although this is not a threat to health, it can cause some discomfort and reduce compliance with a high-fiber diet. The development of flatulence and diarrhea can be minimized by increasing the fiber content of the diet gradually and giving the fiber in divided doses. An increased fluid intake is also helpful.

PROCEDURES FOR DECREASING DIETARY FIBER

Diet Planning
Reduced-fiber diets may be restricted to varying extents. For some patients, the removal of high-fiber foods, such as bran, legumes, corn, and nuts, is sufficient. Other patients may require greater restriction.

In general, fiber-restricted or low-fiber diets avoid raw fruits and vegetables, whole-grain breads and cereals, and nuts, seeds, and legumes. They consist of the following food groups:

1. Refined breads, cereals, and cereal products.
2. Fruits and vegetables, cooked whole, pureed, or as juice, depending on degree of restriction. They should be those without skins, hulls, or seeds.
3. Meat, milk, eggs.
4. Any fat.
5. Desserts without fruits, nuts, or seeds.

Details of foods allowed and not allowed are found in the diet manuals of most institutions.

The minimal residue or strict low-fiber diet restricts foods with even a moderate fiber content. General guidelines for planning this diet are as follows:

1. Use fruit juices and vegetable juices. Prune juice is eliminated.
2. Avoid whole fruits and vegetables.
3. Use refined breads and cereals; avoid whole-grain breads and cereals, seeds, nuts, legumes, potatoes, peanuts, and coconut.

Milk and connective tissue of meat are low in fiber but are believed by some to increase stool volume. There is little scientific evidence to support this, however, and the topic is therefore controversial. In some institutions, the following guidelines are also observed.

4. Limit milk and milk products (ice cream, milk pudding, and cheese) to the equivalent of 2 c of milk per day.
5. Eliminate meat, poultry, or shellfish with tough connective tissue.

For patient requiring a diet free of fiber, a clear liquid diet (see Chapter 12) is sometimes used, but only for a brief period. If a fiber-free diet is needed over a long period, chemically defined formulas should be added (see Chapter 13).

If an absolute minimum of fiber is required, fruits and vegetables are excluded, as is any meat or poultry with tough connective tissue. This diet sometimes excludes milk, which is reputed to be high in *residue, not* fiber.

Side Effects

A strict low-fiber diet will be adequate in most nutrients only if it includes 3 c of milk per day and an adequate amount of meat. It may be inadequate in vitamin A, unless liver is included in the meats, and inadequate in iron for women. It may be inadequate in energy content for patients with high-energy requirements. Patients may thus need supplements of vitamin A and iron if the diet is used for an extended period. High-calorie, fiber-free liquid supplements provide additional energy.

Patients eating a restricted-fiber diet are prone to constipation. Generally, however, the diet is used for only a limited period.

DIETS FOR OSTOMY PATIENTS

Ostomies may be created for feeding and for purposes of excretion. *Gastrostomies* and *jejunostomies*, used for feeding, are discussed in Chapter 13. An *ileostomy* is formed when the ileum is brought out as an opening in the abdominal wall. The colon is removed or bypassed. A *colostomy* consists of an opening of some portion of the colon through the abdominal wall. Both are used for excretion.

Many patients find that their diet can be less restricted following creation of the ostomy than it was prior to the surgery. Nevertheless, patients often benefit from nutritional counseling.

NUTRITIONAL CARE OF THE ILEOSTOMY PATIENT

In the early postoperative period, the patient is usually kept NPO or fed by TPN. When the bowel begins to function again, the patient may be given a clear liquid diet. Additions are made to bring the patient gradually to a low-fiber diet and eventually to an unrestricted diet. During this period, foods are added one at a time so that the source of any problems can be identified. Four general problems can develop:

Disorders of Water and Electrolyte Balance

When the colon is removed, the water, sodium, and potassium normally reabsorbed by the colon are lost in the effluent from the ileostomy. These must be replaced. Adequate fluid must be provided, with special precautions in hot weather and with heavy exercise. Since many patients will restrict their fluid intake in an attempt to decrease the amount of effluent, they should be reminded that excess fluid will not add to the effluent; it is excreted by the kidneys, not the intestine. In addition, foods high in sodium and potassium should be eaten daily (Dietary sodium and potassium modifications are discussed in detail in Chapters 20 and 21).

Danger of Mechanical Blockage

The stoma is smaller in diameter than is the colon. This is not usually a problem, since the ileal content is liquid. However, blockage by large pieces of food can occur when food that has been insufficiently chewed passes intact through the intestine. Therefore, the patient should be instructed to *chew food thoroughly*. In addition, some high-fiber foods pass through the intestine unchanged; it may therefore be necessary to omit or reduce the intake of the following foods:

Corn on the cob	Raw pineapple and other
Coleslaw	raw fruits
Mushrooms	Popcorn
Nuts	Raw celery, carrots, and
Tough meats	relishes
Chinese vegetables such	Spinach
as pea pods, bean	Coconut
sprouts	Skins and seeds of fruits
Bamboo shoots	and vegetables
Orange pulp	

Odor and Flatulence

Some patients are concerned that an unpleasant odor will be noticeable. Others have problems with flatulence and pain. If odor is a problem, it may be helpful to avoid foods that form gas or particularly strong odors. The following are sometimes found to be troublesome:

Cabbage

Broccoli

Onions

Corn

Green peppers

Beans

Nuts

Carbonated beverages

Whips and meringues

Baked beans and
  other legumes

Chocolate

Coconut

Oat bran

Dark rye bread

Pumpernickel bread

Eggs

Fish

Pork

Some cheeses

Alcoholic beverages
  (especially beer)

It is also helpful to advise the patient to avoid habits that result in the swallowing of air, such as chewing gum and using a straw. Yogurt and cranberry juice have been reported to reduce odor.

Excessive Effluent Volume

A large volume of effluent is often inconvenient for the patient, even if fluid and electrolyte balances are maintained. Some foods are reputed to cause an increase in ileal output, while others cause a decrease:

Increasing Output	*Decreasing Output*
Beans	Applesauce
Broccoli	Bananas
Spinach	Boiled milk
Prune juice	Rice
Raw fruits, juices	Peanut butter
Licorice	
Red wine	
Beer	
Highly spiced foods	

It is important for patients to realize that they will not reduce effluent volume by limiting fluid intake: They will simply become dehydrated. If moderate adjustment of intake of the foods just listed is not successful, a low-fiber diet may be helpful. The patient may be advised to keep a diary of food intake and side effects so that troublesome foods may be detected.

NUTRITIONAL CARE OF THE COLOSTOMY PATIENT

The needs of the patient with a colostomy are determined by its location. If the colostomy is in the first part of colon, it will behave much like an ileostomy. When the colostomy is further down, fecal matter is less liquid.

The early postoperative period is handled similarly to that for an ileostomy, as just described. Problems of fluid and electrolyte loss, odor, and excess effluent

may also be handled similarly. There is less tendency to obstruction in a colostomy than in an ileostomy. High-fiber foods may increase fecal volume, however, and the patient may wish to restrict their use. The patient may learn to control volume and thickness of the stool by manipulating intake of foods that cause loose stools and increase effluent volume (raw fruits and vegetables, fruit juices, coffee) and foods that thicken and reduce the volume of effluent.

Ostomy patients are sometimes fearful of abandoning their previous diets even though the diet may no longer be necessary. Patients may need careful counseling in order to liberalize their diets. In counseling these patients, it is important to ensure that a sufficient variety of foods is available to provide an adequate diet. If a food is omitted because it causes a problem in ostomy management, it should be tried again later because some adaptation does occur.

After correction of their digestive disease, some patients tend to become obese. They may need to be counseled on weight control. It is sometimes helpful to refer patients to support groups, which may be found in many cities.

TOPICS FOR FURTHER DISCUSSION

1. What suggestions could be made to a person who complains of chronic constipation? flatulence?
2. Discuss the nutritional care of a patient with acute pancreatitis.

REFERENCES

1. **Slavin, J.A.** Dietary fiber: classification, chemical analyses, and food sources. *J. Am. Dietet. Assoc.* 87:(1987)1164.
2. **Trowell, H.C.** Definitions of fibre. *Lancet* 1:(1974)503.
3. **Marlette, J.A.** Content and composition of dietary fiber in 117 frequently consumed foods, *J. Am. Dietet. Assoc.* 92:(1992)175.

ADDITIONAL SOURCES OF INFORMATION

Pilch, S.M. *Physiological Effects and Health Consequences of Dietary Fiber.* Bethesda, MD: Life Sciences Research Office, Federation of American Societics for Experimental Biology, 1987.

G.A. Spiller, ed. *CRC Handbook of Dietary Fiber in Human Nutrition,* 2d ed., Boca Raton, FL: CRC Press, 1993.

Kritchevsky, D., C. Bonfield, and **J.W. Anderson,** eds. *Dietary Fiber Chemistry, Physiology and Health Effects.* New York:. Plenum, 1990.

Gorman, M.A., and **C. Bowman.** Position of the American Dietetic Association: health implications of dietary fiber. *J. Am. Dietet. Assoc.* 93:(1993)1446.

TO TEST YOUR UNDERSTANDING

1. a. For each of the following foods, give the dietary fiber content (g/100 g) of each, and rank them as sources of fiber on a weight basis, with the most fiber rated as 1. Consult Table B-2.

Banana
Corn, frozen
Cornflakes
Bread, white wheat
Kidney beans, canned

b. Portion sizes for each food are listed below. Calculate the fiber content per serving, and rank the foods again as sources of fiber, with the food containing the most fiber as 1.

Banana	(120 g, 1 med)
Corn	(80 g, 1/2 c)
Cornflakes	(28 g, 1 c)
Bread, white wheat	(25 g, 1 slice)
Kidney beans	(125 g, 1/2 c)

c. How much of each of the foods listed below would be required to provide the same amount of fiber (13.2 g) as 30 g of wheat bran?

Product	Fiber content	Amount required	Serving size
Wheat Bran	44g/100 g	30 g	
Pear, unpeeled			
Cracker, graham			
Peanut, butter			
Brocolli, cooked			

2. Ms. S. is being tube fed over a long period with a low-residue formula. She complains of constipation. Assuming the patient is capable of digesting any formula, list the commercial formulas you might suggest as an alternative to the one presently in use.

3. A high-fiber diet has been recommended for Mr. R., who has diverticulosis. A 24-hr recall gives you the following diet, which he states is typical.

Breakfast:
4 oz orange juice
1 egg
1 slice white bread, toasted
1 t margarine
8 oz low-fat milk
Coffee

Lunch:
3 oz sliced meat
2 slices white bread
1 t mayonnaise
Chopped lettuce salad, French dressing
2 canned peach halves
8 oz low-fat milk

Dinner:
4 oz sliced beef
1/2 c mashed potatoes
1 serving (about 100 g) cooked asparagus
1 white roll
1/2 c butterscotch ice cream
Tea

a. Next to the menu above, write in some alterations you could suggest to this patient to increase his fiber intake to 20 to 30 g.
b. What side effects could occur in this patient as a consequence of this diet?
c. What advice would you give this patient to avoid these side effects and improve compliance?
d. If the patient develops diverticulitis, what diet would be appropriate during the acute phase?

4. a. A patient who has a meal pattern similar to that given in question 3 needs a short-term diet that is more restricted in residue. What alterations in this menu would you suggest?
b. Evaluate the vitamin and mineral adequacy of the resulting diet and suggest care procedures if the patient will have this diet for a month. His milk intake is restricted to 8 oz per day because he has developed lactose intolerance.
c. What advice would you give this patient to avoid these side effects and improve compliance?
d. If the patient develops diverticulitis, what diet would be appropriate during the acute phase?

5. A patient undergoing colon surgery requires a fiber-free diet. He is given a clear liquid diet. After 4 days he is not ready for a more varied diet.
a. Evaluate the nutritional adequacy of the diet.
b. If the restriction were needed for 2 more weeks, and the patient rejects tube feeding, what would you suggest? Be specific about items to be used.

(continued)

TO TEST YOUR UNDERSTANDING *(continued)*

6. Mr. R.R. is a white male, age 68, who has diverticulosis. He is of normal weight. You calculate his protein requirement as 60 g per day and his energy requirement at about 1,900 kcal per day. Using the menu provided by your instructor, modify this menu for a high-fiber diet for the patient.

7. Mr. R.R. later develops diverticulitis. Modify the menu provided by your instructor to provide a low-fiber diet for this patient.

8. Ms. V. has a colon resection, and an ileostomy was created. Following discharge from the hospital, she had difficulty controlling the volume of the effluent.

She returns to the clinic for help. Using the menu provided by your instructor, modify the diet as to demonstrate recommended changes for this patient.

9. If Ms. V. had a sigmoid colostomy and problems with constipation, list some general advice you might give her.

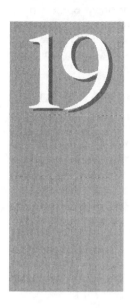

19 Nutritional Care in Diabetes Mellitus

Diabetes mellitus is a common diagnosis with many potential complications over the long term. However, nutrition counseling can significantly contribute to patient well-being, including delay of onset and reduction of severity of complications. Our understanding of diabetes and its care has advanced significantly in recent years. With the development of tissue transplant techniques and greater understanding of the treatment of complications, further advances in nutritional care are certain to come. More immediately, a recent clinical investigation, the Diabetes Control and Complications Trial (DCCT), has had a marked influence on the recommendations for care of diabetic patients (1).

For many years, it was an "article of faith" of many nutritional care specialists that control of blood sugar levels would reduce the incidence of the chronic complications of diabetes (nephropathy, angiopathy, neuropathy, and retinopathy), delay the age of onset, and slow their rate of progression. However, there were few data to support this belief.

The DCCT has now shown strong evidence that treatment to control blood sugar levels at or close to the nondiabetic range results in late onset and slower progression of these complications in insulin-dependent diabetic patients. Therefore, it is now generally accepted that better blood glucose control is important to improve the quality of life and to prolong life of diabetic patients.

The participation of nutritional care specialists in diabetes management is essential in this effort. The principles and recommendations described here are taken from those developed as a result of the DCCT study (1). Although the study did not include noninsulin-dependent subjects, it is believed that the same benefits will accrue to this group of patients in as much as the mechanisms for development of complications are similar.

This chapter provides an introduction to the currently recommended techniques, largely based on the DCCT, for nutritional care of diabetic patients. Before proceeding, you should review the material on diabetes in your textbook.

CLASSIFICATION OF DIABETES

For purposes of this chapter, we will consider spontaneous diabetes mellitus in the following four categories (2):

Type 1, or insulin-dependent diabetes mellitus (IDDM). These patients are usually, but not always, less than 25 years old at onset and are insulin deficient and ketosis prone.

Type II, or noninsulin-dependent diabetes mellitus (NIDDM). These patients are usually, but not always, middle-aged or elderly at onset and are not ketosis prone. This diabetes may be subdivided further into obese or nonobese NIDDM and as maturity-onset DM in the young.

Impaired glucose tolerance (IGT). These patients have some impairment of glucose tolerance. About 20-percent progress to IDDM or NIDDM.

Gestational diabetes. This condition occurs when abnormal glucose tolerance begins during pregnancy and subsides postpartum.

Thus, diabetes consists of a spectrum of disorders. All are characterized by an elevation in blood glucose concentration, and diagnostic procedures focus on this elevation.

DIAGNOSIS

There is a great deal of uncertainty about the diagnostic criteria for diabetes mellitus. This uncertainty is further complicated by the fact that different criteria are used to define the various classifications of the disease.

Patients who have signs and symptoms secondary to hyperglycemia (excessive thirst, frequent urination, increased appetite, ketonuria, glycosuria, and rapid weight loss) are relatively easily diagnosed. For many other patients, however, signs and symptoms are less marked and diagnosis is less certain.

FASTING PLASMA GLUCOSE CONCENTRATION

Glucose concentrations in plasma, serum or whole blood are determined following an 8- to 12-hour overnight fast. A fasting plasma glucose (FPG) concentration over 7.8 mmol/L (140 mg/dL) on at least two occasions in an adult or child is diagnostic of diabetes. Those with FPG levels of 6.1 to 7.8 mmol/L are classified in the IGT category and are considered at risk of developing clinical diabetes. Normal levels for adults over 50 years of age are given in various reports as 3.3 to 5.6, 3.6 to 6.6, or 3.9 to 6.1 mmol per liter. For patients over 50 years of age, FPG is reported to rise 1 to 2 mg/dL for each decade.

You will see FPG recorded in SI units (mmol/L) or conventional units (mg/dL). To convert one form to the other in order to be able to interpret results, use the following equations.

To convert mg/dL to mmol/L:

$$mmol/L = 0.0555 \times mg/dL \qquad \textbf{(19-1)}$$
$$or$$
$$mmol/L = mg/dL \div 18.02 \qquad \textbf{(19-2)}$$

To convert mmol/L to mg/dL:

$$mg/dL = mmol/L \div 0.055 \qquad \textbf{(19-3)}$$
$$or$$
$$mg/dL = mmol/L \times 18.02 \qquad \textbf{(19-4)}$$

Note that any one of the four equations above can be derived from any of the others.

In tables of reference values, such as those in Appendix E, normal values for adults are given. The following are additional useful normal reference values:

Newborn,
premature   1.1–4.4 mmol/L   (20–80 mg/dL) plasma
Full term,
infant   1.1–5.0 mmol/L   (20–90 mg/dL) plasma
Children   3.3–6.4 mmol/L   (60–115 mg/dL) plasma

In interpreting results, it is important to remember that FPG can also be increased in acute pancreatitis; in hyperfunction of the pituitary, adrenal, or hypothalamus; and in patients taking anabolic hormones, epinephrine, norepinephrine, benzothiadiazine diuretics, or diphenyl-hydantoin (phenytoin or Dilantin). FPG may be increased also if the patient is nonfasting, under stress, or receiving IV glucose.

TWO-HOUR POSTPRANDIAL BLOOD GLUCOSE

The *2-hour postprandial* (2hPP) *blood glucose*, that is, 2 hours after eating a meal, is elevated in the diabetic individual. In the normal person, postprandial glucose is usually less than 8.0 mmol/L (145 mg/dL), but may be 8.1 mmol/L (160 mg/dL) in persons over 60 years of age. Higher values are considered diagnostic of diabetes mellitus in the absence of the following: some pituitary, adrenal, or thyroid diseases, advanced liver diseases or pancreatitis, and intake of drugs such as oral contraceptives, thiazides, or phenytoin.

GLUCOSE TOLERANCE TESTS

The *glucose tolerance test* (GTT) is not used alone to diagnose diabetes because it is impaired by increasing age, obesity, inactivity, infection, and drugs such as steroids, thiazides, and phenytoin. It is useful, however, in diagnosing two types of patients:

1. Adults under 50 years of age who are healthy and active and have FPG levels under 7.7 mmol/L (138 mg/dL), but who are suspected to have diabetes because of family history or current symptoms
2. Pregnant women, to screen for gestational diabetes

For the nonpregnant patient, a screening test on a nonfasting patient is often done first. A 75-g glucose load is given. If blood glucose exceeds 7.8 mmol/L (140 g/dL), the GTT is done. For that test, it is sometimes recommended that the patient have a normal- to high-carbohydrate diet (150 g or more per day) for 3 to 7 days prior to the test in order to ensure that liver glycogen is at maximum and that increased glycogen storage does not mask a diabetic response.

On the day of the GTT, a fasting blood sample is taken, and the patient is then given a glucose dose. The usual dose is 1.75 g per kg IBW, to a maximum of 75 g. It is given in an aqueous solution (25 mg/dL, often with lemon juice or in a cola drink) to be taken within 5 minutes. Blood samples are then collected by venipuncture at intervals—usually at 30, 60, 90, and 120 minutes, and sometimes also at 180 minutes (3). The criteria for interpretation of results are given in Table 19-1.

In pregnancy, a 50-g glucose load, non-fasting, is used for screening between the 24th and 28th week of gestation. The results are considered abnormal if the plasma glucose, non-fasting, is 150 mg/dL (8.3 mmol/L) or higher after 1 hour. Other results indicating the need for the 3-hour follow-up are: (1) fasting plasma glucose at 105 mg/dL (5.8 mmol/L) or greater, or (2) 2-hour or longer postprandial plasma glucose at 120 mg/dL (6.6 mmol/L) or higher. This latter value can be a random (non-fasting) sample also.

If the screening test indicates a need for follow-up, the 3-hour glucose tolerance test, with a 100-g glucose dose, is administered. Results are indicative of a diagnosis of GDM if any two values are greater than the following:

GDM	mg/dL (mmol/L)
Fasting	105 (5.8)
1 hour	190 (10.6)
2 hours	165 (9.2)
3 hours	145 (8.1)

ACID-BASE BALANCE

When diabetes is first being diagnosed, or when it is uncontrolled for any reason, it is important to determine the patient's acid-base status. Acid-base balance is discussed in Chapter 4 and should be reviewed, if necessary, before proceeding further with this chapter.

NUTRITIONAL ASSESSMENT

The nutritional assessment procedures described in Chapter 5 are used for diabetic patients, with emphasis

TABLE 19-1 Comparison of Glucose Concentrations in Normal Nonpregnant Adults, Impaired Glucose Tolerance and Diabetes

	Glucose Concentration, mmol/L		
	Normal	Impaired glucose tolerance	Diabetic
Venous plasma			
Fasting	< 6.4	< 7.8	≥ 7.8
30, 60, 90 min	< 11.1	≥ 11.1	
120 min	< 7.8	≥ 7.8 to < 11.1	≥ 11.1 * †
Venous whole blood			
Fasting	< 11.1	< 6.7	>6.7
30, 60, 90 min	< 10.0	≥ 10.0	
120 min	< 6.7	≥6.7 to < 10.0	≥ 10.0 †
Capillary whole blood ‡			
Fasting	< 5.6	< 6.7	≥ 6.7
30, 60, 90 min	< 11.1	≥ 11.1	
120 min	< 7.8	≥ 7.8 to < 11.1	≥ 11.1 †

* Diagnostic of diabetes if seen along with classic symptoms at any time.
† Diagnostic of diabetes if seen at 120 min and one other time in glucose tolerance test.
‡ Diagnostic if noted values are seen at three time periods in glucose tolerance test
Adapted from National Diabetes Data Group. Classification and diagnosis of diabetes millitus and other categories of glucose intolerance. *Diabetes* 28:(1979)1039

on some specific points. Achieving and maintaining normal weight, or at least reducing some of the excess weight, is emphasized for overweight patients. On the other hand, pregnant women or children who are diabetic must be assessed for normal growth and development, as descibed in Chapters 8 and 9.

For patients who have other conditions, such as renal disease, in addition to diabetes, nutritional assessment procedures need to be combined. For example, if the patient has renal or cardiovascular disease, assessment of nutrition status might include the additional procedures described in Chapter 20 or 21. Laboratory values for blood cholesterol and triglycerides, BUN, urine protein, and serum creatinine should be continually monitored in any case.

In general, patients are more likely to follow a diet if it is designed to fit into their current lifestyle. In order to plan such a diet, you must have detailed information about the patient. You must consider income and food budget, as well as cultural, social, religious, and ethnic factors. The home and family should be evaluated. What are the physical facilities for food storage and preparation? Who plans and prepares the food? The diet should accommodate the patient's work and activity schedule, particularly in IDDM, in which diet, insulin, and activity must be integrated. Therefore, the patient's occupation, work hours, and scheduled meal hours and coffee or milk breaks must be known.

It is also important to assess the patient's attitude toward the disease. Is the reaction one of acceptance and compliance or of denial, depression, anxiety, or fear? Also, what is the patient's motivational level? What are the learning capabilities and limitations? What is the patient's reading level? What is the level of current knowledge? When you have all this information, you and the patient *together* would plan a meal pattern with which the patient is willing to comply.

MONITORING CONTROL

Because of the chronic nature of diabetes mellitus, control of the disease is assessed at more frequent intervals than is nutritional status. However, both processes are necessary for appropriate nutritional counseling.

Maintenance of blood glucose levels within normal limits (see Table 19-1) is usually used as the criterion for good control. As part of the health care team, you will need to interpret the results of monitoring procedures. Therefore, it is important that you be familiar with these methods.

BLOOD TESTS

Blood tests include both the measure of blood glucose that has been used for many years and the more recently developed test for glycosylated hemoglobin.

Blood Glucose

Monitoring of glucose levels is considered to be a very effective procedure for monitoring short-term diabetic control. A small drop of blood obtained by finger puncture is placed on a test strip. The test procedure causes a color change in the pad proportional to the blood glucose level; the change is interpreted visually or with a meter. Meters vary in price and some are expensive, but most third-party payers (health insurance) are now willing to cover the cost. *Self blood glucose monitoring*, or SBGM (also called *home blood glucose monitoring* or HBGM), is especially valuable in establishing control. Results of the DCCT study have shown that type I patients who kept blood glucose levels close to normal had a 50 to 75 percent reduction in chronic complications of diabetes.

Results obtained from properly used meters are used as the information base for decisions on altering diet or insulin dose in order to maintain blood glucose within normal limits 80 to 120 mg/dL (4.4 to 6.7 mmol/L) before meals and 100 to 140 mg/dL (5.6 to 7.8 mmol/L) at bedtime. In order to accomplish this, frequent self-monitoring, 3 to 4 times or more per day, is now recommended. An SBGM program may begin with premeal, 2-hour postmeal, and bedtime determinations, 7 times a day for at least a week. It may progress, as control is achieved, to fewer determinations, at fasting, 2-hour postprandial, and at bedtime. The achievement of control is confirmed by determination of glycosylated hemoglobin at intervals of 4 to 12 weeks.

Glycosylated Hemoglobin

The determination of glycosylated hemoglobin, particularly the HbA_{1c} fraction, is very useful. Its use is based on the fact that an irreversible C-N bond can form between the terminal amino group of hemoglobin and the No.-2 carbon atom of glucose. This type of reaction occurs in browning of cooked meat, baking or toasting of baked goods, and browning of sliced fruits. It is known as the *browning reaction* in these situations. When the same reaction occurs in human tissue, it is called the *glycosylation reaction.*

The glycosylation reaction between the red cell hemoglobin and glucose increases when the blood glucose level rises. The reaction is irreversible, but the life span of the red cell averages 120 days. As a result, the amount of glycosylated hemoglobin reflects the average blood glucose level for the previous 120 days, and HbA_{1c} indicates the degree of control of diabetes. Patients cannot then mislead you by being careful about their diets or by taking more insulin only immediately prior to clinic appointments. If hemoglobin A is measured, results are higher than if hemoglobin A_{1c} is measured, since A_{1c} is a fraction of hemoglobin A.

Guidelines for interpretation vary among institutions, but are approximately as follows:

6–7%	Normal
8–9 %	Acceptable
11–13 %	Poor
5.5–6.5 %	For pregnancy

Normal values for the laboratory used by your organization should be consulted.

URINE TESTS

Urine testing is less accurate than blood testing, but it is still used by some patients.

Limitations of Urine Testing

An important limitation of urine testing is the lack of information on specific blood glucose values at levels below renal threshold. Additional sources of error are (1) increased renal thresholds in advancing age or in renal or heart failure and (2) deceased renal threshold in the young, in pregnancy, with severe exercise, and in fever. In addition, the patient needs to provide a "double-voided" urine sample. Urine is voided first, and the urine is discarded. Another sample is then collected after a known interval and used for the testing. Some patients have difficulty with this procedure.

Urine Glucose

If blood glucose rises above the renal threshold, usually 8.8 to 10.0 mmol/L (150 to 180 mg/dL), glucose will appear in the urine. This may be used as a rough indicator of a blood glucose concentration above renal threshold.

Four products are commonly used for urine glucose testing: Chemstrip uG, Clinitest, Diastix, and Tes-Tape. Clinitest may be used with the "5-drop" method (5 drops urine and 10 drops water) or the "2-drop" method (2 drops urine and 10 drops water). Color charts are provided for interpretation of results. Results used to be expressed on the "plus system" —1+, 2+, 3+, and 4+— and some long-term patients will use this terminology. Tests results are now given in percentages. Table 19-2 provides a translation from the plus system to the percentage system.

A number of factors affect the accuracy of tests performed with these products. Diastix and Tes-Tape are less accurate in the presence of ketonuria. False positive Clinitest results may occur in patients receiving barbiturates, L-dopa, or high doses of some antibiotics. The reaction of Diastix is inhibited by L-dopa and high doses of salicylates, such as aspirin. Large quantities of ascorbic acid cause false positive Clinitest results and false negatives with the other three products are shown in Table 19-2. Diabetic patients using urine testing should therefore avoid megadoses of ascorbic acid.

Urine Ketones

Urine ketones can be monitored with Acetest tablets, Ketostix, or Chemstrip uK. The patient should test for the presence of ketones during infections or other illness, when under emotional stress, when there is an increase in glycosuria for any reason, and when blood glucose is consistently above 13.3 mmol/L (240 mg/dL) (2, 3).

TABLE 19-2 Summary of Results of Urine Sugar Tests Comparing Plus and Percent System

Plus System	0	0.1	0.25	0.5	0.75	1.0	2.0	3.0	5.0
Chemstrip uG	neg*	0.1	0.25	0.5	–	1 %	2 %	3 %	5 %
Clinitest, 5 drop	neg	neg	tr	+	+ +	+ + +	+ + + +	–	–
2 drop	neg	neg	tr	1/2	–	1	2	3	5
Diastix	neg	tr*	+	+ +	–	+ + +	+ + + +	–	–
Tes-Tape	neg	+	+ +	+ + +	–	–	+ + + +	–	–

*Neg = negative; tr = trace

MANAGEMENT TOOLS

The four main aspects of management of diabetes mellitus are a blood glucose–lowering agent (not always used), medical nutrition therapy, exercise, and blood glucose monitoring. Because they are interrelated, you need to understand all aspects. Management is provided primarily by the patient with the help of a team consisting, at minimum, of a physician, nurse, pharmacist, and nutritional care specialist. Behavior and exercise specialists may be involved as necessary.

The commonly used levels of management are known as *conventional management, pattern control*, and *intensive insulin therapy* (IIT). Conventional management consists of one or two doses of fixed amounts of insulin per day. Insulin, nutrition, exercise, and blood glucose monitoring should be relatively constant from day to day. Pattern control and intensive insulin therapy are succeeding steps in intensification of therapy. There are more doses of insulin per day or use of an insulin pump. Properly used, these may provide improved control and greater flexibility; however, they require more patient education. The patient must first understand the basic management methods.

BLOOD GLUCOSE–LOWERING AGENTS

There are two types of glucose-lowering agents: insulin and oral hypoglycemic agents (OHAs).

Insulin

The objective of insulin therapy is to mimic insulin delivery by the normal pancreas. Insulin needs are divided into two parts:

1. *Basal insulin* requirement is the amount needed to control blood glucose between meals.
2. *Dietary insulin* requirements are the additional amounts needed before each meal or during exercise.

Insulins are available in the following forms, listed in the order of decreasing tendency to cause insulin resistance or allergy:

1. Improved single-peak with less than 20 ppm of impurities
2. Single monocomponent ("purified") with less than 10 ppm of impurities
3. "Human" insulin prepared by "genetic engineering" methods

Types of Insulin. Insulin dose and time of administration are integrated with food intake on the basis of their speed of onset, time to peak action, and duration of action. The insulins available in the United States and their properties are shown in Table 19-3. Most are available in concentrations of 100 units per mL (U-100), with hypodermic syringe sizes to match. Some are also sold as U-500.

Planning Daily Insulin Injections. Patients routinely give themselves insulin by subcutaneous injection at rotating sites, but insulin may be given to them intramuscularly or intravenously in acute situations. Protocols for self-administered insulin are frequently a mixture of intermediate- or long-acting insulin to provide the basal level, plus regular insulin for the dietary needs.

Patients first diagnosed as having IDDM may be treated in a hospital or on an outpatient basis. Brief hospitalization may be recommended for initial stabilization of IDDM and for pregnant patients; it is more strongly indicated for patients with acute complications such as diabetic ketoacidosis or infection, and for evaluation of patients suspected of having chronic complications.

A number of protocols for insulin administration have been found to be effective. Patients are sometimes given rapid-acting insulin for initial control and later changed to a combination with a longer-acting type. The dosage of insulin of a newly diagnosed patient may start with 0.5 to 1.0 unit per kilogram of body weight per day (4). It is then adjusted based on blood glucose monitoring. The dose varies with the patient's age, severity of symptoms, and the existence of other illnesses. Larger doses may be necessary in growth, pregnancy, adrenal steroid treatment, stress, illness, or increased food intake. Insulin need may decrease with lower food intake and with illnesses such as renal failure. Generally, diabetes is more severe and the dose is increased if the patient is obese. Note that these guidelines do not apply in hyperosmolar nonketotic coma.

Usually, it is recommended that insulin be given 30 minutes prior to food intake. This allows time for insulin

TABLE 19-3 Types of Insulin

Insulin	Onset (hrs)	Peak Action (hrs)	Peak Duration (hrs)	Types Available/ Source [*, †, ‡]			
				Purified		Improved	
				Name	Species [§]	Name	Species [§]
Rapid-acting	1/2–1	2–4	5–7	Regular [*]	b.p.h	Regular [*]	b + p
				Regular [†]	p.h.	Regular [†]	p
				Regular [‡]	p	Semilente [*]	b + p
				Semilente [*]	b + p	Semilente [†]	b
				Semilente [†]	p		
Intermediate-acting	2–4	6–12	18–24	Lente [*]	b + p	Lente [*]	b + p
				Lente [†]	p, h	Lente [†]	b
				NPH [*]	b, p, h	NPH [*]	b + p
				NPH [†]	b, h	NPH [†]	b
				NPH [‡]	p	Globin [†]	b + p
				Mixtard [‡]	p		
				(30 % RI, 70% NPH)			
Long-acting	2–6	18–24	36 +	Ultralente [*]	h	Ultralente [*]	h
				PZI [*]	b + p	Lente [*]	b + p
						PZI [†]	b

[*] Eli Lilly.
[†] Squibb-Novo.
[‡] Nordisk USA.
[§] b = beef; p = pork; h = human; b + p = beef and pork.

absorption and appears to provide for better control of the postprandial rise in blood glucose levels. The blood glucose is monitored and the insulin titrated to produce the desired limitations on blood glucose variations.

The number, size, and timing of doses are scheduled in various ways. Some examples are as follows (5):

1. Once per day of intermediate or premixed insulin in the morning or at bedtime (not usually recommended for IDDM)
2. Twice per day, intermediate-acting insulin, usually 2/3 in the morning and 1/3 before the evening meal.
3. Three injections per day with:
   a. Rapid- and intermediate-acting insulin mixed before breakfast, rapid-acting insulin before the evening meal, and intermediate at bedtime
   b. Human Ultralente plus rapid-acting insulin before breakfast and evening meal; rapid-acting before lunch
   c Rapid-acting insulin before breakfast and lunch. Rapid-acting plus intermediate-acting insulin before evening meal.
4. Four daily injections with:
   a. Rapid-acting insulin before each of three meals, plus intermediate- or long-acting insulin at bedtime
   b. As in 4a above, with addition of intermediate- or long-acting insulin at breakfast
   c. Rapid-acting insulin at 6-hour intervals

Doses must be carefully integrated with the timing of food intake and exercise.

The protocols in which some patients receive *multiple daily insulin injections* are often referred to as MDII. The objective is to mimic the insulin delivery by the normal pancreas. Patients selected for MDII must receive training to become competent in dietary management and must be willing to perform SBGM.

If the patient is skilled in adjusting the diet and performs SBGM properly, it should be possible to:

1. Limit preprandial glucose to 4.4 to 5.5 mmol/L (80 to 100 mg/dL)
2. Limit 2-hour postprandial glucose to less than 11.1 mmol/L (200 mg/dL)

Patients who use an insulin pump receive a *constant subcutaneous insulin infusion* (CSII) to meet basal requirements. Boluses of additional insulin are then given as necessary before meals and for adjustment for activity (6).

Oral Hypoglycemic Agents

Oral hypoglycemic agents (sulfonylureas) are controversial and are not prescribed by all physicians. They are given to NIDDM patients and are most effective for patients who are not obese and have no concurrent disease. They should not be used in IDDM or pregnancy, or for patients with kidney or liver dysfunction. The available products, dosage, and duration of action are given in Table 19-4. Their action is increased by anticoagulants, salicylates, alcohol, and propranolol, and decreased with the use of thyroid drugs, corticosteroids, and thiazide diuretics.

Some NIDDM patients are treated with a combination of insulin and oral hypoglycemic agents if they do not respond adequately to one agent alone. This system is known as BIDS (Bedtime Insulin Daytime Sulfonylureas).

In summary, remember that the overall objective is to control blood glucose within normal limits. To accomplish this, insulin or sulfonylureas must be integrated with food intake and exercise and adjusted as necessary.

MEDICAL NUTRITION THERAPY

In general, the primary goal of medical nutritional therapy is to help the patient improve metabolic control. This is approached by the following:

Balance food intake, insulin, and activity to achieve blood glucose at a level as nearly normal as possible.

Achieve and maintain optimum lipid levels.

Provide energy intake in order to reach and maintain reasonable short- and long-term body weights. Reasonable weight goals may not be ideal weights, as described in Chapter 5, but may be the *achievable* weight.

Reach and maintain normal growth and development in children and adolescents.

Provide for the increased energy needs in pregnancy, lactation, and recovery from catabolic illness.

Prevent or treat acute and chronic complications.

Improve and maintain optimal nutritional status.

Establishing Dietary Goals

The diet prescription. Although the original diet prescription has traditionally been determined by the attending physician, the current trend is toward delegating this procedure to the nutritional care specialist in cooperation with the patient to maximize diabetes control. In establishing nutrition requirements, you might proceed as follows to arrive at some approximations.

Step 1: Establish the total energy content. The energy needs of diabetic patients who are not losing energy via glycosuria do not differ from those of nondiabetics. As in nondiabetics, energy intake must be adjusted for age, activity, physiologic state, and gender. The true test of proper calorie intake is the attainment and maintenance of desirable weight. However, this takes a long time to evaluate. Meanwhile, you have to start somewhere. You might estimate ideal body weight as described in Chapter 5 or estimate the *achievable* weight change. Then, calculate energy requirements based on the weight change goal.

For women *over* 50 years of age, subtract 200 kcal from the total. For men *under* 50, add 200 kcal. If appropriate, add calories for needed weight gain (500 kcal per day for 1 pound of weight gain per week) or for pregnancy or lactation (see Chapter 8).

On the whole, remember that if the patient is currently maintaining an acceptable weight, current intake estimated from the diet history may be used.

Step 2: Establish the protein content. Commonly, 10 to 20 percent of the total energy in the diet is devoted to protein. A 2,000-kcal diet with 10 or 20 percent protein would contain the following:

$$2,000 \times 0.10 = 200/4 = 50 \text{ g protein} \quad \text{or}$$
$$2,000 \times 0.20 = 400/4 = 100 \text{ g protein}$$

An additional 10 g is given in pregnancy and an additional 10 to 15 g in lactation. Protein is also increased in cases of catabolism or metabolic stress (see Chapter 22).

TABLE 19-4   Oral Hypoglycemic Agents

Product	Dosage (mg/day)	Duration of Action (hr)	Half-life (hr)	Doses/day
Tolbutamide (Orinase)	250–3,000	6–12	5	1–3
Acetohexamide (Dymelor)	250–1,500	10–14	5	1–2
Tolazamide (Tolinase)	100–1,100	10–14	7	1–2
Chlorpropamide (Diabinase)	100–500	72	36	1
Glipizide (Glucotrol)	2.5–40	24	3.5–6.0	1–2
Glyburide (Micronase) (DiaBeta)	1.25–10.0	24	3.2+	1–2
Glynase	0.75–12	24	10	1–2
Glipizide xL (extended release)	5.0–20	24		1
Metformin (Glucophage)	500–2500	17.6	17.6	1–2

If the patient has renal disease, which is common in diabetics, the protein allowance is often reduced (see Chapter 21). In addition, patient food preferences and ability to afford the diet should be considered, as should ethnic and religious factors and vegetarianism when indicated.

Step 3: Distribute remaining energy between fat and carbohydrate. The optimum distribution of energy between carbohydrate and fat is unknown and is controversial. Recognizing the tendency of diabetics to develop cardiovascular disease, the lipid content of the diet is usually suggested to provide 30 percent or less of kilocalories. Less than 10 percent of the total kilocalories should be from saturated fats. Less than 300 mg per day of dietary cholesterol is recommended (see Chapter 20). Therefore, diets often consist of 10 to 20 percent of energy derived from protein, 50 to 60 percent from carbohydrate, and 20 to 30 percent from fat (1). The content of a 2,000-kcal diet might then be, for example:

Protein	2,000 kcal × 0.15 = 300/4 = 75 g
Fat	2,000 kcal × 0.3 = 600/9 = 66.7 g
	(usually rounded to 65 g)
Carbohydrate	2,000 kcal × 0.55 = 1,100/4 = 275 g

For patients with NIDDM, the total kilocalorie level is more important than the amount of carbohydrate.

Another controversial matter is the form of carbohydrate to be included. The effects of mono- or disaccharides on blood sugar depend on the amount consumed and the nature of other foods consumed at the same time. Recently, it has been stated that sucrose in the diabetic diet is acceptable in reasonable amounts *provided blood glucose is controlled within normal range*, as indicated by SBGM and by normal HbA$_{1c}$ levels.

There is some evidence that polysaccharides vary in their potential to raise the blood glucose level, that is, in their "glycemic index." At present, however, the potential clinical usefulness of the glycemic index is unknown.

Current recommendations for fiber intake and dietary sodium are the same as those for the general population. Vitamins and minerals do not need to be supplemented as long as the diet is nutritionally adequate, as recommended for the general population.

Step 4: Distribute nutrients among meals and snacks. The nutrients must now be distributed among meals and other feedings, with the primary objective of maintaining blood glucose and lipid levels within normal range. The procedure varies somewhat, depending on the category of the patient.

For NIDDM patients, the primary objective is to avoid wide variations in blood sugar level. Therefore, the restricted amount of kilocalories may be relatively evenly divided among three meals. The ideal division of food intake has not been determined. Therefore, compliance may be promoted by making as few changes as possible in the patient's current dietary habits.

For IDDM patients, meals are planned so that carbohydrate and insulin doses are coordinated to avoid wide fluctuations in blood sugar. The diet must also fit the patient's activity pattern and the patient's customary meal pattern. Results from SBGM are used to indicate changes needed in diet or insulin to achieve control.

Meal-Planning Methods

Once the nutrition assessment has been completed and the goals of the medical nutrition therapy are established, the intervention process to enable patient self-care may begin.

The method chosen for an individual patient should be that with which the patient seems most likely to comply for maximum glycemic control and prevention of complications. Categories of these methods are listed in Table 19-5 and described below (1).

General Guidelines

The Dietary Guidelines for Americans, described in Chapter 6, are useful for diabetic patients to provide general nutritional advice and promote improved diabetes management. Along with the Food Guide Pyramid, also in Chapter 6, they can provide a mind set for promoting weight control and eating a variety of foods. However, they are lacking some specific information needed by diabetic patients, such as knowledge of portion sizes and timing of meals. These and other related needs may be provided by a system referred to as *personal guidelines.* Usually, in this case, emphasis is placed on calorie control, reduction of intake of fat and simple sugars, and other needs of patients who may choose diets suited to their lifestyles. This approach may be successful for patients who are unable or unwilling to accept a more structured plan. These guidelines are especially useful *in combination* with the other planning methods described below (1). Used alone, these methods may be suitable in type II diabetes but not for type I.

Exchange Lists

The exchange list system was first established in 1950 and has undergone a number of revisions since that time, the latest in 1995 (9). The 1986 version, still in use, consists of six categories of food that can be substituted or "exchanged" for each other *within* each category (7, 8).

TABLE 19-5   Methods for Meal Planning for Diabetic Patients

I.	Guidelines
	A. Dietary guidelines for Americans
	B. Personal Guidelines
II.	Exchange systems
	A. Exchange lists ("ADA diet")
	B. High carbohydrate–high fiber (HCF)
	C. Canadian Good Health Eating Guide (GHEG)
III.	Counting systems
	A. Calorie, carbohydrate or fat counting
	B. Point systems
	C. Total available glucose
IV.	Food choice planning using menus (FCP)

Adapted from J.A. Green, Meal planning alternatives in diabetes management *Diab. Care & Education Newsletter* 7:(1986)(9)1.

It is a commonly used tool for developing meal plans for diabetic patients, and is often referred to as the "ADA diet." The 1986 exchange lists are listed in Appendix C, Part I. The newest (1995) version is given in Appendix C, Part II. Both are in current use.

Because of its frequent use, the exchange system is described in detail in the next section. Besides its use in diabetes, it can be useful for planning diets for modifications of energy, fat, fiber, and other individual needs. However, the system is not suitable for all patients. In particular, the amount of structure may not be accepted by some patients. It may be conceptually difficult for those with limited education, and may be excessively structured for those with irregular schedules.

In addition to the lists most closely resembling those given in Appendix C, an alternative exchange list system for a "high carbohydrate-high fiber" (HCF) diet is also available. It consists of ten exchange lists: milk, A vegetables, B vegetables, C vegetables (which vary in carbohydrate content), beans, cereal, bread, fruit, meat, and fat.

The HCF diet plan may be used for patients needing an increase in dietary fiber and may be helpful for patients with hypercholesterolemia and associated cardiovascular disease (see Chapter 20) or with difficulties in diabetes control (1, 10). It is also sometimes helpful for obese patients who need to control food intake and for those who prefer a more "vegetarian-like" diet (see Chapter 10). Also, some patients complain of gastric distress (see Chapter 18). The problems inherent in the structure as described above also apply to the HCF diet.

In Canada, the *Good Health Eating Guide* (*GHEG*) is also an exchange list system for diabetics. The items on each list are called *choices*. The lists are as follows:

1. *Protein foods* (meat, fish, eggs, cheese, tofu) contain 7 g protein, 3 g fat per choice, cooked, on the primary list. A separate list is labeled as containing "extra fat," with a recommendation to be used "less often."
2. *Starchy foods* (bread, cereal, cookies, biscuits, grains, pastas, starchy vegetables) contain 15 g carbohydrate, 2 g protein per choice. A separate list of prepared foods contains, in addition, one "fats and oils" choice.
3. *Milk* choices are 1/2 cup in size and contain 4 g protein, 4 g fat, 6 g carbohydrate of whole milk with adjustments for lower-fat milks as necessary.
4. *Fruits and vegetables* (fruits: fresh, frozen without sugar, water-packed canned, dried, unsweetened juice, and selected vegetables) contain 1 g protein, 10 g carbohydrate in amounts varied to approximate the stated carbohydrate content. In addition, a list of extra vegetables is counted only if eaten in "large quantities," usually 1 cup or more. Another list contains low-calorie vegetables usually not calculated in the meal plan.
5. *Fats and oils* choices contain 4 g fat per choice and include nuts, salad dressings, olives, cream, cheese spreads, and similar high-fat items.
6. A list of *extras* includes some beverages, condiments, herbs, and spices that can be used in unlimited quantities. An additional list can be used in limited quantities. These are mostly condiments.

Counting approaches to meal planning

There are four alternatives included in the counting approaches to meal planning: calorie or carbohydrate counting, total available glucose, and a point system.

The *point system* has been used to count calories, carbohydrate, fiber, fat, or other nutrients. For example, in calorie counting, one point equals 75 calories. In carbohydrate counting, one point equals 15 grams. Therefore, in either case, one slice of bread counts as one point. The patient is given a reference manual that gives the points per serving for the foods in various groups, and is given a "quota" of the nutrient to be counted for each meal. This again provides a reproducible food intake from day to day.

The system has been used successfully for those with limited cognitive skills. It is considered to be useful for those with type II diabetes.

Carbohydrate counting may provide more variety and flexibility than does the exchange system . Amounts of carbohydrate in foods may be taken from values in the exchange lists, from tables of food values, and from nutrition labels on food packages. Carbohydrate counting may be combined with the point system. One point is set as equivalent to 15 g of carbohydrate and is equal to 1 fruit or starch exchange. In this system, 1 milk exchange is also considered as 1 carbohydrate choice. Vegetables from the vegetable exchange list are counted only if the amount eaten is very large. If the patient eats 1 1/2 cups of carrots, for example, that amount would equal 3 exchanges at 5 g each, or 1 carbohydrate point (11).

The meal plan might state that breakfast should contain 4 points (equal to 1 fruit, 1 milk, and 2 bread/starch exchanges). Lunch could contain 4 points (perhaps equal to 1 fruit, 1 milk, 1 or 2 vegetables, and 2 bread/starch exchanges), and at supper, 5 points (2 fruit, 1 milk, 2 vegetables, and 4 bread/starch exchanges, for example).

After the grams of carbohydrate or of carbohydrate points are established, the amount of insulin needed is calculated. Amounts of insulin needed are calculated from carbohydrate intake and SBGM data.

Protein and fat intake are not counted but must be considered. This may become a problem if the patient increases the intake of protein and fat and thereby promotes weight gain. Patients are therefore encouraged to eat about the same amount of protein each day and to choose foods that provide approximately 3 g of fat or less for each point (15 g) of carbohydrate. Thus, if a patient is considering a canned entree containing 30 g (2 points) of carbohydrate, he knows that the food is not a good choice if it contains more than 6 g of fat.

Calorie counting requires that the patient be given lists containing information on the calorie content of foods. The kilocalorie intake per day is agreed upon, and food intake is recorded.

This approach is often useful for patients who need to lose weight, a situation common in NIDDM. For patients using an insulin pump, the amount of regular insulin may be calculated with the equation:

$$\text{Insulin dose(U)} = \frac{\text{blood glucose (mg/dL)}}{25} \\ - \frac{100 + \text{kcal/meal}}{100} \qquad \textbf{(19-5)}$$

Another counting approach is *fat counting*. For this, the patient needs information on fat content of foods after a daily "ration" of fat has been agreed to (1). This procedure is much less frequently used, but it might be useful with the case of a patient with problems of hyperlipidemia.

Total available glucose (TAG) is a more complex method that calculates the glucose available from the diet by calculating:

$$100 \% \text{ of grams of carbohydrate} \\ + \\ 58 \% \text{ of grams of protein} \\ + \\ 10 \% \text{ of grams of fat} = \text{TAG} \qquad \textbf{(19-6)}$$

The insulin dose is calculated by dividing the TAG by the total units of insulin per 24 hours. For example, if TAG equals 200 g and 50 U of insulin are administered daily, the glucose:insulin ratio is 200/50 = 4. Thus, changes in intake can be related to changes in insulin dosages.

Clearly, a major problem with this method is its complexity. In addition, the patient may infer that fat can be taken in large quantities, since only 10 percent will "count." This may lead to large weight gains, undesirable fat intake, and abnormal serum lipid levels.

Menu Approaches

In the *Food Choice Plan* (FCP), the patient chooses the foods and plans menus for 3 days. A dietitian checks portion sizes and energy content for accuracy. The patients use these menus in rotation for about 2 weeks. Then the menus and records of foods eaten and blood glucose levels are reviewed.

This method may be used for type I or II diabetes, especially for patients who do not demand a great deal of variation in their meals or who dislike the decision-making process in planning menus daily.

An alternative for patients who prefer to be given menus to follow is to use a set of published menus. These may also be used temporarily, while education in a more flexible method is undertaken. There are now five sets of these in books entitled *Month of Meals 1* through *Month of Meals 5*, issued by the American Diabetes Association (12). Each volume contains menus for 28 days from which the patient may choose. These may be followed for a time and used as a teaching tool.

Stability of intake is provided because each day's menu is planned to contain 1,500 kcal, and directions are given for adjustments to 1,200 and 1,800 kcal. Each menu consists of three meals of 350, 450, and 550 kcal, along with two 60-kcal snacks or one snack of 125 kcal. Menus are approximately 20 percent protein, 45 to 50 percent carbohydrate, and 30 percent fat. The menus are based on the Exchange Lists for Meal Planning (7).

In summary, regardless of the method used, it is currently recommended that patients monitor their blood glucose on a regular basis and keep a record of food intake. These records are reviewed at regular intervals by the nutritional care specialist. If blood glucose exceeds the desirable range, adjustments in diet patterns or insulin dosage may then be made to bring blood glucose under control. This should be done with the cooperation of the patient. Consideration must be given to the following questions:

What can the patient do? What is the patient willing to do? What does the patient see as problems in compliance?

What is the patient's weight gain or loss, if any, and what might be done? (Remember that increasing insulin to decrease blood glucose may result in weight gain. Consider if this is desirable.)

Is the diet nutritionally adequate? If not, should the diet plan be changed? Does the patient need further education? (Note that the *Dietary Guidelines* and the *Food Guide Pyramid* should be considerations in combination with any of the other planning methods described.)

Procedures for Planning with 1986 Exchange Lists

The planning of diets with exchange lists will now be described in detail, since it involves procedures that are very frequently used, not only for diabetic diets but also for planning for diets for renal disease (see Chapter 21), obesity, and hypoglycemia. The exchange lists—along with the average protein, fat, carbohydrate, and calorie content of each—are listed in Table C-1 (7, 8). Before proceeding, you should stop now and memorize these values. It will save you a great deal of time as you continue with this chapter.

Now, let us look at the individual lists in Tables C-2 through C-9. You will see that many items in each list are set in italics. These are the foods that should be chosen preferentially to reduce the saturated fat in the diet. You will also see that the milk, fruit, and vegetable exchange lists each consist of similar products that have similar uses in meal planning. The meat list consists of meat, poultry, fish, and also cheese and eggs, used similarly in meals. However, the bread/starch exchange list contains not only a variety of breads but also cereals and cereal products, such as breakfast cereals, pastas, crackers, and biscuits. It also contains legumes and starchy vegetables. The fat exchange list consists not only of butter, margarine, solid shortenings, and oils but also nuts, bacon, salt pork, cream, and salad dressings.

In addition, there is a "free" list (Table C-8). These foods contain under 20 calories per serving and can be used freely in addition to the calculated meal plan, if no serving size is specified. No more than 2 to 3 servings per day of free food with specified serving sizes should be eaten. The "free" food list is quite popular with patients, as it provides a relief from the feeling of regimentation.

These lists also contain some items labeled "ethnic foods" and a notation on the ethnic source. These may help in providing additional variety to the diet and in satisfying members of ethnic groups among your patients.

Calculation of the total exchange lists in the diet
Armed with the exchange lists, we will now calculate a meal plan for a patient at IBW. For illustrative purposes, we will assume that after a thorough nutrition history, you arrive at the following diet recommendation:

2,000 kcal; 100 g protein; 70 g fat; 250 g carbohydrate
Divide carbohydrate 1/6, 2/6, 1/6, 2/6. (1/6 of total kcal at breakfast and afternoon snack; 2/6 at lunch and supper)

First, we need to establish the number of each of the exchanges to be included in the diet for the day. Let us see how we could arrive at the calculations given in Table 19-6.

Step I. List the exchanges in the order given—that is, milk, fruit, and vegetables in any order first, followed by the bread exchanges, then the meat exchanges, then the fat exchanges.

Step 2. Based on patient preferences and nutritional needs, estimate the number of milk exchanges that will fit into the diet. For an adult, a minimum of two exchanges to a maximum of one exchange for each meal and snack are often acceptable, while amounts for adolescents and children are adjusted for age.

TABLE 19-6 Calculating a Meal Pattern

Total Calories 2,000
Carbohydrate 250 (g)
Protein 100 (g)
Fat 70 (g)
Division of carbohydrate: 1/6, 2/6, 1/6, 2/6

Daily Meal Pattern

Exchange	# of Exchanges	Protein (g)	Fat (g)	Carbohydrate (g)
* Milk— NF, LF, whole	3	24		36
Fruit	4			60
Vegetable	3	6		15
Subtotal		(30)		(111)
Bread/Starch	9	27		135
Subtotal		(57)		
* Meat——lean, medium, high fat	6	42	30	
Fat	8		40	
TOTAL		99	70	246

* Circle the one used in calculating the meal pattern

Distribution of Exchanges at Meals and Snacks

Exchanges	Total # of Exchanges	Breakfast	AM Snack	Lunch	PM Snack	Dinner	HS Snack
Milk, NF	3	1 (12)	( )	1 (12)	( )	1 (12)	( )
Fruit	4	1 (15)	( )	1 (15)	1 (15)	1 (15)	( )
Vegetable	3	( )	( )	1 (5)	( )	2 (10)	( )
Bread	9	1 (15)	( )	3 (45)	2 (30)	3 (45)	( )
Meat, med.	6	( )	( )	2 ( )	1 ( )	3 ( )	( )
Fat	8	1 ( )	( )	4 ( )	( )	3 ( )	( )
Total		(42)	( )	(77)	(82)	(82)	( )

For purposes of our calculation, we'll assume that our patient wants an 8-oz glass of milk at breakfast, lunch, and supper, for a total of three milk exchanges. Note that we use *skim* milk in the calculation. The three milk exchanges contain 24 g protein and 36 g carbohydrate. If 2-percent or whole milk is used instead of skim milk, the exchanges contain 5 g or 8 g of fat, respectively, in addition.

Step 3. Estimate the number of vegetable exchanges that closely approximate the patient's usual intake. For example, you might use two exchanges, one at midday and one at the evening meal. However, some patients prefer more or less. If a patient is a vegetarian, for example, the number of vegetable exchanges would certainly be increased. Let's assume our patient prefers three vegetable exchanges in the meal plan. These contribute 6 g protein and 15 g carbohydrate to the diet.

Step 4. Estimate the number of fruit exchanges the patient is willing to eat. For example, a plan might include a minimum of one for each meal. If the patient prefers more fruit, additional exchanges could be included.

We'll assume that the patient in our example says he prefers one serving of fruit at each meal and snack. These four servings will then contribute 60 g carbohydrate to the total intake.

Step 5. Total the carbohydrate you have calculated into the diet thus far and subtract from the prescribed amount: $36 + 15 + 60 = 111$; $250 - 111 = 139$.

Step 6. To find the number of bread exchanges needed to provide the total carbohydrate, divide the amount still needed by the amount in one bread exchange: $139 \div 15 = 9$ (rounded to the nearest whole number). Note that nine bread exchanges add 27 g protein and 135 g carbohydrate to the diet plan in Table 19-6.

It may be necessary to remind the patient at this point that this does not mean he should eat 9 slices of bread, but includes breakfast cereals, potatoes, some vegetables, and other items in the starch exchange list. Do his usual food habits coincide with the diet plan thus far?

Step 7. Find the total protein included thus far and subtract from the total needed: $24 + 6 + 27 = 57$. Then, $100 - 57 = 43$.

Step 8. To find the number of meat exchanges needed to fill the prescription, divide the amount needed into the amount in one meat exchange: $43 \div 7 = 6$ (rounded to the nearest whole number).

Note that six medium-fat meat exchanges add 42 g protein and 30 g fat to the diet. It is recommended that meal plans be calculated with medium-fat meats. However, clients should be encouraged to use lean meats whenever possible, and high-fat meats should be limited to not more than 3 servings per week.

Step 9. Total the fat included thus far and subtract from the amount prescribed: $70 - 30 = 40$.

Step 10. To find the number of fat exchanges needed to provide the total fat, divide the amount still needed into the amount in one fat exchange: $40 \div 5 = 8$.

Again, the number of meat and fat exchanges should resemble those recorded in the diet history.

Step 11. Add the total amounts of protein, fat, and carbohydrate. Totals should agree with the prescription within a reasonable range.

The meal plan. The exchanges just calculated must now be distributed among the meals and snacks. The distribution is influenced by the type of insulin the patient is receiving. In NIDDM, the food, or the carbohydrate at least, is divided relatively evenly into meals and snacks in order to keep variations in blood glucose to a minimum.

We'll assume our example patient is taking regular and NPH insulin and needs an afternoon snack. This is reflected in the prescription for part of his carbohydrate at that time. (An example of the procedure is shown in Table 19-6. The diet contains 246 g carbohydrate. Therefore, 41 g ($246 \div 6 = 41$) could be included in the breakfast and afternoon snack, and twice that, or about 82 g, at lunch and dinner. The milk exchanges can be distributed one to each meal, the fruit exchanges distributed one to each meal, and snack as requested by the patient. The vegetable exchanges are scheduled for lunch and dinner. The bread exchanges are then distributed to meet the prescribed distribution of carbohydrate.

Meat and fat exchanges are distributed according to patient preferences. In those institutions where calorie distribution is prescribed, meat and fat could be distributed to meet that requirement.

A final reminder: The diet should be planned to resemble the patient's food habits and preferences in order to achieve the greatest compliance with the diet. Aspects of the existing diet habits that are acceptable should be retained. Necessary changes should be made slowly, that is, at intervals. Also, the primary objective is control of blood glucose. Alteration of the insulin may be more successful than attempting to make major alterations in diet habits.

Planning daily menus. Using the meal plan, a series of daily menus can be planned for or by the patient. For each exchange on the meal plan, a choice is made from the corresponding exchange list. Choices are made within the list, not between lists. A sample menu is shown in Table 19-7.

Some foods are almost free of protein, fat, and carbohydrate. These foods, listed in Table C-8, may be added to the planned diet in reasonable amounts as desired to vary the menu. You will see that coffee, tea, broth, vinegar, dill pickles, and lettuce have been added to the menu in Table 19-7 as "free" foods not calculated into the meal plan.

Expanding the exchange lists. A variety of information sources on food values can be used to expand the

TABLE 19-7   Sample Diabetic Diet Menu

Exchange	Food	Exchange	Food
Breakfast		*Lunch*	
1 Fruit	1/2 Grapefruit	_____	1 c Broth (no fat)
1 Bread	1 Slice whole-wheat bread	1 Bread	6 Saltines
1 Fat	1 t Margarine	2 Meat	2 oz Hamburger patty
1 Milk, skim	1 c Milk, skim	4 Fat	4 t Mayonnaise
	Coffee, black	2 Bread	1 Hamburger bun
			Dill pickles;
		1/2 Vegetable	Leaf lettuce
		1/2 Vegetable	1/4 c Sliced tomato
		1 Fruit	1/4 c Carrot and celery sticks
		1 Milk, skim	4 Fresh apricots
			1 c Milk, skim
		_____	Coffee black
PM Snack		*Dinner*	
1 Fruit	1 Small pear	3 Meat	3 oz Roast pork loin
2 Bread	12 Saltine crackers	1 Vegetable	1/2 c Tomato juice
1 Meat	1 oz Mozzarella cheese	1 Vegetable	1/2 c Broccoli
		2 Bread	2/3 c Sweet potato
		1 Bread	1 Plain roll
		1 Fruit	1/8 Honeydew melon
		3 Fat	3 t Margarine
		1 Milk, skim	1 c Milk, skim
		_____	Tea, black

exchange lists. Table C-9 gives exchange values for various combination foods. A number of fast-food restaurant chains publish the composition of their products in terms of the diabetic exchange lists.

Procedures for Planning with 1995 Exchange Lists

As new information about diabetes and about food composition becomes available, and as new food products are put on the market, exchange lists have been modified. When a new version is released, there is a period when the previous and new editions are both in use. You may currently see patients using either the 1989 or 1995 version

The 1995 version (9) is intended to be compatible with the recent DCCT recommendations. It strongly resembles the 1989 lists. Comparison of the 1989 and 1995 lists given in Parts I and II, respectively, of Appendix C will show the following changes in 1995.

Foods are listed in 3 major categories (see Table C-11): (1) the Meat and Meat Substitutes Group, the supplier of a major portion of the protein in the diet, (2) the Fat Group, and (3) the Carbohydrate Group, which encompasses the main sources of starches and sugars. This approach also makes the exchange list system more closely resemble carbohydrate counting.

The Carbohydrate Group contains lists for starches, fruits, vegetables, and milk, along with "other carbohydrates." The starch exchange contains 3 g protein, 15 g carbohydrate and up to 1 g fat, and averages 80 kcals per serving. It contains sublists of breads, cereals and grains, starchy vegetables, crackers and snacks, dried, peas, beans, and lentils (also counting as one very lean meat exchange), and starchy foods prepared with fat (also counting as one fat exchange) (see Table C-12). Comparison with the 1989 exchange list for breads and cereals shows that the new list is very similar but has been expanded somewhat.

The Fruit List (Table C-13) in the 1995 version is considered to include fruits canned in "very light" syrup and "juice-pack" as equivalent to fresh and canned unsweetened. The items on the list average 15 g carbohydrate. The 1995 Vegetable List (Table C-14) contains cooked (1/2 c) and raw (1 c) vegetables, excluding those in the Starch List. Each serving is estimated to contain 2 g protein, 5 g carbohydrate, and 25 kcals. In planning diets, carbohydrate from vegetables is not included until the daily total reaches to 3 servings or 15 g carbohydrate.

The Milk List (Table C-15) has been rearranged to contain subcategories of skim and very low fat milk (< 1 percent fat), low fat (up to 2 percent fat), and whole milk. All 3 categories contain 8 g protein and 12 g carbohydrate with 0 to 3, 5, or 8 g fat, respectively.

Since 15 g carbohydrate is provided by one item in the Starch or Fruit Lists or by 3 servings from the Vegetable List, they may be exchanged one for another. One milk serving is also considered to be exchangeable for a fruit or a starch serving. For example, if a person's meal plan contains 4 fruits and 5 starches, this can be equal to 3 fruit, 4 starch, 3 vegetables, and 1 milk.

In 1995, a list of "Other Carbohydrates" was also provided (Table C-16). The items on this list can be substituted for 1 starch or 1 fruit or 1 milk in the meal plan. Some also substitute for 1 or more fat exchanges.

TABLE 19-8 Nonnutritive Sweeteners

Product	Brand names	Sweetness (compared to sucrose)	Uses	Acceptability	Acceptable daily intake (mg/kg BW)
Saccharin	Sucaryl Sugar Twin Sweet Magic Sweet'n Low	300–500 ×	Table top Soft drinks	Bitter after taste Do not use in cooking	2.5
Aspartame	Nutrasweet	180 ×	In manufactured foods Soft drinks Chewing gum	Not used in cooking No aftertaste Not for use by PKU pts.	40
	Equal	180 ×	Table top	Has 4 kcal/g	
AcesulfameK	Sunette	200 ×	Table top in manufactured foods	No aftertaste	15
Cyclamate		30 ×		Not available in U.S.	

These changes from the 1989 exchanges allow for more variety and greater flexibility in meal planning as recommended by the DCCT. At the same time, more counseling to assure a nutritionally adequate diet may be required.

Because diabetic patients have a tendency to develop cardiovascular disease, it is useful to provide information on types and amounts of fats in foods. For this purpose, the Meat and Substitutes and the Fat Lists were modified in 1995. In the Meat and Substitutes List (Table C-17) the former low, medium, and high fat categories were altered to create a "very lean" category. All 4 categories contain about 7 g protein plus 0 to 1, 3, 5, or 8 g of fat, respectively. Thus, a patient has more information to help him control his fat intake. The Fat Exchange List (Table C-18) has been subdivided to provide separate lists of monounsaturated, polyunsaturated, and saturated fats. These are also useful for modifying dietary fats. Rationale for these modifications is given in Chapter 20.

The 1995 Exchange Lists also include tables of Free Foods (Table C-19), Combination Foods (Table C-20, and Fat Foods (Table C-21). These are also useful to provide increased variety and flexibility. All lists are contained in Appendix C, Part II

Some Special Problems in Meal Planning

Special foods for diabetic diets. There are a number of products designed for use in diabetic diets. These include sweeteners and foods labeled as "diabetic" or "dietetic" foods.

Sweeteners may be categorized as *nonnutritive* (calorie-free or nearly so) and *nutritive* (calorie-containing). Nonnutritive sweeteners are available in several types and forms. Information on these is contained in Table 19-8. Nutritive sweeteners include sugars such as sucrose, fructose, and glucose (dextrose), and sugar alcohols such as sorbitol and mannitol. These are safe to use, but yield 4 kcal per gram and must be calculated into the diet.

Alcohol use. The energy content of alcohol (7 kcal/g) may be responsible for unwanted weight gain. It may be responsible for hypoglycemia in the IDDM patient, especially if meals are missed or delayed. The hypoglycemia may be difficult to distinguish from alcohol intoxication and may result in a delay in needed treatment. The oral hypoglycemic agents given to NIDDM patients may interact with even very small amounts of alcohol to produce a reaction resembling alcohol intoxication. Despite these contraindications, it must be recognized that alcohol consumption is an important part of the social life of many patients and is likely to continue. Some patients find alcohol consumption a necessary part of their occupations. The patient who has decided to consume alcoholic beverages must be taught about its effects and about setting reasonable limits.

Because alcohol is metabolized in two-carbon fragments similar to fat, it is usually incorporated into diabetic diets in place of the fat exchanges. In fact, it has been suggested that an "alcohol equivalent" be considered to be equal to two fat exchanges if the patient is using exchange lists. Some alcoholic beverages also contain carbohydrate, and some bread exchanges are removed to compensate for this.

The substitution is recommended only for NIDDM patients. No food is removed from the diet of the IDDM patient because of the risk of alcohol-induced hypoglycemia (13). Insulin is not required for alcohol metabolism. In either case, the need for *moderate* intake or less should be emphasized to the patient.

The patient may be given a list of exchange values for alcoholic beverages. A typical list is given in Table C-10.

Eating and travel tips. If diabetic patients are to lead normal lives, they need to know how to order meals in restaurants and how to take care of themselves while traveling.

In restaurants, simple foods that follow the prescribed diet should be ordered. The diabetic should ask that gravies and sauces not be added to food and that salad dressings be served "on the side" so that the amount used can be controlled. Most restaurants serve more food in a meal than a diabetic diet allows, and most are happy to provide a container so that the excess can be taken home.

Travel generally does not present a problem for NIDDM patients. For the patient with IDDM, however, certain precautions may be necessary.

All IDDM patients should be instructed to carry with them at all times some foods that can be used to avoid hypoglycemic reactions. Procedures vary with the means of transportation and length of trip. The following guidelines may be given to the patient:

Car travel—If driving, especially for more than a half hour and if the time is during peak insulin action, have some food, such as a half sandwich (one meat, one bread, one fat) taken from your next meal. Do not have any alcohol before driving; it tends to cause hypoglycemia, which may not be distinguishable from intoxication. Always carry some sugar or candy with you—even if you are just a passenger.

Air travel—Carry an emergency supply of sugar. Find out whether meals will be served. Airlines will serve special diets if ordered well in advance. Carry sandwiches in case there is a mix-up about meals.

Ship travel—Food is usually available. The main problem may be motion sickness. A liquid diet or the diet for "morning sickness" may be helpful.

Rail travel—Long-distance trains usually have food available. It is a good idea to carry some sandwiches and fruit as a precaution in case of problems with the dining car. Commuter-train travel is likely to require only an emergency sugar supply.

Bus travel—Commuter-bus travel is similar to travel by commuter train. Long-distance bus travel is difficult because there is no food on buses and schedules are often erratic. Patients should carry enough food to provide all meals in transit.

Adjusting for illness. Concurrent illnesses sometimes interfere with control of diabetes. Some illnesses, such as infections, increase the demand for insulin, causing hyperglycemia; decreased activity may further increase blood glucose. Patients who are ill should check their blood glucose frequently and be guided primarily by those results.

The ill diabetic may be unwilling or unable to eat part of the food in a meal. If the patient is not receiving a hypoglycemic drug, particularly if obese, substitution may not be necessary. Substitution may be required for a short period in some cases, since some products have a half-life of 1 to 2 days. If the patient has received the prescribed insulin, however, failure to eat food can lead to a hypoglycemic reaction.

All institutions have procedures to deal with such situations. Common procedures are as follows:

1. No substitutions are needed if the uneaten food contains only protein and fat (that is, meat or fat exchanges).
2. No substitution is offered if the uneaten food contains less than a specified amount of carbohydrate. In many institutions, the specified amount is 5 g or less. Thus, 1/4 c milk or a serving of vegetable would not require substitution.
3. Substitutions are offered for foods containing more than 5 g of carbohydrate. Usually, the food offered is in a form easier to eat (or drink) and in a smaller volume than the rejected food.

In institutions, it is common practice to use *unsweetened* fruit juice as the substituted food, using a graduated cylinder to measure.

If the patient refuses the substitute, the nursing staff must be alerted to check the patient frequently for signs of hypoglycemia. If necessary, the physician will order IV glucose or glucagon injections. In some illnesses, the diabetic patient needs additional modifications in the diet. Increases or decreases of major nutrients, such as fat-restricted and protein-restricted diets, can be accommodated by recalculating the meal plan. Other diets, such as low-sodium and soft diets, can be accommodated with appropriate choices from exchange lists and by instructing patients on food preparation.

The diabetic liquid diet. The diabetic patient who has, for example, an upset stomach or a sore throat, may feel more comfortable with a liquid diet. Therefore, patients should be given instructions on how to convert their usual diet to a liquid diet. For a short illness, it is common practice to ensure the carbohydrate intake and to de-emphasize protein and fat. Using exchange grouping as an example, the following procedures can be used.

Milk exchange—Use as is or mixed with other foods.

Vegetable exchange—Use pureed vegetables and mix with the milk exchange to make a cream soup.

Fruit exchange—Use fruit juice.

Bread exchange—Mix refined cooked cereal with milk exchange to make thin gruel. Substitute fruit juice. Substitute 1/2 c ice cream (1 bread and 2 fat).

Meat exchange—Use eggs (coddled, as a precaution against salmonella) plus milk to make eggnog or to make baked custard. Recalculate the diet to substitute milk for bread and meat. (This should be done for the patient, not left for the patient to do.)

Fat exchange—Add butter, margarine, or cream to cereal, gruel, or cream soups.

MANAGEMENT METHODS

The methods of management of medical nutrition therapy in diabetes differ in the amount of control of blood glucose possible, degrees of flexibility, and complexity of the methods.

CONVENTIONAL MANAGEMENT

Conventional management is so-called largely because it has been used for the longest time for the largest number of patients. It consists primarily of prescribed insulin, usually once per day, food, often using the exchange list system or one of the other methods described above, exercise, and sometimes blood glucose monitoring.

These components ideally should be consistent from day to day. The diet should be consistent in amount and timing with meals and snacks taken within an hour of the same time daily.

Insulin is taken once or twice a day at the same times daily. Exercise should be as consistent as possible from day to day in timing, frequency, and intensity. Blood glucose monitoring also should be done at the same time daily. It is also recommended that the patient keep careful records of blood glucose, amount and kinds of insulin taken, ketones if any, and notes of other factors, such as stress, illness, or hormone changes that may affect blood glucose levels.

Even if the patient controls diet and exercise very carefully, blood glucose may not remain within desired limits. As a consequence, the risk of complications increases as shown by the DCCT. However, this type of management may be as far as some patients are willing or able to go.

Some patients will elect to undertake a program to monitor more closely their glucose levels in order to achieve "tighter" blood glucose control. Benefits are reduced occurrence and severity of complications, general improvement in feeling of well-being, and greater flexibility in lifestyle.

PATTERN CONTROL

Once the patient has mastered the information and procedures involved in conventional management, this next step may be undertaken. It demands a commitment to spend more time and effort in controlling blood glucose and may be emotionally draining at first. The patient must be willing to take insulin 3 to 4 times per day, with blood glucose monitoring at least that often. In addition, the risk of hypoglycemia increases with its attendant fear. Thus, this procedure is not for every one.

Let us assume, however, that we have a patient who wishes to undertake this program *and who lives in an area where a support team is available*. The patient is already on some type of insulin regimen with NPH, Lente, or Ultralente insulin for basal and Regular for bolus. The patient also must be skilled in SBGM.

The patient keeps records of blood glucose levels before each meal and snack. These are examined to determine if blood glucose levels are within the target range (70 to 120 mg/dL). For example, let us assume that values obtained are as follows for a patient who is taking NPH insulin at breakfast and supper, and Regular insulin at breakfast, lunch, and supper. Also assume for the moment that diet and exercise are stable from day to day.

The SBGM values for this example patient are as follows:

	Breakfast	Lunch	Supper	Snack
Tues.	86	152	112	99
Wed.	77	220	102	129
Thurs.	93	197	115	168
Fri.	84			

Although the patient's diabetes seems to be reasonably well controlled, examination of these values *vertically* shows a pattern of values exceeding target range daily at lunch time. This pattern of excess is then controlled by adjustment in the dosage of the insulin *acting at that time*.

Some guidelines for insulin adjustments may be given:

1. Limit changes in insulin up or down 1 or 2 units of *one* insulin (basal or bolus) no more frequently than once in 3 or 4 days.
2. Adjust only the insulin that affects the abnormal blood glucose value, increasing insulin if blood glucose values are too high and decreasing insulin if blood glucose values are too low. In the example given, the breakfast insulin could be increased by 1 or 2 units.
3. If blood glucose values are:

Abnormal at	*Then adjust insulin as follows*
Lunch	Regular at breakfast
Supper	NPH at breakfast
Evening snack	Regular at supper

If blood glucose values are elevated at breakfast time, choosing the appropriate action becomes more complex. In order to distinguish the mechanisms involved, it is necessary to determine blood glucose levels at about 3 AM for several days. If the amount of insulin taken at supper or evening snack is insufficient, the blood glucose will rise and be elevated at 3 AM. Therefore, the insulin dose at supper or evening snack needs to be increased.

An alternative situation is the *dawn phenomenon*, in which there is an increase in counterregulatory hormones, such as glucagon, in the early morning. In this case, blood glucose is within acceptable range at 3 AM but high at breakfast time. The NPH insulin at supper should be moved to the time of the evening snack. If it is already taken at that time, increase the dose.

Another alternative is the *Somogyi phenomenon* or *rebound effect*, in which insulin taken at supper time peaks at about 3 AM. Blood glucose is then low, and the liver releases glucose, so blood glucose, is high at breakfast time. For these patients, NPH insulin at supper or evening snack time should be reduced.

4. When one adjustment is made in insulin dose, the results sometimes create a situation in which a second adjustment becomes necessary. Therefore, it is essential that blood glucose levels be followed carefully by SBGM until values stabilize.

In summary, if blood glucose values are elevated before breakfast and

Value at 3 AM is:	*Adjust NPH insulin as follows:*
Elevated	Increase at supper or evening snack
In acceptable range	Change supper dose to evening snack, or
	Increase evening snack dose
Too low	Decrease at supper or evening snack

These procedures result in improved blood glucose control, but still limit flexibility. For some patients, pattern control provides sufficient flexibility and also adequate control. For others, yet another step may provide greater control and allow greater flexibility in lifestyle.

INSULIN INTENSIFICATION THERAPY

In pattern control, as the previous section illustrated, hyperglycemic values can occur, for example, daily at the same time for 3 days before correction is made. In addition, there may be sporadic episodes of high blood glucose for 1 or 2 days. Therefore pattern control is not the ultimate in control.

Patients who desire greater control with a high level of flexibility can undertake *insulin intensification therapy* (IIT). These patients must be highly motivated, must have a health care team available for counseling, and must be extensively and thoroughly educated. IIT procedures make it possible to adjust for high or low blood glucose levels that same day. These adjustments may be one of two types.

Compensatory Insulin Adjustments

The patient may have a high glucose value caused by overeating, lack of exercise, stress, or unknown reasons, and she or he may wish to correct this situation immediately. This is done by increasing the Regular insulin dose at that time.

For example, let us assume that a patient has blood glucose levels obtained by SBGM of 101 mg/dL before breakfast and 149 mg/dL before lunch. Clearly, the breakfast value is within the target range, but the value before lunch is elevated. The patient then compensates for his high value by increasing the dose of Regular insulin by 1 unit at lunch time.

Patients need guidelines to tell them how much insulin to add. In the example above, 1 unit of Regular insulin would be added to the usual dose.

A typical set of guidelines are as follows for breakfast, lunch, or supper:

If blood glucose is:	*Regular insulin dose is:*
71–120 mg/dL	As prescribed
121–150	Increased by 1 unit
151–200	Increased by 2 units
201–250	Increased by 3 units
over 250	Increased by 4 units
less than 70	Decreased by 1 or 2 units

These values are guidelines only and may be individualized based on previous experience.

An example of a compensatory adjustment is as follows: The patient's prescribed insulin is 15 units of Regular insulin and 25 units of NPH insulin before breakfast, 10 units of Regular before lunch, and 10 units of Regular and 25 units of NPH before supper. The patient also has an evening snack, but no insulin. SBGM before meals and snacks gives the following values:

	Breakfast	Lunch	Supper	Snack
Day 1	139	105	95	85
Day 2	50	65	95	108

Because the breakfast blood glucose was high before breakfast the first day, one additional unit of Regular insulin was added. Values at lunch were within the normal range, as were the other two values that day. On the second day, the breakfast value was low; therefore, the insulin dose was reduced by 2 units. At lunch time, blood glucose was still low, and another unit of insulin was taken from the prescribed dose before lunch.

Anticipatory Insulin Adjustments

The patient can also learn to make adjustments when changes in food intake or exercise that can alter blood sugar level can be anticipated but have not yet occurred. This is a more complex procedure, since one must not only anticipate the change but also predict its dimensions. A patient may anticipate a large holiday dinner, a bridal shower, or some other social affair where increased food intake is expected. Conversely, less food, such as missed meals, or less activity might be anticipated. Sometimes additional activity may be predicted, such as an after school game for a child, or an aerobics class or a swimming meet for a college student.

In order to adjust the insulin dose for such events, the patient must be able to estimate the amount of insulin that must be added or subtracted and the appropriate time that this should be done. The carbohydrate content of the extra food items may be obtained from the exchange lists or carbohydrate counting described previously. Other sources of information may be obtained from nutrition labels or from tables of food values.

Next, the amount of insulin to be changed must be estimated. There are two ways this may be done:

1. If most of the prescribed insulin is NPH or Lente, add 1 unit of Regular insulin for each 10 to 15 grams of added carbohydrate. For example, if you wish to add 30 g of carbohydrate to your usual lunch intake, then add 2 units of Regular insulin to your usual dose before lunch.
2. The second method applies only to persons who take multiple injections and who take Regular insulin to cover the greater part of insulin for meals.

The first step of this method is to divide the total carbohydrate in the usual meal by the usual number of units of Regular insulin. If, for example, the breakfast usually contains 1 fruit, 1 milk, and 3 bread exchanges or 72 g carbohydrate, and the usual Regular insulin dose is 6 units, then a unit of Regular insulin will cover $72 \div 6 = 12$ g of carbohydrate.

In the second step, divide the 12 g carbohydrate into the added carbohydrate you anticipate. For example, if the patient expects to eat a dessert adding 24 g carbohydrate to the usual diet, then $24 \div 12 = 2$ units of regular insulin that should be added.

Some cautions must be heeded: Patients should be encouraged to follow their treatment plans closely until blood glucose values are relatively stable within the goal range. Also, these adjustments should be in addition to any adjustments for premeal blood glucose values obtained by SBGM.

ADJUSTMENTS FOR EXERCISE

In addition to a hypoglycemic agent and diet, the person with diabetes is likely to need some advice on exercise from the health care team. This must be integrated with the other aspects of care. Therefore, it is necessary that all team members be knowledgeable in this area.

BENEFITS OF EXERCISE
Most persons with diabetes profit in a variety of ways from an exercise program. Regular exercise results in greater sensitivity to insulin and thus lowers blood glucose levels and increases glucose tolerance. It decreases risk factors related to cardiovascular disease such as hypercholesterolemia, hypertriglyceridemia, excess LDL, high HbA_{1c}, and hypertension, as well as increasing HDL levels. Advantages of exercise include improved overall fitness, with improved cardiovascular and pulmonary function, and greater muscle strength, endurance, and flexibility. Exercise also reduces fat, increases muscle, and thus increases overall physical capacity. It may help with weight control, provided energy intake does not rise in excess, and it also has psychological benefits (4, 10).

When the nutrition counselor and patient are planning the diet and hypoglycemic drug routine, the usual daily activity is considered. This section is devoted to guidelines for those who now wish to begin an exercise program added to their daily activities or for those whose exercise is sporadic.

Side Effects of Exercise
In patients with NIDDM who are controlled by diet and exercise, the exercise may have a sufficient blood glucose–lowering effect to avoid the use of medication. For IDDM or for NIDDM requiring hypoglycemic drugs, a primary side effect may be increased risk of hypoglycemia. In some circumstances, however, hyperglycemia may develop. As a result, patients using these treatments need advice on blood glucose control.

Guidelines for patients
Because exercise can pose risks to some persons with diabetes, it is important to obtain a doctor's approval before beginning an exercise program. Those who are taking insulin or OHA should be sure their diabetes is under good control, that is, blood glucose levels should be 150 to 180 mg/dL or less. It is recommended that blood glucose at 240 to 300 mg/dL or higher is a contraindication to an exercise program (5, 12). Exercise tends to lower blood glucose levels as muscle cells use glucose if the diabetes is well controlled. If the diabetes is not controlled (indicated by blood glucose 240 to 300 mg/dL), more glucose is released from the liver and glucose levels rise, worsening the hyperglycemia. When glucose levels are this high, an exercise program should be delayed until the diabetes is under better control.

Exercise affects the rate of insulin absorption. Therefore, insulin should not be injected into muscles to be exercised. For example, a runner should not inject insulin into a leg muscle before running.

For those using conventional management, a common recommendation is to eat a snack with 10 to 15 g of carbohydrate before the exercise if the exercise is brief (1 hour or less) and moderate. Longer or more strenuous activity requires a greater increase.

Multiple doses of insulin (MDII or CSII) allow for greater flexibility and precision in adjusting for exercise. Patients can make changes in insulin doses and diet at short intervals. Blood glucose levels obtained from SBGM will also provide some guidance (See chart on next page).(14).

Patients taking insulin or an oral hypoglycemic agent should always carry a source of carbohydrate to counteract potential hypoglycemia. In addition, they should continue to monitor their blood glucose every 2 hours for up to 30 hours, especially if the activity has been strenuous and prolonged.

When the activity extends over a long period, such as all day, increased food intake does not always serve to totally avoid hypoglycemia. It may be necessary, in addition, to reduce the type of insulin acting *during the exercise period* by 10 percent of the total daily dose. If both insulins are acting, for example, during an all-day

If blood glucose is:	And exercise is:	Increase carbohydrate intake by:
< 100 mg/dL	Low to moderate intensity	10–15 g carbohydrate per hr of exercise
100 mg/dL	Low to moderate intensity	None needed
< 100 mg/dL	Moderate	25–50 g per hr before and 10–15 g per hr after
100–180 mg/dL	Moderate	10–15 g per hr of exercise
180–300 mg/dL	Moderate	None needed
300 mg/dL or more	Moderate	Do not exercise until better controlled
< 100 mg/dL	Strenuous	50 g and monitor often
100–180 mg/dL	Strenuous	25 –50 g
180–300 mg/dL	Strenuous	10–15 g hr
300 mg/dL or more	Strenuous	Do not exercise until better controlled

hike, the 10 percent insulin reduction should be divided between the two types of insulin during the day.

An SBGM program can provide much guidance. Before undertaking an exercise program, the diabetic person should seek approval of the physician for the duration and intensity of the exercise to be undertaken. SBGM prior to the exercise will indicate the adjustments to be made.

Risks of Exercise in Diabetes Complications
In addition to the risk of hypoglycemia in some patients, complications of diabetes present additional problems. Several precautions must be observed. In the patient with neuropathy, frequently there is decreased feeling. Thus, it is important to provide great care of the feet with appropriate shoes. The patient should walk, not jog, since jogging increases the impact on the feet. Exercises should not be weight bearing. Range-of-motion exercises are useful in preventing injury.

Many diabetic patients develop retinopathy. They should not do exercises that are likely to increase blood pressure in the retinae. Weight lifting should be avoided as should bouncing, as in high-impact aerobics. During exercises, the head should not be allowed to be below the waist.

Since cardiovascular disease is common in diabetic patients, exercise programs should not be so strenuous that they raise blood pressure or increase heart rate beyond a rate specified by the physician. If exercise is undertaken for weight loss, adjustments of food and insulin to compensate for the additional energy used should consist most commonly of decreased insulin, rather than increase in food intake.

DIABETES AND PREGNANCY

Pregnant diabetics may be classified into two groups: the diabetic woman who becomes pregnant (pregestational diabetes) and the patient with gestational diabetes mellitus, that is, the patient who becomes carbohydrate intolerant while she is pregnant. In both cases, the pregnancy is considered high risk; rigid control of the diabetes is therefore required in both cases and requires

great effort. Without adequate control, there is increased risk of preterm delivery, macrosomia, intrauterine growth retardation, newborn hypoglycemia, and newborn hyperbilirubinemia.

THE PREGNANT WOMAN WITH PREGESTATIONAL DIABETES

Patients who are diabetic when they conceive, but who are not well controlled, are often hospitalized for control of diabetes, review and correction of previous education, education on aspects of pregnancy, and self-monitoring techniques as soon as pregnancy is diagnosed. It is preferable that a diabetic patient contemplating pregnancy achieve excellent control before conception. The NIDDM patient who becomes pregnant will usually need insulin during pregnancy. Many of these patients will profit by MDII or CSII while pregnant.

Monitoring
SBGM is considered important, even essential, for successful outcome. Pregnancy is associated with a decrease in fasting blood sugar concentrations and an increase in postprandial blood sugar concentrations compared to the nonpregnant state. Desired glucose levels are 3.3 to 5.6 mmol/L (60 to 100 mg per dL) for fasting levels and a maximum of 7.8 mmol/L (140 mg/dL) 1 to 2 hours after meals. The standards for control are more rigid than are those for the nonpregnant woman. When the patient brings you her SBGM records, it is important to ensure that blood glucose has remained within normal limits.

Medical Nutrition Therapy
The diet should have at least 200 g carbohydrate per day and 1.5 to 2.0 g protein per kg per day. Recommended total energy intakes are 30 kcal per kg IBW in the first trimester and 38 kcal per kg IBW in the 240 and third trimesters, with 50 to 60 percent carbohydrate, 20 to 37 percent fat, and 12 to 20 percent protein. An evening snack, containing a minimum of 25 g complex carbohydrate, is always included in order to avoid hypo-

during the night. It is a common, but not universal practice to give six equal meals, or three meals and three snacks, to the IDDM pregnant diabetic (15).

During the first trimester of pregnancy, food intake may decline with symptoms of nausea and vomiting, and insulin doses may need to be decreased. Starvation ketosis, characterized by hypoglycemia and ketonuria, is common during the first trimester, and it is important to adjust the diet to foods that can be tolerated in order to ensure an adequate caloric intake and avoid ketonuria (see Table 8-6).

Insulin is given by multiple subcutaneous injections (MDII) or by CSII and is carefully balanced with the diet. Long-acting insulins are usually avoided. More rapid-acting insulin in multiple doses or CSII gives better control. In addition, human insulin, not animal insulin, is recommended.

The NIDDM patient is often obese. It must be kept in mind that pregnancy is not the time for stringent weight reduction; however, excessive weight gain should be avoided. There is controversy concerning the optimal energy level to include in the diet. It has been stated that a diet of 1,500 to 1,700 kcal per day will provide for fetal growth (16). Alternatively, it has been suggested that 36 kcal per kg of current, or of ideal, body weight should be used. However, the use of current body weight as a base may result in a large overestimation of energy requirement. In the final analysis, it is necessary to monitor weight gain as discussed in Chapter 8 and adjust the energy content of the diet over the course of gestation.

Careful nutritional counseling and individualized treatment are essential. It is important to keep in mind that the nutritional needs for pregnancy must be met (see Chapter 8). In addition, ketonuria should be carefully avoided since there is evidence of fetal brain damage in ketosis.

GESTATIONAL DIABETES

Gestational diabetes mellitus (GDM) is, by definition, diabetes that begins during the second half of pregnancy and is reversible postpartum. Its diagnosis is important because these patients also have an above-normal risk of complications. Therefore, most obstetricians screen all pregnant women for GDM between the 24th and 28th week of gestation, when the symptoms of pregnancy-induced insulin resistance most often becomes apparent.

PATIENTS AT RISK

Patients at risk of GDM include those with a previous history of GDM, those with glycosuria or other symptoms of DM, or those with fasting plasma glucose levels at or above 6.7 mmol/L (120 mg per dL). Patients who are obese, defined as having a body mass index of greater than or equal to 27 before pregnancy, are also at risk. Previous reproductive history may also reveal risk factors: a previous infant weighing over 4,100 g

(9 pounds) at birth, previous unexplained stillbirth, previous infant with a congenital anomaly, or development of polyhydramnios (16).

TREATMENT

Some GDM patients, but not all, require insulin to control hyperglycemia. OHAs are not used because of the risk of teratogenesis. An appropriate diet is needed by all. The pattern of the diet for the nonobese patient is similar to that described for IDDM and NIDDM patients, except that the patient is usually given three meals and one evening snack, rather than three snacks per day. The desirable weight gain for the obese GDM patient is controversial. It has been suggested that an intake of 25 kcal per kg, or not less than 1,700 to 1,800 kcal per day, is a safe level (16). All GDM patients need extensive instruction because, unlike most pregestational diabetics, they have not had previous instruction.

TOPICS FOR FURTHER DISCUSSION

1. What is the rationale for the increase in dietary carbohydrate prior to a glucose tolerance test?
2. The following drugs affect the results of tests used for urine or blood glucose. Discuss the type of patients for whom these drugs are used and in whom you must be alert for errors in testing results: levodopa, sulfobromphthalein, thiazide diuretics, anticoagulants, propranolol.
3. Why is plasma glucose higher than whole-blood glucose?
4. Why is it recommended that patients check for urine ketones during infections or other stresses?
5. From information obtained in the literature (including advertisements), make a list of the products currently available for home blood glucose monitoring. Note the range of values they will record and compare their advantages and limitations.
6. Why are oral hypoglycemic agents not used in IDDM, pregnancy, and kidney or liver dysfunction?
7. How could one of the diets in this chapter be modified for a strict vegetarian? An Orthodox Jew?
8. Discuss procedures for reducing the cost of a diabetic diet if the patient complains of being unable to afford it.
9. What is the glycemic index and what is its significance in diet planning?
10. Discuss the relative sweetness of artificial sweeteners and the safety of their use.
11. Discuss the metabolism of fructose and its use in diabetic diets.
12. How are diabetic diets modified to increase fiber content?
13. Discuss modification of the diabetic diet for various ethnic groups in your area.
14. Discuss modification of the diabetic diet for various religious groups in your area.

REFERENCES

1. **Pastors, J.G.**, and **H.H. Holler**, eds. *Meal Planning Approaches for Diabetes Management,* 2d ed. Chicago: The American Dietetic Association, 1994.

2. **Anderson, J.W.**, and **P.B. Geil**. Nutrition management of diabetes mellitus. *In* M.E. Shils, J.A. Olson, and M. Shike, eds. *Modern Nutrition in Health Disease,* 8th ed. Philadelphia: Lea & Febiger, 1994.

3. **Orland, M.J.** Diabetes mellitus. *In* M.D. Woodley and A. Whelan, eds. *Manual of Medical Therapeutics,* 27th ed. Boston: Little, Brown, 1992.

4. American Dietetic Association. Nutrition recommendations and principles for people with diabetes mellitus. *J. Am. Dietet. Assoc.* 94: (1994) 504.

5. **Pergallo-Dittko, V.**, **K. Godley**, and **J. Meyer**, Eds. *A Core Curriculum for Diabetic Education,* 2d ed. Chicago: American Association of Diabetic Educators, 1993.

6. **Hollander, P.**, **G. Castle**, **J.O. Joynes**, and **J. Nelson**. *Intensified Insulin Management for You.* Minneapolis: Chronimed Publishing, 1990.

7. Committees of the American Diabetes Association and the American Dietetic Association. *Exchange Lists for Meal Planning.* Chicago: American Dietetic Association and American Diabetes Association, in cooperation with the National Institute of Arthritis, Metabolism, and Digestive Disease and the National Heart, Blood, and Lung Institute. U.S. Department of Health, Education, and Welfare, 1986.

8. **Franz, M.J.**, **P. Barr**, **H. Holler**, **M.A. Powers**, **M.L. Wheeler**, and **J. Wylie-Rosett**. Exchange lists: revised 1986. *J. Am. Dietet. Assoc.* 87: (1987) 28.

9. *Exchange Lists for Meal Planning*, Revised 1995. Alexandria, VA and Chicago IL: American Diabetes Association and American Dietetic Association, 1995.

10. **Anderson, J. W.**, **N.J. Gustafson**, **C.A. Bryant**, and **J. Tietjen-Clark**. Dietary fiber and diabetes, a comprehensive review and practical application. *J. Am. Dietet. Assoc.* 87:(1987) 1189.

11. **Barry, B.**, and **G. Castle**. *Carbohydrate Counting. Adding Flexibility to Your Food Choices.* Minneapolis: International Diabetes Center, 1994.

12. *Month of Meals 1: A Menu Planner.* Alexandria, VA: American Diabetes Association, 1989.

13. **Walsh, D.H.**, and **D.J. O'Sullivan**. Effects of moderate alcohol on control of diabetes. *Diabetes* 23:(1974)440..

14. **Franz, M.J.**, and **B. Barry**. *Diabetes and Exercise.* Minneapolis: International Diabetes Center, 1993.

15. **Fagan, C.**, **J.D. King**, and **M. Erick**. Nutrition management in women with gestational diabetes mellitus: A review by ADA's Diabetes Care and Education dietetics practice group. *J. Am. Dietet. Assoc.* 950:(1995)460.

16. **Hollingsworth, D.R**. *Pregnancy, Diabetes and Birth,* 2d ed. Baltimore: Williams & Wilkins, 1992.

ADDITIONAL SOURCES OF INFORMATION

Tinker, L.F., **J.M. Heins** and **H.H. Holler**. Diabetes Care and Education: a practice group of the American Dietetic Association: *J. Am. Dietet. Assoc.* 94:(1994)507.

Beebe, C.A., **J.G. Pastors**, **M.A. Powers**, and **J. Wylie-Rosett**. Nutrition management for individuals with noninsulin-dependent diabetes mellitus in the 1990's: a review by the Diabetes Care and Education Practice Group. *J. Am. Dietet. Assoc.* 91:(1991)196–202, 205–207.

Franz, M.J. Diabetes mellitus: considerations in the development of guidelines for the occasional use of alcohol. *J. Am. Dietet. Assoc.* 83:(1983)147.

Walsh, D.H., and **D.J. O'Sullivan.** Effects of moderate alcohol intake on control of diabetes. *Diabetes* 23:(1974)440.

Konishi, F. Food energy equivalents of various activities. *J. Am. Dietet. Assoc.* 46:(1965)187.

Zorman, L.R. *Beyond Diet: Exercise Your Way to Fitness and Heart Health,* 20–21. Englewood Cliffs, N.J.: CPC International, 1974.

Leon, A.S. *Nutrition and Athletic Performance,* 233. Palo Alto: Bull Publishing, 1981.

Ruderman, N. et al. *Diet and Exercise: Synergism in Health Maintenance,* 143. Chicago: AMA, 1982.

Zeman, F.J. *Clinical Nutrition and Dietetics*, 2d ed. New York: Macmillan, 1991.

Etzwiler, D.D. Patient education and management: a team approach. *In* H. Rifkin and D. Porte, Jr. *Diabetes Mellitus: Theory and Practice,* 4th ed. New York: Elsevier, 1990.

Albert, S., **P. Shragg**, and **D.R. Hollingsworth**. Moderate caloric restriction in obese women with gestational diabetes. *Obstet. Gynecol.* 65:(1985)487–491.

Cohen, S., **M. Miller**, and **R.L. Sherman**. Metabolic acid-base disorders. *Am. J. Nursing.* Part 1, Oct. 1977; Part 2, Jan. 1978; Part 3, Mar. 1978.

Finer, N. Sugar substitutes in the treatment of obesity and diabetes mellitus. *Clin Nutr.* 4:(1985) 207–214.

Michael, S.R., and **C.E. Sabo**. Management of the diabetic patient receiving nutritional support. *Nutr. in Clin. Pract.* 4:(1989)179.

Campbell, S.M., and **M. Rosita Schiller**. Considerations for enteral nutrition support of patients with diabetes. *Topics Clin. Nutr.* 7:(1991)23.

Bruening, K.S., and **E. Luder**. Nutrition considerations in pediatric insulin-dependent diabetes mellitus. *Topics Clin. Nutr.* 7:(1991)33.

Lyon, R.B., and **D.M. Vinci**. Nutrition management of insulin-dependent diabetes mellitus in adults: Review by the Diabetes Care and Education dietetic practice group. *J. Am. Dietet. Assoc.* 93:(1993)309

TO TEST YOUR UNDERSTANDING

1. Assume that in your institution, normal fasting plasma glucose levels are considered to be 70 to 110 mg/dL. You have a patient whose fasting plasma glucose level is 4.0 mmol/L. By your institution's standard, is this value considered to be within normal limits, high, or low? Show your calculations.

2. In each of the following situations, write down the diagnosis you would expect to see. Use the following code: DM—Diabetes mellitus; IGT—Impaired glucose tolerance; WNL—Within normal limits

a. 8 y.o. girl with FBG 8.0 mmol/L. GTT showed 11.6 mmol/L at 60 min, 10.5 mmol/L at 120 min.

b. Nonpregnant 23 y.o. woman with FBG 5.6 mmol/L GTT showed 8.9 mmol/L at 60 min, 7.5 mmol/L at 120 min, and 6.1 mmol/L at 180 min.

c. 60 y.o. man with FBG 6.7 mmol/L. GTT showed 10.5 mmol/L at 120 min.

3. List some general information that you would need to have in order to plan good nutritional care for each of the following patients. List items other than those that apply to all.

a. 16 y.o. girl, IDDM patient, newly diagnosed.

b. 47 y.o. man, IDDM of 30 years' duration; retinopathy.

c. 82 y.o. woman, NIDDM of 20 years' duration.

4. You are advising a highly motivated IDDM patient who feels it is important to maintain her blood glucose concentration within normal limits. The patient monitors her condition before each meal and at bedtime. Evaluate the following methods for their ability to provide the most accurate information to achieve the closest possible control on a daily basis.

a. Urine glucose

b. Urine ketones

c. Blood glucose

d. Glycosylated hemoglobin

5. Your IDDM patient, using the exchange lists, has a diet containing the following exchanges for lunch and dinner:

4 lean meat,	3 bread,
4 fat,	1 vegetable,
1 fruit,	1 skim milk

He tells you that he has a favorite food, a frozen entree that he would like to include in his diet occasionally. Your information from the manufacturer says that a one-serving package contains 36 g carbohydrate, 14 g protein, and 15 g fat. What would you tell the patient to remove from his exchange lists when he includes this entree in his meal?

6. A patient tells you that she would like to make a "chili" containing beans, ground beef, onions, and tomatoes, plus desired "free" seasoning. Using the meal plan given in question 5, how much of these ingredients could she use to make a mixture that fits into her plan?

7. Visit a nearby supermarket and list below the products available (other than those in question 8) that are labeled "diabetic," "low calorie," "dietetic," or that otherwise imply they are useful for diabetic diets or are reduced in calorie content. Evaluate each as indicated in the table:

Product Label (Brand)	Food Value (g)			Comments (usefulness, desirability, truth in labeling, etc.)
	Protein	Fat	CHO	

8. A patient tells you his favorite restaurant is a "steak house" where the menu consists of:

Steaks (broiled) or roast beef
Baked or French-fried potatoes
Sliced tomato salad with choice of dressings
Assorted rolls, butter
Ice cream
Coffee, tea

The restaurant has a full bar. Describe how you would counsel this patient. (Hint: See Chapter 7.)

9. Mrs. Y. is an insulin-dependent diabetic who received her insulin on schedule but says she is too sick to finish her lunch. She has left 1 1/2 oz of meat, 1/4 cup of noodles, 1/2 cup of green beans, and 1 small roll. She states she thinks she can "keep down some orange juice." What would you do? Show your calculations.

10. Mr. W. is an insulin-dependent diabetic who has left two fat exchanges and half of his green beans on his tray. What would you do? Show your calculations.

11. Mr. Q, who has NIDDM, has left his milk (one exchange) and 1/2 cup mashed potatoes on his tray. What would you do? Show your calculations.

continued

TO TEST YOUR UNDERSTANDING   (*continued*)

12 Your patient's lunch has the following exchanges:

1 skim milk, 2 bread, 2 fat,
1 vegetable, 1 fruit,
3 medium-fat meat.

Plan a liquid lunch menu for this patient.

13. You have a male NIDDM patient who is 60 y.o., 220 pounds, IBW = 160 pounds. He has mild retinopathy and neuropathy. A stress test has shown that he can safely undertake moderate exercise. A urine sample taken during his clinic visit is negative for glucose. His blood sugar level is 5.0 mmol/L. HbA_{1c} is 13.5 percent. The patient says that he follows the 1,200 kcal diet he was given but has not lost weight. He plans to undertake an exercise program of weight lifting and 30 minutes of jogging on alternate days.
a. Evaluate the diabetic control of this patient. Explain your reasoning.
b. What effect would you expect weight lifting to have on his diabetic control?
c. Evaluate the wisdom of his plans to jog.
d. How would you advise this patient? Why?

14. Ms. K is a 37 y.o. obese IDDM patient who has been diabetic for 15 years. She understands her diet and other aspects of treatment, but refuses to follow a diet. She has stated that "It isn't worth it to go through all that, and I'm not going to bother." She has signs of advanced vascular disease for her age but has never been hospitalized for diabetic ketoacidosis.
You take a 24-hr recall, which reveals the following:

Breakfast:

1/2 grapefruit
1 Danish pastry

Coffee break:

1 doughnut
Coffee with cream and sugar substitute

Lunch:

Vegetable-beef soup (canned)
12 Saltines
Vegetable salad/French dressing
Soft drink (artificially sweetened)

Dinner:

3—4 oz serving meat or poultry (no skin)
Potato, rice, or noodles with butter, occasionally gravy
Buttered vegetable or salad with dressing
Tea

Snack:

Fruit, unsweetened, canned, or fresh OR
1/2 c "dietetic" ice cream

You have referred the matter to social services, and they are working with the patient. In the meantime, the patient continues to refuse to follow a more structured diet with exchange lists.
a. List some appropriate objectives for counseling at this time.
b. Choose one of your objectives in item a. What changes in her meals, indicated by her 24-hr recall, would be necessary to accomplish this?

15. Mr. B is a 40 y.o. patient who has been admitted to your hospital for the first time. His surgery for hernia repair was done 2 days ago. The patient is an insulin-dependent diabetic of 25 years' standing.
During your interview, Mr. B is alert and cooperative and says he understands his diet. However, you pick up two pertinent comments:
"My diet has 4 oz of meat at noon and night, but I can never figure out how much 4 oz of meat is, especially if the meat has a bone in it, like a pork chop."
"My diet has three bread exchanges at dinner and two graham crackers in the afternoon snack. I get awfully tired of graham crackers every afternoon. Two slices of bread and a potato every night gets tiresome, too, so I sometimes have baked desserts for more variety."
a. Write a SOAP note in the patient's medical record in which you evaluate his understanding of his diet.
b. The patient is being discharged shortly, but he will return to the diabetic clinic in 2 weeks. You can only deal with one of his problems today. Which would you choose? Why?

Diabetes Mellitus

Part I: Presentation

Present illness: Eileen H. is an 18 y.o. young woman who C/O excessive thirst and frequent urination of 2 weeks' duration, in addition to increased appetite and a weight loss of 8 pounds in 4 weeks. Pt is normally active but indicates minor malaise.

Past medical history: Pt was the product of a normal pregnancy and delivery. She had rubella at age 6, an appendectomy at age 15, and a broken arm 6 months ago.

Family history: Parents L&W. Maternal aunt has IDDM. Paternal grandfather died of cardiovascular disease 2° to NIDDM. Other grandparents L&W.

Social history: 18 y.o. female. Lives with parents, one older brother, and one younger sister.

Review of systems:
  GI: No history of nausea, vomiting, diarrhea.
  GU: No history of any urgency, frequency, or burning except for present complaint.
  CNS: No history of loss of consciousness, convulsions, or difficulty with gait or station.

Physical exam:
  General: Slightly underweight white female: ht 163 cm (50th percentile); wt 57 kg (25th percentile).
  Vital signs: T 98.2° F; P 120; R 27 with fruity odor; BP 110/70 in right arm, supine.
  Lungs: Clear to percussion and auscultation.
  Heart: Normal sinus rhythm, no murmurs.
  Abdomen: Flat, liver not enlarged.
  Genitalia: Normal.
  Extremities: Normal.
  CNS: Normal gait and station; normal deep tendon reflexes.

Laboratory:
  FBG: 24.98 mmol/L
  Urine: 4+ sugar, large acetone
  Serum Acetone: 3.0 mg/dL

Impression: Diabetes mellitus in 18 y.o. underweight female with positive family history of DM.

Plan: Admit and place on RI until stabilized, then adjust to NPH.

Nutritionist to evaluate pt and recommend diet as necessary. Also recommend diet for home use. Begin routine diabetes education of pt and significant others.

QUESTIONS

1. Discuss the significance of the family history.

2. Compare this patient's laboratory values with normal values.
  a. FBG
  b. Urine sugar
  c. Urine acetone
  d. Serum acetone

Part II: Nutritional Consult

During the next 2 days, the patient is given regular insulin t.i.d. You briefly meet with Eileen to offer an introduction and general explanation of a diabetic diet.

The routine nutritional assessment includes the following information on a typical day's intake when she is not hospitalized:

Breakfast:
8 oz orange juice
3/4 c cornflakes
1/2 c whole milk, 1 T sugar
2 eggs, fried
2 slices toast, 4 t margarine,
  4 T jelly
8 oz whole milk
AM Snack:
8 oz whole milk
1 doughnut
Lunch:
Bowl cream of tomato soup
1 tunafish salad sandwich on toast
Chocolate eclair
8 oz whole milk

PM Snack:
12 oz soft drink, sweetened
1 chocolate bar
Supper:
6 oz meat loaf
1 large baked potato,
  2T margarine
1/2 c buttered broccoli
1/2 c molded fruit salad
1/2 c butterscotch ice cream
8 oz whole milk
Evening Snack:
8 oz whole milk
12 butter-type crax
2 oz cheese

Eileen says these are foods she usually eats but that the quantity is much greater than usual because she has felt so hungry lately.

QUESTIONS

3. List some points you would initially make in some discussions with Eileen about the diabetic diet.

4. You plan for a diabetic diet as follows to provide for Eileen while she is hospitalized. Your hospital uses the 1989 exchange lists for planning meals for diabetic in-patients. Diet planned is: P–100: F–85; C–220 with H.S. Fdg.

Develop a meal plan to be used for hospital meals for Eileen. Use Form E in Appendix M.

5. Later, you replan the diet using the 1995 exchange lists. Show the new plan on another copy of Form E.

6. Using a menu provided by your instructor, plan 1 day's menu for this patient while she is hospitalized.

(continued)

7. Based on the information gathered in the nutrition assessment, what points might be important to stress in the diet instruction?

When she is ready for discharge, Eileen is taught about the same diet, how to give herself insulin twice a day in AM and PM, and how to do SBGM.

8. Three months later, Eileen comes to see you in the outpatient clinic. Her SBGM records are showing irregular values. She claims she has been following her diet. Insulin prescribed is 20 U NPH and 10 U Regular before breakfast, and 25 units NPH and 10 Units Regular before supper.

SBGM records for the immediately preceding days are as follows: She says these are typical values.

	Breakfast	Lunch	Supper	HS
Tues.	90	157	115	99
Wed.	85	200	110	127
Thurs.	82	199	112	106
Fri.	92			

  a. Evaluate the SBGM values.

  b. Would you recommend a change in insulin? If so, specify which insulin, how much, when?

  c. If the prelunch values had been obtained at presupper, and the presupper values were prelunch, what action would you recommend? Why?

9. Assume that the high values were obtained before breakfast.

  a. Name three interpretations you might consider.

  b. How could you determine which one was correct?

  c. What is the interpretation and recommended action if the 3 AM values are as follows:

    1. Slightly above evening values?
    2. Markedly above evening values?
    3. Markedly below evening values?

Part III: The Sick Diabetic

When Eileen is 20 years old, she has an episode of sore throat and requires a liquid diet. Her diet plan states that her lunch should contain 1 skim milk, 2 fruit, 1 vegetable, 2 bread, 3 lean meat, and 4 fat.

QUESTIONS

10. Plan a liquid diet compatible with her sore throat.

11. During the sore throat episode, Eileen is eating less and asks if she should reduce her insulin dose.

  a. How would you answer her question? Why?

  b. What additional advice would you give her?

Part IV: Increasing Diet Flexibility

During the summer after her high school graduation, Eileen comes back to you and complains that the diet based on the exchange system is too restrictive during her summer activities.

You suggest that she learn carbohydrate counting, but without making basic changes in her diet since she seems content with the overall pattern. Her diet at this time consists of the following exchanges: 4 milk, 3 vegetables, 3 fruit, 8 bread, 7 meat, and 6 fat.

QUESTIONS

12. How many carbohydrate "points" are in her diet daily?

13. What is the maximum number of grams of fat per day you would recommend?

Part IV: Insulin Intensification Therapy

At the end of the summer, Eileen begins her freshman year at the university. At her next visit to see you, her records indicate that her level of control has deteriorated. When you discuss this with her, she tells you that her classes meet on alternate days, making it difficult to keep her activity constant. She chooses her diet from the cafeteria counter and, in addition, her social life is irregular. As a consequence, her food intake is sometimes irregular, although she tries to keep it constant from day to day.

The health care team instructs Eileen very carefully on the procedures for insulin intensification therapy in order to make her self-care more flexible.

14. Eileen is taking insulin as follows: 20 units NPH and 10 units RI before breakfast, 12 units RI before lunch, and 20 units NPH and 10 units RI before supper. SBGM values are given below. What adjustments should be made? When? Give day and meal.

	Breakfast	Lunch	Supper	Evening Snack
Day 1	94	83	112	102
Day 2	129	106	97	78
Day 3	52	65	95	102

15. At the beginning of the next quarter, Eileen tells you she has signed up for a swimming class each Tuesday and Thursday afternoon, in addition to her previous activities. She asks you how to adjust for this activity. What would you tell her?

Cardiovascular Disease

There has been a significant decline in cardiovascular mortality in recent years, although coronary heart disease is still the number one cause of death in the United States. During the last two decades, the mortality from coronary heart disease has decreased about 50 percent, and that from stroke has fallen 57 percent (1). The risk for coronary heart disease is strongly associated with three variables: high blood cholesterol level, high blood pressure, and smoking.

This chapter focuses on those aspects of cardiovascular disease that have a nutritional component and are commonly seen in a clinical setting: hypertension, hyperlipidemia, myocardial infarction, and congestive heart failure. The emphasis in on evaluation of risk for coronary heart disease, integration of clinical care and nutritional management, and considerations for counseling individuals with these cardiovascular disorders. Before you proceed, you may want to review related chapters in your text.

HYPERTENSION

Hypertension is defined as an arterial blood pressure of greater than or equal to 140/90 mm Hg, or a condition requiring control of blood pressure with medication. Primary or essential hypertension is the most common type of hypertension. The etiology of primary hypertension is unknown. In contrast, secondary hypertension is caused by a specific medical condition and is reversible when the underlying medical problem is treated. Untreated high blood pressure is a major risk factor for coronary heart disease and the most important risk factor for cerebrovascular accident or stroke. In the general population, risk for cardiovascular disease is lowest with an average systolic blood pressure of less than 120 mm Hg and an average diastolic blood pressure of less than 80 mm Hg (1).

Approximately 20 percent of Americans have elevated blood pressure or are taking antihypertensive medications. The prevalence of high blood pressure increases with age, is greater for blacks than for whites, and in both races is greater in less educated than more educated people (1). The southeastern region of the United States has been referred to as the stroke belt because blacks and whites in this area have a greater stroke death rate than do blacks and whites in other areas of the country (2).

CLASSIFICATION, DIAGNOSIS, AND EVALUATION OF HIGH BLOOD PRESSURE

Table 20-1 summarizes current guidelines for the classification of high blood pressure from the National High Blood Pressure Education Program (1). This classification system describes stages of blood pressure with a progressive increase in risk for cardiovascular and renal disease with higher levels of blood pressure. Increased risk of morbidity, disability, and mortality are associated with higher levels of *either* systolic or diastolic blood pressure. Normal adult blood pressure consists of a systolic blood pressure of less than 130 mm Hg and a diastolic blood pressure of less than 85 mm Hg. High normal blood pressure, defined as a systolic blood pressure of 130 to 139 and a diastolic blood pressure of 85 to 89, is associated with a great risk for developing definite hypertension. High blood pressure stage 1 or "mild" hypertension (Table 20-1) is the most common form of high blood pressure in the adult population.

TABLE 20-1 Classification of Blood Pressure for Adults*

Category	Systolic (mm Hg)	Diastolic (mm Hg)
Normal†	<130	<85
High Normal	130–139	85–89
Hypertension‡		
Stage 1 (mild)	140–159	90–99
Stage 2 (moderate)	160–179	100–109
Stage 3 (severe)	180–209	110–119
Stage 4 (very severe)	≥210	≥120

*Not taking antihypertensive drugs and not acutely ill. When systolic and diastolic pressures fall into different caategories, the higher category should be selected to classify the individual's blood pressure status. For instance, 160/92mm Hg should be classified as stage 2, and 180/120 mm Hg should be classified as stage 4. Isolated systolic hypertension (ISH) is defined as systolic blood pressure (SBP) ≥140 mm Hg and diastolic blood pressure (DBP) <90 mm Hg and staged appropriaately (e.g., 170/85mm Hg is defined as stage 2 (ISH).

†Optimal blood pressure with respect to cardiovasculaar risk is SBP<120 mm Hg and DBP<80 mm Hg.

‡Based on the average of two or more readings taken at each of two or more visits following an initial screening.

Adapted from: National Heart, Lung and Blood Institute. Fifth report of the joint national committee on detection, evaluation, and treatment of high blood pressure. NIH Publication No. 93–1088, Jan. 1993.

The diagnosis of hypertension requires more than one measurement of blood pressure. An initial elevation in blood pressure should be confirmed based on the average of two or three measurements taken at each of two or more visits (1). Arterial blood pressure is measured indirectly by an inflatable cuff and pressure manometer.

Clinical evaluation of patients with confirmed primary hypertension s.hould determine if target organ damage is present, because management may be more aggressive in cases where target organ damage exists. In addition it is important to assess whether other cardiovascular risk factors are present besides the hypertension. The presence of a risk factor such as hyperlipidemia may affect both diet and drug therapy for hypertension. Risk factors associated with an increased incidence of coronary heart disease, as defined by the National Cholesterol Education Program, are outlined in Table 20-2.

NUTRITIONAL ASSESSMENT

There are several key features of nutritional assessment for the client with primary hypertension. First is the consideration of changes in body weight and evaluation of healthy body weight, which may include calculation of body mass index or BMI and waist-hip circumference ratio, as discussed in Chapter 5. Second, the usual pattern of physical activity should be considered. Third are possible side effects associated with pharmacologic therapy for hypertension, such as hypokalemia because of diuretic therapy. Fourth is an evaluation of the serum lipoprotein profile, as discussed in the next section, and consideration of other risk factors for coronary heart disease, as outlined in Table 20-2. Lastly, dietary assessment of typical sodium and potassium ingestion, alcohol use and intake of saturated fats and cholesterol is important for subsequent dietary counseling.

TREATMENT

All stages of hypertension warrant effective *long-term* therapy because of the strong association between increased incidence of cardiovascular disease and increased levels of *either* systolic or diastolic blood pressure. The objective of hypertension therapy is to maintain arterial blood pressure below 140 mm Hg systolic blood pressure and 90 mm Hg diastolic blood pressure, while concurrently controlling other modifiable cardiovascular risk factors (1). Treatment of hypertension includes lifestyle modifications or, for those with more severe hypertension, pharmacologic therapy. Research suggests that approximately 39 percent of people with stage-1 hypertension achieve adequate blood pressure control with lifestyle modifications alone (3). In general, a 3- to 6-month trial of lifestyle modifications is initially used, and then if blood pressure is still greater than or equal to 140/90 mm Hg, drug therapy may be added. If target organ damage and/or other known risk factors for cardiovascular disease are present, drug therapy is used more aggressively. Continuation of lifestyle modifications is important during drug therapy because these behavioral changes may reduce the number and doses of antihypertensive medications needed. The preferred drugs for initial therapy of hypertension include diuretics and

TABLE 20-2 Risk Factors for Coronary Heart Disease Other Than Low-Density Lipoprotein Cholesterol*

Age

   Male: ≥45 years

   Female: ≥55 years or premature menopause without estrogen replacement therapy

Family history of premature CHD (definite myocardial infarction or sudden death before 55 years of age in father or other male first-degree relative, or before 65 years of age in mother or other female first-degree relative)

Current cigarette smoking

Diabetes mellitus

Hypertension (≥140/90 mm Hg†, or on anti-hypertensive medication)

Low HDL cholesterol (<35 mg/dL or <0.9 mmol/L‡)

*High risk, defined as a net of two or more coronary heart disease (CHD) risk factors, leads to vigorous intervention. Age (defined differently for men and women) is treated as a risk factor because rates of CHD are higher in the elderly than in the young, and in men than women of the same age. Obesity is not listed as a risk factor because it operates through other risk factors that are included (hypertension, hyperlipidemia, decreased HDL cholesterol, and diabetes mellitus), but it should be considered a target for intervention.

†Confirmed by measurements on several occasions.

‡If the HDL cholesterol is ≥60 mg/dL (1.6 mmol/L) subtract one risk factor (because high HDL cholesterol levels decrease CHD risk).

Adapted from: National Heart, Lung, and Blood Institute. Second report of the expert panel on detection, evaluation, and treatment of high blood cholesterol in adults (Adult Treatment Panel II). MNIH Publication No. 93-3095, Sep. 1993.

beta-blockers, as these drugs have been shown to reduce cardiovascular morbidity and mortality in controlled clinical trials (1).

Lifestyle modifications for hypertension control are outlined in Table 20-3. Four of the five suggested modifications concern dietary intake of the following: alcohol, total energy, sodium, potassium, calcium, and magnesium. In addition, a reduced intake of total fat and saturated fat, and cessation of smoking, are recommended for overall cardiovascular health, although, they do not play a direct role in the control of high blood pressure. Caffeine is not routinely restricted for control of blood pressure, as it does not cause a sustained elevation in blood pressure.

Alcohol

Moderation of alcohol intake is especially important because excessive alcohol intake can raise blood pressure and cause resistance to antihypertensive therapy (1). Many hypertensive patients who regularly consume alcohol will experience a reduction in blood pressure when alcohol intake is limited to 1 oz of ethanol per day; 1 oz of ethanol is contained in approximately 8 oz of wine, 24 oz of beer, or 2 oz of 100-proof whiskey. The alcohol concentration of beer is approximately 4 to 6 percent, of wine is 9 to 12 percent, and of distilled liquor is 35 to 50 percent.

The alcohol concentration of distilled beverages is often expressed as "proof." One proof equals 0.5 percent alcohol. Thus, 80-proof whiskey contains 40 percent alcohol. Distilled alcohol is customarily measured in a "jigger," which is 1 1/2 oz, or 45 mL. Two jiggers, or approximately 3 oz, or 90 mL, of 80-proof whiskey would provide 36 g alcohol and 252 kcal according to the following calculation:

$$3 \text{ oz} \times 30 \text{ mL/oz} \times (40 \text{ g/100 mL}) = 36 \text{ g alcohol}$$

$$36 \text{ g alcohol} \times 7 \text{ kcal/g} = 252 \text{ kcal}$$

TABLE 20-3 Lifestyle Modifications for Hypertension Control

Lose weight if overweight.

Limit alcohol intake to no more than 1 oz of ethanol per day (24 oz of beer, 8 oz of wine, or 2 oz of 100 proof-whiskey).

Reduce sodium intake to less than 100 mmol/day (<2.3 g of sodium or <6 g of sodium chloride).

Maintain adequate dietary intakes of the following:
    potassium, 90–120 mmol or 3.5–4.6 g/day
    calcium, 20–30 mmol or 0.8–1.2 g/day
    magnesium, 11.5–14.4 mmol or 0.28–0.35 g/day

Exercise (aerobic) regularly.

Adapted from National Heart, Lung and Blood Institute. Fifth report of the Joint National Committee on Detection, Evaluation, and Treatment of High Blood Pressure. NIH Publication No. 93–1088, Jan. 1993 and 10th ed. Recommended Dietary Allowances, 1989.

Weight Reduction and Physical Activity

Weight reduction reduces blood pressure in a large proportion of hypertensive individuals who are more than 10 percent above ideal weight (4). Patients should be strongly encouraged to lose weight, as even a small weight loss is beneficial and achievement of ideal weight is not needed to see a reduction in blood pressure. Weight reduction diets can be planned using the exchange lists developed for planning diabetic diets (see Appendix C). A gradual weight loss of 0.5 to 1 pound per week is recommended in conjunction with a program of behavior modification for maintenance of weight loss. Women and men generally require 1,200 and 1,500 kcal per day, respectively, to achieve such a gradual weight loss. Ideally, a weight reduction diet should be combined with a program of regular physical activity. For most sedentary patients, 30 to 45 minutes of brisk walking 3 to 5 times per week will be beneficial (1). Besides enhancing weight loss, exercise can reduce systolic blood pressure in hypertensive patients by approximately 10 mm Hg (5). In order for exercise to be effective in reducing blood pressure, it must be moderately intense or aerobic. Physician approval is needed before initiation of an exercise program in hypertensive patients.

An aerobic exercise program that is adequate to condition the muscles and cardiovascular system usually requires exercising for 15 to 60 minutes 3 to 5 times per week at 60 to 90 percent of maximum heart rate. Maximum heart rate may be estimated by using an age-based average derived by the formula "220 minus one's age." Thus, for a 50-year-old, the predicted maximum heart rate is 170 ± 10 beats per minute, and the target heart rate range for 60 to 90 percent maximum heart rate is 102 to 153 beats per minute.

Potassium, Calcium, and Magnesium

Adequate potassium intake is important for individuals with hypertension for several reasons. First, animal and human studies suggest that a high dietary potassium intake may protect against developing hypertension, and potassium deficiency may increase blood pressure. Second, hypokalemia is a common, potentially dangerous complication of diuretic therapy, as it may induce ventricular ectopy. Thus, normal plasma concentrations of potassium (3.5 to 5 mmol/L) should be maintained during treatment of hypertension. The clinical symptoms of potassium deficiency include anorexia, malaise, and muscle weakness. Dietary intakes of potassium and sodium should approximate a 1:1 ratio. For example, if sodium intake is limited to approximately 100 mmol or 2.3 g per day then potassium intake should be 90 to 120 mmol or 3.5 to 4.6 g per day. Foods high in potassium include milk, meats, nuts and beans, and selected fruits and vegetables. A table listing the potassium content of foods is provided in Appendix B. Potassium containing salt substitutes, e.g., potassium chloride, may be used by some individuals adhering to a low-sodium diet and may provide 30 to 50 mmol of potassium per teaspoon.

Adequate intakes of calcium and magnesium have been suggested to protect from developing hypertension. However, the evidence is not sufficient to recommend supplementation of calcium and magnesium above the levels specified in the RDA. Thus, it is important to ensure that intakes of calcium and magnesium meet the RDA for adults of 20 to 30 mmol or 0.8 to 1.2 g calcium per day, and 11.5 to 14.4 mmol or 0.28 to 0.35 g magnesium per day.

Sodium-Restricted Diets

Some individuals with primary hypertension show a decrease in blood pressure when dietary intake of sodium chloride is limited. Blacks and older people are more likely to show a decrease in blood pressure with sodium restriction (6). However, even in patients who require drugs to control hypertension, sodium is frequently restricted, as this often helps decrease the dose of medication needed. The current recommendation for sodium restriction during treatment of hypertension is a moderate restriction of 100 mmol of sodium per day, which is equivalent to 100 mEq of sodium, 2.3 g of sodium, or 6 g of sodium chloride (1). Sodium-restricted diets are useful in the nutritional care of many conditions besides hypertension, including kidney and liver diseases and congestive heart failure. The following section discusses information needed to plan low-sodium diets.

Commonly Used Diets. Dietary sodium content may be expressed in milligrams (mg), grams (g), milliequivalent (mEq), or millimoles (mmoles). The atomic weight and valence of a number of elements needed to make conversions between these units are given in Appendix E. Sodium chloride is approximately 40 percent by weight sodium. Therefore, 2,500 mg NaCl can be considered to contain $2,500 \times 0.40 = 1,000$ mg Na.

The sodium content of unrestricted American diets has been estimated to be 2,500 to 8,800 mg, a quantity much in excess of the average minimum requirement of 500 mg sodium per day for adults (7). An intake of 2,400 mg of sodium per day is considered to be a safe and reasonable intake for adults (7) and is currently used as the daily reference value for nutrition labeling as defined by the Food and Drug Administration (8).

Most institutions will offer a series of sodium-restricted diets with differing sodium contents. The most common are:

500 mg	22 mmol	Severe restriction
1 g	44 mmol	Strict restriction
2–3 g	87–130 mmol	Mild or moderate restriction
4 g	174 mmol	No added salt

Exchange lists are frequently used for planning sodium-restricted diets. For renal patients, the combined protein, sodium, and potassium exchange lists are useful (Chapter 21). For patients with liver disease, combined protein and sodium exchange lists are useful. Patients with hypertension are frequently given general guidelines on the sodium and calorie content of foods to use in meal planning. Consult a diet manual for specific examples of low-sodium diets.

Dietary Sources of Sodium. Sources of sodium in the diet fall into five categories.

1. Sodium compounds, primarily table salt (NaCl), and including baking soda ($NaHCO_3$), baking powder, monosodium glutamate, and soy sauce.
2. Foods in which sodium is naturally contained. Animal foods—meats, fish, eggs, and dairy products—have a substantial inherent sodium content. Unprocessed fruits, vegetables, legumes, and grains are naturally low in sodium (9).
3. Processed foods with added salt or other sodium compounds.
4. Sodium in the water supply.
5. Medications.

The largest contribution to typical sodium intake comes from processed foods. A recent study demonstrated that 77 percent of dietary sodium intake resulted from sodium added during food processing, whereas naturally occurring sodium in foods contributed 12 percent of dietary sodium intake (10). Thus, in planning low-sodium diets, it is very important to counsel patients to eat primarily fresh rather than processed foods. Processed foods especially important to avoid include condiments such as catsup and mustard, smoked or cured meats such a luncheon meats, canned soups, and prepackaged frozen foods, and packaged mixes. In addition, no salt or salty seasonings such as garlic salt, celery salt, or soy sauce should be added during food preparation or at the table.

A summary of the approximate sodium content of basic foods follows. Consult a handbook of food composition or a computer program with a food composition database for more detailed information about the sodium content of specific foods.

Food	*Amount*	*~mg Sodium*
Milk	8 oz	120
Meat, unsalted	1 oz	25
Egg	1	65
Fat	1 tsp	50
Fruits	1/2 cup	2–5
Vegetables, fresh		
or frozen	1/2 cup	10–40
canned	1/2 cup	250
Bread, yeast,	1 slice	120
baking soda	1 roll	300

The water supply is naturally high in sodium in some areas. Patients requiring 500 mg sodium diets should use bottled, distilled water if the sodium content of their water supply exceeds 40 mg of sodium per liter. Information on sodium in the water is usually available from the Department of Public Health or the local Heart Association.

Water softeners add appreciably to the sodium content of the drinking water. If possible, the water softener should be attached to the hot-water line only, and patients should be advised to use the cold water for drinking and cooking

Patient Counseling. Many patients need a restricted-sodium diet for extended periods. In order to comply with the diet, they may need information on acceptable food products, salt substitutes, food preparation methods, and eating out on a diet.

Some patients find that the use of salt substitutes helps to make the low-sodium diet more acceptable. Most salt substitutes contain less than 1 mmol of sodium per teaspoon but large amounts of potassium (30 to 50 mmol per teaspoon) from potassium chloride. Patients with renal disease should not use salt substitutes, because ingestion of additional potassium could result in hyperkalemia. Salt substitutes that contain ammonium salts are not suitable for patients with hepatic failure because of impaired ability to synthesize urea.

Patients need to understand how to read food labels in order to select foods appropriate for a low-sodium diet. Several references are available that explain the nutrition-labeling regulations (8, 11). The new food labels state the mg of sodium per serving of food and also show the percentage of the daily reference value for sodium that the food provides. Daily reference values refers to a set of dietary references that applies to eight nutrients listed on the food label: fat, saturated fat, cholesterol, carbohydrate, protein, fiber, sodium, and potassium. The daily reference value for sodium is 2,400 mg per day. Note that reference *amount* refers to serving size, which the Food and Drug Administration has defined for over 130 categories of foods for use in food labeling. In addition, several definitions apply to sodium content on the food label (11):

Salt- or sodium-free, less than 5 mg sodium per serving

Low, 140 mg or less sodium per reference amount or 50 g

Reduced/low, at least 25% less sodium per reference amount than an appropriate referenced food

Light in sodium, if food is reduced by at least 50% of reference amount

Very low sodium, 35 mg or less sodium per reference amount or 50 g

Patients should be given information on alternatives to salt for seasoning and flavor. Wines can be used to add flavor in cooking, but those labeled "cooking wine" are high in salt content and should not be used. Various herb combinations, homemade or purchased already mixed, can be used in a shaker.

Many recipe books are available to help patients use herbal seasoning and to provide recipes for low-sodium, low-fat dishes. Another useful product is sodium-free baking powder: 2 tablespoons *each* cream of tartar, potassium bitartrate, arrowroot starch, and potassium bicarbonate (Caution: Sodium-free baking powder is not to be used by patients who are at risk of retaining potassium).

Eating out presents a challenge. Travelers can ask in advance for low-sodium meals on airplanes. Sandwiches for carried lunches can be made with low-sodium bread, pita bread, or unseasoned crisp breads. Cold, sliced roast meats can be used as fillings. Fresh tomatoes, lettuce, and celery can be included, as can fresh fruit.

HYPERLIPIDEMIA

MEASUREMENT OF SERUM LIPID AND LIPOPROTEIN CONCENTRATIONS

The measurement of total serum cholesterol and high density lipoprotein (HDL) cholesterol concentrations is the first step in evaluation of risk for coronary heart disease. Total serum cholesterol concentration is equal to the sum of cholesterol carried by the very low density lipoprotein (VLDL), low density lipoprotein (LDL), and HDL fractions. Clinically, the relative amounts of the lipoprotein classes VLDL, LDL, and HDL are estimated by determining cholesterol content in each of these fractions.

Routine clinical analysis of serum lipoprotein levels requires measurement of *fasting* levels of total cholesterol, total triglyceride, and HDL cholesterol. VLDL cholesterol concentration is estimated as 20 percent of fasting triglycerides when triglyceride concentration is less than 300 mg per 100 ml. HDL cholesterol concentration is measured directly. LDL cholesterol is calculated by difference according to the following equation:

$$\text{LDL Chol} = \text{Total Chol} - (\text{HDL Chol} + 0.2\,\text{TG})$$

(20-1)

Lipoprotein analysis should not be performed when a patient is in the recovery phase from an acute coronary or other medical event, as these circumstances are likely to lower their usual LDL cholesterol level. Note that percentile values from serum lipid and lipoprotein levels in the United States adult population are given in Appendix L, Tables 1 to 3.

A simple technique for determining the abnormal presence of chylomicrons and VLDLs involves allowing a fasting plasma sample to stand for 18 to 24 hours at 4° C, the so-called *refrigerator test*. If abnormal chylomicron metabolism exists, a cream layer will form on top, and elevated VLDL levels will produce turbidity throughout the tube. Thus, from measurement of serum cholesterol, triglyceride, and HDL cholesterol, extrapolation to LDL-cholesterol, and a refrigerator test, a preliminary assessment of the levels of chylomicrons, VLDL, LDL, and HDL can be established. An elevation in plasma cholesterol and triglyceride levels is often further characterized by electrophoresis to provide additional information on the lipoprotein profile.

Hyperlipidemia is defined as an elevation of plasma lipids including cholesterol, cholesterol esters, phospholipids, and triglycerides. When hyperlipidemia is defined in terms of class or classes of elevated plasma lipoproteins the term *hyperlipoproteinemia* is used. The simplest nomenclature for defining the type of lipoprotein(s) present in excess is the *phenotyping* system proposed by Fredrickson and Levy in 1980 (12). Although widely used, this system offers no information about the causes of the different forms of hyperlipoproteinemia. A summary of the lipoprotein phenotypes follows:

Phenotype	Plasma lipoprotein present in excess
I	Chylomicrons
IIA	LDL
IIB	LDL + VLDL
III	Beta VLDL (cholesterol-rich VLDL remnants)
IV	VLDL
V	Chylomicrons + VLDL

EVALUATION: NATIONAL CHOLESTEROL EDUCATION PROGRAM

The National Cholesterol Education Program, Adult Treatment Panel II, provides guidelines for the evaluation and treatment of high blood cholesterol in adults (13, 14). Initial evaluation of risk for coronary heart disease requires an assessment of nonlipid risk factors, as outlined in Table 20-2, and determination of fasting or nonfasting total serum cholesterol and HDL cholesterol concentrations. The following guidelines are used to evaluate these lipid determinations:

Total cholesterol	Classification
<200 mg/dL (5.2 mmol/L)	desirable
200–239 mg/dL (5.2–6.1mm0l/L)	borderline high
≥240 mg/dL (6.2 mmol/L)	high

HDL cholesterol	
<35 mg/dL (0.9 mmol/L)	low
≥60 mg/dL (1.6 mmol/L)	high, negates one risk factor

After initial screening, lipoprotein analysis, as described in the preceding section, is recommended for all individuals with blood cholesterol levels greater than 240 mg/dL (6.2 mmol/L). Individuals whose blood cholesterol levels are greater than 200 mg/dL (5.2

mmol/L) and who also show HDL cholesterol levels of less than 35 mg/dL (0.9 mmol/L) *or* 2 or more risk factors for coronary heart disease (Table 20-2) should also have lipoprotein analysis.

Treatment decisions are based on LDL cholesterol levels and the presence of risk factors for coronary heart disease, as outlined in Table 20-4. Note that the LDL cholesterol level used to determine if diet or drug therapy are needed is lower if risk factors for coronary heart disease are present or if the patient has coronary heart disease. Figure 20-1 provides a flow chart summarizing the steps needed to make treatment decisions for adults based on LDL cholesterol levels and the presence of risk factors for coronary heart disease. Recommendations for treatment of high blood cholesterol in children and adolescents are given in Chapter 9.

DIETARY TREATMENT AND REGULAR PHYSICAL ACTIVITY

Dietary modification of saturated fat and cholesterol intake, weight control, and appropriately increased physical activity are the essential first steps in treatment of high blood cholesterol, as these changes can significantly decrease risk for coronary heart disease in many patients (14). The primary diet recommended for treatment of high blood cholesterol is the *Step One diet* which is described in Table 20-5. The Step One diet limits total fat intake to 30 percent or less of total calories, saturated fat intake to 8 to 10 percent of total calories, and cholesterol intake to less than 300 mg per day. To adopt the Step One diet, the average American will need to reduce total fat intake by about one-fifth, and saturated fat intake by about one-third. *The Step Two diet* further reduces saturated fat intake to less than 7 percent of total calories, and cholesterol intake to less than 200 mg per day. To adopt the Step Two diet, the average American will need to reduce the intake of saturated fat and cholesterol by about one-half.

TABLE 20-4   Treatment Decisions Based on LDL Cholesterol Levels

	Initiate Diet		Consider Drug Treatment	
	(mg/dL)	(mmol/L)	(mg/dL)	(mmol/L)
Without CHD* and with fewer than 2 risk factors	≥160	≥4.1	≥190	≥4.9
Without CHD and with 2 or more risk factors	≥130	≥3.4	≥160	≥4.1
With CHD	>100	>2.6	≥130	≥3.4

*CHD = coronary heart disease. See Table 20-2 for nonlipid risk factors.
Adapted from National Heart, Lung and Blood Institute. Second report of the expert panel on detection, evaluation, and treatment of high blood cholesterol in adults (Adult Treatment Panel II). NIH Publication No. 93–3095, Sep. 1993.

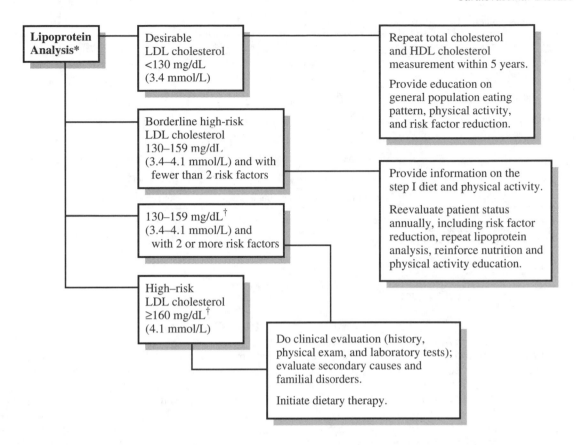

*Fasting 9–12 hours may follow a total serum cholesterol determination or may be done initially.

†On the basis of the average of two determinations. If the first two LDL cholesterol tests differ by more than 30 mg/dL (0.7 mmol/L) a third test should be obtained within 18 weeks, and the average value of the 3 tests used.

Adapted from National Heart, Lung and Blood Institute. Second report of the expert panel on detection, evaluation, and treatment of high blood cholesterol in adults (Adult Treatment Panel II). NIH Publication No. 93–3095, Sep. 1993.

FIGURE 20-1   Flowchart of treatment decisions for adults without evidence of coronary heart disease based on LDL cholesterol.

The Step One diet is similar in nutrient composition to the eating pattern recommended for the general population by the National Research Council and the U.S. Department of Agriculture for prevention of chronic disease (15). In addition, nutrition labeling according to the Food and Drug Administration (8, 11) specifies daily reference values for total fat, saturated fat, and cholesterol intake that are consistent with the nutrient composition of the Step One diet (Table 20-5). For example, the daily reference values for a 2,000 calorie diet are ≤65 g total fat, ≤20 g saturated fat, and ≤300 mg cholesterol.

Examples of daily food choices used to plan a Step One or Step Two diet are shown in Table 20-6. In general, these diets emphasize the use of fruits, vegetables, grains, cereals, and legumes, as well as poultry, fish, lean meats, and low-fat dairy products. Servings of animal protein foods are limited because they contain apprecia-ble amounts of total fat, saturated fat, and cholesterol as shown in Table B-7. Low-fat dairy products are substituted for full-fat dairy products. Added fats such as salad dressing, cream sauce, and gravy are also limited, and foods are cooked with little if any fat. Three plant oils—palm oil, palm kernel oil, and coconut oil—are high in saturated fatty acids and should be avoided. However, animal fats provide the primary source of saturated fat in the American diet. Table 20-7 shows the maximum daily intakes of fat and saturated fatty acids to achieve the Step One and Step Two diets at various dietary energy levels.

The primary goal of diet therapy for high blood cholesterol is to decrease LDL cholesterol levels, as reduction in LDL cholesterol levels in men at high risk for coronary heart disease has been shown to reduce morbidity (14). Information about LDL cholesterol levels indicating the need for initiation of diet therapy and levels used to monitor the progress of diet therapy are

TABLE 20-5 Dietary Therapy of High Blood Cholesterol

Nutrient	Step One Diet	Step Two Diet
Total fat	30% or less of total calories	30% or less of total calories
Saturated fat	8–10% of total calories	Less than 7% of total calories
Polyunsaturated fatty acids	Up to 10% of total calories	Up to 10% of total calories
Monounsaturated fatty acids	Up to 15% of total calories	Up to 15% of total calories
Carbohydrates	55% or more of total calories	55% or more of total calories
Protein	Approximately 15% of total calories	Approximately 15% of total calories
Cholesterol	Less than 300 mg/day	Less than 200 mg/day
Total calories	To achieve and maintain desirable weight	To achieve and maintain desirable weight

Adapted from: National Heart, Lung and Blood Institute. Second report of the expert panel on detection, evaluation, and treatment of high blood cholesterol in adults (Adult Treatment Panel II). NIH Publication No. 93-3095, Sep. 1993. The response to these diets should be determined at 4–6 weeeks and at 3 months. Failure to achieve goal cholesterol levels (Table 20-7) often suggests inadequate dietary compliance.

given in Table 20-8 and Fig. 20-1. The goal of dietary therapy is to reduce LDL cholesterol levels to <160 mg/dL (4.1 mmol/L) in individuals without coronary heart disease who have fewer than two risk factors for heart disease. The goal for individuals without coronary heart disease who have two or more risk factors is an LDL cholesterol level of <130 mg/dL (3.4 mmol/L). Lastly, the goal of therapy for individuals with coronary heart disease is to reduce LDL cholesterol levels to ≤100 mg/dL (2.5 mmol/L). Individuals with established coronary heart disease often require diet and drugs to achieve a reduction in LDL cholesterol levels.

Response to a Step One diet varies depending on inherent biologic responsiveness, baseline cholesterol levels, and baseline dietary habits. However, evidence in free-living subjects suggests that the Step One diet may decrease blood cholesterol by 3 to 14 percent (16, 17). In addition, the response to a Step One diet may be considerably enhanced with weight reduction. The response to the Step One diet should be assessed after 4 to 6 weeks, and again after 3 months. The response to dietary treatment is monitored based on a total cholesterol level (Table 20-8). If problems in dietary adherence are suspected, reinforcement, support, and additional diet counseling should be provided. If dietary adherence is good but blood cholesterol levels are not reduced, the Step Two diet may be initiated. Progressing to a Step Two diet may result in another 3 to 7 percent reduction in cholesterol levels depending in part on the degree to which saturated fats and cholesterol are restricted (13).

Individuals with elevated triglyceride levels (>200 mg/dL or 2.3 mmol/L, fasting) require slight modifications to the Step One diet. Weight reduction as needed to achieve ideal body weight is the most effective dietary treatment for hypertriglyceridemia, as well as promoting a decrease in blood cholesterol level. A restricted intake of alcohol and simple carbohydrates are also useful dietary modifications for individuals with elevated triglyceride levels.

DRUG THERAPY

For most patients at least 6 months of intensive dietary therapy and counseling should be carried out before considering drug therapy. If drug therapy is initiated, dietary therapy should continue. Recommendations for initiation of drug therapy based on LDL cholesterol levels are given in Table 20-4. The goals of drug therapy are the same as those for dietary therapy in terms of reduction in LDL cholesterol levels. Drug therapy generally is indicated in patients with established coronary heart disease if LDL cholesterol levels are 130 mg/dL (3.4 mmol/L) or greater after maximal dietary therapy, i.e., the Step Two diet (14). Initiation of drug therapy in individuals without established coronary heart disease requires clinical judgment. In general, drug therapy is delayed in young adult men (less than 35 years of age) and premenopausal women without other risk factors whose LDL cholesterol levels are in the range of 190 to 220 mg/dL (4.9 to 5.7 mmol/L) (14).

The major classes of drugs used to treat hyperlipidemias include bile acid sequestrants (cholestyramine and colestipol), nicotinic acid, HMG CoA reductase inhibitors (statins, such as lovastatin, pravastatin, and simvastatin), and other drugs such as fibric acid derivatives (gemfibrozil and clofibrate) and probucol. Estrogen replacement in postmenopausal women is an alternative or adjunct to drug therapy in some women with elevated LDL cholesterol levels. Bile acid sequestrants and nicotinic acid are currently the drugs of choice for treatment of hyperlipidemia because of evidence demonstrating efficacy in prevention of mortality due to coronary heart disease and evidence of long-term safety. Consult your textbook or additional references (13) for further information about drug therapy for hyperlipidemia.

Bile acid sequestrants are the drugs of first choice for men less than 45 years and women less than 55 years who have isolated elevations in LDL cholesterol in the 160 to 220 mg/dL (4.1 to 5.7 mmol/L) range. In

TABLE 20-6 Examples of Daily Food Choices for a Step One and Step Two Diet

Food Group	No. of Servings	Serving Size	Some Suggested Foods
Vegetables	3–5	1 cup leafy / raw 1/2 cup other	Leafy greens, lettuce Corn, peas, green beans, broccoli, carrots, cabbage, celery, tomato, spinach, squash, bok choy, mushrooms, eggplant, collard and mustard greens
		3/4 cup juice	Tomato juice, vegetable juice
Fruits	2–4	1 piece fruit 1/2 cup diced fruit	Orange, apple, applesauce, pear, banana, grapes, grapefruit, tangerine, plum, peach, strawberries and other berries, melons, kiwi, papaya, mango, lichee
		3/4 cup fruit juice	Orange juice, apple juice, grapefruit juice, grape juice, prune juice
Breads, cereals, pasta, grains, dry beans, peas, potatoes, and rice	6–11	1 slice 1/2 bun, bagel, muffin 1 oz. dry cereal 1/2 cup cooked cereal 1/2 cup dry beans or peas 1/2 cup potatoes 1/2 cup cup rice, noodles, barley, or other grains 1/2 cup bean curd	Wheat, rye or enriched breads / roll, corn and flour tortillas English muffin, bagel, muffin, cornbread Wheat, corn, oat, rice, bran cereal, or mixed grain cereal Oatmeal, cream of wheat, grits Kidney beans, lentils, split peas, black-eyed peas Potato, sweet potato Pasta, rice, macaroni, barley, tabouli Tofu
Skim / low-fat dairy products	2–3	1 cup skim, 1% milk 1.0 oz low-fat, fat-free cheese	Low / nonfat yogurt, skim milk, 1% milk, buttermilk Low-fat cheeses
Lean meat, poultry, and fish		≤ 6 oz / day Step I Diet ≤ 5 oz / day Step II Diet	Lean and extra lean cuts of meat, fish, and skinless poultry, such as: sirloin, round steak, skinless chicken, haddock, cod
Fats and oils	≤ 6-8*	1 teaspoon soft margarine 1 tablespoon salad dressing	Soft or liquid margarine, vegetable oils
		1 oz nuts	Walnuts, peanuts, almonds, pecans
Eggs		≤ 4 yolks / week-Step I ≤ 2 yolks / week-Step II	Used in preparation of baked products
Sweets and snack foods		In moderation	Cookies, fortune cookies, pudding, bread pudding, rice pudding, angel food cake, frozen yogurt, candy, punch, carbonated beverages Low-fat crackers and popcorn, pretzels, fat-free chips, rice cakes

* Includes fats and oils used in food preparation, also salad dressings and nuts
Reprinted from National Heart, Lung, and Blood Institute. Second report of the expert panel on detection, evaluation, and treatment of high blood cholesterol in adults. NIH Publication No.93-3095, Sep. 1993.

these patients, adequate LDL cholesterol lowering often can be achieved with low doses of sequestrants (8 g of cholestyramine or 10 g of colestipol) when they are combined with maximal dietary therapy (13). When combined with HMG CoA reductase inhibitors, the bile acid sequestrants are highly effective in treating patients with severe hypercholesterolemia.

The bile acid sequestrants are contraindicated as single-drug therapy in patients with hypertriglyceridemia (>500 mg/dL or >5.7 mmol/L) because they tend to raise triglyceride concentrations. Sequestrant therapy may result in gastrointestinal symptoms including constipation, bloating, epigastric fullness, nausea, and flatulence. They may also decrease absorption of fat-soluble vitamins and folic acid with prolonged high doses. However, routine vitamin supplementation is not necessary for otherwise healthy adult patients.

The B vitamin—nicotinic acid or niacin—lowers serum total and LDL cholesterol and triglyceride levels and also raises HDL cholesterol levels (13).

TABLE 20-7 Recommended Intake of Total Fat and Saturated Fat for the Step One and Step Two Diets*

	Total Calorie Level					
	1,600	1,800	2,000	2,200	2,400	2,800
Total fat, g	53	60	67	73	80	93
Saturated fat – Step One, g [†]	18	20	22	24	27	31
Saturated fat – Step Two, g [†]	12	14	16	17	19	22

[*] The average daily energy intake for women is 1,800 calories; for men it is 2,500 calories.
[†] The recommended intake of saturated fat on the Step One diet should be 8–10% of total calories, and less than 7% for the Step Two diet.
Adapted from: National Heart, Lung and Blood Institute. Second report of the expert panel on detection, evaluation, and treatment of high blood cholesterol in adults (Adult Treatment PanelII). NIH Puablication N. 93–3095, Sep. 1993.

Nicotinamide, which also may be referred to as niacin, has no effect on lipid levels and cannot be used in place of nicotinic acid. The disadvantage of nicotinic acid is its high frequency of side effects, including flushing, gastrointestinal symptoms, hyperuricemia and gout, mild hepatotoxicity, and hyperglycemia. Nicotinic acid is used cautiously or not at all in patients with noninsulin-dependent diabetes mellitis because it may reduce glucose tolerance.

PATIENT COUNSELING

Nutritional counseling of patients with risk factors for coronary heart disease or established coronary heart disease involves the guiding of dietary behavior to achieve weight control, often in conjunction with an increase in daily physical activity, and modification in the usual intake of fat or sodium, or a combination of both. The process of changing life-long eating habits is slow. It is usually best accomplished with gradual changes in eating patterns and by enlisting the support of family members to help prevent a relapse in eating patterns. A Dietary Assessment Questionnaire used to assess adherence to a Step One or Step Two diet is provided in Appendix L, Figure 1. Teaching about the composition of processed foods and about how to read food labels are important aspects of counseling patients to modify dietary intakes of fat and sodium. Table 20-9 provides the definition of terms used in food labeling that relate to total fat,

saturated fat, and cholesterol contents. Information needed to plan sodium-restricted diets is provided earlier in this chapter.

MYOCARDIAL INFARCTION

Nutritional care plays a role in both the acute and long-term management of myocardial infarction (MI).

IMMEDIATE POSTINFARCTION CARE

The rationale for nutritional management of an individual in the immediate postinfarction period follows a knowledge of the physiologic response to MI. The objectives of nutritional care during this period include the following:

1. Reduction of potential arrhythmias by elimination of caffeine and use of a liquid diet in the first 24 hours, when nausea and choking are common.
2. Reduction of cardiac workload with small, frequent feedings of soft or liquid foods, 800 to 1,200 kcal per day.
3. Individualization of sodium restriction according to sodium and fluid status.
4. Provision of consistent dietary information as a basis for later education for long-term nutritional management.

TABLE 20-8 Initiation and Goal Cholesterol Levels for Dietary Therapy

	Initiation Level		Monitoring Goal	
	LDL cholesterol		Total cholesterol	
	(mg/dL)	(mmol/L)	(mg/dL)	(mmol/L)
Without CHD* and with fewer than 2 risk factors	≥160	≥4.1	<240	<6.2
Without CHD and with 2 or more risk factors	≥130	≥3.4	<200	<5.2
With CHD	>100	>2.6	≤160	≤4.1

[*] CHD = coronary heart disease. See Table 20-2 for nonlipid risk factors
Adapted from National Heart, Lung and Blood Institute. Second report of the expert panel on detection, evaluation, and treatment of high blood cholesterol in adults (Adult Treatment Panel II). NIH Publication No. 93-3095, Sep. 1993.

TABLE 20-9 Nutrient Content Claims Regarding Fat Composition Approved for Food Labeling

Claim	Total Fat	Saturated Fat	Cholesterol
Free	Less than 0.5 per reference amount and per serving*	Less than 0.5 saturated fat and less than 0.5 *trans-fatty* acid per reference amount and per serving*	Less than 2 g per reference amount and per serving*
Low	3 g or less per reference amount (and per 50 g if reference amount is small)	1 g or less per reference amount and 15% or less of calories from saturated fat	20 mg or less per reference amount (and per 50 g if reference amount is small)
Reduced / Low	At least 25% less fat per reference amount than an appropriate reference food	At least 25% less saturated fat per reference amount than an appropriate reference food	At least 25% less cholesterol per reference amount than an appropriate reference food
Comments	"__%Fat Free" must meet the requirements for "Low Fat." "Light" or "Lite" means ≥50% less fat per reference amount or 1/3 fewer calories if <50% of calories from fat		Cholesterol claims only allowed when food contains 2 g or less saturated fat per reference amount

* If an ingredient is present that is understood to contain this nutrient, it must be followed by an asterisk that refers to a footnote stating that it contains a trivial amount of the nutrient.

Note: Other approved nutrient content claims include "Lean"—on seafood or game meat that contains <10 g total fat, 4.5 g or less saturated fat, and < 95 mg cholesterol per reference amount and per 100 g, and "Extra Lean"—on seafood or game meat that contains <5 g total fat, <2 g saturated fat, and <95 mg cholesterol per reference amount and per 100 g.

Adapted from: Food Labeling Reform. *Nutrition Today* 28:(1993)4–43, and Food and Drug Administration, Focus on Food Labelling, an FDA Consumer Special Report, *FDA Consumer*, 1993.

LONG-TERM MANAGEMENT

Patients most likely to benefit from long-term dietary intervention after an MI are those with the best prognosis: in general, younger patients without functional impairment of the heart. Cardiac rehabilitation programs—which include cessation of smoking, gradual increase in exercise, weight reduction, and adherence to a Step One diet—are felt to be of value in improving the quality of life and arresting, retarding, or reversing the atherosclerotic process.

Patients who have had an MI and have various complications, such as hypertension or diabetes mellitus, should have appropriate nutritional management in addition to the Step One or Two diet. Many cardiologists feel that since congestive heart failure is a common long-term complication of MI, all MI patients should be advised to follow a moderate sodium restriction of 2 to 3 g per day.

For patients with persistent or recurrent angina, slow eating of frequent, small meals may reduce pain. Also, resting before and after a meal may be of benefit. Weight reduction may help decrease angina in the obese patient with significant chest pain.

Programs promoting a rapid weight reduction—a weight loss of greater than 2 pounds per week—should be used with caution in the postinfarction patient. The elevation in plasma free fatty acid levels that accompanies rapid weight reduction can induce cardiac arrhythmias. In addition, the fluid and electrolyte alterations that accompany rapid weight reduction can be particularly dangerous to the post-MI patient maintained on diuretic and digitalis therapy.

CORONARY BYPASS

The patient who has successful coronary bypass surgery also needs appropriate sodium restriction and adherence to a Step One diet. Atherosclerosis may progress more rapidly in bypass graft vessels than in the native circulation. Patients often consider themselves cured because of dramatic relief of symptoms after bypass surgery and must be carefully counseled on their nutritional needs.

CONGESTIVE HEART FAILURE

The nutritional management of congestive heart failure (CHF) comprises several aspects. Sodium restriction to reduce fluid retention and cardiac workload is essential in the management of CHF. A patient in severe cardiac failure may require a sodium restriction of 500 mg per day, while patients with moderate failure may tolerate as much as 2 to 3 g sodium per day. It is important to control obesity with a restricted calorie intake in order to reduce cardiac workload. Diuretic and digoxin therapy are commonly used in the management of CHF, and serum potassium levels are usually followed closely to guard against hypokalemia and associated digitalis toxicity. Small, frequent feedings may be useful in the case of severe cardiac failure. Alcohol depresses myocardial contractility and should not be consumed in excess by the CHF patient. The use of caffeine is controversial, but it should not be used if there is a history of MI or cardiac arrhythmia.

TOPICS FOR FURTHER DISCUSSION

1. The role of antioxidant nutrients such as vitamin C, vitamin E, and carotene in the process of atherosclerosis.
2. The effects of moderate alcohol intake on platelet aggregation and the serum lipoproteins.
3. Describe the principles of nutritional support for a cardiac transplant patient.
4. Discuss and describe procedures for establishing counseling programs on lifestyle modifications for prevention of coronary heart disease.
5. Principles of childhood nutrition for long-term prevention of atherosclerosis.

REFERENCES

1. National Heart, Lung and Blood Institute. *Fifth report of the Joint National Committee on Detection, Evaluation, and Treatment of High Blood Pressure.* NIH Publication No. 93–1088, Jan. 1993.
2. Roccella, E.J. and C. L. Enfant. Regional and racial differences among stroke victims in the United States. *Clin. Cardiol.* 12:(1989) IV-18–IV-22.
3. Stamler, R., J. Stamler, R. Grimm, F. Gosch, et al. Nutritional therapy for high blood pressure. Final report of a four-year randomized controlled trial—the hypertension control program. *J.A.M.A.* 257:(1987)1484–91.
4. Langford, H.G., B.R. Davis, M.D. Blaufox, et al. Effect of drug and diet treatment of mild hypertension on diastolic blood pressure. *Hypertension* 17:(1991)210–17.
5. World Hypertension League. Physical exercise in the management of hypertension: a consensus statement by the World Hypertension League. *J. Hypertens..* 9:(1991)283–87.
6. Flack, J.M., K.E. Ensrud, S. Mascioli, et al. Racial and ethnic modifiers of the salt-blood pressure response. *Hypertension* 17:(1991, supp I) I-115–I-121.
7. Food and Nutrition Board, Commission on Life Sciences, National Research Council. *Recommended Dietary Allowances,* 10th ed. Washington, DC: National Academy Press, 1989.
8. Food and Drug Administration. An FDA consumer special report, Focus on food labeling. *FDA Consumer.* Document number 017-012-00360-5, Pittsburgh: Superintendent of Documents, May 1993.
9. Helmke P.A. and D.M. Ney. Relationships between concentrations of sodium, potassium and chlorine in unsalted foods. *J. Agric. Food Chem.* 40:(1992)1547–52.
10. Mattes, R.D. and D. Donnelly Relative contributions of dietary sodium sources. *J. Am. Coll. Nutr.* 10:(1991)383–93.
11. Wilkening, V.L. FDA'S regulations to implement the NLEA. *Nutr. Today* 28:(1993)13–20.
12. Fredrickson, D.S. AND R.I. Levy. *Dietary Management of Hyperlipoproteinemia: A Handbook for Physicians and Dietitians.* National Heart and Lung Institute. DHEW Publication No. (NIH) 80-110, 1980.
13. National Heart, Lung and Blood Institute. Second Report of the Expert Panel on Detection, Evaluation, and Treatment of High Blood Cholesterol in Adults (Adult Treatment Panel II). NIH Publication No. 93-3095, 1993.
14. Expert Panel on Detection, Evaluation, and Treatment of High Blood Cholesterol in Adults. Summary of the second report of the National Cholesterol Education Program (NCEP) expert panel on detection, evaluation, and treatment of high blood cholesterol in adults (adult treatment panel II). *J.A.M.A* 269:(1993)3015–23.
15. U.S. Departments of Agriculture and Health and Human Services. *Dietary Guidelines for Americans,* 3d ed. U.S. Government Printing Office Document No. 273–930, 1990.
16. Caggiula, A.W., G. Christakis, M. Farrand, et al. The multiple risk factor intervention trial (MRFIT), IV: intervention on blood lipids. *Preventive Medicine* 10:(1981)443–475.
17. Ginsberg, H.N., W. Karmally, M. Siddiqui, S. Holleran, A.R. Tall, S.C. Rumsey, R.J. Deckelbaum, W.S. Blaner, and R. Ramakrishnan. A dose-response study of the effects of dietary cholesterol on fasting and postprandial lipid and lipoprotein metabolism in healthy young men. *Arterioscler. Thrombosis* 14:(1994)576–86.

ADDITIONAL SOURCES OF INFORMATION

Sports and Cardiovascular Nutritionists. A Practice Group of the American Dietetic Association. *Cardiovascular Disease: Nutrition for Prevention and Treatment*, P.M. Kris-Etherton, ed. Chicago, American Dietetic Association, 1990.

National Heart, Lung and Blood Institute. *Step by Step Eating to Lower Your High Blood Cholesterol.* NIH Publication No. 94-2920, Aug. 1994.

National Cholesterol Education Program. *Report of the Expert Panel on Blood Cholesterol Levels in Children and Adolescents.* NIH Publication No. 91-2732, Sep. 1991.

O'Keefe, J.H., C.J. Lavie, and B.D. McCallister. Insights into the pathogenesis and prevention of coronary artery disease. *Mayo Clin. Proc.* 70:(1995)69–79.

Hamet, P. The evaluation of the scientific evidence for a relationship between calcum and hypertension. *J. Nutr.*, supplement 2, 125:(1995)311–400.

TO TEST YOUR UNDERSTANDING

1. Why are increased potassium losses seen with thiazide and loop diuretic therapy?

2. Describe the symptoms of hypokalemia.

3. Why is hypokalemia of particular concern with a combination of digitalis and thiazide or loop diuretic therapy?

4. What is the potassium content of 1 tsp (5 g) salt substitute (assume pure KCl), and what is the sodium content of 1 tsp (5 g) of sodium chloride? Express your answer in both mg and mmol of potassium and sodium

5. List three examples of food choices that would provide 40 mmol of potassium and no more than 300 kcal. List each food's portion, mmol K, and kcal.

6. a. Calculate the amount of cholesterol, total fat, saturated fat, sodium, and kcal in the following menu. For the lunch from McDonald's, obtain nutrients information from your local franchise. Consult a handbook of food composition, or utilize a computer program to complete calculations for the rest of the meals

Breakfast	*McDonald's lunch*	*Supper*
Milk, 2%, 8 oz	Diet Coke	Milk, 2%, 8 oz
Eggs, 2 poached	Quarter Pounder	Potato, baked, 1 med
Toast, 2 slices	French fries, small	Sour cream, 2 T
Butter, 1 T	Salt, 0.5 g	Chicken w/skin, baked, 6 oz
Salt, 0.5 g		Broccoli, 1/2 cup
		Tossed salad, 1 cup
		Bleu Cheese Dressing 2 T
		Butter, 1 T
		Ice cream, 10% 1 cup
		Salt, 0.5 g

b. What changes would be required in this menu to make the food choices consistent with a Step One diet? Assuming a caloric intake of 2,500 kcal per day, how many g of total and saturated fat would be included?

7. What advice could you offer an individual for the selection of a margarine with a high P:S ratio?

8. Visit a local grocery store and name at least two brands of products in each of the following categories that would be acceptable for an individual following the Step One diet.

Crackers	Margarine
Cream Substitute	Oil
Cheese	Frozen meat dish
Egg Substitite	Salad dressing
Dessert	Sauce mix

9. Explain the potential dangers of routinely using a sodium-restricted diet for all MI patients in the acute phase.

10. In physiologic terms, what is the rationale for a sodium-restricted diet in congestive heart failure?

Cardiovascular Disease

Part I: Presentation

Present Illness: Jim. C. is a 42 y.o. engineering technician referred to his family physician for evaluation of arterial hypertension detected during a preemployment examination and confirmed one week later. He relates no prior history of elevated BP but had been warned to "watch his weight." He denies current symptoms of chest pain, shortness of breath (SOB), edema, or visual symptoms. He smokes one pack of cigarettes a day and plays tennis once or twice a week. His body weight has been steadily increasing by 2 to 4 pounds per year for the last ten years.

Past Medical History: He had measles, mumps, and chicken-pox in childhood, and an appendectomy approximately 20 years ago. There is no history of rheumatic fever, diabetes, or kidney disease.

Family History: Father died at 48 years of age from an acute MI, and mother is being treated for essential hypertension.

Social History: Has two children; wife works as a legal secretary.

Review of Systems: Patient has no complaints except for occasional mild tension headaches.

Physical Exam: General: somewhat overweight white male; 5 ft, 10 in, 180#, small frame. BP 155/103, right arm, sitting, without postural changes. P76 and regular. R 15. HEENT-fundoscopic exam revealed normal A-V ratio, no A-V nicking, with flat disc and no hemorrhages or exudates. Neck without thyromegaly, venous distention, or bruits. Lungs clear to P&A. Heart-regular rhythm, without murmur or gallop. Abdomen slightly obese, soft, and without bruit. Extremities revealed no edema. Screening neurological exam, including mental status exam, is completely WNL.

Laboratory: Hct 50%, Hgb 158 g/L, glucose 6.55 mmol/L, BUN 6.43 mmol/L, total cholesterol 7.76 mmol/L, LDL cholesterol 5.17 mmol/L, HDL cholesterol 1.29 mmol/L, triglycerides (fasting) 1.35 mmol/L. U/A negative for glucose, protein, and blood). EKG revealed normal sinus rhythm with a rate of 80, normal intervals, and no evidence of ischemia, strain, or hypertrophy. CXR was unremarkable.

Impression: Essential hypertension and elevated LDL cholesterol in a 42 y.o., slightly obese, otherwise healthy male with a positive family history of CHD.

Plan: Nutrition Clinic referral for instruction in 1,500 kcal, 2-g sodium Step One diet. Encourage cessation of smoking and increase in exercise. RTC in 2 weeks for BP check.

QUESTIONS

You are the dietitian for the nutrition outpatient clinic associated with the local University hospital. Mr. C. comes to you for initial dietary counseling with a physician referral which reads as follows: Instruct In: 1,500 kcal, 2-g-Na, Step One diet. You have access to his medical record as outlined in Part I.

1. List the risk factors for CHD that Mr. C. has (see Table 20-2).

2. You assess Mr. C.'s knowledge of a low-Na, Step One diet which is limited to "just don't add any salt to food and avoid fried foods". List three major points or areas that you will need to explain to Mr. C. in order for him to follow a 2 g-Na diet and 3 major points that he will need to understand in order to follow a Step One diet.

3. Calculate a 1,500 kcal, 2 g-Na, Step One diet meal plan for home use for Mr. C., using Form C in Appendix M and the low-Na exchange lists provided in your diet manual. You may find it helpful to add a column to Form C to summarize the Na content of the exchange lists. Assume that Mr. C. has decided to stop smoking and has no major food preferences other than a distaste for nonfat milk and the need to take a lunch to work.

4. Summarize your observations, assessment and plan of action in a SOAP note.

Part II: Medical Management of Hypertension

Mr. C. keeps his FU appointments and is evaluated several times in the next 2 months. He successfully quits smoking and reduces his sodium intake, but he gains 5 lbs. PE reveals a weight of 185 lb and BP of 152/99. LDL cholesterol is reduced slightly to 5.0 mmol/L. He is considered to have failed nonpharmacologic management of his hypertension and is started on hydrochlorothiazide (HCTZ) 25 mg po qd. He is referred back to the nutrition clinic for FU on his diet, 1,500 kcal, 2 g-Na Step One with a suggested K intake of 125–200 mmol/day. His medical record states:

Problem 1:	essential hypertension
Problem 2:	elevated LDL cholesterol
Problem 3:	excess body weight

QUESTIONS

You see Mr. C. in nutrition clinic for FU 10 wks after your initial consultation. He has started HCTZ, now weighs 186 lb, and has a recent serum K of 4.0 mmol/L. He tells you that he has stopped using salt, but he is always hungry since he quit smoking. A 24-hr diet recall reveals the following intake (assume that no added salt is used in preparation):

Breakfast
    1 c apple juice
    3 c puffed cereal
    1 1/2 c 2% milk
    2 c coffee

Lunch
    2 tuna sandwiches (4 slices bread, 1 c water-packed tuna,
        1/4 c mayonnaise)
    1 large apple
    1 small candy bar
    Diet cola

Dinner
    2 broiled, skinned chicken breasts (7 oz. total meat)
    Large baked potato
    1 T margarine
    1 c green beans
    Tossed salad
    2 T oil for dressing
    1/2 c ice cream

5. a. Compare the content of the 24-hr recall to the diet prescription (1,500 kcal, 2 g-Na, Step One diet, 125 to 200 mmol K/day). Use a handbook of food composition or a computer database to assist with your intake calculations.

b. List the major differences between the prescribed and reported intake.

6. What *positive* feedback can you give Mr. C. regarding his dietary intake? Identify two changes in food intake behavior that Mr. C. could strive to achieve in small steps.

Part III: Angina and Elevated LDL Cholesterol

Mr. C. continues FU with his physician. His BP is maintained with HCTZ at 130–140/86–92 during repeated visits. His LDL cholesterol remains at 4.5–5.1 mmol/L after 6 months on the Step One diet followed by a 3-month trial on the Step Two diet. Weight is stable at 175 lb. He is started on cholestyramine therapy, 8 g/day, for diet-resistant hypercholesterolemia which reduces his LDL cholesterol to 3.5 mmol/L. However, Mr. C. complains of abdominal discomfort and constipation with cholestyramine therapy and does not consistently take the medication. Mr. C. starts smoking again about 4 years after stopping.

Approximately 10 years after his initial presentation, Mr. C. at age 52 begins to notice vague retrosternal discomfort during moderate physical activity, which he describes as a dull, heavy sensation that always subsides after a few minutes of rest. An EKG shows mild left ventricular strain, and a treadmill stress test is considered equivocal. Mr. C. undergoes cardiac catheterization, which indicates a narrowing of a single coronary artery, and he receives balloon angioplasty. Nitroglycerin (NTG), 0.4 mg sublingually prn for chest pain and before exercise, is prescribed. He notices an improved exercise tolerance with NTG. Mr. C.'s medical record now contains the following problem list:

Problem 1:   essential hypertension
Problem 2:   elevated LDL cholesterol
Problem 3:   excess body weight
Problem 4:   angina s/p angioplasty

Part IV: Myocardial Infarction

At age 55, the patient reports a 3-hr history of severe retrosternal pain associated with SOB, which occurred while he was painting a room in his house. This pain is only partially relieved with NTG and radiates to his jaw and left arm. There is also associated diaphoresis, nausea, and light headedness, but he denies palpitations.

On PE he is found to be moderately overweight and extremely anxious. BP is 115/90, P 96, and R 28 and regular. Skin is dusky, cold, and moist. Fine rales are heard in both lung bases, and there is a dyskinetic pulse at the fifth intercostal space lateral to the midclavicular line. Peripheral pulses are symmetrical but of decreased volume. There is an audible fourth heart sound. His EKG reveals ST-segment elevation and a poor R-wave progression in the anterior precordial leads.

Laboratory tests reveal a white count of 12,500, with a normal differential, cholesterol of 5.95 mmol/L, and triglycerides of 4.65 mmol/L. His CPK on admission is 2.1 mmol/L (Normal is less than 2.5).

Mr. C. is admitted to the CCU to R/O MI, and is given oxygen at 2 L per minute by nasal passage prongs, minidose subcutaneous heparin, parenteral morphine sulfate, streptokinase, and a prophylactic lidocaine drip. During his first day in the hospital, his CPK peaks at 677, with an MB isoenzyme fraction of 11 percent, confirming the diagnosis of MI. He has no recurrence of chest pain and only occasional ventricular premature contractions.

Mr. C. medical record now contains the following problem list:

Problem 1:   essential hypertension
Problem 2:   elevated LDL cholesterol
Problem 3:   excess body weight
Problem 4:   angina, s/p angioplasty
Problem 5:   chest pain → MI

His CCU diet orders include the following:

Day 1: 2 g Na, clear liquid, no caffeine, 6 small feedings of no more than 360 mL each.

Day 2: 2 g Na, 1,200 kcal, soft, low cholesterol, low fat (Step One), no caffeine, 6 feedings, with fluids restricted to 360 mL per feeding.

Day 3 and on: 2-g-Na, 1,200 kcal Step One diet, no caffeine.

His activities follow routine protocol with bed rest until he is transferred from the CCU to the general ward on day 2. He then begins a program of rehabilitation, with passive exercises followed by progressive ambulation. He is discharged from the hospital on the sixth day, fully ambulatory, with instructions to limit his activity to leisurely walking with a slowly progressive exercise program. He is again strongly encouraged to stop smoking and told that his prognosis is generally favorable. The patient has lost 5 #

during hospitalization and now weighs 170 #. He is discharged on a 2 g-Na Step One as well as NTG, propranolol, and HCTZ. He returns to work 5 weeks after his MI.

Angiography is performed 2 months after hospital discharge to evaluate the status of the coronary arteries since angioplasty was done. The angiogram reveals a 70% occlusion of the right coronary artery and distal lesions of the left circumflex artery. Mr. C. is not a candidate for coronary artery bypass graft (CABG) because his lesions are not appropriate for surgery. Medical management is continued.

QUESTIONS

7. Discuss the significance of the WBC and CPK levels and the MB isozyme level.

8. Is a cholesterol determination valid in the immediate postinfarction period? Answer yes or no, and explain your answer.

9. Explain the rationale and, where appropriate, the nutritional significance of the following therapies:
    a. Oxygen by nasal prongs
    b. Lidocaine
    c. Morphine sulfate
    d. Heparin
    e. Propranolol
    f. Hydrochlorothiazide
    g. Nitroglycerin
    h. Streptokinase

10. Why is caffeine eliminated from the diet?

11. Explain the rationale for a calorie restriction of 1,200 kcal and small feedings with limited fluids in the post (5–8 days) infarction period.

Part V: Congestive Heart Failure

Over the next 15 months, Mr. C.'s angina is controlled on the above regimen, with pain occurring approximately once every 2 to 3 weeks and easily controlled with sublingual NTG. He then presents with symptoms of increasing SOB and DOE. PE at that time reveals BP of 142/85, with bilateral rales a quarter of the way up from the long bases and 2+ bipedal edema. Cardiac exam reveals an audible third heart sound and evidence of increased CVP. He is felt to have moderate CHF.

The propranolol is stopped, and digoxin 0.125 mg/day is started. Symptoms of SOB and DOE persist, and the HCTZ is stopped and furosemide begun. Mr. C. finally becomes stable on digoxin, with 80 mg of furosemide po every am and continued adherence to a 2 g-Na Step One diet. Routine evaluation, approximately 2 months after initiation of this therapy, reveals a serum K of 3.0 mmol/L. After a trial of increasing dietary K intake, Mr. C. is begun on a 10% KCl solution, 1 T po b.i.d.

QUESTIONS

12. What is the primary nutritional concern with combined use of the drugs digoxin and furosemide?

Part VI: Cardiac Cachexia

Mr. C. decides to retire at age 62 due to increasing weakness and SOB. He succeeds in quitting smoking and generally follows his diet, but he never increased his activity level after his first MI. His weight progressively decreases. At age 66 he weighs 145# and is becoming increasingly weak and losing muscle mass. Medical management with adjustment of drug dosage is continued, as Mr. C. is not a surgical candidate. The diagnosis of early cardiac cachexia is made.

QUESTIONS

13. What is cardiac cachexia, and what are potential mechanisms associated with its occurrence?

14. Describe an appropriate diet for Mr. C. now that he is in the early stages of cardiac cachexia.

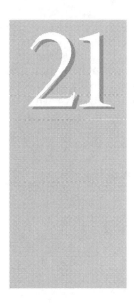

21 Nutritional Care in Chronic Renal Failure

Nutritional care of patients with renal disease is extremely demanding. It requires an understanding of fluid and electrolyte balance, acid-base balance, and nitrogen balance. Since the patient's condition changes with time, the nutritional care specialist must be able to alter the care to meet changing needs. Nutritional care must also be adjusted to the type of treatment afforded to the patient, including drug treatment, hemodialysis, peritoneal dialysis, and renal transplant. Before proceeding, you may need to review the material on kidney disease in your text.

Chronic renal failure (CRF), the presence of irreversible nephron damage, may develop either relatively rapidly or slowly, over periods varying from months to decades. In fact, the kidneys have a large reserve capacity, and patients are often unaware of the existence of renal disease until it is quite advanced.

The severity of the disease is often clinically defined in terms of decreases in creatinine and urea clearances and corresponding increases in serum concentrations of creatinine and urea nitrogen. If managed properly, patients may remain symptom-free until glomerular filtration rate (GFR) has decreased from a normal level of 80 to 120 mL per minute to less than 10 mL per minute, and sometimes to less than 5 mL per minute. The condition at this point is called *endstage renal disease* (ESRD). In this advanced stage of the disease, patients have lost their ability to cope with stresses such as dehydration, overhydration, large amounts of nitrogenous waste products, limited or excessive amounts of electrolytes, hypertension, infection, or the presence of a renal toxin. Proper management then becomes even more important.

The general objectives of nutritional care are to:

1. Maintain optimal quality of life for the patient as the disease progresses, including reduction of the severity of symptoms
2. Minimize secondary effects, such as renal osteodystrophy
3. Retard progression of renal failure if possible
4. Delay the necessity for dialysis for some patients, as long as possible
5. Maintain life for some patients, until a kidney for transplant is available.

Treatment of CRF may be divided into three phases. The first phase consists of *conservative management,* primarily using diet and drugs. The diet consists of changes in intake of protein, sodium, potassium, phosphorus, and fluid. Many of the drugs interact with certain foods, as we shall see.

As renal function declines, a second phase develops, during which the patient is *dialyzed*. The diet changes somewhat, but the same nutrients are the major concerns. During the third phase, the patients receives a *transplanted* kidney. Some patients go through all phases, while others skip some phases. Each phase varies markedly in length and has some unique requirements for nutritional care.

NUTRITIONAL ASSESSMENT

MODIFICATIONS IN ROUTINE PROCEDURES
Nutritional assessment is important in renal disease because these patients have a high incidence of

malnutrition. The procedures for assessment described in Chapter 5 are generally applicable to the renal disease patient; however, some differences in methods and interpretation must be taken into account. In addition, since CRF is a long-term, progressive disease, the assessment must be repeated at intervals to evaluate changes in the patient's condition, the effectiveness of the diet, and compliance with the diet. Some of the procedures therefore monitor not only the patient's nutritional status but also the response to and adequacy of the diet as it relates to the progress of the disease. Some special considerations follow.

Anthropometric Measurements

Weight and height. Body weights of renal patients should be obtained after the bladder has been emptied and with similar clothing at each weighing. For patients who tend to become edematous, calculations involving body weight are usually based on dry weight, that is, weight at normal hydration. A patient is assumed to be at dry weight when blood pressure is normal, there is no evidence of edema, and serum sodium is within normal range. Dry weight in the dialyzed patient is the weight at the end of a dialysis treatment when normal blood pressure is reached.

The weight best used as the standard for interpretation in renal patients is not known. *Usual weight*, that is, the weight before the onset of illness, is often used as the standard for adults. Alternatively, the patient's weight is compared to ideal body weight (see Chapter 5).

Another possibility is the *adjusted ideal body weight* (AIBW). In obese patients, the excess weight is sometimes assumed to contain a lesser proportion of lean tissue, 36 to 38 percent for men and 22 to 32 percent for women. The AIBW is then calculated as follows:

Men: AIBW
= IBW + [(actual weight − IBW) × 0.38]   **(21-1)**

Women: AIBW
= IBW + [(actual weight − IBW) × 0.32]   **(21-2)**

See Chapter 5 to find the IBW.

Once the actual and desired dry weights have been established, subsequent changes compared with previous weights will indicate the direction of changes in nutritional status. Rate of weight loss is also important. Rapid weight loss is considered to be more clinically significant than a slow loss. Standards for interpretation are given in Table 21-1.

Height is a special concern in children; it is often severely affected by renal disease. It is therefore important to monitor height in children and compare it to standard height for age, as described in Chapter 9.

It is also suggested that weight and other anthropometric measures are best compared with subgroups of similar age, race, sex, treatment modality, and concurrent diabetes. For example, one subgroup might be black,

females, age less than 40, diabetic, and on hemodialysis. Unfortunately, standards for many such subgroups are not available (1, 2)

Muscle mass and body fat. Midarm muscle circumference and triceps skinfold measurements may be useful in evaluating the extent of the wasting syndrome frequently seen in CRF and in monitoring the efficacy of nutritional care. Thus, they should be repeated at intervals separated by at least 2 weeks. Useful values are given in Table 21-1, but it is important to keep in mind that standards for triceps skinfold for uremic patients are based on few data. However, serial measurements are useful in determining *direction of change*. Comparison with appropriate subgroups, as described above, is helpful in distinguishing the effects of malnutrition from the effects of uremia (1, 2).

When MAMC is measured in hemodialysis patients, the use of the "nonaccess" arm is recommended—that is, the arm that is *not* attached to the dialyzer. Some degree of error is introduced if the nonaccess arm is the dominant arm, but sequential measurements may still be useful to indicate direction of change. Arm anthropometry is not used if both arms contain access sites. Suggested values for interpretation are given in Table 21-1. The extent to which these measurements are altered by edema is unknown. As a consequence, some treatment centers do not use them in evaluating edematous CRF patients.

Biochemical Measurements

In this chapter, rather than using S.I. units, laboratory values are given in conventional units, since these are primarily used in monitoring renal patients. If S.I. units are desired, conversion factors may be found in Appendix E.

Serum albumin is a poor early indicator of malnutrition since it has a long half-life and a large pool in the body. It also generally does not respond well to supplementary feeding. Nevertheless, serum albumin is extensively used because its determination is inexpensive and

TABLE 21-1   Standards for Interpretation of Nutritional Assessment in Chronic Renal Failure

	Deficit		
Nutritional Parameter	Normal/Mild	Moderate	Severe
Dry weight as % of usual relative body weight	85–95	75–85	< 75
Triceps skinfold (mm)			
Men		4–6	< 4
Women		8–12	< 8
Arm muscle circumference (cm)			
Men		22–24	< 22
Women		18–20	< 18
Serum albumin (g/dL)		2.8–3.3	< 2.8
Serum transferrin (mg/dL)		150–180	< 150

readily available, and because CRF is a long-term disease. Serum albumin is frequently decreased in the patient with CRF, but it should be maintained within normal range, if possible.

Insulinlike growth factor(IGF-I) in the serum has been reported to decrease in malnutrition well before changes in anthropometric measurements were detected (3). Thus, IGF-I may be a promising indicator for early malnutrition.

Diet Assessment
The diet history obtained from the patient with chronic renal disease must be detailed if it is to be useful, and must consider intakes of fluid and electrolytes, as well as protein, fat, and carbohydrate. A 24-hour recall is often insufficient for this type of patient. A food intake record kept by the patient for 3 to 4 days is more appropriate, and it should be redone every few months. In addition, the patient's family, social worker, and primary care-givers are often good sources of information.

Diet analysis should include the proportion of protein that is of high biological value, as well as total protein and estimates of intake of sodium, potassium, calcium, phosphorus, iron, ascorbic acid, and fluids.

You will need to inquire about the use of various types of special products. For example, it is important to know whether the patient is using salt substitutes, and if so, the brand and the amount. In addition, you should inquire as to whether the patient is using any "special diet" products, the type, nutritional value, and amount. The use of vitamin and mineral supplements should also be determined along with the brand, content, and dose.

Other sources of both nutrients and losses must also be considered, including losses in hemodialysis and the additional calories from peritoneal dialysis.

MONITORING PROCEDURES FOR RENAL PATIENTS

In addition to the above routine procedures, the following can be especially useful in monitoring the efficacy of nutritional care in renal disease and, in some cases, the patient's adherence to the various aspects of the prescribed diet, which may include restrictions of protein, Na, fluid, K, or P.

Monitoring Protein Homeostasis
Serum creatinine is used to measure the extent of renal failure at the time of diagnosis and to monitor the efficacy of treatment. Creatinine is produced at a fairly constant rate from metabolism of muscle creatine and is excreted by the kidneys. The amount of creatinine in the serum is thus directly related to the amount of muscle mass and the inability of the kidney to excrete creatinine. It may be useful as an indicator of an increase or decrease in muscle mass, but only if values are obtained over a long period during which treatment has not changed markedly, and if the adequacy of renal function had not changed in the interim. It is not diet-related unless the patient has a diet with a high meat intake.

Creatinine clearance (Cl_{CR}) is an indicator of the GFR and serves as a measure of renal damage. It is not diet related. Creatinine clearance is depressed in renal failure; consequently, serum creatinine is elevated. Creatinine clearance (Cl_{CR}) may be calculated with the following equation:

$$Cl_{Cr}(ml/min) = \frac{(140 - age\ in\ years)(wt\ in\ kg)}{72 \times serum\ creatinine\ in\ mg/dL}$$

$$(21-3)$$

Blood urea nitrogen (BUN) may also be an indicator of the extent of renal failure but is affected by many other factors. If the renal disease patient is stable, that is, in nitrogen balance with BUN and body weight relatively constant, BUN is closely correlated with protein intake. While increased BUN may be associated with excessive protein intake, it can also be caused by dehydration, catabolic states, such as surgery, infections, burns, or other trauma, the intake of catabolic medications, such as steroids, in high doses, and gastrointestinal bleeding. Levels of 60 to 80, or sometimes up to 100, mg/dL are considered acceptable for the patient with CRF since uremic symptoms generally do not develop until BUN is 80 mg/dL or more. If values are less than 40 mg/dL, the patient should be checked for malnutrition.

Urea clearance (Cl_{UREA}) may also be used to indicate renal filtration ability. True GFR or inulin clearance is difficult to measure directly in clinical settings. Cl_{CR} tends to overestimate GFR, whereas Cl_{UREA} tends to underestimate it. In clinical settings, GFR may be obtained by averaging Cl_{CR} and Cl_{UREA}. The estimate obtained is most accurate in patients with severe renal disease.

Urinary urea nitrogen (UUN) can be used to assess recent protein intake in clinically stable, chronically uremic patients, and thus to monitor adherence to the diet (4). The amount of urea in the urine per day is obtained in the laboratory and recorded in the patient's chart. In assessing protein intake, recent nitrogen intake is first calculated from the equation.

$$Recent\ mean\ N\ intake = 10/9\ x\ UUN + 1.8$$

$$(21-4)$$

where all values are given in g per day. The value 1.8 is for fecal, respiratory, and integumental losses. Protein is then calculated from nitrogen. Protein intake can also be calculated directly, with the equation

$$Protein\ intake = 7.0 \times (UUN) + 11 \quad (21-5)$$

where all values are in g per day. If a protein-restricted diet has been prescribed, estimated intake can be compared with the prescription to assess compliance. If, for example, the results from Eq. (21-5) indicate that intake is 70 g protein per day for a patient whose prescribed intake is 40 g, it is clear the patient is not complying with the prescribed diet.

Traditional nitrogen balance is not useful in assessing protein requirements in patients with compromised renal function because of the patient's tendency to accumulate, rather than excrete, end-products of protein metabolism and fluid. In these patients (with creatinine clearance less than 50 mL/min) *urea kinetics* provide a useful alternative tool making it possible to determine protein requirements and to evaluate compliance and adequacy of hemodialysis.

Urea kinetics are based on the assumptions that (1) urea freely crosses membranes and is thus present in all body fluids at the same concentrations, (2) short-term changes in body weight are composed of fluid, and (3) there is a direct linear relationship between the urea generation rate and protein catabolic rate (5, 6).

There are a number of advantages to this method:

1. Urea kinetics take into account changes in serum urea levels.
2. In stable patients, that is, those in protein balance with stable body weights and urea levels, it is not necessary to calculate protein intake from diet records because, in these patients, protein catabolic rate equals daily protein intake:

$$PCR = DPI \qquad (21\text{-}6)$$

3. Protein catabolic rate can be used to verify intake and thus monitor compliance.
4. Protein catabolic rate can be used to identify patients at nutritional risk and identify protein deficiency or excess.
5. Catabolic demands can be quantified.

The abbreviations used in urea kinetics are listed in Table 21-2, which should be consulted in this discussion.

There are several steps in the calculations:

1. *Determine urea volume distribution.* The volume of fluid through which the urea is distributed corresponds to total body water, since urea diffuses freely across cell membranes. For clinical purposes, it is considered sufficient to use 58 percent of *lean tissue weight* for males and 55 percent of *lean tissue weight* for females (7, 8) to represent total body water.

2. *Calculate the urea generation rate.* When the patient is anuric, the changes in levels of BUN and urea volume distribution are used to calculate the urea nitrogen generation rate (GUN) (9, 10). The time interval used is the time in minutes between the end of one dialysis period, where the volume of body water is V_1, and the beginning of the next, where the volume of body water is V_2.

Using symbols listed in Table 21-2, the calculation is as follows:

$$GUN = [(BUN_2 \times V_2) - (BUN_1 \times V_1)]\theta \qquad (21\text{-}7)$$

TABLE 21-2 Useful Abreviations in Urea Kinetics

G	Urea generation rate	g/24 hr
GUN	Urea nitrogen generation rate	mg/min
BUN_1	Blood urea nitrogen, postdialysis	mg/mL
BUN_2	Blood urea nitrogen, predialysis	mg/mL
V_1	Total body water (in "dry weight")	mL
V_2	V_1 plus fluid weight gain	mL
t	Time between urine collections	minutes
UUN	Urine urea nitrogen	mg/mL
UV	Urine collection volume	mL
t	Time interval between dialyses or time of urine collection	minutes
KrUN	Residual urea cleaarance	mL/min
SUN	Mean SUN = $\dfrac{(SUN_1 + SUN_2)}{2}$	mg/mL
θ	Time interval between blood samples	minutes
Vu	Estimated urea volume of body water	mL
PCR	Protein catabolic rate	g/24 hr

3. *Calculate residual clearances.* If the patient has some residual renal function, the amount of excreted urea in the urine must be included. This residual urea clearance (KrU) is calculated with the equation:

$$KrU = \frac{UUN}{BUN} \times \frac{UV}{t} \qquad (21\text{-}8)$$

Note that BUN, in this case, is the mean of the beginning and ending BUN values for the test interval.

Example: This female patient is anuric and weighs 60 kg at dry weight. Intake provides 60 g protein and 2,000 kcal/day. Dialysis schedule is:

Postdialysis (V_1): 4 PM Monday, weight = 60 kg, BUN = 25 mg/dL

Predialysis (V_2): 10 AM Wednesday, weight = 64 kg, BUN = 75 mg/dL

Total body water (V_1) = 60 × 0.55 = 33 kg or 33,000 mL.
(V_2) = 33000 + 4000 = 37,000 mL

$$
\begin{aligned}
GUN &= [(37{,}000 \times 0.75) - (33000 \times 0.25)]/2520 \\
&= (27{,}750 - 8250)/2520 \\
&= 19{,}500/2520 \\
&= 7.7 \text{ mg nitrogen/min}
\end{aligned}
$$

4. *Calculate the protein catabolic rate.* Using the value for GUN, the protein catabolic rate, in grams of protein catabolized per day, can be calculated. The formula can also be adjusted for body size and an allowance for non-urea nitrogen excretion in g/24 hours.

$$PCR = 9.35\ GUN + 0.294\ V_1 \text{ (in liters)} \quad \textbf{(21-9)}$$

5. *Convert the protein catabolic rate to nitrogen balance.* The PCR may be used to estimate protein balance in the usual way:

$$\text{Protein balance} = \text{Protein intake} - (\text{PCR} + \text{protein losses}) \quad \textbf{(21-10)}$$

where all values are in grams/day.

The procedure above may be modified for patients who are stable vs. catabolic, and for patients who are dialyzed vs. nondialyzed. In summary, the equations are (11):

A. Stable, nondialyzed

$$GUN = KrUN \times BUN \quad \textbf{(21-11)}$$

B. Catabolic, nondialyzed

$$GUN = \frac{[(BUN_2 - BUN_1)(Vu)]}{\theta} + KrUN \times BUN \quad \textbf{(21-12)}$$

C. Dialyzed, anuric

$$GUN = \frac{[(Vu_2 \times BUN_2) - (Vu_1 \times BUN_1)]}{\theta} \quad \textbf{(21-13)}$$

D. Dialyzed with some urea losses in urine

$$GUN = [(Vu_2 \times BUN_2) - (Vu_1 \times BUN_1)] + (KrUN \times BUN) \quad \textbf{(21-14)}$$

In dialysis units, computer programs are now used to reduce the need for burdensome calculations and to make possible refinements of these general methods. One of the refinements includes adjustment for the efficiency of the dialyzer. The program provides a value of $\frac{Kt}{V}$ where K is the clearance of the dialyzer, t is time of dialysis, and V is the volume of distribution of urea in the body. A ratio of pre- and post-dialysis BUN of 0.4 yields a $\frac{Kt}{V}$ of 1.0 and is considered to be minimal. Larger values are believed to improve survival rates.

Monitoring Sodium Homeostasis and Fluid Balance

Serum sodium concentration is an indicator of the balance between sodium and water. Used alone, it does not give information on deficiency or excess: it must be combined with other indicators of hydration status.

If weight is stable, *urinary sodium* is an indicator of sodium intake. In nonsteady state, when weight is changing, it may indicate sodium retention with concurrent, fluid retention or sodium wasting.

Daily *urine volume* does not always change with changes in fluid intake in renal disease. It is important that daily volume be known, as well as *any change in volume*. Urine volume should be compared with *fluid intake* and changes in body weight. Intake and output (I & O) of inpatients are recorded in the patient's medical record by the nursing staff.

Blood pressure may also be a useful guide to hydration status. In the absence of hormonal or other lesions, decreased blood pressure may indicate dehydration, while an elevated blood pressure may result from overhydration. Ideally, treatments related to body weight should be based on dry weight—that is, body weight in the absence of excess fluid and the weight above which the patient becomes hypertensive.

Monitoring Potassium Homeostasis

Serum potassium concentration may not rise until the creatinine clearance falls to 20 mL per min or less. However, potassium levels may be increased if the patient takes potassium-containing medications or salt substitutes containing potassium, in severe catabolic disease, in metabolic acidosis, or following blood transfusion. It may rise with very high potassium intake, very low sodium intake, or both.

Monitoring Serum Calcium and Phosphate Homeostasis

Serum ionized calcium is often depressed and serum *phosphate*, elevated in CRF patients. Because these changes lead to severe bone disease, normalization of these values is important. *Increased serum alkaline phosphatase* often signals early renal bone disease. Serum *parathyroid hormone* (PTH) is also monitored. The results must be interpreted in relation to serum calcium. Normal serum calcium and serum PTH of 100 to 600 pg per ml are consistent with normal parathyroid function. In chronic renal disease, secondary hyperparathyroidism is indicated by a serum calcium level less than 9.4 mg per dL and a serum PTH level over 800 pg per mL.

Monitoring Effects of Medications

Renal patients often take substantial amounts of a variety of medications. These may be prescribed or may consist of self-medications with nonprescription drugs. The intake of medications containing sodium or potassium or those affecting phosphate absorption and excretion are of particular interest in nutritional monitoring. Some patients are given phosphate binders by prescription. Patients who become acidotic have increased protein catabolism. This can be corrected by administration of sodium bicarbonate (12, 13). Corticosteroids will also increase protein catabolism in these patients (13). You should inquire about the amount and the time at which these are taken in relation to the time of food intake. Poor compliance with the medication regimen is a common problem and should be investigated.

The composition and function of medications taken

by renal patients should be familiar. Some of the references listed at the end of the introduction of this volume are useful sources of this information.

PREDIALYSIS NUTRITIONAL CARE IN CHRONIC RENAL FAILURE

Depending on the etiology of the disease, the stage of progression of renal failure, and medications being used, CRF patients may require either increases or decreases in dietary protein, sodium, potassium, and fluid. Although energy requirements are not increased, appetite is often depressed, and a concerted effort must be made to ensure normal energy intake. For some patients, phosphorus restriction may also be necessary. You must be able to recognize the indications for the specific modifications and to manipulate the diet to meet these requirements.

PROTEIN MODIFICATIONS

As CRF progresses, the ability of the kidneys to excrete nitrogen metabolites declines, and the concentration of these metabolites in the blood rises, indicating the need for *protein restriction*. On the other hand, patients whose renal disease includes nephrotic syndrome lose protein and may need to *increase* their protein intake. Nitrogen retention and proteinuria can coexist.

Protein restriction is a major, and usually earliest, part of a modified diet for the patient with chronic renal insufficiency (CRI) and then for those with CRF. Some evidence suggests that early restriction of dietary protein slows the progression of renal disease; however, other investigations have indicated that protein restriction is ineffective. The conflicting evidence on this point has been reviewed (14).

A common recommendation for CRI or CRF patients is 0.6 to 0.8 g protein per kilogram of body weight (14, 15). The higher levels within this range are recommended for patients who are malnourished, diabetic, or who have difficulty complying with a more restricted diet. The diets of patients with nephrotic syndrome generally have the amount of their daily urinary protein loss added to the above.

Diets with even lower protein content have been recommended in the past but are no longer commonly used. Occasionally, diets with protein levels as low as 0.3 g/kg body weight are used along with supplements of essential amino acid or their nitrogen-free ketoanalogs.

In addition to the quantity of protein, its quality must be considered. Therefore, 70 to 80 percent of the protein in the diet should be high-biological-value (HBV) protein. HBV proteins are those that contain all essential amino acids in concentrations proportional to the minimum daily amino acid requirements and in which most of the nitrogen is in the form of essential amino acids. When sufficient HBV protein is provided, the patient can meet needs for essential amino acids and use the remaining nitrogen to synthesize those that are nonessential, thus reducing the amount of urea to be excreted.

Egg protein has the highest biological value: 0.94 on a scale of 0 to 1.0. Milk, lean meat, poultry, and fish are also HBV proteins. Eggs and milk have a greater proportion of essential amino acids than do meats, so 10 to 15 g of HBV protein should come from these sources. Gelatin and the plant proteins in grains and vegetables are low in biological value and make up the remaining 20 to 30 percent of the diet protein.

ENERGY INTAKE

The energy needs for CRF patients are highly variable and must be estimated on an individual basis. Sufficient energy must be provided to prevent catabolism of protein for energy in the patient on a protein-restricted diet. If possible, sufficient energy must also be provided to maintain the patient at ideal weight. Calculations of BEE (see Chapter 5) may be used as a baseline and adjusted for activity, the patient's present weight, and stress factors. In general, at least 35 kcal per kg ideal body weight is recommended for patients consuming low-protein diets.

Fewer kcals are given if the patient is *obese*, defined as body weight at least 120 percent of normal weight. Deficient energy intake is common in CRF since patients are often anorectic. Many patients have been found to be malnourished and need an increase in energy intake (16).

Since most staple foods contain protein and cannot be used in larger quantities, additional calories must be derived from those sources of carbohydrate and fat that have been separated from their natural food source. These may be categorized as high-carbohydrate foods lacking in protein and as concentrated fats. Patients frequently complain that the diet is "too sweet and too greasy."

If the patient's fluid prescription will allow, high-carbohydrate, low-protein, low-electrolyte liquid supplements can be used. (Some of these are listed in Table K-2) You must keep in mind, however, that as fluid is restricted, the fluid content of these formulas must be included within the prescribed amount.

Commercial formula products designed to provide energy sources without adding protein or unacceptable amounts of electrolytes are CalPower, Controlyte, Hycal, Maxijul, Moducal, Polycose, Sumacal, Lipomul, and Microlipid. Products designed particularly for use by the renal patient are Alterna, Travasorb Renal, Amin-Aid, Nepro and Suplena. They contain a small amount of protein. These products, including their sodium and potassium content, are described in further detail in Tables K-2 and K-3. In addition, a number of mixtures developed by renal dietitians are valuable for increasing patients' intakes of protein and energy. They provide various levels of sodium, phosphorus, and potassium and thus must be chosen with the patient's total needs in mind. When you counsel renal patients, you will find it useful to make a collection of these recipes.

It is particularly important to provide specific suggestions for increasing energy intake to patients who are underweight. Some examples of strategies for increasing the content of the diet include the following:

1. Add allowed butter or margarine to cooked cereals, vegetables, rice, potatoes, and pasta products.
2. Use butter generously on bread, toast, and rolls.
3. Use cream in place of milk on cereals and in cooking.
4. Use the higher-calorie foods from each choice list.
5. Sweeten beverages, such as tea and coffee, and unsweetened soft drinks in place of water.
6. Add powdered supplements like Polycose or Sumacal to cooked dishes such as casseroles, puddings, and cereals.

All the suggestions listed are not always useful to every patient. You will need to choose those compatible with the limitations of the individual patient's diet.

SODIUM

Sodium-Restricted Diets. The healthy kidney can reabsorb about 99 percent of the sodium filtered by the glomerulus, adjusting the amount reabsorbed to the need. As renal failure progresses, however, the ability to adapt to changes in sodium intake is lost. The objective then becomes to make daily sodium intake equal to daily loss. In practice, dietary intake is adjusted to urinary sodium excretion.

The sodium content of the diet is established at a level to avoid either a large fluid excess or volume depletion. A large fluid excess, with attendant edema, can lead to pulmonary edema and congestive heart failure (CHF). Volume depletion can reduce renal blood flow and further compromise renal function. Therefore, patients are commonly maintained in a slightly edematous state to achieve the maximum possible GFR while avoiding CHF.

A reduction in weight or a drop in blood pressure can indicate the need for a higher sodium intake, provided the patient is not overloaded with fluid. Accompanying decreases in serum or urinary sodium, or both, may also indicate sodium deficit. On the other hand, a sudden increase in body weight or development of hypertension may indicate developing edema and the need to reduce sodium intake to prevent CHF. These may be accompanied by increases in serum or urinary sodium or both.

Most conservatively managed renal patients are maintained on mild sodium restrictions of 2 to 3 g per day. As renal failure progresses, however, the sodium intake may have to be further restricted. For predialysis patients who are not hospitalized, diets containing 1,000 to 3,000 mg per day are commonly recommended as a starting point. See Chapter 20 for information on planning sodium-restricted diets.

Increased Sodium in the Diet

Some patients have a decreased capacity to conserve sodium and a resultant need for increased intake. For these "salt losers," additional sodium can be provided with more highly salted foods, with bouillon cubes (2,500 mg Na per cube), and by generously salting their food. Some patients are given sodium chloride as medication. If a patient becomes severely depleted, the sodium and fluid balance must be corrected intravenously.

MODIFICATIONS IN FLUID INTAKE

The fluid needs of renal disease patients also vary widely. In patients who have lost renal concentrating ability and have polyuria, intake requirements may be 3,000 mL per day to excrete the solute load. If thirst does not stimulate this intake, the prescription may state "force fluids" or "encourage fluids."

If sodium balance is properly maintained, the patient's thirst mechanism may control water balance appropriately (commonly at 1,500 to 3,000 mL of fluid) until the GFR falls to 5 mL per minute or less. It eventually becomes necessary to monitor fluid intake to prevent fluid overload. For the patient who is not dialyzed, the volume of urine output in 24 hours, plus 500 to 750 mL for replacement of insensible losses plus abnormal losses (like vomiting), is considered an appropriate fluid intake once the patient is brought to normal hydration (as indicated by approximately normal blood pressure, normal serum sodium, and absence of edema). Insensible losses may also be estimated as 10 mL per kg body weight. This intake will usually maintain a stable weight. It should be adjusted as necessary if the patient gains or loses weight in a short period. Patients should weigh themselves daily and measure urine output. Each 1,000 mL of retained fluid will add a kg of body weight.

Any intake of 2,000 mL fluid or less per day is considered a restriction. In planning for fluid content of the diet, the following sources of fluids must be counted:

1. Obvious sources of fluids such as drinking water, milk, juices, soups, gruels, coffee, tea, soft drinks, and alcoholic beverages.
2. Syrup or juice served with canned fruit.
3. Foods that are liquid at body temperature, even if they are relatively solid as served, such as gelatin, ice cream and other frozen desserts, and ice; the following are used as the approximate fluid contents of these products:

1/2 c ice cream, ice milk, or sherbet	70 mL
1/2 c Jello or other gelatin	100 mL
1 ice cube	30 mL

4. Foods containing the normal fluid allowance, such as milk in puddings and sauces.

Another source of fluid is the water content of solid food, which can be estimated as 14 mL per 100 kcal. This is considered only if the patient's condition demands a severe fluid restriction with very careful control. This amount is ordinarily considered to counterbalance the insensible losses. Water from metabolism of protein, fat, and carbohydrate is not included in these calculations.

Careful compliance with the sodium restriction tends to limit the feeling of thirst. Some patients do complain of thirst, however, particularly at the more restricted levels. The problem may be worsened when part of the fluid ration must be used for liquid medication or to swallow medications in solid form. For hospitalized patients, the fluid ration for each patient is divided between the dietary department for use in meals and the nursing service for use in administering drugs. If increasing the energy intake is a concern, medications may be taken with the high-calorie, low-protein, low-electrolyte liquids previously described.

The following suggestions can be made to ease the discomfort of the nonhospitalized patient:

Suck on sliced lemon wedges to stimulate saliva.

Use sour hard candy or chewing gum to stimulate saliva.

Rinse the mouth with water but do not swallow it, or use a spray mouth wash.

Freeze allowed fruit juices or water in ice cube trays. Ice is more satisfying because it stays in the mouth longer.

Put lemon juice in ice cubes (a half lemon per tray)

Freeze lemonade into individual popsicles in an ice cube tray.

When thirsty, eat something allowed from the diet. This food may alleviate the dry mouth.

Try eating allowed fruits and vegetables ice cold between meals.

If possible, take medications with liquids allowed at mealtime.

Use very small cups and glasses.

Avoid very-high sodium foods.

POTASSIUM INTAKE

Serum potassium levels that are abnormally low (*hypokalemia*) or abnormally high (*hyperkalemia*) can occur in patients with renal disease. Either can be life-threatening.

Hypokalemia

Hypokalemia as a consequence of inadequate intake is unlikely because potassium is present in most foods. It is more often the consequence of (1) increased losses due to vomiting and diarrhea, or (2) the use of diuretics that cause the kidney to excrete potassium.

Diuretic medications are classified into three categories:

1. Thiazides, which principally decrease sodium reabsorption in the distal tubules

2. Loop diuretics, which decrease NaCl reabsorption in the ascending limb of the loop of Henle and in the proximal tubule

3. Potassium-sparing diuretics, used to prevent the potassium-losing effects of the other two types

Diuretics are used not only in the treatment of renal disease, but also in cardiovascular disease and liver disease.

In general, in nutritional care of the CRF patient receiving diuretics, you need to have information on baseline body weight, BUN, serum creatinine, and serum electrolytes. Fluid intake and output should be monitored, as should body weight. Some considerations are specifically related to the type of diuretic used. Thiazide and loop diuretics can result in hypokalemia. Thiazide diuretics are less frequently used in renal disease since they become ineffective in renal insufficiency at a GFR below 30 mL per minute. Loop diuretics are more commonly used.

If the patient has a tendency to become hypokalemic, treatment is preferably via oral intake, and a potassium supplement is usually prescribed. The least expensive forms of these are the potassium-containing salt substitutes. Some patients on sodium-restricted diets are already using these. An appreciable amount of fluid is needed for the administration of potassium-supplement medications since potassium salts are gastric irritants; this can be an important consideration if the diet is fluid-restricted.

An increase in dietary potassium alone is sometimes sufficient. High-potassium foods that are particularly useful for this purpose are listed in Appendix B, Table 6. It is also helpful to ensure that patients limit their sodium intake since excess sodium excretion increases potassium loss. Precautions must also be taken to ensure that energy intake does not become excessive when foods are added to the diet for the primary purpose of supplying potassium

Hyperkalemia

The kidney maintains its potassium-excreting ability until GFR is severely compromised. Patients who have a Cl_{Cr} over 30 mL per minute usually will not become hyperkalemic, especially if they maintain sufficient urine output. There are exceptions, however; patients who have a catabolic illness in which catabolized cells release intracellular potassium into the extracellular fluid, patients who are acidotic or oliguric, and occasionally, those with a very high potassium intake. Hyperkalemia as a consequence of excess intake alone is unlikely, however. Some drugs, such as penicillin, have a high potassium content. Triamterene (Dyrenium) and spironolactone (Aldactone), the "potassium-sparing" diuretics, can cause severe hyperkalemia and are not used for patients in renal failure.

It is important that serum potassium be kept within normal limits. If necessary, an exchange resin, sodium polystyrene sulfonate (Kayexalate), may be given by mouth. One t contains 7 to 12 g of resin, and each g exchanges approximately 1 mEq of potassium for 1.3 to 1.7 mEq sodium. Since it contributes sodium, it is used cautiously in patients who are volume overloaded. Also, Kayexalate is constipating and is therefore given with an osmotically active substance, such as sorbitol.

Potassium-restricted diets are used to prevent potassium accumulation. In severe failure, patients generally do not receive more than 70 mEq of potassium per day, and some diets are restricted to 40 mEq. Lower levels than these are not achievable over an extended period since potassium is present in most foods. Hyperkalemia which persists when the diet is at 40 mEq per day is an indication for dialysis.

The usual daily intake of potassium is estimated to vary from 2,000 to 6,000 mg per day (50 to 150 mEq). Since meats, milk, vegetables, and fruits are the most concentrated sources, they are the most often restricted.

The potassium content of foods can be altered in processing. In general, more highly refined foods, such as refined cereals, are lower in potassium than are whole grains. Bran and germ are even higher. Similarly, among dairy products, butter and cream products are lower than cheeses, other than cream cheese, while fluid, dried, evaporated, and condensed milk are highest.

Higher-potassium forms of fruits are whole fruits, including raw, dried, or frozen fruits. The potassium level is lowered when fruit is canned if the surrounding liquid, into which potassium is leached, is discarded. The same principle applies to vegetables. The high potassium concentrations in vegetables present a problem in menu planning since only limited amounts of vegetables can be used. This tends to limit vitamin intake from food. In addition, vegetables contribute greatly to the color and general appearance of food. In their absence, the aesthetic value of meals is reduced.

The high potassium content of strong, brewed coffee can be moderated by using a weak, instant coffee. Candies can be low in potassium if they consist primarily of refined sugar and do not contain additions such as chocolate, nuts, coconut, and raisins:

Some other pointers in diet planning:

1. Be certain that energy intake is adequate. Cell breakdown as a consequence of energy deficit releases potassium
2. Distribute potassium-containing foods evenly throughout the day.

Patients should also be encouraged to exercise to the extent possible in order to prevent cell breakdown and promote movement of carbohydrate into cells.

Because potassium restriction becomes necessary only late in renal failure, it is seldom the only diet modification. Instead, it is often combined with protein, sodium, and fluid restriction

PHOSPHORUS, CALCIUM, AND

VITAMIN D INTAKE

Phosphorus is present almost entirely as phosphate and is excreted primarily in the urine. The elevated phosphate and reduced calcium levels in the serum of patients with a GFR less than 20 mL per minute must be controlled in order to avoid renal osteodystrophy. Average adult daily phosphorus intake in the United States is 1.0 to 1.8 g/day (17). In order to control serum phosphorus levels by diet, commonly recommended intakes are 8 to 12 mg/kg ideal body weight (15).

Phosphorus is contained primarily in protein foods; therefore, low-protein diets tend to be low in phosphorus. Conversely, it becomes more difficult to control phosphorus levels in the diet if the protein level is higher.

The following are some general guidelines for planning a phosphorus-controlled diet:

1. Omit milk, yogurt, and ice cream. Substitute nondairy cream products, such as Mocha Mix, Poly-Perx, Coffee-Rich, Cool Whip, Dessert Whip, or Rich's Whip Topping.
2. Use meat, fish, poultry, and egg only in amounts compatible with reduced protein intake.
3. Exclude whole-grain cereals or breads and any products containing bran.
4. Exclude dried beans and peas.
5. Omit beverages made with milk, cola beverages, and powdered fruit beverage mixes.

A diet containing 50 g protein will contain 700 to 800 mg phosphorus with the above guidelines. A 40 g protein diet contains 500 to 600 mg phosphorus (18). Efforts to restrict phosphorus intake further interfere with the ability to reach desired protein and energy intakes. In addition, the diet becomes unpalatable since so many foods must be excluded. Therefore, as renal function falls to 60 to 30 ml/minute and phosphate levels continue to rise, phosphate-binding compounds are used to decrease phosphate absorption from the gastrointestinal tract.

When phosphate binders are prescribed, calcium-containing products are used initially. The products used are calcium acetate or calcium carbonate. Citrate is not used because it increases aluminum absorption from the gut.

These binders should be taken with meals, and the total daily dose should be distributed, as is the phosphorus in the meals in order to avoid hypercalcemia. The nutritional care specialist should monitor the serum calcium level until a stable level is reached.

Other phosphate binders are aluminum-based. These are usually less often used because aluminum accumulates and becomes toxic to the nervous and skeletal systems. However, they may be prescribed for a short period for patients with severe hyperparathyroidism and a high calcium-phosphorus product. It is important that these patients avoid citrate (calcium citrate, Alka-Seltzer, *and fruit juices*). Constipation is a common side effect, so patients may also be given a bulk laxative and a stool softener.

Calcium intake in CRF patients is usually low because of the restriction of calcium-rich foods containing large amounts of protein, phosphorus, and sometimes fluid. In addition, intestinal absorption of calcium is defective in renal failure (17), in part because of a low level of vitamin D.

In order to correct the calcium deficiency, the first step is to reduce serum phosphorus to avoid soft tissue calcification. Then, a calcium supplement, usually 1 to 2 g per day, is given. A common dose for undialyzed patients with GFR between 40 and 10 mL/minute is 1.2 to 1.5 g calcium carbonate b.i.d. with meals to provide 40 percent calcium (1,200 mg per day) (17). Alternatives are calcium acetate, calcium citrate (but not given to patients receiving aluminum salts), calcium chloride (not used in acidosis), calcium lactate, calcium gluconate, or calcium gluconogalactogluconate (useful for small children but costly).

Vitamin D is also given in some form. Vitamin D_3 as it first appears in serum is cholecalciferol or 7-dehydrocholecholesterol. Hydroxylation in the liver forms 25-hydroxycholecalciferol, also known as 25-hydroxyvitamin D, $25(OH)D_3$, 25-HCC. Further hydroxylation in the kidney forms the active metabolite, 1,25-dihydroxycholecalciferol, also known as 1,25-dihydroxyvitamin D, $1,25$-$(OH)_2D_3$, 1,25-DHCC, or calcitriol.

Treatment with the active form of the vitamin, calcitriol (Rocaltrol), is postponed until serum phosphorus is normalized. It then begins with 0.25 to 0.5 μg/day by mouth. Serum calcium levels are monitored. If they do not rise to normal within 4 to 6 weeks, the 1,25-DHCC dose is increased by similar increments until serum calcium is normal. It is also important to monitor serum phosphorus levels to be sure that the calcium-phosphorus product (mg serum Ca/mL $\times$ mg serum P/mL) does not exceed 55 (17).

IRON INTAKE

Anemia almost always occurred in patients with CRF and was treated with blood transfusion. The patients then became iron overloaded. Since 1985, recombinant human erythropoietin (rH-EPO) has been available for treatment, and transfusions are less often given. With the use of EPO, iron stores must be monitored since erythropoietin is not effective in iron deficiency. If iron supplements are needed, they are preferably given orally. Parenteral iron increases the risk of iron overload because the intestinal barrier mechanisms are bypassed. Serum ferritin assay is used to monitor iron stores. Serum ferritin >300 μg/mL indicates overload. For a uremic patient, 50 to 100 μg/mL is normal. In nonuremic persons, normal is 12 to 30 μg/mL.

LIPIDS

A variety of hyperlipidemias may develop in CRF patients. The most common type is hypertriglyceridemia. Its management is described in Chapter 20. The mechanisms involved are not well understood (19).

VITAMINS

Vitamin A is not given, since vitamin A does not dialyze, resulting in elevated serum vitamin A levels. Vitamin E may not need to be supplemented.

Water-soluble vitamins are supplemented daily as follows (20); 1.5 mg thiamin, 1.8 mg riboflavin, and 60 to 100 mg ascorbic acid. Sometimes, but not always, 1 mg folic acid, 20 mg niacin, 5 mg pantothenic acid, and 3 μg vitamin B_{12} are also prescribed.

ALKALINIZING AGENTS

Many CRF patients develop mild metabolic acidosis due to a decreased ability to excrete hydrogen ions, loss of bicarbonate, and retention of fixed anions, such as sulfate and phosphate. The restricted dietary protein reduces acid production. Calcium carbonate to correct calcium deficiency and to bind intestinal phosphate also contributes to correction of acidosis. Some patients require sodium bicarbonate medications in addition.

PROCEDURES IN CALCULATING RENAL DIETS

The steps in planning renal diets are similar in principle to those for planning diabetic diets, but are more complex. Renal diets must consider more nutrients simultaneously. In addition, the diets often must be adjusted more frequently as the disease progresses. To provide uniformity and guidance, *The National Renal Diet* (NRD) has been developed for use by patients with renal disease and by health professionals who care for or counsel these patients.

The NRD consists of a professional guide (15) along with six booklets for clients. These booklets are for pre-end stage renal disease (20), hemodialysis (21), and peritoneal dialysis (22). Since more than 30 percent of renal failure patients are diabetic, the three other booklets (23–25) are for patients at the same three stages of renal disease, but with accompanying diabetes.

The NRD divides foods into groups according to their nutrient content, in a manner similar to that used for the diabetic exchange lists. The lists are referred to as *choices* rather than *exchanges*. The values for the lists of choices for renal disease patients are given in Table 21-3 for nondiabetics and Table 21-4 for diabetics.

The list of *milk choices* is given in Table 21-5. Because these foods are high in potassium and phosphorus, the serving size is 1/2 cup rather than the whole cup usually used as a diabetic exchange.

As an alternative to milk in meal planning, a list of *nondairy milk substitutes* (Table 21-6) is given. These items contain less protein, phosphorus, and potassium, compared to the milk choices, and are useful to increase the energy content of the diet.

The *meat choice* list (Table 21-7) contains meats, poultry, fish, and eggs. *All are prepared without adding salt.* In addition, some items are prepared with salt and count as a meat choice *plus* one salt choice. These are

TABLE 21-3   Average Calculation Figures for Nondiabetic Renal Diets

Food Choices*	kcal	Pro (g)	CHO (g)	Fat (g)	Na (mg)	K (mg)	P (mg)
Milk	120	4.0	12	6	80	185	110
Nondairy Milk Substitute	140	0.5	12	10	40	80	30
Meat	65	7.0	—	4	25	100	65
Starch	90	2.0	18	1	80	35	35
Vegetable							
Low K	25	1.0	5	Trace	15	70	20
Medium K	25	1.0	5	Trace	15	150	20
High K	25	1.0	5	Trace	15	270	20
Fruit							
Low K	70	0.5	17	—	Trace	70	15
Medium K	70	0.5	17	—	Trace	150	15
High K	70	0.5	17	—	Trace	270	15
Fat	45	—	—	5	55	10	5
High-Calorie	100	Trace	25	—	15	20	5
Beverage	Varies	Varies	Varies	Varies	Varies	Varies	Varies
Salt	—	—	—	—	250	—	—

*Serving sizes for each choice are shown in the client booklets.
Reprinted with permission from: Renal Dietitians Dietetic Practice Group of The American Dietetic Association. *National Renal Diet*. Chicago,: American Dietetic Association, 1993.

TABLE 21-4   Average Calculation Figures for Diabetic Renal Diets

Food Choices*	kcal	Pro (g)	CHO (g)	Fat (g)	Na (mg)	K (mg)	P (mg)
Milk	100	4.0	8	5	80	185	110
Nondairy Milk Substitute	140	0.5	12	10	40	80	30
Meat	65	7.0	—	4	25	100	65
Starch	80	2.0	15	1	80	35	35
Vegetable							
Low K	25	1.0	5	Trace	15	70	20
Medium K	25	1.0	5	Trace	15	150	20
High K	25	1.0	5	Trace	15	270	20
Fruit							
Low K	60	0.5	15	—	Trace	70	15
Medium K	60	0.5	15	—	Trace	150	15
High K	60	0.5	15	—	Trace	270	15
Fat	45	—	—	5	55	10	5
High-Calorie	60	Trace	15	—	15	20	5
Beverage	Varies	Varies	Varies	Varies	Varies	Varies	Varies
Salt	—	—	—	—	250	—	—

*Serving sizes for each food choice are shown in the client booklets.
Reprinted with permission from: Renal Dietitians Dietetic Practice Group of The American Dietetic Association. *National Renal Diet*. Chicago,: American Dietetic Association, 1993.

indicated by a symbol representing a saltshaker. Items particularly high in phosphorus (>100 mg) are indicated with a symbol representing a bone. The decision to use sparingly or to avoid high-sodium and high-phosphorus items should depend on an individual patient's condition. Foods particularly contraindicated for most patients include dried peas and beans and legumes, bacon, sausages, prepared luncheon meats such as cold cuts, nuts, nut butters, and any cheese, with the exception of cottage cheese.

Starch choices (Table 21-8) include breads, crackers, cereals, pastas, high carbohydrate vegetables, and most flour-based baked goods. Because of the high-phosphorus content of whole grains, the items on the list are highly refined. High-phosphorus (>70 mg) and high-sodium items are indicated with the same symbols used in the list of meat choices. All items should be prepared without salt.

Vegetable choices (Table 21-9) for nondialyzed patients lists vegetables in three serving sizes. Items relatively low in potassium are listed in one-cup servings; medium-potassium choices are listed in 1/2-cup servings, and higher-potassium choices are in 1/4 cup servings. All but a few are prepared or canned without added salt.

Vegetables canned with salt are counted as a vegetable choice plus one salt choice. Other exceptions are:

TABLE 21-5   Milk Choices

	choices per day
Average per choice: 4 g protein, 120 calories, 80 mg sodium, 110 mg phosphorus	
Milk (nonfat, low fat, whole)	1/2 cup
Lo Pro	1 cup
Buttermilk, cultured	1/2 cup
Chocolate milk	1/2 cup
Light cream or half-and-half	1/2 cup
Ice milk or ice cream	1/2 cup
Yogurt, plain or fruit flavored	1/2 cup
Evaporated milk	1/4 cup
Sweetened condensed milk	1/4 cup
Cream cheese	3 tablespoons
Sour cream	4 tablespoons
Sherbet	1 cup

Reprinted with permission from: Renal Dietitians Dietetic Practice Group of The American Dietetic Association. *National Renal Diet*. Chicago: American Dietetic Association, 1993.

TABLE 21-6 Nondairy Milk Substitutes

	choices per day
Average per choice: 0.5 g protein, 140 calories, 40 mg sodium, 30 mg phosphorus	
Dessert, nondairy frozen	1/2 cup
Dessert topping, nondairy frozen	1/2 cup
Liquid nondairy creamer, polyunsaturated	1/2 cup

Reprinted with permission from: Renal Dietitians Dietetic Practice Group of The American Dietetic Association. *National Renal Diet.* Chicago: American Dietetic Association, 1993.

> 1/2 cup sauerkraut = 1 vegetable plus 3 salt choices
> 1/2 cup tomato juice canned with salt = 1 vegetable + 2 salt choices
> 1/2 cup vegetable juice cocktail canned with salt = 1 vegetable + 2 salt choices

Symbols also indicate that parsnips and rutabagas are particularly high in phosphorus.

For dialysis patients, the lists of vegetable choices are more detailed to allow for closer limits on potassium intake (Table 21-10). All serving sizes are 1/2 cup for each choice. Vegetables are then reclassified in three groups. These are low potassium (0 to 100 mg) or medium potassium (101 to 200 mg) with corn, canned mushrooms, green peas, and snow peas indicated as high phosphorus, and sauerkraut again including three salt choices. The third group of choices are high in potassium (201 to 300 mg) and include those that are high in phosphorus (> 40 mg): asparagus, Brussels sprouts, mushrooms, okra, parsnips, rutabaga, spinach, and sweet potatoes. High-salt items are indicated, as they are for nondialyzed patients.

In addition, some vegetables listed in the starch choices for nondialyzed patients are included as vegetables for patients whose renal disease has progressed sufficiently to require dialysis. Potatoes, squashes, some greens, and a few other vegetables are marked with a symbol showing they are "very high potassium" (301 to 350 mg).

Fruit choices (Table 21-11) are listed for nondialysis patients in subcategories similar to those used for vegetables, that is, in 1 cup, 1/2 cup, and 1/4 cup servings. In cases where cup measures are inappropriate, measures are given by the piece or fraction thereof (e.g., 5 prunes, 1/8 small cantaloupe, 1/2 grapefruit).

For dialyzed patients, fruits (Table 21-12) are divided into the same three categories of low (0 to 100 mg), medium (101 to 200 mg), and high (201 to 300 mg) potassium. Most servings are 1/2 cup, with the few exceptions indicated in the table. Symbols also indicate that 1/2 medium banana, 1/2 cup prune juice, and 5 prunes are "very high potassium" (301 to 350 mg).

Fat choices (Table 21-13) list items as unsaturated or saturated fats. Further discussion of fat saturation and its significance is contained in Chapter 20.

High-calorie choices (Table 21-14) provide about 100 kcal each with little protein. Since many CRF patients

TABLE 21-7 Meat Choices*

	choices per day
Average per choice: 7 g protein, 65 calories, 25 mg sodium, 65 mg phosphorus	
Prepared without added salt	
Beef	1 ounce
Round, sirloin, flank, cubed, T-bone, and porterhouse steak; tenderloin, rib, chuck, and rump roast; ground beef or ground chuck	
Pork	1 ounce
Fresh ham, tenderloin, chops, loin roast, cutlets	
Lamb	1 ounce
Chops, leg, roasts	
Veal	1 ounce
Chops, roasts, cutlets	
Poultry	1 ounce
Chicken, turkey, Cornish hen, domestic duck and goose	
Fish	
Fresh and frozen fish	1 ounce
Lobster, scallops, shrimp, clams	1 ounce
Crab, oysters	1 1/2 ounce
Canned tuna, canned salmon (canned without salt)	1 ounce
Sardines (canned without salt)	1 ounce
Wild game	1 ounce
Venison, rabbit, squirrel, pheasant, duck, goose	
Egg	
Whole	1 large
Egg white or yolk	2 large
Low-cholesterol egg product	1/4 cup
Chitterlings	2 ounce
Organ meats	1 ounce
Prepared with added salt	
Beef	
Deli-style roast beef	1 ounce
Pork	
Boiled or deli-style ham	1 ounce
Poultry	
Deli-style chicken or turkey	1 ounce
Fish	
Canned tuna, canned salmon	1 ounce
Sardines	1 ounce
Cheese, Cottage	1/4 cup

The following are high in sodium, phosphorous, and/or saturated fat. They should be used in your diet only as advised by your dietitian.

> Bacon
> Black beans, black-eyed peas, great northern beans, lentils, lima beans, navy beans, pinto beans, red kidney beans, soybeans, split peas, turtle beans
> Frankfurters, bratwurst, Polish sausage
> Luncheon meats, including bologna, braunschweiger, liverwurst, picnic loaf, summer sausage, salami
> Nuts and nut butters
> All cheeses except cottage cheese

*High sodium: each serving counts as 1 meat choice and 1 salt choice.

High phosphorus

Reprinted with permission from: Renal Dietitians Dietetic Practice Group of the American Dietetic Association. *National Renal Diet.* Chicago, IL: American Dietetic Association, 1993.

TABLE 21-8 Starch Choices*

Average per choice: 2 g protein, 90 calories, 80 mg sodium, 35 mg phosphorus

Breads and rolls

Bread (French, Italian, raisin, light rye, sourdough, white	1 slice, (1 ounce)
Bagel	1/2 small
Bun, hamburger or hot dog type	1/2
Danish pastry or sweet roll, no nuts	1/2 small
Dinner roll or hard roll	1 small
Doughnut	1 small
English muffin	1/2
Muffin, no nuts, bran, or whole-wheat	1 small (1 ounce)
Pancake	1 small (1 ounce)
Pita or "pocket" bread	1/2 6-in diameter
Tortilla, corn	2 6-in diameter
Tortilla, flour	1 6-in diameter
Waffle	1 small (1 ounce)

Cereals and grains prepared without added salt

Cereals, ready-to-eat, most brands	3/4 cup
Puffed rice	2 cups
Puffed wheat	1 cup
Cereals, cooked	
Cream of Rice or Wheat, Farina, Malt-O-Meal	1/2 cup
	1/2 cup
Oat bran or oatmeal, Ralston	1/3 cup
Cornmeal, cooked	3/4 cup
Grits, cooked	1/2 cup
Flour, all-purpose	2 1/2 tablespoons
Pasta (noodles, macaroni, spaghetti), cooked	1/2 cup
Pasta made with egg (egg noodles), cooked	1/3 cup
Rice, white or brown, cooked	1/2 cup

Starchy vegetables prepared or canned without added salt

Corn	1/3 cup or 1/2 ear
Green peas	1/4 cup
Potatoes, boiled or mashed	1/2 cup
Potatoes, baked, white or sweet	1 small (3 ounces)
Potatoes, French fried	1/2 cup or 10 small
Potatoes, hashed brown	1/2 cup
Squash, butternut, mashed	1/2 cup
Squash, winter, baked (all other varieties), cubed	1 cup

Crackers and snacks

Crackers: saltines, round butter	4 crackers
Graham crackers	3 squares
Melba toast	3 oblong
RyKrisp	3 crackers
Popcorn, plain	1 1/2 cup popped
Potato chips	1 ounce, 14 chips
Tortilla chips	3/4 ounce, 9 chips
Pretzels, sticks or rings	3/4 ounce, 10 sticks
Pretzels, sticks or rings, unsalted	3/4 ounce, 10 sticks

Desserts

Cake, angel food	1/20 cake or 1 ounce
Cake	2x2-in square or 1 1/2 ounce
Sandwich cookie	4 cookies
Shortbread cookie	4 cookies
Sugar cookie	4 cookies
Sugar wafer	4 cookies
Vanilla wafer	10 cookies
Fruit pie	1/8 pie
Sweetened gelatin	1/2 cup

(continued)

TABLE 21-8 *(continued)*

The following foods are high in poor-quality protein and/or phosphorus. They should be used only when advised by your dietitian. Bran cereal or muffins, Grape-Nuts cereal, granola cereal or bars; boxed, frozen, or canned meals, entrees, or side dishes

Black beans, black-eyed peas, great northern beans, lentils, lima beans, navy beans, pinto beans, red kidney beans, soybeans, split peas, turtle beans; Pumpernickel, dark rye, whole-wheat, or oatmeal bread, Whole-wheat cereals, Whole-wheat crackers

*High sodium—each serving counts as 1 Starch choice and 1 Salt choice

High phosphorus

Reprinted with permission from: Renal Dietians Dietetic Practice Group of The American Dietetic Association. *National Renal Diet.* Chicago, IL: American Dietetic Association, 1993.

are malnourished with poor appetites, these items may be included in the diet to provide additional energy. Categories included are candies and other sweets, frozen desserts, and beverages that must be included in the fluid ration if fluid is restricted.

Salt choices (Table 21-15) average 250 mg of sodium for each. It is assumed that salt is not used in food preparation. These choices may be used to provide controlled amounts of sodium and are particularly useful for "salt losers."

Beverage choices (Table 21-16) are included in the diet for patients who must restrict fluid, potassium and phosphorus, that is, patients who are on dialysis.

Alternative protein sources (Table 21-17) are listed for patients who are strict vegetarians. These items are not recommended for nonvegetarians since they contain incomplete proteins with high levels of nonessential amino acids. The legumes on the list are cooked without salt, with a 1/2 cup serving in each choice. If cooked with salt, the 1/2 cup also counts for two salt choices.

A few nuts, *unsalted*, are also listed as choices in the amounts given in the table. If salted, they also count as one salt choice.

CALCULATING THE DIET PLAN

The process of calculating the renal diet often requires more trial and error than is the case with the diabetic exchange lists described in Chapter 19. However, the following sequence of steps is usually effective:

1. Calculate the desired amount of HBV protein.
2. Using the average values for each group in Table 21-5, determine the number of choices of meat, egg, and milk from each group (meat and dairy lists) to provide the HBV protein. Remember that one egg is usually included because of the high biological value of eggs.
3. Using the average values for each group, determine the number of choices of fruits, vegetables, starch and nondairy milk substitutes to provide the LBV protein, sodium, potassium and phosphorus. (Acceptable range: Na ± 10 mg; K ± 5 mg.)
4. Add to find totals of kilocalories, protein, sodium, potassium, phosphorus, and fluid. Alter step 3 if any

TABLE 21-9   Vegetable Choices for Nondialysis Patients[*]

choices per day

See Starch Choices for other vegetables
Average per choice: 1 g protein, 5 g carbohydrate, 25 calories,
   15 mg sodium, 20 mg phosphorus

Prepared or canned without added salt unless otherwise indicated

1-cup serving

Alfalfa sprouts	Escarole
Cabbage	Lettuce, all varieties
Celery	Pepper, green, sweet
Cucumber (or 1/2 whole)	Radishes, sliced (or 15 small)
Eggplant	Turnips
Endive	Watercress

1/2-cup serving

Artichoke	Onions
Bamboo shoots	Parsnips ↗
Bean sprouts	Pumpkin
Beans, green or wax	Rutabagas ⬥
Beets	Sauerkraut ⬥ ⬥ ⬥
Carrots (or 1 small)	Squash, summer
Cauliflower	Tomato (or 1 medium)
Chard	Tomato juice, unsalted
Chinese cabbage	Tomato juice, canned with salt ⬥ ⬥
Collards	Tomato puree
Kale	Turnip greens
Kohlrabi	Vegetable juice cocktail, unsalted
Mushrooms, fresh raw	Vegetable juice cocktail, canned
(or 4 medium)	with salt ⬥ ⬥

1/4-cup serving

Asparagus (or 2 spears)	Mushrooms, fresh, cooked
Avocado (1/4 whole)	Mustard greens
Beet greens	Okra
Broccoli	Snow peas
Brussels sprouts	Spinach
Chili pepper	Tomato sauce

Prepared or canned with salt
Vegetables canned with salt (use serving size listed above) ⬥

⬥   [*] High sodium: each serving counts as 1 vegetable choice and 1 salt choice

⬥ ⬥   High sodium: each serving counts as 1 vegetable choice and 2 salt choices

⬥ ⬥ ⬥   High sodium: each serving counts as 1 vegetable choice and 3 salt choices

↗   High phosphorus

Reprinted with permission from: Renal Dietitians Dietetic Practice Group of The American Dietetic Association. *National Renal Diet.* Chicago, IL: American Dietetic Association, 1993.

values are in excess of prescription or are insufficient.
5. Add sources of additional kcals from fat choices and high-calorie choices.
6. Add items from among the "salt" choices if necessary to reach the prescribed sodium intake.
7. Add desired beverages, if possible, within prescribed fluid intake.
Note: For patients who are not restricted in fluid and potassium, that part of the above may be disregarded.
   In calculating the menu pattern, a small amount of variation from the prescribed diet is allowable for ease of calculation. The amount varies from one center to

TABLE 21-10   Vegetable Choices for Dialysis Patients[*]

choices per day

Average per choice: 1 g protein, 5 g carbohydrate, 25 calories,
   15 mg sodium, 20 mg phosphorus

1/2 cup per choice unless otherwise indicated

Prepared or canned without added salt unless otherwise indicated

Low potassium (0-100 milligrams)

Alfalfa sprouts (1 cup)	Cucumber, peeled
Bamboo shoots, canned	Endive
Beans, green or wax	Escarole
Bean sprouts	Lettuce, all varieties (1 cup)
Cabbage, raw	Pepper, green, sweet
Chinese cabbage, raw	Water chestnuts, canned
Chard, raw	Watercress

Medium potassium (101-200 milligrams)

Artichoke	Mustard greens
Broccoli	Onions
Cabbage, cooked	Peas, green ↗
Carrots, raw (1 small)	Radishes
Cauliflower	Sauerkraut ⬥ ⬥ ⬥
Celery, raw (1 stalk)	Snow peas ↗
Collards	Spinach
Corn (1/2 ear) ↗	Turnip greens
Eggplant	Turnips
Kale	
Mushrooms, canned ↗	
or fresh raw	

High potassium (201-350 milligrams)

Asparagus (5 spears) ↗	Tomato puree (2 tablespoons)
Avocado (1/4 whole	Tomato sauce (1/4 cup)
Beets ↗	Vegetable juice cocktail unsalted
Brussels sprouts	Vegetable juice cocktail
Celery, cooked	cannned with salt ⬥ ⬥
Kohlrabi	Bamboo shoots,
Mushrooms, fresh cooked ↗	fresh cooked ☙
Okra ↗	Beet greens (1/4 cup) ☙
Parsnips	Chard, cooked ☙
Pepper, chili	Chinese cabbage, cooked ☙
Potato, boiled or mashed	Potato, baked (1/2 medium) ☙
Pumpkin ↗	Potato, hashed brown ☙
Rutabagas	Potato chips
Tomato (1 medium)	(1 ounce, 14 chips) ☙
Tomato juice, unsalted	Spinach, cooked ↗ ☙
Tomato juice,	Sweet potato ↗ ☙
canned with salt ⬥ ⬥	Tomato paste (2 tablespoons ☙
	Winter squash (1/4 cup) ☙

Prepared or canned with salt
Vegetables canned with salt (use serving size listed above) ⬥

⬥   [*]High sodium: each serving counts as 1 vegetable choice and 1 salt choice.

⬥ ⬥   High sodium: each serving counts as 1 vegetable choice and 2 salt choices.

⬥ ⬥ ⬥   High sodium: each serving counts as 1 vegetable choice and 3 salt choices.

↗   High phosphorous
☙   Very high potassium

Reprinted with permission from: Renal Dietitians Dietetic Practice Group of The American Dietetic Association. *National Renal Diet.* Chicago, IL: American Dietetic Association, 1993.

another and also with the condition of the patient. For example, the policy at a given center might be to allow

TABLE 21-11 Fruit Choices for Nondialysis Patients

choices per day

Average per choice: 0.5 g protein, 70 calories, 20 mg phosphorus

1-cup serving

Apple (1 medium)	Papaya nectar
Apple juice	Peach nectar
Applesauce	Pear nectar
Cranberries	Pear, canned or fresh (1 medium)
Cranberry juice cocktail	Tangerine (1 medium)

1/2-cup serving

Apricot nectar	Lemon (1/2 medium)
Banana (1/2 small)	Lemon juice
Blueberries	Mango (1/2 medium)
Figs, canned	Nectarine (1/2 medium)
Fruit cocktail	Orange (1/2 medium)
Grapes (15 small)	Peach, canned or fresh (1/2 medium)
Grape juice	Pineapple
Grapefruit (1/2 medium)	Plums, canned or fresh (1 medium)
Grapefruit juice	Rhubarb
Gooseberries	Strawberries
Kiwifruit (1/2 medium)	Watermelon

1/4-cup serving

Apricots (2 halves)	Honeydew melon (1/8 small)
Apricots, dried (2)	Orange juice
Blackberries	Papaya (1/4 medium)
Cantaloupe (1/8 small)	Prune juice
Cherries	Prunes, cooked (5)
Dates (2 tablespoons)	Raisins (2 tablespoons
Figs, dried (1 whole)	Raspberries

Reprinted with permission from: Renal Dietitians Dietetic Practice Group of The American Dietetic Association. *National Renal Diet*. Chicago, IL: American Dietetic Association, 1993.

TABLE 21-12 Fruit Choices for Dialysis Patients[*]

choices per day

Average per choice: 0.5 g protein, 70 calories, 15 mg phosphorous

1/2 cup per choice unless otherwise indicated

Low potassium (0–100 milligrams)

Applesauce	Lemon (1/2)
Blueberries	Papaya nectar
Cranberries (1 cup)	Peach nectar
Cranberry juice cocktail (1 cup)	Pears, canned
Grape juice	Pear nectar

Medium potassium (101–200 milligrams)

Apple (1 small, 2 1/2-in diameter)	Mango
Apple juice	Papaya
Apricot nectar	Peach, canned
Blackberries	Peach, fresh (1 small, 2-in diameter)
	Pineapple, canned or fresh
Cherries, sour or sweet	Plums, canned or fresh (1 medium)
Figs, canned	Raisins (2 tablespoons)
Fruit cocktail	Raspberries
Grapes (15 small)	Rhubarb
Grapefruit (1/2 small)	Strawberries
Grapefruit juice	Tangerine (2 1/2-in diameter)
Gooseberries	Watermelon (1 cup)
Lemon juice	

High potassium (201–350 milligrams)

Apricots, canned or fresh (2 halves)	Nectarine (1 small, 2-in diameter)
Apricots, dried (5)	Orange juice
Cantaloupe (1/8 small)	Orange (1 small, 2 1/2-in diameter)
Dates (1/4 cup)	Pear, fresh (1 medium) ☙
Figs, dried (2 whole)	Banana (1/2 medium) ☙
Honeydew melon (1/8 small)	Prune juice ☙
Kiwifruit (1/2 medium)	Prunes, dried or canned (5) ☙

☙ , [*] Very high potassium

Reprinted with permission from: Renal Dietitians Dietetic Practice Group of The American Dietetic Association. *National Renal Diet*. Chicago, IL: American Dietetic Association, 1993.

the protein intake to differ from the prescription by ± 2 g for nondialyzed patients and ± 5 g for hemodialysis patients. On the other hand, if a patient has a problem controlling the urea level, perhaps only the prescribed amount or 5 g less, but not more, would be acceptable. The proportion of HBV should vary toward the high side.

After calculations described above, a meal plan should be planned for the patient. The plan should be based as much as possible on the patient's preferences and usual eating habits.

An example of a prescription and calculation of the exchanges is shown in Table 21-18.

NUTRITIONAL CARE IN HEMODIALYSIS

The same nutrients are of concern in hemodialysis (HD), but the requirements vary, as do the standards used in monitoring the patient. The same methods for planning the diet and the same lists of choices are used.

PROTEIN MODIFICATION

Hemodialysis patients are often malnourished when they begin dialysis. Many are also debilitated because they

have concurrent catabolic conditions (26). The hemodialyzed patient also loses amino acids and peptides to the equivalent of 10 to 13 g of amino acids (27) per dialysis. As a consequence, one common recommendation for protein intake, provided body weight is within the normal range, is 1.2 to 1.4 g per kg body weight, with 50 percent of HBV protein (28). This recommendation is based on *dry* body weight, that is, body weight postdialysis. Higher levels are used for repletion.

In monitoring the patient, a common objective is to maintain the BUN at 60 to 80 mg per dL following the longest interdialytic interval. Some dialysis centers aim for values under 100 mg per dL. In the stable patient, BUN will correlate with protein intake, but it is not expected that BUN levels will be normal.

The following are some useful guidelines for patient monitoring:

A BUN value over 100 mg/dL and maintenance of weight suggest excess protein intake.

If BUN is unusually elevated, but other values are as

TABLE 21-13 Fat Choices*

	choices per day
Average per choice: trace protein, 45 calories, 55 mg sodium, 5 mg phosphorus	
Unsaturated fats	
Margarine	1 teaspoon
Reduced-calorie margarine	1 tablespoon
Mayonnaise	1 teaspoon
Low-calorie mayonnaise	1 tablespoon
Oil (safflower, sunflower, corn, soybean, olive, peanut, canola)	1 teaspoon
Salad dressing (mayonnaise-type)	2 teaspoons
Salad dressing (oil-type)	1 tablespoon
Low-calorie salad dressing (mayonnaise-type)	2 tablespoon
Low-calorie salad dressing (oil-type)	2 tablespoons
Tartar sauce	1 1/2 teaspoon
Saturated fats	
Butter	1 teaspoon
Coconut	2 tablespoons
Powdered coffee whitener	1 tablespoon
Solid shortening	1 teaspoon

* High sodium: each serving counts as 1 fat choice and 1 salt choice
Reprinted with permission from: Renal Dietitians Dietetic Practice Group of The American Dietetic Association. *National Renal Diet.* Chicago, IL: American Dietetic Association, 1993.

expected, the patient is probably taking too much low-biological-value (LBV) protein.

If BUN and phosphate are elevated without other increases, look for excessive cheese intake.

Increased BUN, potassium, and phosphate are usually the result of too much total protein, often in the form of meat and milk.

Weight loss with high BUN indicates protein catabolism.

If BUN is relatively low for a CRF patient, and if serum albumin is also low, inadequate protein intake may be indicated. Weight should be checked, and the degree of edema should be noted.

If a patient is inadequately dialyzed, there is a tendency to anorexia. The resulting decrease in food intake leads to protein malnutrition and a lower BUN. In these circumstances, dialysis may be increased and often results in a spontaneous increase in protein intake (29).

ENERGY INTAKE

Energy requirements do not differ from those recommended during predialysis management, that is, 35 to 40 kcal per kg ideal body weight. The energy intake must be sufficient to spare protein for tissue formation and to maintain normal dry body weight. Wasting often continues in dialysis patients, not only from loss of nutrients in the dialysis fluid but also because some patients are nauseated during and for several hours after dialysis and are unable to eat. If the amount of activity changes when

TABLE 21-14 High Calorie Choices*

	choices per day
Average per choice: trace protein, 100 calories, 15 mg sodium, 5 mg phosphorus	
Beverages	
Carbonated beverages (fruit flavors, root beer; colas or pepper-type)	1 cup
Kool-Aid	1 cup
Limeade	1 cup
Lemonade	1 cup
Cranberry juice cocktail	1 cup
Tang	1 cup
Fruit-flavored drink	1 cup
Wine †	1/2 cup
Frozen desserts	
Fruit ice	1/2 cup
Popsicle (3 ounces)	1 bar
Juice bar (3 ounces)	1 bar
Sorbet	1/2 cup
Candy and sweets	
Butter mints	14
Candy corn	20 or 1 ounce
Chewy fruit snacks	1 pouch
Cranberry sauce or relish	1/4 cup
Fruit chews	4
Fruit Roll Ups	2
Gumdrops	15 small
Honey	2 tablespoons
Hard candy	4 pieces
Jam or jelly	2 tablespoons
Jelly beans	10
LifeSavers or cough drops	12
Marmalade	2 tablespoons
Marshmallows	5 large
Sugar, brown or white	2 tablespoons
Sugar, powdered	3 tablespoons
Syrup	2 tablespoons
Special low-protein products	
Ask your dietitian for information on how to obtain these products	
Low-protein gelled dessert	1/2 cup
Low-protein bread	1 slice
Low-protein cookies	2
Low-protein pasta	1/2 cup
Low-protein rusk	2 slices

*The following foods are high in poor-quality protein and/or phosphorous. They should be used only when advised by your dietitian.
   Beer†
   Chocolate
   Nuts and nut butters
   High phosphorus
† Check with your physician before using alcohol

Reprinted with permission from: Renal Dietitians Dietetic Practice Group of The American Dietetic Association. *National Renal Diet.* Chicago, IL: American Dietetic Association, 1993.

the patient is being dialyzed, energy intake must also be modified.

To replace lost glucose, it is common to include 200 mg of glucose per deciliter of dialysis solution. To

TABLE 21-15   Salt Choices

	choices per day
Average per choice: 250 mg sodium	
Salt	1/8 teaspoon
Seasoned salts (onion, garlic, etc.)	1/8 teaspoon
Accent	1/4 teaspoon
Barbecue sauce	2 tablespoons
Bouillon	1/3 cup
Catsup	1 1/2 tablespoons
Chili sauce	1 1/2 tablespoons
Dill pickle	1/6 large or 1/2 ounce
Mustard	4 teaspoons
Olives, green	2 medium or 1/3 ounce
Olives, black	3 large or 1 ounce
Soy sauce	3/4 teaspoon
Light soy sauce	1 teaspoon
Steak sauce	2 1/2 teaspoons
Sweet pickle relish	2 1/2 teaspoons
Taco sauce	2 tablespoons
Tamari sauce	3/4 teaspoon
Teriyaki sauce	1 1/4 teaspoons
Worcestershire sauce	1 tablespoon

Reprinted with permission from: Renal Dietitians Dietetic Practice Group of The American Dietetic Association. *National Renal Diet*. Chicago, IL: American Dietetic Association, 1993.

TABLE 21-16   Beverage Choices

	cups per day
The following beverages may be used as desired within your daily fluid allowance	
Carbonated beverages (except Moxie, colas, and pepper-type)	Lemonade, sugar-free / Limeade, sugar-free / Mineral water
Ice	Water
The following beverages contain moderate amounts of potassium and/or phosphorus. They should be used in your diet only as advised by your dietitian.	
Beer *	
Cola or pepper-type carbonated beverages, sugar-free	
Coffee, regular or decaffeinated	
Coffee substitute (cereal-grain beverage)	
Kool-Aid, sugar-free	
Tang, sugar-free	
Tea	
Thirst-quencher beverages, sugar-free	
Wine*	
The following liquids are very high in sodium, potassium, and/or phosphorus. They should be used in your diet only as advised by your doctor or dietitian.	
Broth	Salt-free broth or bouillon
Bouillon	containing potassium chloride
Consomme	(KCl)

Remember: Anything that is liquid or melts at room temperature must also be counted in your fluid allowance (for example, ice cream, Popsicles, sherbet, gelatin).

* Check with your physician before using alcohol.
Reprinted with permission from: Renal Dietitians Dietetic Practice Group of The American Dietetic Association. *National Renal Diet*. Chicago, IL: American Dietetic Association, 1993.

monitor the adequacy of the energy intake, the patient's dry weight should be recorded at the end of dialysis. If energy intake is inadequate, calorie supplements may be helpful. The severely malnourished patient may be fed intravenously during the dialysis treatment (28, 30).

GLUCOSE

Blood glucose levels are usually normal in nondiabetics, but over 30 percent of patients with endstage renal disease (ESRD) are diabetic. When monitoring blood glucose, the following should be kept in mind:

The normal kidney degrades insulin; therefore, in ESRD, the half-life of insulin is prolonged, reducing the needed insulin dose in diabetic patients.

Predialysis blood samples are usually not fasting samples.

Dialysis removes glucose and will therefore transiently lower blood sugar.

Increased glucose may result in fluid retention, diluting blood chemistries. For example, a normal BUN in a hyperglycemic patient may actually be elevated when the hyperglycemia is corrected. Hyperglycemia may also affect values associated with acid-base balance (31).

For further discussion of diabetes, see Chapter 19.

PROPORTION OF MACRONUTRIENTS

Hemodialysis does not improve a patient's hyperlipi-demia, but a diet high in omega (n-3) polyunsaturated fatty acids may help normalize serum lipids (32). Therefore, recommended energy distribution is usually 15 percent of kilocalories from protein; 35 percent from fat, with emphasis on polyunsaturated oils; and 50 percent from carbohydrate, primarily polysaccharides (26).

SODIUM, FLUID INTAKE AND WEIGHT GAIN

Sodium and fluids are restricted to a level that will limit weight gain between dialyses to 1.0 kg per day (31). A patient who is dialyzed on Monday, Wednesday, and Friday could gain 2.0 kg between Monday and Wednesday, and between Wednesday and Friday, and 3.0 kg between Friday and Monday.

To maintain this limit, a common recommendation is 1 to 2 g sodium per day (40 to 80 mEq) and 1,000 mL of fluid, not including the fluid content of solid food if the patient is anuric (28). If the patient is not anuric, the urinary excretion of sodium and fluid are added to this allowance. A common allowance is 1 g plus 2 g of sodium per liter of urine output per day (28). The success of this regimen is determined by monitoring serum sodium, blood pressure, body weight, and, particularly, weight change between dialysis treatments.

TABLE 21-17 Alternative Protein Sources*

Legumes		choices per day
Average per choice: 8 g protein, 20 g carbohydrate, 110 calories, trace sodium, 340 mg potassium, 130 mg phosphorus		

Cooked; prepared or processed without salt

1/2-cup serving

Black beans	Lima beans	Soybeans
Black-eyed peas	Navy beans	Split peas
Great northern beans	Pinto beans	Turtle beans
Lentils	Red kidney beans	

* 1 serving of beans canned with salt also counts as 2 salt choices

Nuts	choices per day
Average per choice: 7 g protein, 7 g carbohydrate, 200 calories, trace sodium, 250 mg potassium, 140 mg phosphorus	

Unsalted

Peanuts and almonds	1 ounce
Cashews and walnuts	1 1/2 ounce
Pecans	2 1/2 ounce
Peanut butter	1 1/2 tablespoon

* 1 ounce of salted nuts also counts as 1 salt choice

Reprinted with permission from: Renal Dietitians Dietetic Practice Group of The American Dietetic Association. *National Renal Diet.* Chicago, IL: American Dietetic Association, 1993.

The following are some additional guidelines:

Excess weight gain (over 1.0 kg per day) with normal serum sodium indicates excessive intake of both salt and water.

Excessive weight gain with low serum sodium suggest excess fluid but not salt.

Excess sodium intake can result in edema, hypertension, and congestive heart failure.

Weight loss, hypotension, decreased urine output (if the patient is not anuric), and an increasing BUN suggest inadequate salt intake.

POTASSIUM

If the hemodialysis patient has a substantial residual urine output or is adequately dialyzed and does not have metabolic acidosis, no potassium restriction is necessary. In a few patients, a mild restriction of potassium is necessary, possibly 2 g (50 mEq)/day. One gram (25 mEq) is added for each liter of urine output/day. In fact, if the patient's protein and potassium intake is low, the intake of more potassium-containing foods may be required.

If predialysis serum potassium is greater than 6 mmol per liter, a potassium-restricted diet may be required. Potassium-binding resins are rarely necessary.

The objective, as with the conservatively managed patient, is to maintain serum potassium within normal range. An elevated potassium level suggests increased potassium intake by ingestion of too many fresh fruits and vegetables or the use of salt substitutes. Acidosis

may also contribute to hyperkalemia. It will be seen with reduced serum bicarbonate values.

CALCIUM, PHOSPHORUS, AND VITAMIN D

Hemodialysis does not diminish the tendency to bone disease in the CRF patient because phosphate is not removed efficiently by dialysis. In addition, the increased protein in the diet of hemodialysis patients tends to increase phosphorus intake.

Elevated serum phosphate may reflect excess phosphorus intake or failure to take phosphate binders. High serum alkaline phosphatase levels indicate bone demineralization. Hence, the use of phosphate binders and restriction of dietary phosphate continues. Once serum phosphate is normalized, patients are usually given a calcium supplement of 1,200 mg per day.

The diet restrictions that reduce phosphorus intake will also lower calcium intake. In order to achieve calcium balance, the hemodialysis patient is usually given calcium and vitamin D supplements. The phosphate binder given is calcium-containing and the dialysate typically contains 6 to 7 mg/dL of calcium. Serum calcium levels must also be monitored, with observation of the Ca × P product.

High serum calcium with normal serum phosphate may occur in patients on vitamin D therapy or oral calcium supplements. Reduced calcium with normal phosphate suggests the patient is not taking the prescribed vitamin D or calcium. Calcium and phosphate levels are affected by acidosis and by parathyroid hormones.

IRON

Anemia begins to develop when GFR falls below 20 to 30 mL/min. In these patients, the production of erythropoietin by the tubulointerstitial cells falls as other functions decline. For comparison, in a patient with normal renal function, if hematocrit falls to 20 percent, the plasma erythropoietin (EPO) rises from normal 10 mU/mL to 1,000 mU/mL. In an anemic dialysis patient, EPO level is more commonly 20 mU/mL.

When dialysis is begun, anemia may improve on the removal of uremic toxins that inhibit endogenous EPO. However, residual blood loss in the dialyzer (1 mL blood loss = 1 mg Fe loss), iron deficiency and decreased erythrocyte survival time serve to increase anemia (31).

EPO therapy is ineffective if the patient is iron deficient as it is in the predialysis stage. Therefore the first step is assessment of the patient's iron stores.

If iron deficiency is documented, its correction should begin a month before EPO therapy is started. Preferably, iron is given orally. Preparations often used are ferrous sulfate, ferrous fumarate, or ferrous gluconate. If gastrointestinal upset occurs, a polysaccharide-iron complex or a sustained release ferrous fumarate or sulfate may be used, but these are more expensive. In either case, dosage is usually in the 100 to 150 mg elemental iron/day range (33).

TABLE 21-18 Example of Calculation of a Renal Diet

Assume that the following diet is prescribed:

Energy, kcal	2,350	
Protein, g	75	HBV (70–80% of total pro = 54–60 g)
Sodium, mg	1,600	
Potassium, mg	2,250	
Phosphorus, mg	950	

Choices	Number	kcal	Pro (g)	Na (mg)	K (mg)	P (mg)
Milk	1	120	4.0	80	185	110
Non-dairy milk sub	1	140	0.5	40	80	30
Meat	7	455	49	175	700	455
Starch	8	720	16	560	280	280
Vegetable Lo K	0					
Med K	1	25	1	15	150	20
Hi K	1	25	1	15	270	20
Fruit Lo K	0					
Med K	1	70	0.5	—	150	—
Hi K	2	140	1.0	—	270	—
Fat	8	360	—	440	80	—
HiCal	3	300	—	45	60	15
Salt	1	—	—	250	—	—
Total		2,355	73	1,620	2,225	930

Sample Menu:

Breakfast

1 meat	1 egg poached		
1 starch	1 slice white toast		
1 starch, 1 salt	1 c cornflakes		
1 med K fruit	1/2 grapefruit		
2 fat	2 tsp margarine		
1 hi Cal	1 c cranberry jc. cocktail		
1/2 milk sub	1/4 c non-dairy creamer		

Lunch

3 meat	3 oz sliced turkey
2 starch	2 slices light rye bread
Lettuce	
1 med K veg	1 med tomato, sliced
2 fat	2 tsp mayonnaise
1 hi K fruit	1 fresh pear
1 hi cal	1 c fruit-flavored drink

Dinner

3 meat	3 oz roast lamb
2 starch	1/2 c mashed potato
	1 small hard roll
1 hi K veg	5 spears asparagus
2 fat	2 tsp margarine
1/2 milk sub	1/4 c frozen dessert topping
1 hi K fruit	1/8 cantaloupe

Snacks

1 starch	1 sweet roll
1 milk	1/2 c milk
1 fat	1 tsp margarine
1 starch	1 1/2 c popped corn
1 fat	1 tsp margarine
1 hi cal	1 c lemonade

Food and phosphate binders interfere with iron absorption. Therefore, the dose is preferably given between meals. In GI upset, it may be given with meals, in an elixir in multiple small doses, or as a single bedtime dose. Oral iron also has a constipating effect that may be treated with sorbitol. Patients who cannot tolerate these side effects may be given iron parenterally after a test dose to check for hypersensitivity (33).

When iron stores are repleted, EPO therapy may begin. It takes the lifetime of the RBC (50 to 90 days in uremia) to reach a steady state. Monitoring reticulocyte count, hemoglobin, and hemocrit will indicate to the nephrologist the need to adjust the dose. Iron stores must be monitored via serum ferritin levels, since iron may become depleted as new hemoglobin is formed.

VITAMINS

Water-soluble vitamins are lost in dialysis. Therefore, patients are given a multivitamin supplement containing the RDA of thiamine, riboflavin, niacin, pantothenic acid, and vitamin B_{12}. In addition, 5 to 10 mg pyridoxine, 1 mg folate, and 60 to 100 mg ascorbic acid are given (31). Large quantities of ascorbic acid should not be given in order to avoid accumulation of oxalates in soft tissues (31). Vitamin preparations should not be taken within several hours prior to dialysis, or the vitamins may be removed. Vitamin A is not given because it is not dialyzed; serum levels thus tend to remain high. The vitamin preparation given should not contain nondialyzable substances such as magnesium and other trace elements

OTHER MEDICATIONS

In addition to phosphate binders, calcium and vitamin D supplements, iron, anabolic steroids, and vitamin supplements, patients with renal disease may be given other drugs of nutritional significance. Hypertension often cannot be controlled by sodium or fluid restriction or by dialysis, so the patient may be given antihypertensive drugs. Side effects include nausea, vomiting, and abdominal distress. CRF patients with congestive heart failure may be given digitalis therapy. Digitalis is not significantly removed by dialysis. Patients can be susceptible to digitalis toxicity, which is exacerbated by hypokalemia. In addition to cardiac arrhythmias and visual disturbances, signs of digitalis toxicity include nausea and vomiting.

INDICATIONS FOR NUTRITIONAL CONSULTATION

The patient load often is such that it is impossible for you, as the provider of nutritional care, to see each patient each time he or she is dialyzed. Instead, many dialysis centers set criteria to indicate the need for nutritional consultation. Typical criteria consist of the following:

Serum sodium, mEq/L	<132, > 148
Serum potassium, mEq/L	<3.0, >6.0
Predialysis BUN, mg/dL	<40, >100
Serum creatinine, mg/dL	>20
Serum calcium, mg/dL	<8.0, >11.0
Serum phosphate, mg/dL	>5.0
Serum albumin, g/dL	<3.0
Dry weight, kg	Any unexplained weight change
Weight change over longest interdialytic interval	>1 kg/day
Other	New diet order Patient dissatisfaction

It is important to note that many values are not expected to stay within the range of what is normal for those with normal renal function.

NUTRITIONAL CARE IN PERITONEAL DIALYSIS

The diet for the patient who is undergoing *peritoneal dialysis* (PD) is, in general, less restricted than that required in hemodialysis. It varies slightly depending on the dialysis protocol in use. The possibilities include intermittent (IPD), now rarely used, and continuous ambulatory (CAPD). In addition, automated dialysis (APD) may be continuous cyclic (CCPD) or nocturnal (NPD), in which a machine does the dialysis automatically. In tidal peritoneal dialysis (TPD) and CCPD, some part of the exchange volume is left during the day, while in NPD, the patient is dry during the day.

PROTEIN

About 1.5 to 3.5 g per day free amino acids are removed by peritoneal dialysis. In addition, patients lose about 9 g of amino acid in 24 hours of CAPD. Below-normal serum albumin levels are common. The usual recommendation for protein intake is 1.2 to 1.5 g per kg IBW. Of the total, 50 percent should be of high biological value (15). The higher protein intake should be used for the patient who needs to rebuild muscle or following an episode of peritonitis. For repletion, protein intake is based on desired, rather than actual, body weight.

ENERGY

Energy intake is generally recommended to be 25 to 35 kcal per kg IBW. It must be increased for patients who are malnourished or who are catabolic from an intercurrent disease (31).

In calculating the energy intake of the patient, the absorption of glucose from the dialysate must be included. Several facts must be kept in mind:

1. The dialysis fluid contains glucose monohydrate. Since the attached water molecule does not yield kilocalories, the yield is 3.74 kcal/g of glucose, not 4 kcal/g.
2. Dialysate fluids for peritoneal use are available in the following concentrations of glucose monohydrate: 1.5, 2.5, 3.5, and 4.25 percent.

The available energy can be calculated from the

volume and concentration of the dialysis fluid, but the permeability of the patient's peritoneal membrane is variable (31). Therefore, the caloric gain is unknown. Therefore, the patient's body weight should be monitored often.

Precautions must be taken to ensure that the patient does not become obese. Obesity is a particular hazard in PD since the glucose in the dialysate is absorbed and contributes to the patient's energy intake. It is also necessary to adjust the level for differences in activity.

SODIUM, FLUID, AND POTASSIUM

In anuric patients, 2.5 kg of fluid per day can be removed rather easily, but the dialysis solutions used must be at the high end of the range of dextrose concentrations.

If this higher range can be used, the patient may be able to tolerate as much as 3 to 4 g (130 to 170 mEq) per day, of sodium, and 2 to 2.5 L of fluid. However, if the patient is obese, diabetic, or hypertriglyceridemic, the dextrose concentration may need to be at minimal level (1.5 percent). The sodium and fluid level should be restricted to 1 to 2 g sodium and 1L of fluid.

These patients usually do not become hyperkalemic. Therefore, the potassium intake can be liberalized, possibly to 75 to 100 mEq (3 to 4 g) per day. Many patients need no potassium restriction (21, 33).

CALCIUM AND PHOSPHORUS

Serum phosphorus levels remain elevated in PD. Dietary phosphorus restriction of 600 to 1,200 mg per day is commonly used, but more is sometimes permitted to allow for the increase in dietary protein. If that is the case, phosphate binders continue to be used. The increased dietary protein may provide additional calcium so that a supplement may be unnecessary. In addition, calcium-containing phosphate binders and calcium in the dialysis solution provide calcium. If a supplement is necessary, it should not be given until serum phosphate is reduced to 4 to 5.5 mg. The patient may also need a vitamin D supplement, but care must be taken to avoid hypercalcemia (33).

IRON

PD patients are routinely prescribed a daily intake of 10 to 15 mg of iron. If the diet history indicates that the patient does not take this amount in the diet, a supplement is given (29).

VITAMINS

Water-soluble vitamins are lost in PD. Vitamin supplements are given in doses similar to those given to hemodialyzed patients. If patients are receiving antibiotics, they may need a vitamin K supplement.

In summary, in monitoring the dialysis patient, regardless of method, the following may be considered acceptable: Serum levels of sodium, potassium, calcium,

phosphorus, total protein, albumin, and serum ferritin, as well as body weight, should be in normal range, or may be slightly higher for diabetics. BUN is high, but should be under 100 mg per dL. Serum creatinine is high, at 10 to 15 mg per dL. Total CO_2 may be lower, indicating some acidosis. Hematocrit is usually lower than normal.

THE DIABETIC PATIENT IN RENAL FAILURE

A third or more of renal patients are diabetic. Therefore, nutritional care for the two conditions must be combined.

Usually the same nutrient limitations recommended for nondiabetic predialysis, hemodialysis, and peritoneal dialysis patients are used when the patient is diabetic. In addition, carbohydrate and fat are added to the calculations, as they are in diabetic diets without renal failure (see Chapter 19).

Saturated fats are limited if possible. In the NRD, some changes are made in the lists of choices in order to make that possible. The amounts of a few choices vary from the lists for nondiabetic changes. The greatest difficulty may be presented by the diabetic patient on peritoneal dialysis, since the dialysate contains a large amount of glucose that must be subtracted from the total carbohydrate prescribed for oral intake.

In the uremic diabetic patient, insulin secretion and peripheral tissue response to insulin are reduced. On the other hand, the rate of insulin catabolism and excretion are reduced. The overall effect may be to intensify the effect of exogenous insulin and to reduce the required dose. In peritoneal dialysis patients, insulin is added to the dialysis solution. Oral hypoglycemic agents are rarely used.

NUTRITIONAL CARE FOLLOWING RENAL TRANSPLANT

Renal transplantation is a major surgical procedure. The nutritional care of the prospective patient should be targeted toward maintaining the patient in the best possible condition prior to surgery. Immediate postoperative feeding will include the clear liquid and transitional diets described in Chapter 12. The patient should advance rapidly to solid food. Thereafter, there are 2 post-transplant phases. The *acute phase* lasts one to two months and the *chronic phase* continues thereafter.

In the acute phase, infection and transplant rejection are major concerns. To prevent rejection, immunosuppressive drugs are given. Ideally, the tendency of the body to reject transplanted organs is suppressed, while the immune system is still sufficiently functional to be able to fight infection.

There are a number of compounds that attempt to achieve these purposes. Unfortunately, all have side effects, many of which are nutrition-related. A summary of immunosuppressive drugs, their mechanism of action, side effects, and nutritional management is contained in Table 21-19. Other products are being investigated,

In the renal transplant patient, a common procedure is

TABLE 21-19 Nutrition Effects of Immunosuppressive Drugs ($\uparrow$ = increase; $\downarrow$ = decrease)

Drug	Mechanisms of Action	Possible Side Effects	Management
Corticosteroids (Prednisone) (Solu-Medrol)	Antiinflammatory Inhibits antibody production Suppresses cell-mediated hypersensitivity Enhances action of other immunosuppressives	Hyperphagia Weight gain Sodium and fluid retention Excretion of K, Zn, N, ascorbic acid $\uparrow$Appetite GI ulceration $\uparrow$HCl Impaired glucose tolerance Hyperglycemia Accelerates protein catabolism, muscle wasting Ca and phosphate wasting Osteoporosis; calciuria Redistribution of adipose tissue to produce cushingoid appearance Hypercholesterolemia Impaired wound healing	Control calories Restrict dietary Na, $\uparrow$K intake, $\uparrow$Calcium, $\uparrow$Dietary protein, $\downarrow$Carbohydrate, esp. concentrated sweets (Need diabetic diet?) $\downarrow$Total fat, cholesterol P:S ratio >1 Avoid gastric irritants (black pepper, chili powder, caffeine, alcohol, nutmeg, mustard seed) Encourage exercise
Azathioprine (Imuran)	Antiinflammatory $\downarrow$delayed hypersensitivity Purine antagonist $\downarrow$nucleic acid synthesis $\downarrow$circulating lymphocytes Phagocytosis by neutrophils	Nausea and vomiting, diarrhea Anorexia Mouth ulceration; stomatitis Esophagitis Increased risk of infection Altered taste acuity Bone marrow depression Anemia, leukopenia, thrombocytopenia	Lipid or soft diet? Diet as tolerated Small, frequent feedings Folate supplementation?
Cyclosporine (Sandimmune) (CsA)	Cyclic polypeptide antibiotic Decreases IL-2 production $\downarrow$Cell-mediated immunity Spares T-suppressor cells	Nephrotoxicity, hepatic toxicity Hypertension Hyperkalemia Hypomagnesemia Hyperuricemia Gingival hypertrophy Nausea, vomiting, diarrhea Anorexia Hiccups Hyperglycemia Hyperlipidemia	Restrict dietary Na$^+$ Restrict K$^+$ Monitor serum Mg, $\uparrow$kcal and protein Diet as tolerated
Antithymocyte Globulin (ATG) (ATGAM)	Inhibits cell-mediated immunity $\downarrow$Circulating lymphocytes	Nausea, vomiting, diarrhea Fever Stomatitis	Diet as tolerated
OKT3 (Arthoclone) (Muromonab)	Inhibits C-cells effector function	Nausea, vomiting, diarrhea Anorexia Fever, chills Fluid retention Hypertension $\uparrow$Risk of infection Respiratory compromise?, pulmonary edema?	Monitor intake Diet as tolerated
FK 506	$\downarrow$IL-2 production $\downarrow$Cell-mediated immunity	Nausea, vomiting Abdominal pain Hyperglycemia Hyperkalemia Pancreatitis? Neurotoxicity? $\uparrow$Serum amylase $\uparrow$Serum uric acid	Monitor intake Diet as tolerated $\downarrow$Dietary K Control kcal
Rapamycin	Inhibits T-cell proliferation		(Under investigation)
RS-61433 (MCA)	Inhibits DNA production Inhibits antibody production		(Under investigation)

the use of a combination of prednisone and azathioprine, the so-called *conventional treatment*.. An alternative is a combination of prednisone, azathioprine, and cyclosporine, the *triple treatment*.

Patients receiving corticosteroids have a high protein catabolic rate. Therefore, a protein intake of 1.3 to 2.0 g/kg body weight is recommended, along with 30 to 35 kcal/kg or 1.3 to 1.5 times the basal energy requirement.

Corticosteroid therapy and stress often promote glucose intolerance. Simple carbohydrates may then need to be limited. Some patients require a diabetic diet. For normoglycemic patients, the diet may be 50 to 70 percent of total calories from carbohydrate, and 30 percent from fat, mostly unsaturated.

Sodium restriction of 2 to 4 g per day may be necessary if fluid is retained. Cyclosporine use may cause hyperkalemia, while refeeding syndrome or the use of potassium-wasting diuretics can result in hypokalemia. Potassium intake should be modified as necessary. If hypophosphatemia and hypomagnesemia are present, the intake of these elements should be increased with selected foods or mineral supplements. Vitamins and other minerals should be supplemented to RDA levels. Some patients may profit from high-protein supplements. Tube feedings or parenteral feedings are not usually necessary.

In the chronic posttransplant phase, the immunosuppressive drug dosage and their catabolic effects decrease. The patient's nutritional needs are reduced, but other problems arise.

A very common problem is excessive *gain in weight* as a consequence of hyperphagia from corticosteroid therapy, lack of activity, and loosening of previous diet restrictions. Therefore, close monitoring and control of body weight is essential.

A second problem is *hyperlipidemia*, thought to result from corticosteroid and cyclosporine therapy, along with age, weight gain, and glucose intolerance. For information on nutritional care in hyperlipidemia, see Chapter 20.

Hypertension is also common in renal transplant patients, resulting fom corticosteroid or cyclosporine therapy and possible rejection, renal artery stenosis, or the presence of the patient's diseased kidneys if they have not been removed. Approaches to treatment have included sodium restriction (2 to 4 g/day), along with medications for hypertension.

Another posttransplant problem is *steroid-induced diabetic mellitus,* which is also affected by hereditary predisposition and the use of diuretics. Approaches to treatment include decreasing corticosteroid dose if possible, reducing diuretic dose, weight reduction if indicated, a diabetic diet, exercise, and use of oral hypoglycemic agents.

Finally, the posttransplant patient is at risk of advancing *osteoporosis*. Bone mineral loss should be monitored closely and treated as necessary. Serum calcium and vitamin D, as well as exercise and estrogen levels, must be monitored.

In summary, the recommended diet for long-term posttransplant patient is approximately as follows:

1 g protein/kg body weight/day

120 to 130 percent BEE for maintenance, adjusted for activity level and current vs. desired body weight

50 to 70 percent of kilocalories as carbohydrate with limited concentrated sweets

<30 percent of kilocalories as fat with <10 percent as saturated fat

1,000 to 1,500 mg calcium/day (plus vitamin D and estrogen medications if indicated)

3 to 4 g sodium/day

Encourage intake of foods high in Mg and P. Supplement if needed.

Adjust K intake as indicated by serum levels.

Supplement vitamins and other minerals to RDA levels.

TOPICS FOR FURTHER DISCUSSION

1. If a growing child has CRF, how would her protein and energy needs per kg of body weight compare to those of an adult?
2. How is nutritional status assessed in a child with CRF?
3. List and price some special low-protein products and low-sodium products. Compare cost per serving with the regular, salted counterpart. If products are available for tasting, compare their acceptability.
4. A 14 y.o CRF patient has a height-age of 9 years and a bone age of 12 years. Is this patient's final height likely to be shorter, taller, or normal for age? Describe the physiological basis for your answer.
5. In nutritional care of the pregnant dialysis patient, what changes are made in the laboratory criteria for control? Discuss potential necessary changes in the diet.
6. Discuss adjustment of TPN procedures for renal patients.
7. Using the menu from a local restaurant, choose some meals for renal patients requiring various diet restrictions.
8. If a patient in renal failure were also diabetic, demonstrate how the diet plan would be altered.

REFERENCES

1. **Nelson, E.E., C.D. Hong, A.L. Pesce, D.W. Peterson, S. Singh and V.E. Pollak.** Anthropometric norms for the dialysis population. *Am. J. Kidney Dis* 16:(1990)32.
2. **Nelson, E.E.** Anthropometry in the nutritional assessment of adults with end-stage renal disease. *J. Renal Nutr.* 1:(1991)162.
3. **Jacob, V., J.E. Lecarpentier, S. Salzano, V. Naylor et al.** IGF-

I, a marker for undernutrition in hemodialysis patients. *Am. J. Clin. Nutr.* 52:(1990)39.

4. **Kopple, J.D.** Significance of diet and parenteral nutrition in chronic renal failure. *In* N.S. Bricker and M.A. Kirschenbaum, eds..*The Kidney: Diagnosis and Management.* New York: Wiley, 1984, 333–52.

5. **Borah, M.F., P.Y. Schoenfeld, F.A. Gotch, J.A. Sargent, M.W. Alfson,** and **M.H. Humphreys.** Nitrogen balance during intermittent dialysis therapy of uremia. *Kid. Internat.* 14:(1978)491.

6. **Sargent, J.A., and F.A. Gotch,** Nutrition and treatment of the acutely ill patient using urea kinetics. *Diab. & Trans.* 23:(1983)5–19.

7. ——— Control of dialysis by a single-pool urea model: The National Co-operative Dialysis Study, *Kid Internat.* 23:(1983)5–19.

8. **Keshavich, P., R. Davis-Pollack, D. Luhring,** and **P. Lee.** *A Practical Guide to Rapid High Efficiency Dialysis.* Minneapolis: Minneapolis Medical Research Foundation, Inc., 1987.

9. **Sargent, J., Gotch, F. Borsh, M. Piercy, M. Spinozzi, N., Schoenfeld, P.** and **M. Humphreys,** Urea kinetics: a guide to nutritional management of renal failure. *Am. J. Clin. Nutr.* 31:(1978)1696.

10. ——— **and F.A. Gotch.** Nutrition and treatment of the acutely ill patient using urea kinetics. *Diab. & Trans* 23: (1983)5–19.

11. **Murray, R.** Protein and energy requirements. *In* S.H. Krey and R. Murray, eds. *Dynamics of Nutrition Support.* Norwalk, CT: Appleton-Century Crofts, 1986.

12. **Hara, Y. et al.** Acidosis, not azotemia, stimulates branched-chain amino acid catabolism in uremic rats. *Kidney Internat.* 32:(1987)868.

13. **May, R.C., R.A. Kelly,** and **W.E. Mitch.** Mechanisms for defects in muscle protein in rats with chronic uremia. The influence of metabolic acidosis. *J. Clin. Invest.* 79:(1987)1099.

14. **Mitch, W.E.** Restricted diets and slowing the progression of chronic renal insufficiency. *In* W.E. Mitch and S. Klahr, eds. *Nutrition and the Kidney,* 2d ed. Boston: Little, Brown. 1993.

15. Renal Dietitian's Dietetic Practice Group of the American Dietetic Association and Council on Renal Nutrition of the National Kidney Foundation. *National Renal Diet: Professional Guide.* Chicago: American Dietetic Association, 1993.

16. **Maroni, B.J.** Requirements for protein, calories, and fat in the predialysis patient. *In* W.E. Mitch and S. Klahr, eds. *Nutrition and the Kidney,* 2d ed. Boston: Little, Brown, 1993.

17. **Massry, S.G., and J.D. Kopple.** Requirements for calcium, phosphorus, and vitamin D. *In* W.E. Mitch and S. Klahr, eds. *Nutrition and the Kidney,* 2d ed. Boston: Little, Brown, 1993.

18. **Walser, M., and E.C. Chandeler.** Phosphorus. *In* M. Walser, A. Imbembo, S. Margolis, and G.A. Eefert, eds. *Nutritional Management.* Philadelphia: Saunders, 1984.

19. **Klahr, S.** Management of lipid abnormalities in the renal patient. *In* W.E. Mitch and S. Klahr, eds. *Nutrition and the Kidney,* 2d ed. Boston: Little, Brown, 1993.

20. American Dietetic Association. *A Healthy Food Guide. Kidney Disease.* Chicago: The American Dietetic Association, 1993.

21. ——— *A Healthy Food Guide. Hemodialysis.* Chicago: The American Dietetic Associaton, 1993.

22. ——— *A Healthy Food Guide. Peritoneal Dialysis.* Chicago: The American Dietetic Association, 1993.

23. ———. *A Healthy Food Guide. Diabetes and Kidney Disease.* Chicago: The American Dietetic Association, 1993.

24. ———. *A Healthy Food Guide. Diabetes and Hemodialysis.* Chicago: The American Dietetic Association, 1993.

25. ——— *A. Healthy Food Guide. Diabetes and Peritoneal Dialysis.* Chicago: The American Dietetic Association, 1993.

26. **Bergstrom, J.** Nutritional requirements of hemodialysis patients. *In* W.E. Mitch and S. Klahr, eds. *Nutrition and the Kidney,* 2d ed. Boston: Little, Brown, 1993.

27. **Wolfson, M., M.R. Jones,** and **J.D. Kopple.** Amino acid losses during hemodialysis with infusion of amino acids and glucose. *Kidney Internat.* 21:(1982)500.

28. **Bilbrey, G.L., and T.L. Cohen.** Identification and treatment of protein-calorie malnutrition in chronic hemodialysis patients. *Dial. Transplant.* 18:(1989)669..

29. **Kopple, J.D.** and **R. Hirschberg,** Nutrition and Peritoneal Dialysis. *In* W.T. Mitch and S. Klahr, eds. *Handbook of Dialysis,* 2d ed. Boston: Little, Brown, 1993.

30. **Cano, N., et al.** Predialytic parenteral nutriton with lipids and amino acids in malnourished hemodialysis patients. *Am J. Clin. Nutr.* 52:(1990) 726.

31. **Blumenkrantz, M.J.** Nutrition, *In* J.T. Daugirdas and T.S. Ing, eds. *Handbook of Dialysis,* 2d ed. Boston: Little, Brown, 1994.

32. **Bilo, H.G.J.** Omega-3 polyunsaturated fatty acids in chronic renal insufficiency. *Nephron* 57:(1991)385.

33. **Paganini, E.P.** Hematologic abnormalities. *In*: J.T. Daugirdas and T.S. Ing, eds. *Handbook of Dialysis,* 2d ed. Boston: Little, Brown, 1994.

ADDITONAL SOURCES OF INFORMATION

Schrier, R.W. and **C.W. Gottschalk,** eds. *Diseases of the Kidney,* 5th ed. Boston: Little, Brown, 1994.

Greenberg, A. ed., *Primer in Kidney Diseases.* San Diego: Academic Press, 1994.

☑ TO TEST YOUR UNDERSTANDING

1. A renal patient's weight was 160 lb prior to his current illness. Four months later, the patient weighs 128 lb. He is 5 ft, 10 in tall.

    a. Calculate his weight as a percentage of usual weight.

    b. How would you interpret his nutritional status based on weight only?

    c. How would you alter your interpretation in the following circumstances? (Explain your reasoning for each.)

        1. The patient's weight has increased 10 lb in 2 weeks. Blood pressure is 135/95.

        2. You obtain a 3-day diet record and find that the patient's fluid intake is 1,500 mL per day. His medical record says his maximum urine output is 1,200 mL per day.

2. An obese male patient with CRF has the following laboratory values:

	Patient	Normal
BUN, mg/dL	80	___
Serum creatinine, mg/dL	10	___
Urinary urea nitrogen, g/24	4.1	___

His body weight is 30 lb in excess of IBW of 150 lb. A 40-gram protein diet has been prescribed.

    a. In the space provided, fill in the normal values.

    b. Calculate his adjusted ideal body weight

    c. Calculate the patient's intake from the UUN.

    d. Does the value obtained in part c indicate that the patient is complying with the diet?

3. If a patient's diet contains 50 g protein, what is the nitrogen content of the diet?

4. You have the following data on Mr. L., a CRF patient who is not being dialyzed:.

Initial BUN, mg/dL	60.0
BUN, 72 hrs. later, mg/dL	100.0
Initial body weight, kg (IBW)	70.0
Body weight, 72 hrs. later, kg	75.0

    a. Calculate the volume of fluid in which urea is distributed in this patient.

    b. Calculate the urea generation rate.

    c. Calculate the protein catabolic rate.

5. You have a patient for whom a 40-g-protein diet has been prescribed. Using Form F, make a list of the exchanges and the number of exchanges that would fill this prescription.

6. Using the choice lists from the NRD diet, plan the menu for a patient whose diet contains the following choices:

    1 egg
    4 oz meat
    1 c milk, whole
    2 vegetables
    2 fruit
    1 starch
    10 fat
    1 high calorie

7. A female patient weighing 110 lb was at her ideal weight. She had a GFR of 15 mL/min. The prescribed diet contained 40 g protein. Estimate her energy requirement.

8. An adult male patient weighing 72 kg has a GFR of 12 mL/min, BUN of 80 mg per dL, and serum albumin of 4.8 g/dL. He has nephrotic syndrome and is losing 20 g protein per day in his urine.

    a. What protein intake would you recommend?

    b. What protein intake would you recommend if the GFR were 40 mL/min, BUN was 18 mg/dL, and serum albumin 1.5 g/dL?

9. A diet containing 1.0 g protein/kg body weight/day with 75 percent HBV protein is prescribed for an adult male patient. The medical record gives the following values:

Body weight, kg	70.0
Body weight prior to illness, kg	64.0
Urine volume/day, mL	800.0
Creatinine clearance, mL/min	15.0
Serum creatinine, mg/dL	8.0
BUN, mg/dL	100.0
Blood pressure	140/90
Serum albumin, mg/dL	2.0
Urine protein, g/day	20.0

(continued)

✓ **TO TEST YOUR UNDERSTANDING** *(continued)*

a. List normal values.

b. List the values that are compatible with a diagnosis of CRF and indicate how they compare to normal values.

c. List the values that are compatible with a diagnosis of nephrotic syndrome, and indicate how they compare with normal values.

10. A patient's normal dry weight is 145 lb. The patient's energy intake is adequate for weight maintenance. In each of the following circumstances, all of which developed in a short period, would you consider the sodium intake too low, too high, or about right? Describe your reasoning.

a. Body weight is 135#; BP 115/75

b. Body weight is 150#; BP 122/79

c. Body weight is 160#; BP 130/90

d. Weight gain of 3 kg in 2 days

11. You have a prescription for a diet as follows: Protein, 40 g; sodium, 600 mg

a. Using Form F and the NRD, plan a meal pattern for this patient

b. Using a menu assigned by your instructor, plan the day's diet for this patient.

c. The patient tells you of a canned tuna product he enjoys and asks if he can use it on his diet. He says it is labeled "low source of sodium." What would you tell him?

12. Calculate the fluid content of the following menu for a renal patient:

1 c cream of tomato soup

2 oz beef patty

1/2 c buttered green beans

Molded vegetable salad on lettuce (1/3 c gelatin, 2T chopped vegetables)

3/4 c ice cream

6 oz iced tea with 2 ice cubes and 2 t sugar

13. You have a patient who is using a potassium-losing diuretic. How would you modify a menu to increase the potassium content without increasing its kcal content?

14. You have a patient whose diet prescription is as follows:

Protein	40 g
Sodium	40 mEq
Potassium	40 mEq
Fluid	1,000 ml
Kcal	1,500

Using the NRD, calculate a meal plan for this patient on Form F.

15. You have an adult female patient whose diet prescription reads as follows:

Protein	50 g
Sodium	3 g

Her medical record lists the following values:

	Current	Normal
Fluid intake, mL	2,000	___
Fluid output, mL	1,000	___
BUN, mg/dL	120.0	___
Serum creatinine, mg/dL	5.0	___
Serum sodium, mEq/L	140.0	___
Serum, potassium, mEq/L	6.5	___
Creatinine clearance, mL/min	20.0	___
Body weight change, 1 week, kg	6.0	___
BP	140/92	___

a. Fill in normal values in the spaces provided.

b. Which values are expected to remain high? What values would be your objective for these?

c. What changes, in your opinion, should be made in the diet prescription, assuming you are satisfied that the patient is complying with the currently prescribed diet? Explain your answer.

16. Your patient is complying with a diet containing 40 g protein, 40 mEq Na, and 40 mEq K. Serum phosphate is elevated, and the attending physician asks you to ensure that phosphorus intake is under 1,000 mg per day.

a. What modification in the diet is indicated?

b. The physician prescribes a phosphate binder for the patient. What nutrition-related problems might you anticipate, and what action on your part do these suggest?

c. The patient complains that the diet is tasteless. She asks whether she can use a salt substitute. What is your response?

17. When you are monitoring a hemodialysis patient's progress, what data would you look for to determine whether intakes of the following are at appropriate levels?

a. Protein

b. Sodium

c. Potassium

d. Fluid

18. You have a patient whose diet prescription reads as follows:

> 1 g protein/kg, 50 percent HBV; 2,800 kcal; 1,500 mL fluid; 55 mEq Na; 70 mEq K

a. What changes would you suggest if the patient's predialysis lab values are as follows? (Assume for this and succeeding parts of this question that the patient is complying with the diet.)

BUN	100 mg/dL
Serum Na	WNL
Serum K	WNL
Serum albumin	2.9 g/dL
MAMC	19.8 unchanged
TSF	10.1 unchanged
Body wt (estimated dry)	70 kg
Ideal body wt	84 kg
Urine output	200 mL/day
Weight gain between dialyses	1.5 kg/3 days
No edema	

b.

BUN	180 mg/dL
Serum Na	WNL
Serum K	WNL
Serum albumin	3.1 g/dL
MAMC	21.4 cm
TSF	11.2 mm
Body weight (estimated dry)	72 kg
Blood pressure	140/92
Weight gain between dialyses	3 kg/3 days
Edema	3+, pitting

Explain the basis for your answer.

c.

BUN (increase of 30 from previous months	150 mg/dL
Serum Na	130 m Eq/L
Serum albumin	3.3 mg/dL
TSF	11.2 mm
Body weight (estimated dry)	68 kg
Blood pressure	112/70
Weight gain between dialyses	0.5 kg/3 days
Edema	None

Explain the basis for your answer.

Chronic Renal Failure

Part I: Presentation

Present Illness: Ellen R. is a 20 y.o. university student referred to the Renal Clinic from the university's student health center for evaluation of renal function. She had come to the health center C/O fatigue, weakness, anorexia, periobital and pedal edema, and sudden weight gain. The health center reports data listed below.

Past Medical History: T&A at age 7; streptococcal infection of throat at age 11, followed by glomerulonephritis; fractured arm at age 14.

Family History: Parents are a&w. Brother age 16 a&w.

Social History: Single. Resides in university residence hall.

Review of Systems: Patient C/O mild, intermittent headache; nocturia 1-2 times/night; fatigue; anorexia; mild pruritis.

Examination: General: White female; 5 ft, 7 in; 57 kg; medium frame. BP 128/85, right arm, sitting. P 72, regular. R 15. T 37 C. Fundi normal. Lungs clear. Heart without murmur or gallop. Extremities show 2+ pedal edema. Rest of exam WNL.

Impression: Nephrotic syndrome with renal insufficiency in 20 y.o. normal-weight female with medical history of post-streptococcal glomerulonephritis.

Plan: Nutrition Clinic referral for instruction on 4 to 6 g salt diet.

Rx: Furosemide (Lasix) 60 mg q.d., RTC in 1 wk for BP check and serum K assay, renal biopsy.

BP	135/90
Albuminuria	3+
BUN	50 mg/dL
Serum albumin	2.8 g/dL
Current body wt	140#
Pre-illness wt	128#

Laboratory	Units	Normal	Patient	Interpretation
BUN	mg/dL	—	50	—
Serum creatinine	mg/dL	—	2.2	—
Creatinine clearance	mL/min	—	40	—
Serum sodium	mEq/L	—	138	—
Serum potassium	mEq/L	—	4.0	—
Serum albumin	g/dL	—	2.0	—
Urine pH		—	6.2	—
24-hr urine protein	g/24 hr	—	7.00	—
Urine specific gravity		—	1.004	—
Urine volume	mL/24 hr	—	2,000	—
Hgb	g/dL	—	9.8	—
Hct	%	—	33	—
Rheumatology W/U		NL	broad casts	—

QUESTIONS

1. The patient's complaint of anorexia and weight gain and the fact that she is at approximately normal weight seem incompatible. Explain how these conditions can coexist.

2. In the above column headed *Normal*, write in the normal values.

3. In the above column headed *Interpretation*, write P for any value that suggests the kidney disease is affecting Ellen's protein and nitrogen homeostasis.

4. In the same column, write *S* for any value that indicates the disease is affecting the kidney's ability to conserve or excrete solutes.

5. In the same column, write *F* for any value that suggests that the disease is compromising the kidney's ability to maintain fluid balance.

6. In the same column, write *B* for any value suggesting that the patient might develop skeletal abnormalities.

7. Explain why a protein restriction was not ordered.

8. a. Would you suggest any other diet modification? If so, what? Explain your reasoning.

    b. If you answered positively to part *a*, describe in general terms the content of your suggestions to the patient.

Part II. Medical Management of Renal Insufficiency

Ellen continued on this program of conservative management for the next 3 years. During this time she graduated from college, began her career as an elementary school teacher in a rural community, and was married. She was followed by her personal physician and was not seen in the renal clinic for several years.

Three years later, she was again referred to the renal clinic. She C/O more frequent headaches, nausea and vomiting, severe itching, and an unpleasant taste in her mouth. She also C/O muscle cramps and twitching, weight loss, weakness, and drowsiness, with difficulty concentrating. The examination and interview provided the following information:

BUN	100 mg/dL
Serum creatinine	4.89 mg/dL
Creatinine clearance	10.0 mL/min
Urea clearance	16 mL/min
Serum sodium	142 mEq/L
Serum potassium	5.7 mEq/L
Serum albumin	2.8 g/dL
Hgb	19.2 g/dL
Hct	28%

Serum transferrin   150 mg/dL
BP   160/100, standing, right arm
Proteinuria   Negative
Urine pH   7.31
Serum alkaline
   phosphatase   18 units/dL (King-Armstrong)
Blood CO_2 14.8 mEq/L
Urine volume   500 mL/24 hr
Dry weight   52 kg (estimated by urologist)

Impression: Chronic renal failure in a 23 y.o. underweight female with history of renal insufficiency and nephrotic syndrome.

Plan: Nutrition clinic referral for advice on diet: protein, 40 g; Na, 1,000 mg; K, 40 mEq; fluid, output +500 ml.

Rx: furosemide (Lasix), 60 mg t.i.d.; methyldopa (Aldomet), 250 mg t.i.d.; sodium bicarbonate, 1 g t.i.d.; 4 × 500 mg tab t.i.d.

QUESTIONS

9. From the laboratory values given, calculate Ellen's GFR.

10. Explain the purpose of each of the following, and list the data indicating the need for the treatment.
   a.   Methyldopa
   b.   Sodium bicarbonate
   c.   Protein restriction
   d.   Sodium restriction
   e.   Potassium restriction
   f.   Fluid restriction

11. When you see Ellen in the Nutrition Clinic, you note that the diet prescription does not specify a calorie content.
   a. How many kcals would you try to include in her diet? Show your calculations and explain your reasoning.
   b. On Form F, calculate a diet plan for this patient.

12. The patient tells you she has a salt substitute which she uses "sparingly." What action would you take at this point?

13. When Ellen comes to see you again, you find the following data in her medical record:

	March 5	March 7
BUN, mg/dL	95.0	98.0
Body wt, kg	52.0	52.0
UUN, g/24 hr	4.3	4.3

You interview Ellen at some length. She assures you she is following her diet. You take a 24-hr recall, and your calculations show that her diet contained approximately 40 g protein.
   a. Calculate her nitrogen intake.
   b. Calculate the protein catabolic rate.
   c. Calculate the nitrogen balance
   d. Is the protein content of her diet sufficient to avoid tissue catabolism? Explain your answer.

14. Ellen tells you that she feels thirsty all the time. She would like to have more fluid, but the attending physician is reluctant to allow this. She says that she needs most of her fluid allowance to take her medications. What procedures could you suggest to her?

Part III: Hemodialysis

Ellen is no longer able to keep up her work at the school. Her GFR is 16 mL/min. Her physician recommends a transplant, but a kidney is not immediately available. As a consequence, hemodialysis is recommended.

An arteriovenous fistula was surgically created in Ellen's left forearm. A month later, she is admitted to the hospital. Her serum potassium level has risen further and BUN is 110 mg/dl. Her BP has also risen. She is started on hemodialysis 5 hr, 3 times a week.

Her diet prescription now reads: protein, 1 g/kg; Na, 55 mEq; fluid, 1,500 mL; K, 70 mEq; phosphate, 1,200 mg. She was given prescriptions for a phosphate binder and calcium supplement and was instructed to discontinue previously prescribed bicarbonate and steroid. She was also given vitamin supplements.

Her postdialysis weight was 50 kg.

QUESTIONS

15. How much protein per day would you recommend for Ellen? Explain your reasoning.

16. At one time, Ellen's laboratory values were as follows:

BUN (predialysis)	110 mg/dL
Serum sodium	140 mEq/L
Serum potassium	4.6 mEq/L
Serum albumin	3.1 g/dL
BP	145/95
Interdialytic weight gain/day	3 kg
MAMC	19.5
TSF	13.2

   a. How would you interpret the data?
   b. What action would you take?
   c. Which values would you monitor to determine the long-term adequacy of the diet?

17. Explain the rationale for the following:

    a. Phosphate binders, calcium supplement, and dietary phosphate restriction

    b. Water-soluble vitamin supplements

18. Why are the following not given:

    a. Vitamin A

    b. Bicarbonate

Part IV: Peritoneal Dialysis

The three trips a week to the dialysis center from her rural community become a hardship for Ellen as months pass, and a kidney for transplant is still not available. Her physician considers home hemodialysis, but they are concerned that the power and water supplies are not sufficiently reliable. In addition, her husband's work does not allow him to be of enough help in the process.

A decision is made to have Ellen use continuous ambulatory peritoneal dialysis. She and her husband are both carefully instructed in the procedures.

The diet prescription is as follows: protein, 120 g; kcal, 2,100; Na, 3 g; fluid, 2,000 ml; phosphate, 1,200 mg.

QUESTIONS

19. **a.** What nutritional problems might arise?

    b. Describe the nutritional care procedures indicated.

Part V: Renal Transplant

One day, Ellen receives a telephone call telling her that a kidney is available for her transplant. She leaves for the hospital immediately and receives her transplant late that evening. She is given a clear liquid diet for 3 days and then advanced to a more adequate diet. She is given immunosuppressants, and a diet is prescribed. Six months later, you see Ellen for the last time. She reports that she is teaching again and is expecting her first child.

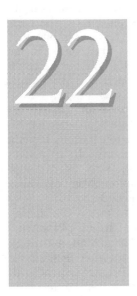

Nutritional Care of the Critically Ill Patient

Critically ill patients are in the acute stages of trauma or disease. These individuals require specialized medical management and nutritional support in order to sustain life. Critical illness can occur in a variety of disease states and conditions, including gastrointestinal, cardiac, hepatic, or renal disease, cancer, burns, trauma, sepsis, and associated surgeries. The degree of stress associated with an illness is an indication of the level of nutritional support that may be needed. Full-thickness burns, trauma, and sepsis are considered to be the most catabolic or stressful injuries. Nutritional support for the critically ill patient often requires parenteral nutrition or tube feeding because of poor appetite or a reduced digestive capacity.

The catabolic response to injury is mediated by neurohormonal events that include activation of the sympathetic nervous system and release of catecholamines, stimulation of glucocorticoids, growth hormone and cytokines, and an increase in the secretion of glucagon relative to that of insulin. These neurohumoral signals result in the clinical symptoms and metabolic events that characterize the stress response: tachycardia, tachypnea, hyperglycemia, mobilization of body fat, and net breakdown of skeletal-muscle protein (1). Aggressive nutritional support during catabolic illness will reduce, but not prevent, the loss of body protein (1). Thus, current research seeks to optimize the response to nutritional support by modulating the catabolic response to injury (2). Several approaches are being studied to modify the body's catabolic response to injury: use of monoclonal antibodies that block cytokine responses, such as anti-tumor necrosis factor alpha and interleukin-1 receptor antagonists (3); provision of specific amino acids such as glutamine, arginine, or branched-chain amino acids (4); modification of immune responses by use of n-3 fatty acids; and administration of growth factors such as growth hormone or insulinlike growth factor 1, to promote protein synthesis (5). Depending on the results of current clinical trials, future nutritional therapy for patients with critical illness may include a variety of compounds designed to combat the catabolic response to injury and ultimately optimize the response to nutritional support.

In this chapter we will focus on the following areas: nutritional assessment of the critically ill patient, multiple organ systems failure, nutritional support of the critically ill pulmonary patient, nutrition and burn trauma, and nutrition during cancer, including human immonodeficiency virus infection.

NUTRITIONAL ASSESSMENT

Nutritional assessment of the critically ill patient follows the general principles of anthropometric, biochemical, clinical, and dietary evaluation outlined in Chapters 4, 5, and 6. Many of the standard nutritional assessment tests are affected by stress, however, making their interpretation difficult.

The timing of the nutritional assessment is an important consideration in the critically ill patient (6). An initial assessment within 5 days of admission usually coincides with the peak metabolic response to injury and is thus of limited value, other than in identifying the high-risk patient and in establishing an estimate of calorie and nutrient needs. The stress response to injury usually subsides by the fifth to tenth postinjury day, allowing for a more complete and meaningful "postcatabolism" nutritional assessment. Serial assessment of nutritional status is important during convalescence to adjust nutritional intake as requirements subside with time and healing.

The clinical course of a patient's illness and the degree of stress imposed on the patient determine his nutritional needs. For example, the patient who develops a fistula or becomes septic after surgery is more stressed and requires greater nutritional support than the patient who experiences an uncomplicated postoperative recovery period. Another example would be a patient undergoing therapy for cancer who requires surgery compared to an individual who undergoes the same surgery without a recent history of serious illness. If a comprehensive nutritional assessment cannot be completed on a critically ill patient, an examination of the history of the patient's illness often forms the basis for determination of nutritional needs.

The nutritional evaluation of the critically ill patient will be considered from the standpoint of the following: an initial postinjury assessment and estimation of nutrient needs, a more in-depth postcatabolism evaluation, and long-term serial assessment of the adequacy of the nutritonal care plan.

INITIAL POSTINJURY ASSESSMENT

Many of the common anthropometric measurements cannot be used in the five-day postinjury period. A statement of usual preinjury body weight from the patient or family is probably the most useful. Roy and colleagues (7) suggest that percentage of usual body weight is a valid predictor of surgical risk in individual patients. In Roy's sample of 46 high-risk surgical patients, no complications or deaths occurred when the percentage of usual body weight was 94 percent or greater. Measurement of triceps skinfold and arm circumference can provide information on somatic protein and subcutaneous fat stores. However, many serious accidents involve injuries to the upper arm, thus often making these measurements impossible to perform.

During the first few days postinjury, the results of various standard biochemical tests used to assess nutritional status are not valid. For example, the creatinine-height index (CHI) is not useful because creatinine excretion is increased by trauma and stress, and creatinine excretion becomes an indicator of the degree of catabolism rather than of depletion of somatic protein stores (8). Measurement of serum concentrations of transport proteins such as albumin, transferrin, prealbumin, and retinol-binding proteins is also invalid. The sudden increase in protein catabolism that occurs in stress and increased levels of mediators of the inflammatory response decrease serum concentrations of these proteins, in particular albumin (6, 9). Evaluation of visceral protein status by measurement of serum concentrations of transport proteins may not respond to nutritional intervention for up to 20 days postinjury. Other factors that will alter serum protein concentrations include administration of blood products (such as albumin, fresh frozen plasma, or whole blood) and iron deficiency.

Indicators of immunocompetence, such as lymphocyte count and delayed cutaneous hypersensivity testing, are also affected by stress and injury. The presence of a large wound or burn may reduce lymphocytes in the serum, and sepsis can cause an elevation in the WBC count so that the absolute total lymphocyte count is invalid (6). Anergy has been associated with trauma, burn injury, and surgery (10).

The initial postinjury assessment should include an estimate of energy and nutrient requirements and an evaluation of the patient's ability to tolerate various feeding regimens. Feeding regimens for the critically ill patient may include oral intake, tube feeding, TPN, use of a supplemental feeding, or any combination of these approaches, as discussed in Chapters 13 and 14.

Various methods can be used to assess the energy needs of the critically ill patient (see Chapter 14 for a discussion of energy needs during parenteral nutrition). Indirect calorimetry is the most accurate method for determining energy expenditure in the critically ill patient, and it is being used with increased frequency in the intensive care unit setting. *Maintenance* energy needs in the critically ill adult patient can be established as 1.2 times *resting* energy expenditure (REE, as measured by indirect calorimetry) and as 1.35 times REE for children (9). Nutritional *repletion* of the critically ill patient should not be attempted until the initial hypermetabolism associated with the injury subsides.

If indirect calorimetry is not available, the Harris-Benedict equation can be used to calculate BEE with adjustment for activity and injury, as explained in Chapter 5: Eqs. (5-19) to (5-21). For the critically ill patient, however, use of an injury factor may overestimate energy needs, when compared to true energy needs as measured by indirect calorimetry (6, 11). The choice of body weight to use in the calculation of BEE will affect the accuracy of the calculation. If the patient is edematous, usual or preinjury weight should be used to calculate BEE, and if the patient is obese, an adjusted body weight should be used.

POSTCATABOLISM ASSESSMENT

A more comprehensive and accurate nutritional assessment can be completed once the initial period of peak catabolism subsides, often by the sixth to tenth postinjury day. In many severe illnesses, such as full-thickness burns, trauma, and sepsis, the catabolic phase may last longer that 10 days. Bistrian (12) has described a catabolic index (CI) based on urinary urea excretion to assess the stress response to an injury. The CI is calculated as follows:

$$CI = UUN - 1/2 \text{ dietary nitrogren} + 3 \qquad \textbf{(22-1)}$$

where UUN (urinary urea nitrogen) and dietary nitrogen are in g per day. It is interpreted as follows: CI of 0 = no significant stress, CI of 1–5 = mild stress, and CI of > 5 = moderate to severe stress. The calculation of the CI compares actual nitrogen excretion with expected nitrogen excretion. The equation assumes that 50 percent of dietary nitrogen is utilized, 50 percent is converted to urea, and 3 g, known as the obligatory nitrogen loss, is excreted even if the patient consumes no protein. Thus, the extent to which the measured UUN exceeds 50 percent of nitrogen intake is an index to assess the degree of stress imposed by an illness. A postcatabolism nutritional assessment could be performed when the CI is less than 5, suggesting that the stress response has subsided.

SERIAL NUTRITIONAL ASSESSMENT

The best continuing evaluation of adequacy of the nutritional care plan consists of a monitoring of daily calorie and nutrient intake coupled with a recording of changes in body weight. Serial evaluation of body weight should be compared with usual preinjury, or postcatabolism, weight to eliminate the effect of fluid resuscitation. A weight change greater than 1 pound per day, or 0.5 kg per day, suggests fluid imbalance that will usually negate the interpretation of serum protein concentration values.

Indicators of lean body mass, such as arm muscle area and creatinine-height index, are not highly sensitive to changes in somatic protein and need be measured no more than every 10 days. If the patient is immobile and physical therapy is not given, lean body mass will probably not increase in spite of aggressive nutritional support (6).

Immunocompetence usually returns after 7 to 10 days in anergic patients when nutritional support is given. A poor prognosis may be anticipated when anergy persists despite aggressive nutritional support.

Nitrogen retention, which reflects adequacy of protein intake, can be estimated by measuring urea nitrogen in a 24-hour urine collection and calculating nitrogen balance using Eqs.(5-22) and (5-23). However, this formula does not take into account abnormal extrarenal nitrogen losses such as commonly occur with burns, extensive soft tissue damage, fistulas, or severe vomiting or diarrhea. The formula can thus underestimate nitrogen losses in critically ill patients who experience abnormal nitrogen losses, and can result in an invalid value for nitrogen retention. Monitoring of daily weight change and of fluctuations in plasma albumin and transferrin levels every 10 to 14 days will help indicate adequacy of protein intake in cases in which calculation of nitrogen balance is not feasible.

MULTIPLE ORGAN SYSTEM FAILURE

Patients who survive the immediate effects of severe trauma and those who develop postoperative complications may experience a syndrome known as *multiple organ system failure* (MOSF). MOSF may include a functional collapse of the following systems (13):

1. The lungs, resulting in acute respiratory distress syndrome (ARDS).
2. The kidneys, resulting in acute oliguric renal failure.
3. The liver, resulting in cholestatic jaundice and hepatocyte failure.
4. The GI tract, resulting in ileus and stress ulceration.

MOSF is frequently seen with septic complications following surgery. An individual is more susceptible to MOSF if underlying factors that decrease the body's functional capacity are present. These factors may include nutritional depletion, systemic disease, immune deficits, chronic illness, and a history of smoking or alcohol abuse. Guidelines for the nutritional management of GI, renal, and liver failure which may occur in MOSF are discussed in preceeding chapters.

THE CRITICALLY ILL PULMONARY PATIENT

Respiratory or pulmonary failure is a clinical diagnosis confirmed by alterations in arterial blood gases (ABGs). *Acute respiratory failure* occurs when the partial pressure of oxygen in arterial blood (PaO_2) is less than 60 mm Hg, and the $PaCO_2$ is greater than 50 mm Hg with an arterial pH of less than 7.30 (14). Normal values are as follows: PaO_2 of 80 to 100, $PaCO_2$ of 35 to 45 mm Hg, and pH of 7.35 to 7.45. Acute respiratory failure is most commonly seen in critical illness or with chronic obstructive pulmonary disease (COPD). *COPD* refers to a group of diseases, including chronic bronchitis and emphysema, which are characterized by irreversible airway obstruction resulting in resistance to airflow during expiration. COPD is the most common form of chronic respiratory illness and the primary cause of death from lung disease.

MALNUTRITION AND PULMONARY FUNCTION

The basic problem in respiratory failure is insufficient oxygenation of the tissues coupled with retention of carbon dioxide. With increasing calorie intake and the oxidation of nutrients, both oxygen demand and carbon dioxide production are increased. On the other hand, discontinuation of, or a great reduction in, feeding decreases oxygen demand and carbon dioxide production and reduces the burden on the respiratory system. However, malnutrition further compromises respiratory insufficiency and should be avoided, especially in the ventilator-dependent patient (9).

With malnutrition, the muscles of breathing—that is, the diaphragmatic, intercostal, and accessory muscles—are catabolized for energy, resulting in a decrease in inspiratory capacity. The decrease in serum albumin level which occurs with inadequate protein intake, if sufficiently severe, may cause a decrease in oncotic pressure, leading to pulmonary edema. The central nervous system control of respiration can be impaired by the hypoxia which accompanies starvation.

Malnutrition also depresses clearance of bacteria from the lungs and predisposes to pulmonary infection, to which pulmonary patients are already susceptible. In fact, pneumonia is the most frequent immediate cause of death in starvation. Lung surfactant production is reduced in malnutrition, which can result in decreased compliance, pulmonary collapse, and pneumonia. All these factors suggest that adequate nutritional support is especially important to maintain normal pulmonary function.

Respiratory Quotient

The *respiratory quotient* (RQ) is defined as the ratio of carbon dioxide produced to oxygen consumed. The higher the RQ, the more carbon dioxide is produced to be expired, and the greater the demand on the respiratory system. The RQ is an indication of the type of substrate being metabolized for energy. Protein, carbohydrate, and fat have characteristic RQs when metabolized. Recall the equation for the oxidation of glucose:

$$C_6H_{12}O_6 + 6O_2 \rightarrow 6CO_2 + 6H_2O$$

Thus, 6 molecules of oxygen are used to produce 6 molecules of carbon dioxide. The RQ of glucose oxidation is thus 6/6, or 1.0, a higher amount of carbon dioxide production than is seen with other nutrients. Fat is oxidized with an RQ of 0.7 and is associated with a lesser degree of carbon dioxide production than glucose, while protein has an intermediate RQ value of 0.80. The RQ of a mixed diet is approximately 0.825.

It is also possible for the RQ to be higher than 1, putting an even greater strain on the respiratory system. Triglyceride synthesis from carbohydrate is associated with an RQ greater than 1. Table 22-1 summarizes the RQ of various metabolic fuels.

Increased carbon dioxide production caused by either excessive administration of total calories or adequate administration of total calories composed primarily of glucose will increase the workload of the lungs. When excess calories are reduced or fat replaces carbohydrate as a calorie source, production of carbon dioxide is decreased, and the demands on pulmonary function are also decreased.

MECHANICAL VENTILATION

The patient with respiratory failure requires mechanical ventilation in order to maintain a blood volume of oxygen that meets tissue needs. In order to place a patient on a respirator or mechanical ventilator, intubation or establishment of an airway via the trachea to the lungs is required. The common means of establishing an airway for mechanical ventilation are placement of an orotracheal tube or a nasotracheal tube. A tracheostomy is used when a patient requires mechanical ventilation for longer than 1 to 2 weeks. If an orotracheal tube or a nasotracheal tube is used the patient cannot speak or swallow. Depending on the type of tracheostomy, the patient may be able to speak; a fenestrated tracheostomy permits speaking.

Adequate oxygenation on a respirator is accomplished by manipulation of the concentration of inspired oxygen (FiO$_2$) and, in some cases, use of *positive end-expiratory pressure* (PEEP). PEEP prevents alveolar collapse and enables a lower FiO$_2$ to be used.

TABLE 22-1 Respiratory Quotient of Metabolic Fuels

Substrate	Respiratory Quotient (RQ) [*]
Carbohydrate	
glucose oxidation	1.00
Fat	
triglyceride oxidation	0.71
triglyceride synthesis from:	
glucose	8.70
triglyceride	1.00
amino acids	0.74
Protein	
amino acid oxidation	0.80
Mixed Diet	
carbohydrate, protein, and fat	0.825

[*]RQ = ratio of the amount of CO$_2$ expired to the amount of O$_2$ inspired. An RQ of greater than 1 is considered medically dangerous.

Weaning a patient from a respirator is a gradual process that eventually leads to the patient's breathing independently. The PEEP must be 5 cm of H$_2$O or less before weaning can start, as breathing against PEEP requires extra effort during expiration. The FiO$_2$ is decreased at a rate of 5 to 10 percent per hour, and PEEP is also gradually decreased. The FiO$_2$ of room air is approximately 21 percent oxygen.

Many approaches are used in weaning from mechanical ventilation. One approach involves removing the patient from the ventilator for progressively longer intervals. Another approach involves the use of synchronized intermittent mandatory ventilation (SIMV), which allows the patient to breathe independently as the ventilator delivers a preset number of machine breaths in synchrony with the patient's breaths (14). SIMV serves as a form of graduated active exercise for the respiratory muscles. The patient's progress is monitored by *arterial blood gas* (ABG) determinations throughout the weaning process.

Nutritional Considerations in Weaning from the Respirator

Nutritional support plays an important role in weaning a patient from a respirator. In one report (15), 86 percent of ventilator-dependent patients who had received some degree of nutritional support, compared to only 22 percent of those patients who had received only 5 percent dextrose in water, were able to be weaned from mechanical ventilation.

Provision of a calorie level above the maintenance requirement will result in increased carbon dioxide production and difficulty in weaning a patient from a ventilator. For the nutritionally depleted patient on a respirator, such as commonly occurs with COPD, it is sometimes considered to be preferable to continue the patient on the respirator for a longer period, providing a higher level of caloric support for repletion. This allows for restoration of lean body mass, including the muscles of respiration. As a result, respiratory function would be improved and weaning from the respirator would be facilitated.

For both the nutritionally depleted patient and the hypermetabolic patient, a consideration of calorie level and proportion of calories as glucose is essential to facilitate weaning. Monitoring of ABG determinations and RQ values, if available, during the weaning process can be used as a guideline for making changes in the nutrient intake.

NUTRIENT REQUIREMENTS

Calorie needs for *maintenance* in the ventilator-dependent patient can be established as 1.2 times the measured REE if indirect calorimetry is available (9). Calculation of *maintenance* energy expenditure as BEE × 1.2 to 1.5 is recommended depending on the estimated severity of the disease (9, 11). In one study where indirect calorimetry was compared with calculation of energy expenditure as BEE × 1.2, 70 percent of patients were within values determined by indirect calorimetry (9). Alternatively, 30 to 35 kcal/kg body weight is sufficient for maintenance in most patients with mild to moderate stress, as discussed in Chapter 14. For *replenishment* of undernourished, *stable* respiratory patients, energy needs may be established as 1.5 × REE or BEE.

The proportion of calories to provide as fat or carbohydrate is an important consideration in the ventilator-dependent patient. To reduce carbon dioxide production, lipid should provide 30 to 50 percent of total calories. A continuous infusion of parenteral lipid is preferred in order to minimize the proinflammatory and vasoconstriction responses associated with rapid parenteral infusion of lipid. Parenteral glucose infusion should not exceed 4 to 6 mg per kg per minute. A protein intake of 1.2 to 1.5 g per kg per day or 0.2 g N per kg per day is usually adequate. A protein intake of 2.0 to 2.5 g protein per kg per day may be needed in patients experiencing severe stress due to sepsis, trauma, or burns. Excess protein intake should be avoided when attempting to wean a patient from mechanical ventilation. Patients receiving high protein intakes have been observed to have an increased ventilatory drive, resulting in dyspnea (9, 11).

Adequate provision of minerals, vitamins, and trace elements is also important. Phosphate depletion can result in respiratory failure due to decreased levels of 2, 3-diphosphoglycerate concentration in red blood cells. This decrease in 2, 3-diphosphoglycerate concentration can cause an increase in oxyhemoglobin affinity and a decrease in oxygen delivery to tissues. Serum phosphorus levels should be monitored at all times, but especially during nutritional repletion when phosphorus requirements increase. Low levels of magnesium and calcium will also affect respiratory muscle strength and should be monitored (16). Magnesium depletion is more common during TPN, in conditions of malabsorption or alcoholism, and when drugs such as cisplatin and diuretics are used (17).

METHODS OF NUTRITIONAL SUPPORT

Enteral or parenteral feeding can be used to provide nutritional support for the ventilator-dependent patient. Nutritional support is instituted after the patient has stabilized on mechanical ventilation. Many patients become agitated when placed on a respirator and require sedation. Drugs that are selective neuromuscular blocking agents, such as pancuronium and vecuronium, are often required to intubate and maintain a patient with mechanical ventilation. At common clinical doses these drugs do not interfere with intestinal motility, so that enteral feeding can be used depending on the patient's overall condition.

Enteral Feeding
Enteral feeding, rather than TPN, is indicated when the gut is functioning. The long-term tracheostomy patient is usually able to eat but may have difficulty swallowing. A swallow study should be performed to confirm that swallowing is not associated with an increased risk of aspiration in these patients. Tracheal tube cuffs should be inflated during feeding to seal off the trachea and reduce the risk of aspiration. Consuming a large meal can result in exertion, abdominal distention, and considerable dyspnea for a pulmonary patient. Resting before and after meals may help with fatigue, and eating six small meals per day may reduce respiratory distress. The patient should also be instructed to eat slowly and be given soft, easy-to-chew foods to avoid overexertion during meal times.

In ventilator-dependent patients with an orotracheal or nasotracheal tube and a functioning gut, tube feeding is necessary. Nasoduodenal or jejunal feeding is often used to reduce the risk of aspiration. Bolus feeding of formulas is associated with a higher incidence of vomiting, reflux, and aspiration. Continuous feeding is preferred in the patient on a respirator if tube feeding is necessary.

Parenteral Feeding
TPN is required when maximal rest of the intestinal tract is indicated. A nearby tracheostomy can increase septic risk at a subclavian catheter insertion site. Special dressings may be used to protect the catheter insertion site, or the catheter may be tunneled under the skin away from the tracheostomy.

Transitional Feeding
Patients maintained on mechanical ventilation frequently experience several transitions in feeding technique (see

Chapter 14 for a detailed discussion of transitional feeding). A transition from TPN to tube feeding is probably the most common type of change in feeding technique in ventilator-dependent patients. At a later point, most patients maintained on tube feedings eventually consume an oral diet with discontinuation of their tube feedings. When a respirator patient is changed from tube feeding to an oral diet, an important consideration is the texture of the diet. A soft diet is usually better tolerated because the patient will probably have a sore throat, which often occurs with intubation for a period of time.

BURNS

A severe burn is an extremely catabolic injury, resulting in higher energy requirements than any other condition. Burns are associated with increased risk of sepsis, and multiple surgical procedures for skin grafting are usually required during recovery. Vigorous nutritional support of the burn patient is essential for wound healing and survival.

The severity of the burn injury determines nutrient requirements and the techniques required for nutrition support. Burns are classified as minor, moderate, or major, depending on the percentage of the total body surface area (TBSA) burned and the thickness of the burn. The epithelium is not completely destroyed with a *partial-thickness burn* (formerly called *second-degree burn*) and, thus, these wounds regenerate without grafting. A *full-thickness burn* (formerly called *third-degree burn*) results in complete destruction of the epithelium and requires skin grafting. A minor burn includes partial-thickness burns of less than 15 percent TBSA and full-thickness burns of less than 2 percent TBSA in adults, and partial-thickness burns of less than 10 percent TBSA in children. The classification of moderate and major burns as percentage TBSA is summarized below (18):

	Moderate (%)	Major (%)
Partial-thickness		
Adults	15–25	>25
Children	10–20	>20
Full-thickness		
Adults	2–10	>10
Children	<10	>10

NUTRIENT REQUIREMENTS

Ideally, REE should be measured by indirect calorimetry 2 to 3 times per week in the patient with moderate to major burns. Assuming light activity, energy needs can then be determined as REE times 1.2 for adults and REE times 1.35 for children to account for light activity (19).

If indirect calorimetry is not available, a formula can be used to predict energy expenditure for adult burn patients. The energy needs of children with burns can be estimated as twice their predicted BEE (17). The Matsuda formula is based on data from indirect calorimetry and includes a factor of 20 percent to account for energy expenditure in daily physical therapy and dressing changes (20). The Harris-Benedict equation is first used to calculate BEE and then the following factors are applied according to the percentage of TBSA burned when using the Matsuda formula:

Percent TBSA Burned	Daily Energy Needs
0–10	BEE × 1.5
10–30	BEE × 1.6
>30	BEE × 1.7

The Curreri formula is thought to be the best formula for estimating *peak* energy expenditure in burn patients (21). However, the Curreri formula may result in overfeeding as the catabolic response subsides and skin grafting occurs. Daily energy needs are calculated as follows:

$$\text{Daily energy needs} = (25 \text{ kcal} \times \text{kg preburn body wt})$$

$$+ (40 \text{ kcal} \times \% \text{ TBSA burned}) \quad \textbf{(22-2)}$$

For burns over 50 percent TBSA, a constant of 50 percent TBSA is used to prevent overestimation of energy needs.

Protein requirements also reflect the extent and severity of burn injury, as protein is lost through the burn wound itself. Protein should comprise 20 percent of total daily energy intake for adults and children with greater than 10 percent TBSA burned and 15 percent of total daily energy intake if the burn wound size is 1 to 10 percent TBSA (17). This results in a nonprotein calorie to nitrogen ratio of 100–150:1 g nitrogen.

There is controversy regarding the proportion of energy to provide as fat or carbohydrate to burn patients. Recent evidence suggests that the usual provision of 25 to 40 percent energy from fat may produce hyperlipidemia and be immunosuppressive, especially when linoleic acid intake is high (22). Gottschlich and Alexander recommend that enteral or parenteral nutrition for adults and children with burn injury should provide 10 to 15 percent of nonprotein calories from lipid, and approximately 5 percent of nonprotein calories from linoleic acid (22). Further research is needed to resolve this issue; parenteral nutrition and tube feedings can be easily adjusted to limit fat intake, (see Chapters 13 and 14).

Some studies suggest that vitamin and mineral requirements increase with burn injury (23). Vitamin C is usually supplemented to provide 1.0 to 1.5 g per day, and zinc is frequently provided at a level of 2 to 3 times the RDA. There is some evidence to suggest that the requirements for niacin, biotin, pyridoxine, thiamin, and folate are increased with burns. With the exception of vitamin C and zinc, commercial tube feedings and supplemental parenteral-feeding solutions will provide an adequate intake of vitamins and minerals for the burn victim. If the patient is consuming an oral diet, a daily multiple vitamin-mineral supplement should be included.

METHODS OF NUTRITIONAL SUPPORT

The real challenge of providing nutritional care to a burn victim is in devising feeding regimens that can provide large calorie and protein intakes. The first 24 hours after a moderate to major burn are used to fluid resuscitate the patient. After hemodynamic stability is achieved, nutrition support, either enteral or parenteral, is begun as soon as possible. Recent evidence suggests that early enteral feeding in the burn patient may actually decrease the hypermetabolism associated with burn injury (24). Criteria for selecting the method of nutrition support include age, percentage and location of burn, total estimated calorie and protein needs, ability to ingest an oral diet, gastrointestinal tract function, fluid balance, liver and renal function, respiratory status, previous nutritional status, and the surgical plan (17). In the patient who is able to eat, a high-calorie, high-protein diet is indicated. Small frequent meals and oral nutrition supplements are usually needed to meet energy needs.

Enteral Feeding
Tube feeding is often required in patients with moderate or major burns in order to meet energy and protein needs or to augment oral feeding. For example, if a patient cannot consistently consume 75 percent of calorie and protein needs by oral feeding, supplemental tube feeding at night is indicated. In patients with burns of the face and mouth, an adequate oral intake is difficult to achieve, and tube feeding is essential. Continuous enteral tube feeding (with or without oral intake) is indicated for patients who are unable to meet at least 75 percent of calorie and protein needs via oral diet plus nocturnal tube feedings (17). A tube feeding with a calorie density of 1.5 to 2.0 kcal per mL is often utilized to meet energy needs in burn patients. A tube feeding with an elemental formula may be useful in patients who have burns on the buttocks and thighs, in order to reduce contamination from stool. Procedures for initiating and monitoring tube feeding are discussed in Chapter 13.

Parenteral Feeding
Parenteral feeding (with or without oral intake) is used for patients with a persistent or recurrent paralytic ileus or intractable diarrhea. It is also indicated for patients with the following gastrointestinal complications associated with moderate to major burns (17): stress ulceration of the stomach and duodenum (Curling's ulcer), pancreatitis, acalculous cholecystitis, nonocclusive ischemic enterocolitis, superior mesenteric artery syndrome, or pseudo-obstruction of the colon. Access sites for a TPN catheter can be limited when a burn covers a large area of the body. Of greatest concern is the increased risk of sepsis in burn patients when TPN is used. Special precautions must be observed when changing dressings at the catheter site. Despite the risk of infection, peripheral or central parenteral nutrition is frequently used because nutritional support is essential for these patients' survival.

CANCER

In general, the purpose of nutrition intervention in the patient with cancer is to maintain optimal nutritional status in order to maximize the benefits of cancer therapy (25). Rapid loss of body weight is associated with decreased treatment effectiveness and increased mortality. The nutritional care of cancer patients often involves the use of several different feeding techniques and a wide variety of dietary modifications. The diverse nature of nutritional problems and the high frequency of anorexia make the delivery of nutritional care to cancer patients one of the most challenging and demanding areas of work for a nutritional care specialist.

The following information is needed to conduct a thorough nutritional assessment for the patient with cancer:

1. Primary site and type of tumor; presence of metastases.
2. Surgery-type, extent, and findings.
3. Chemotherapy-type, dose, frequency and duration.
4. Radiation-site, dose, duration, and the effect of treatment on gastrointestinal tract function.

A careful assessment of the patient's ability to tolerate food is also needed; this would include the following:

1. The physical ability to ingest food—chewing and swallowing ability, dryness, and soreness or inflammation of oral mucosa secondary to tumor or therapy.
2. Specific food tolerances—anorexia, appetite fluctuation, nausea, and vomiting, allergies, food preferences and aversions, taste changes, and relation of food tolerance to treatment.
3. Bowel habits—diarrhea, steatorrhea, constipation, and presence of an ostomy.

A careful assessment of a patient's specific dietary intolerances and response to cancer therapy will allow for the development of an individualized nutritional care plan. An individualized approach to each patient's specific food intolerances is one of the most important aspects of successful nutritional management of the cancer patient.

EFFECTS OF CANCER THERAPY

Surgery, chemotherapy, and radiation therapy produce a wide variety of effects that influence eating patterns. Anorexia, nausea or vomiting, diarrhea, constipation, taste alterations and aversions, and subsequent weight loss are commonly seen with all three types of therapy. General recommendations for nutrition intervention in the patient with cancer are given in Table 22–2.

Food Preferences
Several generalizations can be made about food preferences in cancer patients. There is an increased sensitivity to the tastes of sweet and bitter, resulting in an aversion to sweet foods and hot meats. If meats are poorly tolerated, alternative sources of protein such as cheese and other dairy products, cooked eggs, tofu, or peanut butter may be acceptable. Liquid beverages and supplements are also popular. In general, cancer patients seem to prefer cold foods or foods served at room temperature to hot foods that formerly were favorites. Experimentation with seasonings and flavorings may improve food acceptance.

Surgery
The location and extent of a surgical procedure determines the appropriate diet. Resections in the head and neck area often result in impaired chewing and swallowing and may require tube feeding. An esophagectomy may decrease gastric motility and acid production and lead to esophageal stenosis. A gastrectomy or

TABLE 22-2   Recommendations for Nutritional Intervention in Patients with Cancer

Symptom	Recommendation
Anorexia	Adjust meal size to appetite. Provide favorite foods. Use wine as an appetite stimulant, if allowed. Use prescribed drugs to stimulate appetite (dexamethasone, tetrahydrocannabinol).

Weight loss	Provide high-calorie and protein-dense foods:
	    Add powdered milk to foods and beverages to increase protein.
	    Add a glucose polymer supplement to beverages, soups, or gravies.
	    Use high-fat or high-calorie forms of foods such as ice cream, whole milk, or fruit packed in "heavy" syrup.
	    Add diced meat or cheese to foods.
	    Encourage between-meal snacks and commercial supplements.

Stomatitis and mucositis	Avoid crisp or rough-textured foods. Avoid salty, spicy, and acid foods. Try bland, soft, or liquid consistency diets served at room temperature. Use warm saline solution or mouth washes with local anesthetics, such as lidocaine HCl, before meals.
Chewing and swallowing difficulty, xerostomia	Drink liquids with meals. Soften consistency of foods to the thick liquid, such as milkshake, or semisolid, such as mashed potatoes. Add sauces, gravies, and fats. Use synthetic saliva. Use a straw to ease swallowing. Try frozen popsicles to numb sore throat.
Nausea or vomiting	Use prescribed antiemetic drugs prior to meals (metoclopramide, chlorpromazine, prochlorperazine maleate, trimethobenzamide, and thiethylperazine). Avoid serving favorite foods during "bad times" to avoid inducing a negative response to favorite foods. Try small frequent meals. Avoid liquid with meals.. Eat cold or room temperature foods rather than hot foods. Avoid serving foods with strong odors or flavors. Avoid foods that are greasy, spicy, or very sweet.
Diarrhea	Increase fluid intake to replace losses. Use antidiarrheals, such as Lomotil or Kaopectate. Increase potassium-rich foods. Adjust fat and lactose content of diet as needed.
Constipation	Increase fluid and fiber intake.

Adapted from A. Gormican, Influencing food acceptance in anorexic cancer patients. *Postgraduate Medicine* 68: (1980) 145–152, and American Dietetic Association. *Manual of Clinical Dietetics*, 4th ed., 1992

vagotomy may require a diet for "dumping syndrome." Gastrectomy may also result in deficiencies of iron, calcium, fat-soluble vitamins, and vitamin B_{12}. Massive resection of the small intestine can result in loss of bile salts and subsequent fat malabsorption, vitamin B_{12} deficiency, metabolic acidosis, and increased risk of renal stones. Parenteral nutrition may be required after radical intestinal resection, and a colostomy or ileostomy may be needed. (See Chapaters 16, 17,and 18.)

Chemotherapy and Radiation Therapy

Chemotherapy will often accentuate preexisting anorexia and nausea. Mucositis, stomatitis, candidiasis, diarrhea, constipation, lactose intolerance, fluid retention, and an increasing number of food aversions are common. Food aversion may be worsened when strongly flavored foods are served before chemotherapy or radiation therapy. Offering blandly flavored foods before treatment may reduce the frequency of food aversions (26).

Radiation therapy is a localized treatment that usually damages normal tissues surrounding the tumor. Irradiation of the oropharyngeal area results in changes in taste buds and taste perception. Reduced salivation, sore throat, dysphagia, and dental deterioration compound eating problems in these patients. Teeth may become overly sensitive to cold, heat, and sweet flavors. Irradiation of the abdomen and pelvis may produce chronic diarrhea, malabsorption, fluid and electrolyte imbalances, stenosis, and obstruction. A diet restricted in lactose, fat, or fiber may be needed.

HUMAN IMMUNODEFICIENCY VIRUS INFECTION

The term *human immunodeficiency virus* (HIV) infection is used to refer to all phases of the disease process culminating in acquired immunodeficiency syndrome (AIDS) (27). AIDS is caused by the HIV, which selectively attracts and depletes CD4+ and T lymphocytes, causing a predisposition to opportunistic infections and malignancies. Persons with HIV infection experience a progressive depletion in acquired immunity and, in the majority of cases, AIDS develops within 7 to 10 years of initial infection. Profound weight loss and tissue wasting are characteristic of HIV infection. The etiology of this malnutrition is multifactorial and is thought to result from (28): decreased food intake, malabsorption secondary to gastrointestinal problems, and increased energy or nutrient requirements as a consequence of changes in intermediary metabolism initiated and possibly mediated by the HIV. Current understanding of the mechanism of malnutrition in HIV infection is incomplete.

Dietary Recommendations

HIV infection is a complex disease associated with a wide array of complications including opportunistic infections, malignancies, and neurological abnormalities. Dietary recommendations should be individualized for patients with HIV infection because patients tend to develop unique complications as they progress through the disease process. Nutritional problems experienced by patients with HIV infection which are similar to those experienced by all cancer patients include anorexia, chewing and swallowing difficulty, nausea or vomiting, and diarrhea and malabsorption. The nutritional management of these problems is outlined in Table 22–2.

Diarrhea and malabsorption are often associated with infections of the gastrointestinal tract due to immunosuppression. Specific pathogens common in HIV patients include cytomegalovirus, *mycobacterium avium intracellulare, giardia lamblia*, and *cryptosporidium*. One study identified the cytomegalovirus in 90 percent of patients with AIDS at autopsy (29). This virus results in ulcerative lesions throughout the entire gastrointestinal tract, but especially in the esophagus, stomach, small intestine, colon, and biliary tract. The symptoms of cytomegalovirus infection may include esophagitis, retrosternal pain, gastritis, enteritis, colitis, proctitis, watery or bloody diarrhea, or biliary disease (17). In some cases parenteral nutrition may be required if the diarrhea is prolonged and severe. If the patient is able to tolerate an oral diet, a low-fat, low-residue, lactose-free or low-lactose, caffeine-free diet is suggested (17). Alternatively, a pectin-containing bulking agent may reduce mild diarrhea.

New drugs for the treatment of HIV infection are continually being released. Many of these drugs have nutritional side effects, such as nausea, vomiting, and altered taste perception, and also result in drug-nutrient interactions. The nutrition care specialist should routinely obtain *recent* information about specific drugs used to treat the symptoms of HIV infection.

Food-Handling Practices

Safe food-handling practices and adequate sanitation are essential for the patient with HIV infection in order to avoid foodborne infections. Food poisoning, especially salmonella, can lead to serious illness and death for someone with HIV infection. Meats, poultry, or fish should be cooked well-done, raw eggs should be avoided, dairy products made from milk that is not pasteurized should be avoided, and raw fruits and vegetables should be carefully washed before eating.

It may be necessary to educate the patient with HIV infection about proper preparation, cleaning, and storage of food, and to stress the importance of thorough hand washing before food preparation or eating (30). To date, there is no evidence that HIV infection can be transmitted through food or handling of trays and silverware. Thus, isolation procedures are not routine for hospitalized patients with HIV infection. However, protective isolation may be required for those patients who are severely immunosuppressed.

Methods of Nutritional Support

Malnutrition is very common in patients with HIV infection; however, the efficacy of nutrition support in these patients has not been clearly demonstrated. Evidence suggests that early nutrition intervention and increased target levels for energy intake are needed for patients with HIV infection (31). In general, patients with more than 10 percent weight loss should be refed utilizing either enteral or parenteral feeding (28, 30). Enteral nutrition support via oral or tube feeding is preferred if the gastrointestinal tract is functional. Home enteral supplementation via a permanently placed feeding tube is a useful approach for some patients. For the HIV patient with mild to moderate diarrhea, characteristics of an acceptable enteral formula include moderate fat content with medium-chain triglycerides, high nitrogen content, and reduced lactose content (17). Research is ongoing to determine if nutritional pharmacological modules such as adding n-3 fatty acids, glutamine, arginine, or structural lipids will be useful in patients with HIV infection (32).

Parenteral nutrition is indicated when gastrointestinal disease is severe and diarrhea and malabsorption persist. Peripheral parenteral nutrition is typically used as an adjunct to enteral nutrition for periods of fewer than 7 days. Central parenteral nutrition is used when long-term nutrition support is needed. Home TPN is also an option for patients with HIV infection.

REFERENCES

1. **Wilmore, D.W.** Catabolic illness-strategies for enhancing recovery. *N. Eng. J. Med.* 325:(1991)695–702.

2. **Moldawer, L.** Nutritional pharmacology. *Support Line* 16:(1994) 1–5

3. **Fisher, C.J., S.M. Opal, J.F. Dhainaut, S. Stephens, J.L. Zimmerman, P. Nightingale, S.J. Harris, R.M. Schein, E.A. Panacek,** and **J.L Vincent.** The influence of anti-tumor necrosis factor monoclonal antibody on cytokine levels in patients with sepsis. The CB006 sepsis syndrome study group. *Crit. Care Med.* 21:(1993)318–27.

4. **Ziegler, T. R., L.S. Young, K. Benfell, M. Scheltinga, K. Hortos, R. Bye, F.D. Morrow, D.O. Jacobs, R.J. Smith, J.H. Antin,** and **D.W. Wilmore.** Clinical and metabolic efficacy of glutamine-supplemented parenteral nutrition after bone marrow transplantation. *Ann. Int. Med.* 116:(1992)821–828.

5. **Yang, H., M. Grahn, D.S. Schalch,** and **D.M. Ney.** Anabolic effects of IGF-I coinfused with total parenteral nutrition in dexamethasone-treated rats. *Am. J. Physiol.* 266:(1994)E690–E698.

6. **McMahon, M.M., M.B. Farnell,** and **M.J. Murray.** Nutritional support of critically ill patients. *Mayo Clin. Proc.* 68:(1993)911–20.

7. **Roy, L.B., P.A. Edwards,** and **L.H. Barr.** The value of nutritional assessment in the surgical patient. *JPEN* 9:(1985)170–72.

8. **Gray, G.E.,** and **L.K. Gray.** Anthropometric measurements and their interpretation: Principles, practices, and problems. *J. Am. Dietet. Assoc.* 77: (1980)534–939.

9. **DeMeo, M.T., W. VanDeGraaff, K. Gottlieb, P. Sobotka,** and **S. Mobarhan.** Nutrition in acute pulmonary disease. *Nutr. Rev.* 50:(1992)320–28.

10. **Twomey, P., D. Siegler,** and **J. Rombeau.** Utility of skin testing in nutritional assessment: A critical review. *JPEN* 6:(1982)50–58.

11. **Deitel, M., V.P. Williams,** and **T.W. Rice.** Nutrition and the patient requiring mechanical ventilatory support. *J. Am. Coll. Nutr.* 2:(1983)25-32.

12. **Bistrian, B.R.** A simple technique to estimate severity of stress. *Surg. Gynecol. Obstet.* 148:(1979)675–78.

13. **Borzotta, A.P.,** and **H.C. Polk.** Multiple-system organ failure. *Surg. Clin. N. Amer.* 63:(1983)315–36.

14. **Shapiro, B.A.** Airway pressure therapy for acute restrictive pulmonary pathology. In W.C. Shoemaker, W.L. Thompson, and P.R. Holbrook, eds. *Textbook of Critical Care,* Philadelphia: Saunders, 1984, 224–36.

15. **Barrocas, A., R. Tretola,** and **A. Alonso.** Nutrition and the critically ill pulmonary patient. *Resp. Care* 28:(1983)50–60.

16. **Landon, R.A.,** and **E.A. Young.** Role of magnesium in regulation of lung function. *J. Am. Dietet. Assoc.* 93:(1993)674–77.

17. American Dietetic Association. *Manual of Clinical Dietetics,* 4th ed., Chicago: 1992.

18. **Choctaw, W.T., M.E. Eisner,** and **T.L. Wachtel.** Causes, prevention, pre-hospital care, evaluation, emergency treatment and prognosis. *In* B.M. Achauer, ed. *Management of the Burned Patient.* Norwalk, CT: Appleton & Lange, 1987.

19. **Long, C.L., N. Schaffel,** and **J.W. Geiger.** Metabolic response to injury and illness: estimation of energy and protein needs from indirect calorimetry and nitrogen balance. *JPEN* 3:(1979)452–56.

20. **Matsuda, T., N. Clark, G.D. Hariyani,** and **R.S. Bryant.** The effect of burn wound size on resting energy expenditure. *J. Trauma* 27:(1987)115–20.

21. **Curreri, P.W., D. Richmond, J. Marvin,** and **C.R. Baxter.** Dietary requirements of patients with major burns. *J. Am. Dietet. Assoc.* 65:(1974)415–17.

22. **Gottschlich, M. M.,** and **J.W. Alexander.** Fat kinetics and recommended dietary intake in burns. *JPEN* 11:(1987)80–85.

23. **Gottschlich, M.M.,** and **G.D. Warden.** Vitamin supplementation in the patient with burns. *J. Burn Care Rehabil.* 11:(1990) 275–88.

24. **Chiarelli, A., G. Enzi, A. Casadei, B. Baggio, A. Valerio,** and **F. Mazzoleni.** Very early nutrition supplementation in burned patients. *Am. J. Clin. Nutr.* 51:(1990)1035–39.

25. **Klein, S.,** and **R.L. Koretz.** Nutrition support in patients with cancer: what do the data really show? *Nutr. in Clin. Prac.* 9:(1994) 91–100.

26. **Gormican, A.** Influencing food acceptance in anorexic cancer patients. *Postgraduate Med.* 68:(1980)145–52.

27. Report of the Presidential Commission on the Human Immunodeficiency Virus Epidemic, Washington DC: Government Printing Office, 1988.

28. **Singer, P., D.P. Katz, L. Dillon, O. Kirvela, T. Lazarus,** and **J. Askanazi.** Nutritional aspects of the acquired immunodeficiency syndrome. *Am. J. Gastroen.* 87:(1992)265–73.

29. **Bartlett, J., B. Loughbon,** and **T. Quinn.** Gastrointestinal complications of AIDS. *In* V.Devita, S. Hellman, and S Rosenberg, eds. *AIDS Etiology, Diagnosis, Treatment and Prevention.* Philadelphia: Lippincott, 1988.

30. Position of The American Dietetic Association and The Canadian Dieteic Association: Nutrition intervention in the care of persons with human immunodeficiency virus infection. *J. Am. Dietet. Asssoc.* 94:(1994)1042-45.

31. **Chlebowski, R.T., M. Grosvenor, L. Lillington, J. Sayre,** and **G. Beall.** Dietary intake and counseling, weight maintenance, and the course of HIV infection. *J. Am. Dietet. Assoc.* 95:(1995)428–35.

32. **Trujillo, E.B., B.C. Borlase, S.J. Bell, K.J. Guenther, W. Swails, P.M. Queen,** and **J.R. Trujillo.** Assessment of nutritional status, nutrient intake, and nutrition support in AIDS patients. *J. Am. Dietet. Assoc.* 92:(1992)477–78, .

TO TEST YOUR UNDERSTANDING

1. Rank the following conditions according to the degree of stress and need for nutritional support; 1= most stressful, in need of aggressive nutritional support, and 5 = least.

a. A healthy, young, well-nourished patient is scheduled for an elective surgical procedure

b. A well-nourished patient with recently discovered cancer is admitted to begin aggressive chemotherapy.

c. A 14-year old male with third-degree burns over 20 percent of his body is admitted to the burn unit.

d. A middle-aged moderately wasted patient with severe emphysema is admitted with pneumonia.

e. An otherwise healthy patient with multiple injuries enters the intensive care unit.

2. Tell why the following parameters of nutritional assessment are not of value in the described situations.

a. A young comatose male with fractures of both arms secondary to a motorcycle accident, and who has recently received 2 units of whole blood.

Midarm muscle circumference
Dietary interview
Serum transport proteins

b. A septic patient on TPN with a draining abdominal fistula.

Nitrogen balance based on urinary urea excretion
Total lymphocyte count
Daily serum albumin levels

c. A burn victim 5 days postinjury.

Body weight
Creatinine-height index
Delayed cutaneous hypersensitivity testing

3. A trauma victim who has undergone several surgeries for compound fractures is now 8 days postinjury. The patient has an intake of 100g of protein per day with a 24-hr UUN excretion of 20 g per day.

a. Calculate the patient's CI.

b. Would it be appropriate to perform a postcatabolism nutritional assessment at day 8 postinjury for this patient? Explain.

4. You are monitoring the nutritional status of a young woman who has recovered from many of the injuries sustained in a car accident, but who is still comatose. The patient receives 1,600 kcal per day from Osmolite in an intermittent tube feeding. How do you monitor the patient's long-term nutritional status in the following areas:

a. Overall adequacy of nutrient intake

b. Lean body mass

c. Visceral protein

5. A fifty y.o. male is admitted to the emergency room (ER) following a motor vehicle accident. The patient has a history of alcoholism and has smoked two packs of cigarettes per day for the past twenty years. He weighs 55 kg and is 5 ft, 10 in tall. The patient undergoes surgery shortly after admission to the ER. By the third postoperative day, evidence of pulmonary edema and sepsis is present. The patient is started on 24 percent oxygen delivered by a face mask. The following parameters are noted in the chart:

Mental status: disoriented
P: 150
R: 45
BP 170/100
ABG on 24 percent oxygen:
    pH = 7.25
    $PaCO_2$ = 68 mm Hg
    PaO_2 = 43 mm Hg

The patient is diagnosed as having acute respiratory failure. He is intubated and placed on a mechanical ventilator set to provide full ventilatory support. Representative ABGs obtained once the patient is settled on mechanical ventilatory support with 40 percent oxygen are as follows: pH = 7.42, $PaCO_2$ = 53 mm Hg, and PaO_2 = 71 mm Hg.

a. Suggest three factors that most likely contributed to the patient's acute respiratory failure.

b. Why was the patient disoriented and why did he demonstrate an elevated heart and respiratory rate before being intubated and placed on mechanical ventilation?

6. List three enteral feeding products that could be used to provide a respiratory patient with 35 percent of total calories as fat.

7. a. What does the RQ indicate?

b. Can the RQ be used to assess the degree of hypermetabolism that a patient is experiencing? Answer yes or no, and explain your answer.

8. The following situations are associated with difficulty in weaning from mechanical ventilation. Explain how nutrition may affect the weaning process in each case.

a. A cachectic patient with a 10-year history of COPD develops acute bacterial pneumonia and is placed on mechanical ventilation. The patient develops an ileus and is maintained on peripheral TPN. The solution infused includes 250 ml per day 10 percent fat emulsion and 1 L per day composed of 5 percent amino acids and 10 percent dextrose. A serum phosphorus value of 20 mg/L is determined at the time of weaning.

(continued)

b. A young, otherwise healthy near-drowning victim is placed on mechanical ventilation and maintained with a tube feeding that provides 45 kcal per kg per day. The RQ is greater than 2.0.

c. A patient is receiving 30 kcal per kg per day of Vivonex TEN tube feeding while being maintained on mechanical ventilation. The RQ is 1.0.

9. A patient on a respirator has been maintained with TPN for the past 15 days. His GI tract is now functioning and the physician asks that you make recommendations to initiate tube feeding. Circle your choices and explain why in the following areas:

a. Tube placement: nasogastric or nasoduodenal. Why?

b. Method of infusion: bolus, intermittent, or continuous. Why?

c. Choice of formula: Isocal, Vivonex, or Sustacal. Why?

d. Strength, rate: full str, 50 ml per hr; 1/2 str, 25 ml per hr; full str, 25 ml per hr. Why?

e. What clinical signs will you watch for to evaluate tolerance of the tube feeding?

f. When should the TPN be decreased?

10. Mr. G. a 32 y.o. industrial chemist, was severely burned over much of the trunk, arms, and back in an accident at the chemical plant where he works. After emergency first aid at the plant, he was transported by ambulance to the university hospital burn center. Mr. G. was admitted to the burn center in shock.

Physical Exam: Patient is experiencing pain, but no respiratory distress. Unburned skin is pale and cool. 5 ft, 10 in; 165# (preinjury); BP 90/60; P 110, weak and thready; R 22 and regular.

Laboratory: The following laboratory tests were ordered: CBC, blood type and cross-match, broad-spectrum screening panel, ABGs, and UA.

Impression: 30 percent TBSA, partial and full-thickness burns over lower part of the face, neck, arms, hands, and upper thighs.

Plan: IV therapy was initiated with Ringer's lactate. A Foley catheter was inserted, and urinary output, P and BP were monitored hourly. Mr. G. was NPO for the first 24 hours of hospitalization. A nasogastric tube was passed to the stomach for decompression. Maalox was given every 2 hours through the tube.

As soon as the shock was under control, Mr. G.'s wounds were washed with soap and saline, debrided, and dressed with silver sulfadiazine using a fine-mesh gauze. He was given a tetanus shot, and 600,000 U of procaine penicillin were administered every 12 hours.

After 2 days, Mr. G.'s urinary output was 40 to 50 ml per hour, and peristalsis had resumed. NG feedings of 50 ml per hour 1/2-strength Ensure Plus were initiated. These were advanced to 100 ml per hour full strength Ensure Plus. Mr. G. was encouraged to eat whatever he could.

a. Why was Mr. G. NPO for the first 24 hours after admission to the hospital?

b. Why was an NG tube necessary for decompression?

11. Calculate Mr. G.'s calorie requirements by the following methods. Show your calculations.

a. Curreri formula   _____ kcal/day
     Matsuda formula   _____ kcal/day

b. Estimate Mr. G.'s protein requirement
     _____ g/day

c. What is the best method for determining whether calorie and protein intake are adequate for a burn patient?

12. Assume that Mr. G. is trying to eat orally despite the burns on his face and hands. How could his Ensure Plus tube feeding be changed in order to provide approximately 2,400 additional kcal per day and not interfere with his intake at meal times?

13. Assume that Mr. G. is undergoing skin grafting and is generally recovering from his burn injury. By 28 days postburn, his weight is 68 kg and he is no longer receiving a tube feeding. Plan a menu for Mr. G. that includes three meals and three snacks, and provides approximately 3,000 kcal and 150 g protein per day.

14. A description of common problems experienced by patients undergoing cancer therapy follows. Suggest diet modifications you might recommend in each case.

a. A patient with HIV infection experiences chronic mild diarrhea and nausea.

b. A patient receiving chemotherapy for breast cancer develops mucositis and stomatitis.

c. A patient undergoes surgery for head and neck cancer and then receives radiation to the oropharyngeal area. Tube feeding is used initially, but when oral intake eventually resumes, the patient experiences a general lack of taste associated with eating.

The Critically Ill Patient

Part I: Presentation

Ms. C. is a 50 y.o. telephone operator who is admitted to university hospital with a 2-week history of constipation, decreased appetite, nausea, vomiting, and progressive abdominal distention.

Past medical history: Remarkable for 10 years of hypertension, moderate alcohol consumption, and 30 years of smoking two packs of cigarettes per day.

Physical exam: Unremarkable except for a pelvic mass discovered on bimanual examination. Subsequent evaluation by barium enema demonstrated an obstructed sigmoid colon at 35 cm.

Impression: Colon cancer.

Plan: The patient is scheduled for surgery on the third day of hospitalization for tumor resection and temporary colostomy.

The patient's immediate postop period is characterized by hypotension and tachycardia. By the second postop day, she has developed frank pulmonary edema and evidence of sepsis. On the third postop day, the patient is intubated and placed on a ventilator due to deteriorating pulmonary status. A trial of tube feeding is given, but there is evidence of gut dysmotility, probably due to an abdominal abscess, and enteral feeding cannot be used to meet energy needs in this patient. Central parenteral feeding is started on the fourth postop day. A nutritional consult is requested from the nutrition support team. The consult reads "Advise on appropriate CPN regimen for 50 y.o. septic female, s/p CA surgery with ARDS."

QUESTIONS

1. You are the dietitian member of the hospital nutrition support team, which also includes a surgeon, a nurse, and a pharmacist. You visit Ms. C., who is intubated with an orotracheal tube, review her medical record, and speak with her daughter. You complete an initial postinjury nutritional assessment based on the following available information: 5 ft, 6 in; 135# (usual), 120# (preinjury); serum albumin 25 mg/L; WBC 25,000/mL.

   a. You estimate a calorie and protein intake sufficient to *minimize* further loss of body weight in this moderately stressed patient based on her preinjury weight. Assume Ms. C. has normal hepatic and renal function. Show your calculations.

1.   BEE = _____ kcal.
2.   _____ × BEE = _____ kcal/day.
3.   _____ kcal/kg = _____ kcal/day.
4.   _____ g pro/kg = _____ g pro/day.

   b. Should daily calorie needs be calculated as total calories or nonprotein calories? Explain your answer.

   c. After the nutrition support team evaluates the patient, you establish recommendations for composition and delivery of CPN as a TNA with a total fluid volume of 2 L. Summarize your observations and recommendations in a SOAP note.

Part II: Transition from CPN to Tube Feeding

Ms. C.'s condition deteriorates, requiring surgical reexploration of the abdomen with drainage of an abdominal abscess. A tracheostomy is placed, and she remains on mechanical ventilation. After 20 days of hospitalization, motility is returning to the gastrointestinal tract. Theoretically, Ms. C. could receive foods by mouth; however, a modified barium swallow study indicates a risk of aspiration, so the transition to tube feeding is initiated. Body weight has decreased from 120# to 110#. A nutrition support team consult is again requested. The consult reads: "Advise on appropriate transition to enteral feeding for pt presently maintained on CPN and mechanical ventilation."

QUESTIONS

2. Assume that the hypermetabolic response to injury has subsided and that the prognosis for this patient is good, as there is no evidence of metastases. State the current goal of nutritional therapy and the rationale for this goal.

3. Suggest a target intake of calories and protein consistent with the goal of nutritional therapy. Should daily calorie needs be calculated as total or nonprotein calories? Explain your answer.
   a. _____ g protein/day
   b. ._____ kcal/day

4. Assume that a nasoduodenal feeding tube is placed.
   a. Select an appropriate tube feeding and provide a rationale for your choice.
   b. How much of this tube feeding would be needed to provide for the nutrient needs outlined in question 3?

(continued)

5. a. What progression of continuous feeding would you recommend?

Day   TF rate, cc/hour   kcal

b. When could CPN be decreased and then discontinued?

c. List five clinical parameters that you will monitor to ensure adequacy and tolerance of the tube feeding.

Part III: Weaning from the Respirator and Initiation of Oral Feeding

The patient's clinical status gradually improves. After 40 days of hospitalization, the serum albumin concentration is 30 mg/L, and body weight is 117#. At this time, several unsuccessful attempts are made to wean Ms. C. from the ventilator.

QUESTIONS

6. Discuss what role Ms. C.'s nutritional support may play in the failure to wean her from mechanical ventilation.

7. Assume that Ms. C. is successfully weaned from the ventilator. A modified barium swallow study indicates little risk of aspiration and oral feeding is started. How would you initiate and monitor the transition from tube feeding to oral feeding?

23 Nutrition Support of Inborn Errors of Metabolism

Phyllis B. Acosta, Dr PH, RD

Nutrition support of infants, children, and adults with inborn errors of metabolism requires in-depth knowledge of metabolic processes: the science and application of nutrition, growth, development, normal feeding behaviors, and food science. When providing nutrition support for patients with inborn errors, the specific nutrient needs of each patient, based on his or her individual genetic and biochemical constitution, must be considered. Nutrient requirements established for normal populations may not apply to individuals with inborn errors of metabolism, not only because of the metabolic error but also because of the use of chemically defined or elemental diets. Some chemical compounds, normally not considered "essential" because they can be synthesized *de novo*, cannot be synthesized in patients with some metabolic defects. In some inborn errors, metabolites accumulate, resulting in organ damage and loss of specific chemicals from the body. Certain compounds may then become "conditionally" essential. Among these are the amino acids arginine, cystine, taurine, and tyrosine, and the "vitamins" carnitine, lipoic acid, and tetrahydrobiopterin. Failure to adapt nutrient intake to the individual needs of each patient can result in mental retardation, metabolic crises, neurologic crises, growth failure, and, with some inborn errors, death. Quality care is best achieved by an experienced team of specialists in a genetic/metabolic center.

Many inborn errors of metabolism respond to nutrition support. While it is not possible to describe nutrition support for all inborn errors, we will reiterate general principles and practical considerations of nutrition support that, with the present state of knowledge, cover all inborn errors and provide two examples of general principles. Before proceeding further, you should review the related chapter in your text. In addition, you should review, if necessary, the material on feeding of infants and children in Chapter 9.

PRINCIPLES AND PRACTICAL CONSIDERATIONS OF NUTRITION SUPPORT

PRINCIPLES OF NUTRITION SUPPORT

Eight approaches to nutrition support of inborn errors of metabolism are presently available. The appropriate approach is dependent on the biochemistry and pathophysiology of disease expression, and several of the following therapeutic approaches may be used simultaneously (1, 2):

1. *Correct the primary imbalance in metabolic relationships.* This correction involves reduction, through diet restriction, of accumulated substrate(s) that are toxic. Some examples of inborn errors of metabolism and their restricted substrate(s) are phenylketonuria (PKU), phenylalanine; maple syrup urine disease (MSUD), leucine, isoleucine, and valine; and galactosemia, galactose.

2. *Provide alternative metabolic pathways to decrease accumulated toxic precursors in blocked reaction sequences.* For example, in isovaleric acidemia, a disorder of leucine catabolism, innocuous isovaleryl-carnitine is formed from accumulating isovaleric acid if supplemental carnitine is provided. Isovaleryl-carnitine is excreted in the urine.

3. *Supply products of blocked primary pathways.* Some examples are arginine in disorders of the urea cycle, except arginase deficiency; cystine in homocystinuria;

tyrosine in PKU; and tetrahydrobiopterin in biopterin synthetic defects.

4. *Supplement "conditionally essential" nutrients.* Examples are carnitine, cystine, and tyrosine in secondary liver disease or with excess excretion of carnitine in organic acidemias.

5. *Stabilize altered enzyme proteins.* The rate of biologic synthesis and degradation of holoenzymes is dependent on their structural conformation. For some holoenzymes, saturation by coenzyme increases their biologic half-life—thus, overall enzyme activity at the new equilibrium. Pharmacologic intake of pyridoxine in homocystinuria and thiamine in maple syrup urine disease increases intracellular pyridoxal phosphate and thiamine pyrophosphate, and increases the specific activity of cystathionine ß-synthase and branched-chain α-ketoacid dehydrogenase complex, respectively.

6. *Replace deficient cofactors.* Many vitamin-dependent disorders are due to blocks in coenzyme production and are "cured" by pharmacologic intake of a specific vitamin precursor. This mechanism presumably involves overcoming a partially impaired enzyme reaction by mass action. Impairment of reactions required to produce either methylcobalamin and/or adenosylcobalamin result in homocystinuria and/or methylmalonic aciduria. Daily intakes of appropriate forms of milligram quantities of vitamin B_{12} may "cure" the disease.

7. *Induce enzyme product.* If the structural gene or enzyme is intact, but suppressor, enhancer, or promoter elements are not functional, abnormal amounts of enzyme may be produced. The structural gene may be "turned on" or "turned off" to enable normal enzymatic production to occur. In the acute porphyria of type I tyrosinemia, excessive delta-aminolevulinic acid (ALA) may be reduced by suppressing transcription of the delta-ALA synthase gene with excess glucose.

8. *Supplement nutrients that are inadequately absorbed or not released from their apoenzyme.* Examples are zinc in acrodermatitis enteropathica and biotin in biotinidase deficiency.

PRACTICAL CONSIDERATIONS IN NUTRITION SUPPORT (2)

Nutrients. Diet restriction required to correct imbalances in metabolic relationships in disorders of amino acid and nitrogen metabolism usually requires the use of chemically defined or elemental medical foods. These chemically defined products are normally supplemented with small amounts of whole natural protein that supply the restricted amino acid(s). Natural foods seldom supply more than 25 percent of the protein requirements of patients with disorders of amino acid metabolism. Nitrogen-free natural foods that provide energy are limited in their range of nutrients. Consequently, care must be taken to provide nutrients

often considered to be food contaminants, because their essentiality has been demonstrated through long-term use of total parenteral nutrition. Thus, in addition to nutrients for which Recommended Dietary Allowances (RDA) (3) are established, other nutrients must be supplied in adequate amounts. These include the trace minerals chromium, copper, manganese, and molybdenum; and the vitamins biotin, pantothenic acid, choline, and inositol. Other possible conditionally essential nutrients must be considered, depending on the specific enzyme deficiency.

Osmolality. Chemically defined diets consist of small molecules that may provide an osmolality greater than the physiologic tolerance of the patient. Abdominal cramping, diarrhea, distention, nausea, and vomiting have resulted from use of hyperosmolar formulas. Aside from gastrointestinal distress, more serious consequences, such as hypertonic dehydration, hypovolemia, hypernatremia, and death can occur in infants. The neonate *should not* be fed an elemental formula that contains an osmolality greater than 450 mOsm/kg water, while adults seldom tolerate an osmolality greater than 1,000 mOsm/kg water.

Maillard reaction. Medical foods for most inborn errors of amino acid or nitrogen metabolism are formulated from L-amino acids or hydrolysates and free sugars. The Maillard reaction is a name given to a complex group of chemical reactions in foods in which reacting amino acids, peptides, and protein condense with sugars, forming bonds for which no digestive enzymes are available. The Maillard reaction is accelerated by heat and is characterized in its initial stage by a light-brown color, followed by buff yellow and dark brown in the intermediate and final stages. Caramel-like and roasted aromas develop. Those who prepare medical foods need to be able to recognize the Maillard reaction because it causes loss of some sugars and amino acids. For this reason, medical foods should not be heated beyond 100° F. Thus, terminal sterilization of formulas containing L-amino acids or hydrolysates is contraindicated.

Introduction of natural foods. Natural foods should be introduced into the diet of the infant at about 3 to 4 months of age if the infant shows developmental readiness by a decrease in tongue thrust. Natural foods are important in the diet as sources of unidentified nutrients, to provide fiber, to enhance the child's acceptance of a variety of tastes and textures, and, when solid foods are eaten, to develop jaw muscles important for speech.

Changes in nutrition support prescription. As soon as nutrition requirements are well established in an infant, child, or adult, the prescription should be fine-tuned routinely and frequently. Small, frequent changes in prescription work better than large, infrequent changes. Small, frequent changes prevent "bouncing" of amino acids, glucose, organic acids, or ammonia concentrations and allow the intake to grow with the child, thus precluding the child's "growing out of the prescription."

Monitoring. Successful management of inborn errors of metabolism requires frequent monitoring. Frequent monitoring gives the nutritional care specialist data that verify the adequacy of the nutrition support prescription. These data are also useful in motivating patient/parent compliance with the prescription. Patients with insulin-dependent diabetes often monitor blood glucose 3 times daily, so frequent monitoring of plasma amino acids or other indicated analytes should pose no major problem, except for cost. Some centers may wish to draw blood when the patient is fasting to monitor plasma amino acids. Prolonged fasting (> 6 to 8 hours) may cause spurious elevations of plasma amino acids that could lead to unwarranted diet changes, and blood drawn 15 minutes to 1 hour after a meal may also yield spuriously high values.

Protocol for treatment. The problem of ensuring adequate nutrition for infants, children and adults with inborn errors of metabolism may be decreased by the use of a protocol—plan for treatment. Each patient requires *individualized* nutrition care. When specific amino acids or nitrogen require restriction, total deletion for 1 to 2 days *only* is the best approach to initiating therapy. Longer-term deletion or overrestriction may precipitate deficiency of the amino acid(s) or protein. The most limiting nutrient determines growth rate, and over-restriction of an amino acid, nitrogen, or energy will result in further intolerance of the restricted nutrient. Only *frequent* monitoring of plasma amino acids, nutrient intake, and growth can verify the adequacy of intake of restricted amino acids.

Protein requirements of infants, children, and adults with inborn errors of amino acid metabolism are normal if liver or renal function is not compromised. However, the form in which the protein is administered must be altered in order to restrict specific amino acids. Consequently, medical foods formulated from L-amino acids, specially treated protein hydrolysates, or soy protein isolate must be used with very small amounts of natural protein to provide amino acid and nitrogen requirements. Because utilization of L-amino acid mixes may differ somewhat from use of amino acids derived from whole protein during digestion and absorption, recommended protein intakes of infants with inborn errors of amino acid metabolism are greater than RDA.

Energy intakes of individuals with inborn errors of metabolism must be adequate to support normal rates of growth for infants and children and weight appropriate for height in adults. Provision of apparently adequate amino acids and nitrogen without sufficient energy will lead to growth failure or weight loss. Pratt et al. (4) suggested that energy requirements may be greater than normal when L-amino acids supply the protein equivalent. Maintenance of adequate energy intake is essential for normal growth and development and to prevent catabolism. If energy for normal growth of children or weight maintenance of adults cannot be achieved through oral feeding, nasogastric, gastrostomy, or parenteral feeding must be used.

Major, trace, and ultra-trace mineral and vitamin intakes should meet RDA and Safe and Adequate Daily Dietary Intakes for age (3). If the medical food mixture fails to supply 100 percent of RDA for patients, and if plasma or whole blood concentrations fall below the lower limit of normal, appropriate supplements should be given.

CORRECTING THE PRIMARY IMBALANCE IN METABOLIC RELATIONSHIPS

GALACTOSEMIAS

Galactosemia may occur due to at least seven different defects in the gene for galactose-1-phosphate uridyl transferase and because of defects in galactokinase and uridine diphosphate galactose-4-epimerase (UDP-Gal-4-epimerase) (5). Patients with no UPD-Gal-4-epimerase activity cannot synthesize galactose, but some exogenous galactose is required for synthesis of glycoproteins and galactolipids. The amount of galactose required for these patients is not known. Elimination of human milk, lactose-containing formulas, and cow and goat milks from the diet of the patient with galactokinase deficiency may be adequate galactose restriction. However, no long-term studies have been completed on these patients, and greater restriction may be required.

Patients with ≤ 10 percent of galactose-1-phosphate uridyl transferase activity require therapy with a galactose-"free" diet. Sources of galactose are both endogenous and exogenous. Endogenous sources include lactose synthesized by the maternal mammary gland, available to the fetus in utero, synthesis by UDP-Gal-4-epimerase from UDP-glucose, and from normal turnover of the body's glycoproteins and galactolipids. Exogenous sources of galactose include human milk, infant formulas with added lactose, cow and goat milks and any products derived from them or to which they or their products are added, organ meats (glycoproteins and galactolipids), some fruits and vegetables, legumes (dried beans and peas), some drugs, including most oral contraceptive agents, and artificial sweeteners to which lactose is added as an excipient and Neocalglucon® (Table 23-1).

For many years, foods containing bound galactose in various forms were believed to be safe for use, since human enzymes were thought not to digest these compounds. Some carbohydrates in foods that contain bound galactose are arabinogalactans I and II, feruloylated D-galactose, galactan, galactinol, galactolipids, galactopinitols, raffinose oligosaccharides (raffinose, stachyose, verbascose), and rhamnogalacturonans I and

TABLE 23-1 Foods, Drugs, and Supplements That Should Be Deleted from a Galactose "Free" Diet

Foods

Fermented foods	Bacterial fermentation of miso, natto, pickles,
Fruits	sauerkraut, soy sauce, tempeh, etc.
Legumes	See Table 23-4 and Table 23-5
Milk, milk products, and foods containing milk	Dried beans and peas See Table 23-3
Organ meats	Brain, heart, intestines, kidney, liver, pancreas (sweetbreads), tongue
Vegetables	See Tables 23-4 and 23-5

Drugs

Oral contraceptive agents and any prescription and nonprescription medications to which lactose is added as an excipient. (Check with manufacturers frequently.)

Supplements

Minerals, vitamins	Those to which lactose is added as an excipient. (Check with manufacturers frequently.)
Neocalglucon ®	Contains 625 mg galactose per 5 ml.

stachyose, verbascose), and rhamnogalacturonans I and II (6). Recent data suggest that plant enzymes *may* release free galactose from these carbohydrates (7). Consequently, use of foods listed in Table 23-2 is presently questioned, and awaiting further research.

Infant formulas made with soy protein isolate may be

TABLE 23-2 Some Food Sources of Bound Galactose (6)

Carbohydrate	Food Choices
Arabinogalactan I	Beans (mung, snap, soy), carrots, eggplant, garlic, onions, papaya, pectin, potato (white, sweet)
Arabinogalactan II	Asparagus, bamboo shoots, beans (lima, soy), fruits, leaves, maple syrup, oats, rice bran, roots, seeds, tomato, wheat
Feruloylated D-galactose	Spinach
Galactan	Acacia gum, beans (snap, soy), potatoes (white), snails
Galactinol	Beans (chick pea, cow pea, fava, field pea, lentil, lima, lupine, mung, navy, northern, snap, soy), potatoes (white), safflower kernels
Galactolipids	Beans (chick pea, mung), cereals (corn, oats, rice, wheat), muskmelon seed kernels, potatoes (white), spinach leaves, tomatoes
Galactopinitols	Beans (chick pea, cow pea, fava, lentil, mung, snap, soy)
Raffinose oligosaccharides	Beans (chick pea, cow pea, fava, field pea, green pea, lentil, lima, lupine, mung, navy, northern, snap, soy), cocoa beans, flour (cottonseed, sunflower seed), safflower kernels, wheat
Rhamnogalacturonan I	Beans (kidney, peas, snap), apples, cabbage, carrots, cereals (barley, wheat), onions, pectin, potatoes (white)
Rhamnogalacturonan II	Beans (peas, pinto), oats, pectin

used. These are Isomil®, Nursoy®, Prosobee®, and RCF®, and contain about 14 mg bound galactose per liter. See Appendix H for ingredients and composition. If a soy protein isolate formula that is adequately fortified with calcium, vitamin D, and other nutrients normally supplied by milk is not continued for life, appropriate galactose-free supplements must be administered. Casein hydrolysate formulas should be avoided since they contain 60 to 75 mg galactose/L.

As solid foods are added to the diet, labels must be carefully read, and foods containing milk in any form (Table 23-3), legumes, fruits and vegetables containing >10 mg free galactose/100g (Tables 23-1, 23-4, 23-5), and organ meats containing glycoproteins should also be excluded. Prescription drugs such as oral contraceptive agents and over-the-counter drugs should be evaluated for lactose content before they are used. The diet, with lactose-free vitamin and mineral supplements, especially calcium, should be continued for life. Neocalglucon® should never be used as a calcium supplement, since 5 mL provides about 625 mg galactose (8).

Monitoring. Traditional methods of monitoring dietary control of galactose intake include erythrocyte galactose-1-phosphate (nondetectable in fasting normal children) and urinary galactose excretion (normally < 10 mg/dL). Unfortunately, longitudinal erythrocyte galactose-1-phosphate concentrations are unrelated to long-term outcomes in patients. Other analytes, such as erythrocyte UDP-galactose, UDP-glucose, and urinary galactitol excretion might provide information useful to management. Frequent monitoring of analytes and evaluation of nutrient intake are essential to management. Other indices of nutrition status as described in Chapter 9 should be routinely assessed.

TABLE 23-3 Milk and Milk Products Excluded from the Galactose-Free Diet

Butter
Buttermilk
Casein
Caseinates
Casein hydrolysates
Cheeses: aged (ripened), cottage, cream, processed, unripened
Cream: imitation, sweet, sour, whipping
Curds
Ice cream, ice milk
Lactalbumin (milk albuminate)
Lactoglobulin
Lactose (milk sugar)
Margarine with milk solids, whey or butterfat
Milk: cow, human, goat, condensed, evaporated, skim, 1 %, 2 %, whole, chocolate, malted, filled, imitation, enzyme-treated
Milk fat
Milk solids: nonfat, whole
Sherbet
Skim milk powder
Whey, whey solids, whey protein
Yogurt

PHENYLKETONURIA

Phenylketonuria is an inherited disorder of phenylalanine (PHE) metabolism. More than 100 gene mutations have been found which lead to alterations in PHE hydroxylase structure and activity. Nutrition support is presently the only method of therapy available to prevent mental retardation, seizures, and hyperactivity.

Initial screening. In all states, newborn infants are routinely screened for elevated blood PHE with a bacterial inhibition assay or fluorimetric test. The blood sample should be drawn at least 24 hours after the start of milk feeding, if possible. If results are equivocal, or the sample is obtained before 24 hours of milk ingestion, the test is repeated within 24 to 48 hours. Positive results that indicate the need for a diagnostic workup are any values ≥ 2 mg/dL before 24 hours of life and ≥ 4 mg/dL after 24 hours. The plasma PHE value in normal infants is usually < 1 mg/dL.

If the screening test is positive for PHE, and plasma tyrosine (TYR) is normal (0.6 to 2.9 mg/dL), a diagnostic workup *must* be completed to identify the type of PKU, since therapy differs depending on the enzyme defect present. Methods of differential diagnosis include determination of blood and/or urinary pterins, biopterin load test, culture of skin fibroblasts for dihydropteridine reductase, and determination of neurotransmitters or their metabolites in the urine (9). A phenylalanine challenge test is seldom used due to possible neurological damage from such a test.

Nutrition support. Patients with plasma PHE concentrations of greater than 300 µmol/L (5 mg/dL) and plasma TYR concentrations below 35 µmol/L (0.6

TABLE 23-4 Mean mg Free Galactose per 100 g Strained Fruits and Vegetables (19)*

Product	Company		
	Beech Nut	Gerber	Heinz
Applesauce	10	14	16
Apricots	2	none detected	none detected
Banana	3	4	5
Peaches	none detected	<1	none detected
Pears	3	2	1
Beets	not available	3	1
Carrots	1	4	<1
Green beans	<1	<1	1
Peas	1	<1	<1
Potatoes, sweet	1	4	1
Spinach, creamed	not available	13	not available
Squash	1	59	6

* Other strained and baby foods may contain free galactose, but analyses are not yet available

TABLE 23-5 Free Galactose Content (mg per 100 g Fresh Weight ± SE) of Various Fruits and Vegetables (19)

Fruit/Vegetable	Content
Apple	8.3 ± 0.7
Apricot	1.1 ± 0.6
Asparagus	1.2 ± 0.6
Avocado	<0.5
Banana	9.2 ± 0.8
Bean sprouts, green	4.3 ± 0.2
Beet, red	0.8 ± 0.2
Broccoli	6.8 ± 0.7
Brussels sprouts	9.2 ± 0.7
Cabbage, common	3.3 ± 0.2
Cantaloupe	4.3± 0.2
Carrot	6.2 ± 0.4
Cauliflower	4.3 ± 0.3
Celery	2.4 ± 0.1
Corn, sweet	3.7 ± 0.3
Cucumber	4.0 ± 0.3
Date	11.5 ± 0.6
Eggplant (aubergine)	4.7 ± 0.2
Grape, green	2.9 ± 0.1
Grapefruit	4.1 ± 0.1
Kale	2.3 ± 0.2
Kiwi	9.8 ± 0.4
Lettuce, garden	3.1 ± 0.3
Onion. yellow	5.1 ± 0.3
Onion, bunching	6.1 ± 0.3
Orange, sweet	4.3 ± 0.4
Papaya	28.6 ± 1.9
Pea, sweet	4.9 ± 0.8
Pear	7.3 ± 1.4
Pepper, bell	10.2 ± 0.4
Pepper, cayenne	9.7 ± 4.0
Persimmon, American	35.4 ± 2.5
Potato, white	1.2 ± 0.3
Potato, sweet	7.7 ± 0.7
Pumpkin	9.9 ± 2.5
Radish, red	0.5 ± 0.3
Spinach	0.1 ±0.1
Tomato	23.0 ± 2.0
Turnip	4.9 ±0.6
Watermelon	14.7 ± 2.0
Zucchini squash	3.3 ± 0.1

mg/dL) require prompt treatment with a PHE-restricted, TYR-supplemented diet. The objective of nutrition support in a child with phenylalanine hydroxylase deficiency is to maintain plasma PHE and TYR concentrations that will allow optimal growth and brain development by supplying adequate energy, protein, and other nutrients while restricting PHE to the patient's tolerance and supplementing TYR intake as necessary (1).

Therapy of the child with biopterin-deficient forms of hyperphenylalaninemia requires administration of tetrahydrobiopterin and use of the PHE-restricted, TYR-supplemented diet in combination with L-DOPA and carbidopa. Serotonin that is derived from tryptophan may also improve behavior if tryptophan hydroxylase is secondarily impaired by the absence of tetrahydrobiopterin (9).

Initiation of nutrition support. Rapid decline of blood PHE concentration at the time of diagnosis may be obtained by feeding the infant a 20 kcal/ounce (67 kcal/dL) PHE-free or low-PHE formula. Within a mean of 4 days (SD±3), blood PHE concentration should drop to treatment range. Treatment should be initiated in hospitalized infants to obtain adequate information to serve as a basis for counseling and to monitor plasma amino acids daily. Laboratory results should be available promptly to prevent precipitation of PHE deficiency and to enable rapid return of PHE and TYR to optimum blood concentrations.

In the event that the infant or child is not hospitalized for initiation of nutrition support, or if only weekly blood PHE concentrations are obtained, a maintenance formula containing adequate PHE from an appropriate source (Table 23-6) should be prescribed. Blood PHE concentration will fall to treatment range within a mean of 10 days (SD ± 5) with this approach. Choice of initial nutrition support should be predicated on producing blood PHE concentrations in the treatment range no later than the third week of life. Evaporated milk and whole cow milk should not be used as a source of PHE for the infant because of their low iron content.

Chronic care: nutrient requirements. Long-term care of the patient with classic PKU dictates that proprietary, chemically defined products (medical foods), and natural foods provide all nutrients in required amounts. Data in Table 23-7 outline the suggested ranges of PHE, TYR, protein, energy, and fluid to offer. A formal prescription must be written that is individualized to the specific degree of impaired enzyme activity, growth rate, and consequent needs of each patient. Weekly adjustments in the diet prescription may be necessary, particularly during the first 6 months of life, based on hunger, growth, development, and laboratory analyses of plasma PHE and TYR concentrations. The PHE provided should maintain the 2 to 4 hour postprandial blood PHE concentration between 120 and 300 µmol/L (2 to 5 mg/dL). PHE is an essential amino acid and cannot be eliminated from the diet. Excess restriction produces

TABLE 23-6 Serving Lists for PHE-Restricted Diets: Approximate PHE, TYR, Protein, and Energy Content Per Serving (1)

List	Nutrients			
	PHE (mg)	TYR (mg)	Protein (g)	Energy (kcal)
Breads/cereals	30	20	0.6	30
Fats	5	4	0.1	60
Fruits	15	10	0.5	60
Vegetables	15	10	0.5	10
Free foods A	5	4	0.1	65
Free foods B	0	0	0	55
Similac with iron RTF* (100 mL)	71	66	1.45	68
Milk, whole (100 mL) (20)	160	160	3.4	62

* RTF = Ready to Feed.

growth failure, skin rashes, bone changes, and mental retardation.

PHE required for growth by the infant with classical PKU is between 25 and 70 mg/kg of body weight. PHE requirement declines rapidly between 3 and 6 months of age as growth rate plateaus. Requirement for PHE in the 6- to 12-month old patient with classical PKU may fall to 15 mg/kg/day, but varies considerably. Frequent monitoring of blood PHE concentration and intake is required to prevent excess intake when growth rate decelerates, and inadequate intake when growth rate is at its peak.

TYR is an essential amino acid for children with PKU. For this reason, plasma TYR values must be monitored. and if they are low, L-TYR supplements given. The supplement required, in addition to that already present in medical and natural food, should be adequate to provide 10 percent of the total protein as TYR. TYR supplements alone will not prevent mental retardation in classic phenylketonuria.

The protein content of the diet for infants with PKU has traditionally been greater than normal. Protein requirements are increased when either an L-amino acid mix or a protein hydrolysate is the primary protein source rather than natural protein. Thus, recommendations for protein for nutrition support of infants are greater than the RDA. Recommendations for energy and fluid intake (Table 23-7) are the same as those for normal infants and children.

Phenylalanine-free and low-phenylalanine, chemically defined medical foods. Adequate protein cannot be obtained from natural foods without ingesting excess PHE. Natural proteins contain 2.4 to 9 percent by weight of phenylalanine. Thus, special proprietary chemically defined medical foods are used to provide protein. Formulations and major nutrient composition of these products are given in Table 23-8. Lofenalac®,

TABLE 23-7 Recommended Daily Nutrient Intakes (range) for Infants, Children, and Adults with PKU (20–22)

Age	Nutrients				
	PHE [*],[†] (mg/kg)	TYR [*] (mg/kg)	Protein (g/kg)	Energy (kcal/kg)	Fluid [‡] (mL/kg)
0 < 3 mo	25–70	300–350	3.50–3.00	120(145–95)	160–125
3 < 6 mo	20–45	300–350	3.50–3.00	115(145–95)	160–130
6 < 9 mo	15–35	250–300	3.00–2.50	110(135–80)	145–125
9 < 12 mo	10–35	250–300	3.00–2.50	105(135–80)	135–120
Female & Male	(mg/day)	(g/day)	(g/day)	(kcal/day)	(mL/day)
1 < 4 yr	200–400	1.72–3.00	30	1,300(900–1,800)	900–1,800
4 < 7 yr	210–450	2.25–3.50	35	1,700(1,300–2,300)	1,300–2,300
7 < 11 yr	220–500	2.55–4.00	40	2,400(1,650–3300)	1,650–3,300
Females					
11 < 15 yr	250–500	3.45–4.60	50	2,200(1,500–3,000)	1,500–3,000
15 < 19 yr	230–500	3.45–4.60	50	2,100(1,200–3,000)	1,200–3,000
≥ 19 yr	220–500	3.75–5.00	50	2,100(1,400–2,500)	1,400–2,500
Males					
11 < 15 yr	225–450	3.38–5.50	55	2,700(2,000–3,700)	2,000–3,700
15 < 19 yr	295–590	4.42–6.50	65	2,800(2,100–3,900)	2,100–3,900
≥ 19 yr	290–580	4.35–6.50	65	2,900(2,000–3,300)	2,000–3,300

[*] Initiate prescription with lowest value in patient's age range. *Modify prescription based on frequent blood and/or plasma values and growth in the infant and child.*

[†] PHE requirements of premature infants may be greater than highest value noted.

[‡] At least 1 mL of fluid should be administered per kcalorie.

formulated from a specially treated enzymatic hydrolysate of casein, is low in PHE (approximately 80 mg/100 g) and contains fat and carbohydrate. Minerals, vitamins, and four L-amino acids are also added. Lofenalac has no added chromium, molybdenum, or selenium. Phenex™-1, designed for infants and toddlers, consists of L-amino acids, a blend of fats and carbohydrate, minerals, trace minerals (including selenium), and vitamins. Carnitine and taurine are added. Phenex-1 is free of PHE and high in tyrosine (Table 23-8). Phenex™-2 is an L-amino acid mix free of PHE and high in TYR, designed for children, adults, and pregnant women. Fat (15.5 g/100 g), carbohydrate, minerals, trace minerals (including selenium), and vitamins are added in amounts that supply requirements of children and adults. Phenyl-Free® is an L-amino acid mix containing carbohydrate, fat, minerals, trace elements (except added chromium and molybdenum), and vitamins. It is designed for children, adults, and pregnant women. Chromium and molybdenum are not added to Phenex-1, Phenex-2, or Phenyl-Free, because these ultra-trace minerals are naturally occurring in the ingredients. PKU1, PKU2, and PKU3 are L-amino acid mixes that are low in carbohydrate and free of added fat, chromium, and selenium. PKU1 is designed for the infant, PKU2 for the child, and PKU3 for the adult and pregnant women. XP Analog®,

designed for infants, consists of L-amino acids, a blend of fat and carbohydrate that produces a fatty acid profile similar to human milk, minerals, trace elements (including chromium, molybdenum, and selenium), and vitamins. Carnitine and taurine have also been added. XP Analog is free of PHE (Table 23-8). XP Maxamaid®, designed for 1- to 8-year-old children, is an orange-flavored powder free of PHE that contains L-amino acids, carbohydrate, minerals, trace elements and vitamins. It contains no added fat. XP Maxamum® is formulated for individuals 8 years of age or older and for pregnant women. It is fat-free, but has added carnitine, taurine, chromium, molybdenum, selenium, and vitamin K.

Natural foods. Serving lists are available to simplify the PHE-restricted diet for families and professional persons guiding them (Table 23-6). The lists are similar to diabetic exchange lists, in that foods of similar PHE content are grouped together and can be exchanged one for another within a list to give variety to the diet. Natural foods should be prescribed in numbers of servings and introduced at the appropriate ages and in the usual textures. as they would be for any child. Children should be given a variety of foods at the appropriate age, so that these foods may be included in the diet later in life. In this way, increasing total PHE requirements may be met.

TABLE 23-8 Formulation and Major Nutrient Composition of Medical Foods for Phenylketonuria

Products	Modified Nutrients (mg/100g)	Protein Equiv. g Source (g/100 g)	Fat, g Source (g/100 g)	Carbohydrate, g Source (g/100 g)	Energy (kcal/100g)	Minerals not added	Vitamins not added
Lofenalac *	PHE-80; TYR-800; TRP-195; added L-carnitine, taurine	15.0 Enzymatically hydrolyzed casein, L-amino acids	18.0 Corn oil	60.0 Corn syrup solids, modified tapioca starch	460	Chromium, molybdenum	None
Phenex-1 †	PHE-0; TYR-1500; TRP-170; added L-carnitine, taurine	15.0 L-amino acids	23.9 Palm oil, coconut oil, soy oil	46.3 Cornstarch, hydrolyzed	480	Chromium, §, molybdenum§	None
Phenex-2 †	PHE-O; TYR-3000; TRP-340; added L-carnitine, taurine	30.0 L-amino acids	15.5 Palm oil, coconut oil, soy oil	30.0 Cornsstarch, hydrolyzed	410	Chromium, §, molybdenum§	None
Phenyl-Free *	PHE-0; TYR-940; TRP-280	20.0 L-amino acids	6.8 Corn oil, coconut oil	66 Sucrose, corn syrup solids, modified tapioca starch	410	Chromium,§, molybdedum§	None
PKU1 *	PHE-0; TYR-3400; TRP-1000	50.0 L-amino acids	0 None added	19 Sucrose	280	Chromium, selenium	None
PKU2*	PHE-0; TYR-4500; TRP-1400	67.0 L-amino acids	0 None added	7 Sucrose	300	Chromium, selenium	None
PKU3 *	PHE-0; TYR-6000; TRP-1400	68.0 L-amino acids	0 None added	3 Sucrose	290	Chromium, selenium§	None
Pro-Phree ™ *	Protein; added L-carnitine, taurine	0.0	31 Palm oil, coconut oil, soy oil	60 Cornstarch, hydrolyzed	520	Chromium, molybdenum §	None
Protein Free Diet Powder *	Protein; added L-carnitine, taurine	0.0	23 Corn oil	72 Corn syrup solids, modified tapioca starch	500	Chromium, molybdenum	None
XP Analog ‡	PHE-O, TYR-1370; TRP-300; added L-carnitine, taurine	13.0 L-amino acids	20.9 Peanut oil, refined lard, coconut oil	59.0 Corn syrup solids	475	None	None
XP Maxamaid ‡	PHE-0; TYR-2650; TRP-570; added L-carnitine, taurine	25.0 L-amino acids	<1.0 None added	62 Sucrose, hydrolyzed corn starch	350	None	None
XP Maxamum ‡	PHE-0; TYR-4030; TRP-890; added L-carnitine, taurine	39.0 L-amino acids	<1.0 None added	45 Sucrose, hydrolyzed corn starch	340	None	None

* Distributed by Mead Johnson Nutritionals, Evansville, IN 47721
† Distributed by Ross Products Divisions, Abbott Laboratories, Columbus, OH 43215
‡ Distributed by Scientific Hospital Supplies, Inc., Gaithersburg, MD 20879.
§ Amount naturally occurring in raw ingredients is adequate to maintain normal blood concentration

Management problems. Management problems described for children with PKU occur in other children with inherited disorders of metabolism as well. Maintenance of an adequate intake of protein and energy is important for the patient with PKU, even though PHE must be restricted. Protein equivalent is obtained from chemically defined medical foods; therefore, the amount of chemically defined medical food offered must be varied to provide the protein needed. Nonprotein sources of energy, such as corn syrup, Moducal®, Polycose®, sugar, Protein-Free Diet Powder®, Pro-Phree™ (Table 23-8), and pure fats can be added to maintain energy intake and to satisfy the child's hunger without affecting blood PHE concentrations. A variety of factors may influence blood PHE levels. Causes of an elevated blood PHE concentration include acute infections with concomitant tissue catabolism, excessive or inadequate PHE intake, and inadequate protein or energy intake. Infection affects plasma amino acids in well-nourished, normal persons. Similar increases in blood PHE occur in febrile, well-nourished, treated PKU patients. Because of this fact, any infection should be promptly diagnosed and appropriately treated. The best approach to nutrition support during short-term infections is to increase the intake of fluids and carbohydrates through use of tolerated fruit juices; high-carbohydrate, protein-free beverages; and soft drinks that do not contain caffeine or Nutrasweet®.

Excess PHE intake is the most common cause of elevated blood PHE concentration in the older child with PKU. This condition may be due to overprescription, misunderstanding of the diet by the caretaker, or "snitching" of food by the child. Frequent evaluations of blood PHE with accompanying accurate diet records for calculation of intake are used to determine the dietary PHE prescription. Diet records are also useful in determining parental understanding. Misunderstanding of diet requires additional education of parents and patient. "Snitching" of food by the child is the most difficult problem to handle. Children should be given sound reasons for avoiding foods not allowed on their diets, and this responsibility should be shifted to the child by 4 to 6 years of age. Lifetime nutrition support should be emphasized to the parents at the onset of therapy and at recurring intervals to both parents and the child.

PHE deficiency associated with inadequate PHE intake has three specific stages of development. The first stage is characterized biochemically by decreased blood and urine PHE (10). Clinically, the child may appear lethargic or anorectic. Failure to gain length or weight may occur. In the older child, increases in blood alanine and mild lactic and ß-hydroxybutyric acidemia occur as a consequence of muscle alanine production and ß-lipolysis (1). In the second stage, blood PHE is increased as a result of muscle protein degradation. Increased branched-chain amino acid concentrations with decreases in other plasma amino acids occur. Aminoaciduria appears as a consequence of renal tubular malabsorption. In this stage, body protein stores are catabolized. Eczema is common. In the third stage of

PHE deficiency, blood PHE is decreased below normal, as are all other amino acids. Accompanying clinical manifestations include failure to gain weight, failure to gain height, osteopenia, anemia, sparse hair, and finally, death, if the deficiency is not corrected by supplements of dietary PHE. Insufficient protein intake results in an inadequate supply of essential amino acids and/or nitrogen for growth. When protein synthesis is decreased, PHE is no longer used for growth and accumulates in the blood. If catabolism occurs due to prolonged lack of nitrogen and/or amino acid intake, blood PHE concentration increases because tissue protein contains some 5.5 percent PHE. In case of protein insufficiency, chemically defined medical food should be increased to supply the required nitrogen and/or essential amino acids.

Energy, the first requirement of the body, is necessary for growth. When energy is provided as carbohydrate, and if adequate nitrogen is available, nonessential amino acids may be synthesized from the keto-acid metabolites. Further, carbohydrate ingestion leads to insulin secretion, and insulin promotes amino acid transport into the cell and consequent protein synthesis. When energy intake is inadequate, tissue catabolism occurs to meet energy needs. Such catabolism releases PHE, leading to elevated blood PHE concentrations. Provision of sufficient energy through generous use of nonprotein and low-protein foods is important in order to ensure a normal growth rate and to prevent weight loss in the adult.

Low blood PHE concentration (< 120 μmol/L; < 2 mg/dL) may lead to depressed appetite, decreased growth, and, if prolonged, mental retardation. Low blood PHE concentrations are often due to inadequate prescription of PHE for the affected child. In such cases, the prescription for PHE can be increased by addition of measured amounts of infant formula for the infant, and milk and/or solid foods for the child and adult.

In some situations, chemically defined medical food may be diluted to a volume that is too great for the child to consume in the allotted time. The volume will need to be decreased to the amount the child is able to ingest. Concentrated, chemically defined medical foods are frequently used without any untoward side effects in children and adults. They may be mixed as a paste and spoon-fed, even to the infant. The practice could begin at 3 to 4 months of age when tongue thrust is no longer evident. Extra fluid must then be offered between feedings to maintain appropriate water balance.

Assessment of nutrition support. Along with biweekly assessment of growth through measurement of length/height, weight, and head circumference, and evaluation of development by appropriate developmental scales, the adequacy of PHE and TYR intake is determined by twice-weekly quantitation of the blood PHE and TYR concentrations. The first year is the period of most rapid growth and of greatest vulnerability to nutrition insult. Therefore, blood tests are suggested 2 times weekly during the first 6 months of life. After 6 months of age, weekly blood tests may be sufficient for monitoring the diet. If, however, blood PHE concentrations are greater than 300 µmol/L (5 mg/dL), more frequent determinations should be obtained. Where indicated, the prescription for PHE is decreased, and frequent blood tests are obtained until blood PHE concentrations are 120 to 300 µmol/L. In order for blood tests to be of use in adjusting the prescription, laboratory methods must be both accurate and prompt. Quantitative methods of PHE and TYR determination using automated ion-exchange chromatography, fluorimetry, or high-performance liquid chromatography and liquid blood are preferable. This method allows for evaluation of all amino acids. The microbiological (Guthrie) method is acceptable for screening, but it is nonquantitative at elevated concentrations and invalid if antibiotics are used. Fluorimetric methods are quantitative and preferred to the Guthrie test to monitor blood PHE. If properly instructed, parents may be given responsibility for obtaining the specimens on filter paper or in microcapillary tubes and mailing them to a central laboratory.

A record of food ingested before and during blood sampling for blood PHE measurements is essential and should be kept by the child's caregiver. The correlation between the child's intake of PHE, TYR, protein, and energy, his growth and clinical status, and blood PHE and TYR concentrations is considered when the diet is altered.

The success of early diet management rests with the parents and depends on their understanding of the disease and their ability to cope with the diet. Later, the child's understanding of the disease and his or her ability to assume responsibility for it are critical. These factors in turn are related to the support the parents and patients receive from various professional members of the genetic/metabolic team.

Diet discontinuation. A number of clinicians have suggested that diet might be discontinued at 4, 6, or 12 years of age with no adverse effects. Investigators have questioned this possibility, because studies have shown significant differences in performance and intelligence in children who discontinued the diet at or above 6 years of age compared to those who continued on the diet (11). In studies using the same patient as his or her own control, elevated plasma PHE concentrations prolonged the performance time on neuropsychological tests of higher integrative function, produced abnormal electroencephalograms, and decreased urinary dopamine excretion and plasma L-DOPA in older treated patients with PKU (12). A correlation was found between high plasma PHE concentration, prolonged performance time on the neuropsychological tests, and decreased urinary dopamine (13). These effects were reversible when plasma PHE was reduced. Severe neurological deterioration and/or psychiatric problems have occurred in many off-diet patients with PKU (14–16). Reversal of most of the symptoms is possible with return to a strict diet.

For the female with PKU, diet discontinuation poses special problems. Few women with PKU, untreated before and during pregnancy, who carried the fetus to term have delivered normal infants. Congenital malformations, microcephaly, and retarded growth and development are associated with in utero elevations of PHE (17). Active transport of amino acids by the placenta to the fetus leads to a fetal blood PHE concentration 2 to 3 times that found in the maternal blood. Thus, it is extremely important to maintain normal plasma PHE concentrations in the reproductive female before and after conception.

Filling the diet prescription. Assume that you have a diet prescription for a 2-week-old female (Joannie R) who weighs 3 kg and whose diagnostic plasma PHE was 25 mg/dL (1,513 µmol/L). Prescription is: 50 mg PHE/kg = 150 mg; 300 mg TYR/kg = 900 mg; 3.0 g protein/kg = 9.0 g; 120 kcal/kg = 360 kcal; 158 mL fluid/kg = 474 mL or water to make a 20 kcal/oz formula = 18 oz or 530 mL.

Step 1: Fill the PHE prescription.
A. Calculate the amount of infant formula with iron required to fill the PHE prescription (Table 23-6).

1. For illustration, Similac® with Iron, Ready-to-Feed, which contains 71 mg PHE/100 mL is used.
   a. Example:

$$\frac{71 \text{ mg}}{100 \text{ mL}} = \frac{150 \text{ mg}}{X}$$

$$71 \text{ mg } X = 150 \text{ mg} \times 100\text{mL}$$

$$X = \frac{15,000}{71 \text{ mL}}$$

X = 211 mL Similac with Iron, Ready-to-Feed

   b. Measure infant formula with a large disposable syringe or volumetric flask.

Step 2: Fill the protein prescription.
A. Calculate the amount of protein provided by infant formula with iron required to fill the PHE prescription.

1. See Table 23-6 for protein in Similac with Iron, Ready-to-Feed.

$$\frac{1.45 \text{ g}}{100 \text{ mL}} = \frac{X \text{ g}}{211 \text{ mL}}$$

$$100 \text{ mL } X = 1.45 \text{ g} \times 211 \text{ mL}$$

$$100 X = 305.95$$

$$X = 3.06 \text{ g protein}$$

B. Subtract the amount of protein provided by Similac with Iron Ready-to-Feed, from the total protein prescription.

$$9.00 \text{ g protein} - 3.06 \text{ g protein} = 5.94 \text{ g protein}$$

C. Supply the remaining prescribed protein with Phenex™-1 (Table 23-8).

$$\frac{5.94 \text{ g protein}}{15.00 \text{ g protein}} \times 100 = 40 \text{ g Phenex–1}$$

Step 3: Fill the TYR prescription.
A. Subtract the TYR in the Similac used to fill the PHE prescription plus that in the Phenex-1 used to fill the protein prescription from the TYR prescription (Table 23-8)

1. Total TYR prescription   = 900 mg

   Similac with Iron, RTF
     66 mg per 100 mL × 2.11   = -139 mg

   Phenex-1: 1,500 mg × 0.40   = <u>-600 mg</u>

   Remainder   = 161 mg

B. Supply any remaining required TYR with pure L-TYR.

1. 322 mL of L-TYR solution containing 50 mg L-TYR per 100 mL.

Step 4: Fill the energy prescription.
A. Subtract the number of kcalories provided by Similac used to fill the PHE prescription plus the number of kcalories provided by the Phenex-1 from the total energy prescription (Table 23-7).

1. Total energy prescription   = 360 kcal

   Similac with Iron, RTF
     68 kcal/100 mL × 2.11   = -143 kcal

   Phenex-1: 480 kcal/100g × 0.40   = <u>-192 kcal</u>

   Remainder   = 25 kcal

B. Supply the remaining energy needs (if any) with table sugar (48 kcal/tbsp).

1. 1/2 tbsp sugar

Step 5: Fill the fluid prescription.
A. Subtract the milliliters of Similac used to fill the PHE prescription and the milliliters of L-TYR solution from total fluid prescribed.

1. 530 mL − 211 mL Similac
    − 322 mL L-TYR solution = 0 mL

B. Supply remaining fluid needs with room temperature, boiled water.

1. None required
The diet is summarized below:

Food	PHE (mg)	TYR (mg)	Protein (g)	Energy (kcal)
211 mL Similac with Iron RTF	150	139	1	143
40 g Phenex-1	0	600	6.0	192
322 ml L-tyrosine solution	0	161	0	0
1/2 tbsp sugar	0	0	0	24
Water to make 530 ml (18 oz)	0	0	0	0
Total	150	900	9.1	359
Prescribed	150	900	9.0	360

Feed 2 1/4 ounces every 3 hours

As the child with PKU grows and becomes developmentally ready, baby foods and, later, table foods, are added to the diet in prescribed amounts to supply the PHE provided by infant formula. Serving lists, similar in principal to the Diabetic Exchange lists, but with serving sizes based on PHE content, are available to simplify diet planning (Table 23-6). Eggs, fish, legumes, meat, milk products, poultry, and regular breads are not included in these lists due to their high PHE content. Serving lists contain some special very low protein foods that are important to provide energy.

Aspartame® (a methyl ester of aspartic acid and PHE) is an artificial sweetener used widely in foods. Blood PHE concentrations increase in a dose-dependent fashion following the ingestion of foods and beverages containing aspartame (Nutrasweet®). Consequently, patients with PKU and PKU heterozygotes must not use foods containing aspartame.

Monitoring the patient with PKU. Ideally, following a positive newborn screening test and after a differential diagnosis, the child is hospitalized and fed Phenex-1 or equivalent medical food at 20 kcal/oz without added PHE after diagnostic samples are obtained. A record is kept of medical food intake and 2- to 4-hour postprandial plasma PHE concentrations. In addition, plasma TYR is determined. With careful monitoring, the plasma PHE can be lowered to the treatment range within about 4 days. When plasma PHE has been lowered to an acceptable concentration, a diet containing PHE should be instituted. Remember that the long-term objectives of the diet are to maintain plasma PHE within specified limits and to support normal growth and development. Although normal plasma PHE is around 1 mg/dL (60 µmol/L), control is considered adequate if plasma PHE is in the range of 2 to 5 mg/dL (120 to 300 µmol/L). Plasma PHE should remain ≥ 2 mg/dL (120 µmol/L) to prevent PHE deficiency.

Protein and iron nutrition status should be assessed at regular intervals. Albumin, plasma ferritin, and hemoglobin are used for this purpose. Growth and development are monitored carefully during clinic visits. Methods

described in Chapter 9 for measures of physical development. The dietitian must examine growth evaluations and laboratory data in relation to nutrient intake. Diet diaries and blood samples are submitted at intervals by the parents. The diet must then be adjusted as indicated by these results. When the infant is growing rapidly, weekly diet adjustments are necessary. The child is evaluated at intervals for psychological and neurological development by other members of the health care team, and an electroencephalogram (EEG) to evaluate brain electrical activity is obtained at intervals. The dietitian evaluates the development of feeding skills in relation to age. The skills listed in Table 9-2 can be used as a guide.

The schedule of assessments vary from clinic to clinic, but are approximately as follows: Diet and serum PHE are monitored between clinic visits from materials submitted by parents, often by mail.

	0 < 6 months	6 < 12 months	1 < 4 years	4 < 7 years	> 7 years
Clinic visits	Monthly	At 9 & 12 months	3/year	2/year	1/year
Length/height, weight, head circumference	Weekly	1/week	1/week	2/month	2/month
Diet assessment	2/week	2/week	1/week	2/month	2/month
Plasma PHE and TYR	2/week	2/week	1/week	2/month	2/year
Hemoglobin and ferritin	At 3 & 6 months	At 9 & 12 months	3/year	2/year	2/year
Plasma albumin	At 3 & 6 months	At 9 & 12 months	3/year	2/year	2/year
EEG	At diagnosis	At 1 year	Alternate years	Alternate years	Alternate years
MRI*			1 year	Every 2–3 years	Every 2–3 years
Psychological assessment			Alternate years	Alternate years	Alternate years

* MRI = magnetic resonance imaging

Counseling parents and patients with PKU. Feeding problems arise in all children, but most are minor and are handled by the parents. In the child with PKU, however, even minor problems can be the source of great anxiety to the persons caring for the child. The dietitian can be helpful in making suggestions for dealing with some problems or can provide referrals for other forms of counseling where that is appropriate. The following are some guidelines that may be used in counseling:

If	Consider that
Child seems unduly hungry.	Prescribed diet may be inadequate Child is refusing medical food, and solid foods do not satisfy appetite. Prescribed foods are being refused to obtain sweet foods.
Child has loss of appetite.	There may be too many sweet "free" foods in diet. Medical food may be excessive, reducing the appetite for solid foods. Child may be ill, e.g., infection. Plasma PHE may be deficient. Plasma zinc may be deficient. Growth rate has slowed normally.
Child is refusing medical food.	There may be a normal fluctuation of appetite. Medical food may be too dilute, making volume excessive. Child may be offered too many other calorie-containing beverages. Medical food may be too concentrated, becoming too thick and unpalatable. Child may be manipulating parents. Refer parents for counseling.
Child refuses solid foods.	Child may have a normal fluctuation of appetite. Child may be refusing prescribed foods in order to obtain free foods. Medical food may be overprescribed. Child may be manipulating parents; refer parents for counseling.

Many of the above problems suggest that the diet should be recalculated. In some cases, recommendations for changes in the diet prescription may be made to the physician.

The problem of the child who refuses medical food is a common one. In this case, several techniques can be used to manage the child:

- Remove all foods and energy-containing beverages from the diet until the medical food is accepted (appropriate only for PKU and homocystinuria).
- Add protein-free flavorings, such as Flavonex™ Flavored Energy Supplement, sugar, honey, Kool-aid®, Strawberry-Quik®, or Tang®.
- Mix PHE-free powder with fruit juices and fruit purees.
- Reduce water in formula and use it as a pudding, or add a Rennet tablet and freeze.
- Add PHE-free powder to soups or cereals after cooking.

PKU can precipitate stressful situations and you may be particularly helpful in allaying parents' anxieties. If these become serious problems, parents should be referred for behavioral counseling.

TOPICS FOR FURTHER DISCUSSION

1. Discuss diet modifications in hereditary fructose intolerance.
2. Discuss management of the diet of the infant with PKU if the mother wishes to breast feed.
3. Demonstrate calculation of the diet for an infant with MSUD.
4. Fill the diet prescription for the infant in this chapter using PKU1 and Lofenalac in place of Phenex-1; use Phenex-2 for the child and adult.

REFERENCES

1. **Elsas, L.J., and P.B. Acosta.** Nutrition support of inherited metabolic disease. *In* M.E. Shils, V.R. Young eds *Modern Nutrition in Health and Disease.* 6th ed. Philadelphia: Lea & Febiger, 1994.

2. **Acosta, P.B.** Nutrition support of inborn errors of metabolism. *In* P. Queen, and C.L.Lang eds *Handbook of Pediatric Nutrition.* Gaithersburg: Aspen Publ Inc., 1992.

3. Committee on Dietary Allowances, Food and Nutrition Board: *Recommended Dietary Allowances*, 9th rev. ed. Washington, DC: National Academy of Sciences, 1980.

4. **Pratt, E.L., S.E. Snyderman, M.W. Cheung, P. Norton,** and **L.E. Holt.** The threonine requirement of the normal infant. *J. Nutr.* 56:(1955)231–51.

5. **Segal, S.** Disorders of galactose metabolism. *In* C.R. Scriver, A.L. Beaudet, W.S. Sly, and D. Valle eds *The Metabolic Basis of Inherited Disease*, 6th ed. New York: McGraw-Hill 1989.

6. **Acosta, P.B, and K.C. Gross:** Hidden sources of galactose in the environment. *Eur. J. Pediatr.* Suppl. 2, 154:(1995)S87–S92.

7. **Gross, K.C., and S.J. Wallner.** Degradation of cell wall polysaccharides during tomato fruit ripening. *Plant Physiol* 63:(1979)117-26.

8. **Budavarl, S.**. ed *The Merck Index*, 11th ed. Rahway, NJ: Merck & Co., 1989, 843.

9. **Scriver, C.R., S. Kaufman, and S.L.C. Woo.** The hyperphenylalaninemias. *In* C.R. Scriver, A.L. Beaudet, W.S. Sly, and D. Valle eds *The Metabolic Basis of Inherited Disease*, 6th ed. New York: McGraw-Hill, 1989.

10. **Umbarger, B., H.K. Berry,** and **B.S. Sutherland** Advances in the management of patients with phenylketonuria. *JAMA* 193:(1965)128–34.

11. **Schuett, V.E., E.S. Brown,** and **K. Michals** Reinstitution of diet therapy in PKU patients from twenty-two US clinics. *AJPH* 75:(1985)39-42.

12. **Epstein, C.M., J.F. Trotter, A. Averbook S. Freeman, M.H. Kutner,** and **L.J. Elsas.** EEG frequencies are sensitive indices of phenylalanine effects on normal brain. *Electroencephal. Clin. Neurophysiol.* 72:(1989)133–39.

13. **Krause, W., C. Epstein, A. Averbook, P. Dembure,** and **L. Elsas.** Phenylalanine alters the mean power frequency of electroencephalograms and plasma L-DOPA in treated patients with phenylketonuria. *Pediatr. Res.* 20:(1986)1112–116.

14. **Villasana, D., I.J. Butler, J.C. Williams,** and **S.M. Roongta.** Neurological deterioration in adult phenylketonuria. *J. Inher. Metab. Dis.* 12:(1989)451–52.

15. **Thompson, A.J., I. Smith, D. Brenton et al.** Neurological deterioration in young adults with phenylketonuria. *Lancet* 336:(1990)602–05.

16. **Waisbren, S.E.,** and **H.L. Levy** Agoraphobia in phenylketonuria. *J. Inher. Metab. Dis.* 14:(1991)755–64.

17. **Lenke, R.R.,** and **H.L.Levy** Maternal phenylketonuria and hyperphenylalaninemia. *N. Engl. J. Med.* 303:(1980)1202–208.

18. **Gropper, S., J. Olds,** and **K.C. Gross.** The galactose content of selected fruit and vegetable baby foods; implications for infants on galactose-restricted diets. *J. Amer. Dietet. Assoc.* 3:(1993)328–330.

19. **Gross, K.C.,** and **P.B. Acosta.** Fruits and vegetables are a source of galactose: implications in planning diets of patients with galactosemia. *J. Inher. Metab. Dis.* 14:(1991)253–58.

20. **Posati, L.P.,** and **M.L. Orr.** *Composition of Foods: Dairy and Egg Products,* Agriculture Handbook No. 8–1. U S Dept of Agriculture, ARS, 1976.

21. **Acosta, P.B., C. Trahms, N.S. Wellman,** and **M. Williamson** Phenylalanine intakes of 1 to 6-year-old children with phenylketonuria undergoing therapy. *Am. .J Clin. Nutr.* 38:(1983)694–700.

22. ———, **E. Wenz,** and **M. Williamson** Nutrient intake of treated infants with phenylketonuria. *Am. J. Clin. Nutr.* 30:(1977)198–208.

23. ———. The contribution of therapy of inherited amino acid disorders to knowledge of amino acid requirements. *In* R.A. Wapnir ed *Congenital Metabolic Diseases.* New York: Marcel Dekker, 1985.

TO TEST YOUR UNDERSTANDING

1. Why is tyrosine an essential amino acid in patients with PKU?

2. You have a PKU patient, Susan W., who is 1 year old. Her plasma PHE has been stable for several months; however, the plasma PHE concentration of her latest sample was elevated to 15 mg/dL. Susan's mother insists that her food intake has been the same as usual. What information would you seek in order to determine the cause of the problem?

3. A mother with a 6-month-old male infant (birth weight of 3.5 kg.) diagnosed as a neonate to have galactose-1-phosphate uridyl transferase deficiency, is referred for a nutrition consultation. The patient has an erythrocyte galactose-1-phosphate concentration of 6 mg/dL. The infant weighs 4 kg and is 60 cm in length. Development is lagging by 1 month. Physical examination is normal. The problems listed in the medical record are galactose-1-phosphate uridyl transferase deficiency and possible developmental delay. The mother has maintained a 1-day diet record that included the following foods:

Food	Amount	Protein (g)	Energy (kcal)
Isomil (20 kcal/oz)	720 mL	_____	_____
Gerber's Rice Cereal, dry	4 tbsp	_____	_____
Gerber's Applesauce	6 tbsp	_____	_____
Gerber's Chicken	4 tbsp	_____	_____
Gerber's Squash	8 tbsp	_____	_____
Total		_____	_____

a. What problem would you suggest be added to the medical record? Explain the basis for your answer.

b. Calculate the protein and energy content of the diet, using any food tables you wish. Record your calculations.

c. In the diet record above, circle the items that surely or possibly contain galactose.

d. For those items you circled as possibly containing galactose, what procedures would allow you to investigate their galactose content?

e. What general principles would you follow in counseling this patient? Show the calculations that serve as the basis for your recommendations concerning nutrient content.

f. Write a day's menu, suitable for age, for this patient.

Phenylketonuria

Part I:

At the age of four months, Joannie R, and her mother are referred for a nutrition consult because Joannie's blood PHE is 12 mg/dL. At this time, Joannie weighs 5 kg and her nutrient intake is 250 mg PHE, 1000 mg TYR, 10.0 g protein and 575 kcal. Joannie has no tongue thrust. She presently has no solid foods in her diet plan.

QUESTIONS

1. The physician asks you for your recommendation for the nutrition support prescription and asks you to work with the mother to fill the prescription. Show your calculation below.

2. Show the recipe for the medical food mixture, the number and size of feedings of medical food mixture, and number of servings of foods also on this form.

Part II.

At the age of 6 years, Joannie weighs 20 kg and is in the first grade at school. Her mother is working outside the home. Joannie carries her lunch to school. The school provides time for a midmorning snack during which the children are given 8 oz of milk and a graham cracker. Blood PHE is 4 mg/dL.

QUESTION

3. On Form G in Appendix M, give the nutrition support prescription you would recommend and show the meal plan.

Part III:

Joannie remains on diet through high school and college. After finishing college, she is married at the age of 22 years and becomes pregnant almost immediately. Her blood PHE at the time of conception is 8 mg/dL. Her height is 168 cm; her weight is 56.8 kg. The prescription for nutrition support is as follows: PHE, 220 mg; TYR, 6.0 g; Protein, 60 g; Energy, 2,500 kcal. Joannie works as an accountant and must carry her lunch.

QUESTION

4. Fill the diet prescription on Form G, Appendix M, providing a lunch that can be eaten at a local restaurant if the medical food mixture is carried in a thermos.

Phenylalanine-Restricted Diet Calculation

Weight _____ kg   Name _____

Recommended nutrients:

Phenylalanine	_____ mg/kg	×	_____ kg	=	_____ mg
Tyrosine	_____ mg/kg	×	_____ kg	=	_____ mg
Protein	_____ g/kg	×	_____ kg	=	_____ g
Energy	_____ kcal/kg	×	_____ kg	=	_____ kcal

Medical Food Mixture	*Measure/Weight*	*PHE (mg)*	*TYR (mg)*	*Pro (g)*	*Energy (kcal)*
Phenex ™	_____	_____	_____	_____	_____
Similac with Iron, RTF	_____	_____	_____	_____	_____
Sucrose or Polycose ® (circle one)	_____	_____	_____	_____	_____

Add water to make _____ oz

Foods

Breads/cereals	_____ servings	_____	_____	_____
Fruits	_____ servings	_____	_____	_____
Vegetables	_____ servings	_____	_____	_____
Total		_____	_____	_____

Number and size of formula feedings: _____ oz × _____ bottles

Recommended Nutrient Intakes

TABLE A-1 *Recommended Dietary Allowances,* [*] *Revised 1989*, Designed for the Measurement of Good Nutrition of Practically All Healthy People in the United States

Category	Age (years) or condition	Weight[†] (kg)	Weight[†] (lb.)	Height[†] (cm)	Height[†] (in.)	Protein[*] (g)	Fat-Soluble Vitamins — Vitamin A (µg RE)[*]	Vitamin D (µg)[‡]	Vitamin E (mg α-TE)[‖]	Vitamin K (µg)
Infants	0.0–0.5	6	13	60	24	13	375	7.5	3	5
	0.5–1.0	9	20	71	28	14	375	10	4	10
Children	1–3	13	29	90	35	16	400	10	6	15
	4–6	20	44	112	44	24	500	10	7	20
	7–10	28	62	132	52	28	700	10	7	30
Males	11–14	45	99	157	62	45	1,000	10	10	45
	15–18	66	145	176	69	59	1,000	10	10	65
	19–24	72	160	177	70	58	1,000	10	10	70
	25–50	79	174	176	70	63	1,000	5	10	80
	51+	77	170	173	68	63	1,000	5	10	80
Females	11–14	46	101	157	62	46	800	10	8	45
	15–18	55	120	163	64	44	800	10	8	55
	19–24	58	128	164	65	46	800	10	8	60
	25–50	63	138	163	64	50	800	5	8	65
	51+	65	143	160	63	50	800	5	8	65
Pregnant						60	800	10	10	65
Lactating	1st 6 months					65	1,300	10	12	65
	2d 6 months					62	1,200	10	11	65

Reproduced with permission from *Recommended Dietary Allowances*, 10th edition, © 1990, by the National Academy of Sciences, National Academy Press, Washington, DC.

[*] The allowances, expressed as average daily intakes over time, are intended to provide for individual variations among most normal persons as they live in the United States under usual environmental stresses. Diets should be based on a variety of common foods in order to provide other nutrients for which human requirements have been less well defined.

[†] Weights and heights of Reference Adults are actual medians for the U.S. population of the designated age, as reported by NHANES II. The median weights and heights of those under 19 years of age were taken from Hamill, P.V.V., Drizd, T.A., Johnson, C.L., Reed, R.B., Roche, A.F., and Moore, W.M. Physical growth: National Center for Health Statistics percentiles. *Am J. Clin. Nutr.* 32:607, 1979. The use of these figures does not imply that the height-to-weight ratios are ideal.

(continued)

TABLE A-1   (*continued*)

| Water-Soluble Vitamins | | | | | Minerals | | | | | | |
Ribo-flavin (mg)	Niacin (mg NE)[f]	Vita-min B$_6$ (mg)	Fo-late (µg)	Vitamin B$_{12}$ (µg)	Cal-cium (mg)	Phos-phorus (mg)	Mag-nesium (mg)	Iron (mg)	Zinc (mg)	Iodine (µg)	Sele-nium (µg)
0.4	5	0.3	25	0.3	400	300	40	6	5	40	10
0.5	6	0.6	35	0.5	600	500	60	10	5	50	15
0.8	9	1.0	50	0.7	800	800	80	10	10	70	20
1.1	12	1.1	75	1.0	800	800	120	10	10	90	20
1.2	13	1.4	100	1.4	800	800	170	10	10	120	30
1.5	17	1.7	150	2.0	1,200	1,200	270	12	15	150	40
1.8	20	2.0	200	2.0	1,200	1,200	400	12	15	150	50
1.7	19	2.0	200	2.0	1,200	1,200	350	10	15	150	70
1.7	19	2.0	200	2.0	800	800	350	10	15	150	70
1.4	15	2.0	200	2.0	800	800	350	10	15	150	70
1.3	15	1.4	150	2.0	1,200	1,200	280	15	12	150	45
1.3	15	1.5	180	2.0	1,200	1,200	300	15	12	150	50
1.3	15	1.6	180	2.0	1,200	1,200	280	15	12	150	55
1.3	15	1.6	180	2.0	800	800	280	15	12	150	55
1.2	13	1.6	180	2.0	800	800	280	10	12	150	55
1.6	17	2.2	400	2.2	1,200	1,200	320	30	15	175	65
1.8	20	2.1	280	2.6	1,200	1,200	355	15	19	200	75
1.7	20	2.1	260	2.6	1,200	1,200	340	15	16	200	75

§ Retinol equivalents. 1 retinol equivalent = 1 µg retinol or 6 µg β-carotene.
‖ As cholecalciferol. 10 µg cholecalciferol = 400 IU of vitamin D.
α-Tocopherol equivalents. 1 mg d-α Tocopherol = 1 α-TE
  1 NE (niacin equivalent) is equal to 1 mg of niacin or 60 mg of dietary tryptophan.

TABLE A-2 Median Heights and Weights and Recommended Energy Intake

Category	Age (years) or condition	Weight (kg)	Weight (lb)	Height (cm)	Height (in)	REE (kcal/day)	Multiples of REE	Average Energy Allowance (kcal)* Per kg	Average Energy Allowance (kcal)* Per/day†
Infants	0.0–0.5	6	13	60	24	320		108	650
	0.5–1.0	9	20	71	28	500		98	850
Children	1–3	13	29	90	35	740		102	1,300
	4–6	20	44	112	44	950		90	1,800
	7–10	28	62	132	52	1,130		70	2,000
Male	11–14	45	99	157	62	1,440	1.70	55	2,500
	15–18	66	145	176	69	1,760	1.67	45	3,000
	19–24	72	160	177	70	1,780	1.67	40	2,900
	25–50	79	174	176	70	1,800	1.60	37	2,900
	51+	77	170	173	68	1,530	1.50	30	2,300
Females	11–14	46	101	157	62	1,310	1.67	47	2,200
	15–18	55	120	163	64	1,370	1.60	40	2,200
	19–24	58	128	164	65	1,350	1.60	38	2,200
	25–50	63	138	163	64	1,380	1.55	36	2,200
	51+	65	143	160	63	1,280	1.50	30	1,900
Pregnant	1st trimester								+0
	2d trimester								+300
	3d trimester								+300
Lactating	1st 6 months								+500
	2d 6 months								+500

Reproduced with permission from *Recommended Dietary Allowances*, 10th edition, © 1990, by the National Academy of Sciences, National Academy Press, Washington, DC.
* In the range of light to moderate activity, the coefficient of variation is ± 20%.
† Figure is rounded.

TABLE A-3 Estimated Safe and Adequate Daily Intakes of Selected Vitamins and Minerals[*]

		Vitamins	
Category	Age (years)	Biotin (µg)	Pantothenic acid (mg)
Infants	0–0.5	10	2
	0.5–1	15	3
Children and adolescents	1–3	20	3
	4–6	25	3–4
	7–10	30	4–5
	11+	30–100	4–7
Adults		30–100	4–7

		Trace Elements[†]				
Category	Age (years)	Copper (mg)	Manganese (mg)	Fluoride (mg)	Chromium (µg)	Molybdenum (µg)
Infants	0–0.5	0.4–0.6	0.3–0.6	0.1–0.5	10–40	15–30
	0.5–1	0.6–0.7	0.6–1.0	0.2–1.0	20–60	20–40
Children and adolescents	1–3	0.7–1.0	1.0–1.5	0.5–1.5	20–80	25–50
	4–6	1.0–1.5	1.5–2.0	1.0–2.5	30–120	30–75
	7–10	1.0–2.0	2.0–3.0	1.5–2.5	50–200	50–150
	11+	1.5–2.5	2.0–5.0	1.5–2.5	50–200	75–250
Adults		1.5–3.0	2.0–5.0	1.5–4.0	50–200	75–250

Reproduced with permission from *Recommended Dietary Allowances*, 10th edition, © 1990, by the National Academy of Sciences, National Academy Press, Washington, DC.

[*] Because there is less information on which to base allowances, these figures are not given in the main table of RDA and are provided here in the form of ranges of recommended intakes.

[†] Since the toxic levels for many trace elements may be only several times usual intakes, the upper levels for the trace elements given in this table should not be habitually exceeded.

TABLE A-4 Estimated Sodium, Chloride, and Potassium Minimum Requirements of Healthy Persons[*]

Age	Weight (kg)[*]	Sodium (mg)[*,†]	Chloride (mg)[*,†]	Potassium (mg)[‡]
Months				
0–5	4.5	120	180	500
6–11	8.9	200	300	700
Years				
1	11.0	225	350	1,000
2–5	16.0	300	500	1,400
6–9	25.0	400	600	1,600
10–18	50.0	500	750	2.000
>18 [§]	70.0	500	750	2,000

Reproduced with permission from *Recommended Dietary Allowances*, 10th edition, ©1990, by the National Academy of Sciences, National Academy Press, Washington,DC.

[*] No allowance has been included for large, prolonged losses from the skin through sweat.

[†] There is no evidence that higher intakes confer any health benefit.

[‡] Desirable intakes of potassium may considerably exceed these values (~3,500 mg for adults).

[§] No allowance included for growth. Values for those below 18 years assume a growth rate at the 50th percentile reported by the National Center for Health Statistics (P.V.V. Hamill, T.A. Drizd, C.L. Johnson, R.B. Reed, A.F. Roche, and W.M. Moore. Physical growth: National Center for Health Statistics percentiles. *Am. J. Clin. Nutr.* 32:(1979)607.

TABLE A-5 Recommended Nutrient Intakes (RNI), Canada, 1990, Based on Age. Energy, and Body Weight Expressed as Daily Rates *

Age	Sex	Energy (kcal)	Weight (kg)	Thiamin (mg)	Ribo-flavin (mg)	Niacin (NE) [†]	n-3 PUFA (g)	n-6 PUFA (g)	Protein (g)	Vit. A (RE)[§]	Vit. D (μg)	Vit. E (mg)
Months												
0–4	Both	600	6.0	0.3	0.3	4	0.5	3	12 [I]	400	10	3
5–12	Both	900	9.0	0.4	0.5	7	0.5	3	12	400	10	3
Years												
1	Both	1,100	11	0.5	0.6	8	0.6	4	13	400	10	3
2–3	Both	1,300	14	0.6	0.7	9	0.7	4	16	400	5	4
4–6	Both	1,800	18	0.7	0.9	13	1.0	6	19	500	5	5
7–9	Male	2,200	25	0.9	1.1	16	1.2	7	26	700	2.5	7
	Female	1,900	25	0.8	1.0	14	1.0	6	26	700	2.5	6
10–12	Male	2,500	34	1.0	1.3	18	1.4	8	34	800	2.5	8
	Female	2,200	36	0.9	1.1	16	1.2	7	36	800	2.5	7
13–15	Male	2,800	50	1.1	1.4	20	1.5	9	49	900	2.5	9
	Female	2,200	48	0.9	1.1	16	1.2	7	46	800	2.5	7
16–18	Male	3,200	62	1.3	1.6	23	1.8	11	58	1,000	2.5	10
	Female	2,100	53	0.8	1.1	15	1.2	7	47	800	2.5	7
19–24	Male	3,000	71	1.2	1.5	22	1.6	10	61	1,000	2.5	10
	Female	2,100	58	0.8	1.1	15	1.2	7	50	800	2.5	7
25–49	Male	2,700	74	1.1	1.4	19	1.5	9	64	1,000	2.5	9
	Female	1,900	59	0.8	1.0	14	1.1	7	51	800	2.5	6
50–74	Male	2,300	73	0.9	1.2	16	1.3	8	63	1,000	5	7
	Female	1,800	63	0.8[‡‡]	1.0 [‡‡]	14[‡‡]	1.1[‡‡]	7 [‡‡]	54	800	5	6
75+	Male	2,000	69	0.8	1.0	14	1.1	7	59	1,000	5	6
	Female[§§]	1,700	64	0.8[‡‡]	1.0 [‡‡]	14[‡‡]	1.1 [‡‡]	7 [‡‡]	55	800	5	5
Pregnancy (additional)												
1st Trimester		100		0.1	0.1	1	0.05	0.3	5	0	2.5	2
2d Trimester		300		0.1	0.3	2	0.16	0.9	20	0	2.5	2
3d Trimester		300		0.1	0.3	2	0.16	0.9	24	0	2.5	2
Lactation (additional)		450		0.2	0.4	3	0.25	1.5	20	400	2.5	3

* From Recommended Nutrient Intakes for Canadians, Bureau of Nutritional Sciences, Ottawa, 1990, and Corrected summary tables of the Recommended Nutrient Intakes, 1990. *J. Canal. Dietet A.* 51(1990:394-395. Reproduced with the permission of the Minister of Supply and Services, Canada, 1994.
[†] NE = Niacin Equivalents
[‡] PUFA = polyunsaturated fatty acids
[§] RE = Retinol Equivalents
[I] Protein is assumed to be from breast milk and must be adjusted for infant formula

(continued)

TABLE A-5 *(continued)*

Vit. C (mg)	Folate (µg)	Vit.B$_{12}$ (µg)	Calcium (mg)	Phosphorus (mg)	Magnesium (mg)	Iron (mg)	Iodine (µg)	Zinc (mg)
20	25	0.3	250¶	150	20	0.3¤	30	2¤
20	40	0.4	400	200	32	7	40	3
20	40	0.5	500	300	40	6	55	4
20	50	0.6	550	350	50	6	65	4
25	70	0.8	600	400	65	8	85	5
25	90	1.0	700	500	100	8	110	7
25	90	1.0	700	500	100	8	95	7
25	120	1.0	900	700	130	8	125	9
25	130	1.0	1,100	800	135	8	110	9
30	175	1.0	1,100	900	185	10	160	12
30	170	1.0	1,000	850	180	13	160	9
40††	220	1.0	900	1,000	230	10	160	12
30††	190	1.0	700	850	200	12	160	9
40††	220	1.0	800	1,000	240	9	160	12
30††	180	1.0	700	850	200	13	160	9
40††	230	1.0	800	1,000	250	9	160	12
30††	185	1.0	700	850	200	13	160	9
40††	230	1.0	800	1,000	250	9	160	12
30††	195	1.0	800	850	210	8	160	9
40††	215	1.0	800	1,000	230	9	160	12
30††	200	1.0	800	850	210	8	160	9
0	200	0.2	500	200	15	0	25	6
10	200	0.2	500	200	45	5	25	6
10	200	0.2	500	200	45	10	25	6
25	100	0.2	500	200	65	0	50	6

¶ Infant formula with high phosphorus should contain 375 mg calcium
¤ Breast milk is assumed to be the source of the mineral
†† Smokers should increase vitamin C by 50%
‡‡ Level below which intake should not fall
§§ Assumes moderate physical activity

Tables of Food Values

TABLE B-1 "Rough" Food Value Table for Crude Assessment of Vitamin and Mineral Content of Diets

Iron
8 mg in
  ½ c Cream of Wheat or Malt-O-Meal
  26 oz commercial infant formula, fortified
7 mg in
  6 T infant cereal (dry)*,†
5 mg in
  ½ c prune iuice
  2 oz beef liver
3 mg in
  3 oz cooked beef, pork (not ham), turkey
  ½ c raisins
  ½ c cooked cereal
  ⅔ c ready-to-eat cereal
  1 waffle
  1 slice pizza
  1 tortilla
  1 T molasses
2 mg or more in
  ¾ c cooked leafy greens, asparagus
  1 c leafy greens, raw
  ½ c dry beans, split peas
  3 oz shellfish, ham
  2 eggs
  3½ T strained liver (infant)
  7 T strained meat (not liver) (infant)
1 mg in
  9 T strained infant dinner ("high meat")
  9 T strained green vegetables (infant)
0.5 mg in
  1 slice whole-grain or enriched bread
  ½ c fruit or vegetable, other than dark greens

  1 T peanut butter
  2 dried prunes or apricot halves
  9 T strained fruit (infant)
  9 T strained vegetables (except green) (infant)
  9 T strained vegetables with meat "dinners" (infant)

Calcium
300 mg in
  1 c of milk or buttermilk (8 oz)
  1 c yogurt (8 oz)
250 mg in
  1 oz Swiss cheese
  ½ c red salmon (with bone)
200 mg in
  1 oz Cheddar cheese
  1 c raw oysters (13–19)
150 mg in
  1 oz American processed cheese
  ½ c dark greens (except spinach, chard, beet greens)
100 mg in
  ⅓ c cottage cheese
  ½ c ice cream or ice milk
  ½ c spinach
300 mg calcium in rest of diet

Phosphorus
300 mg in
  2 oz sardines, beef liver
200 mg in
  1 c whole milk or yogurt
  3 oz turkey
  1 oz cheese
  ½ c cauliflower

*Same nutrient values are used for homemade or commercial infant foods.

†Approximate quantities in commercial infant food jars—Strained meat: 7 T; Strained fruit, vegetables, and "dinners": 9 T.

(continued)

TABLE B-1 *(continued)*

150 mg in
  1 oz cooked calf liver
  ½ c beans, kidney or white, cooked
  ⅓ c cottage cheese
100 mg in
  1 egg
75 mg in
  1 oz broiled cod, halibut
  1 oz cooked lean pork or beef
  1 T peanuts, roasted or butter
  ½ c lima beans; peas, cooked
50 mg in
  1 slice bread
  ½ c fruit
  ½ c other vegetables

Magnesium
70 mg in
  ½ c cooked dry beans
  ½ c dark leafy greens
50 mg in
  1 oz nuts
  2 T peanut butter
30 mg in
  3 oz fish or shellfish
  1 T wheat germ
  1 c cooked pasta
  1 c milk
20 mg in
  1 slice whole-wheat bread
15 mg in
  3 oz meat
  1 oz Cheddar cheese
  ½ c other vegetables

Zinc
2.0 mg in
  3 oz roast beef
  3 oz pork liver
1.0 mg in
  1 egg
  1 c milk
  3 oz other meat, poultry, fish
  ¾ c legumes, cooked
  1 oz whole-grain dry cereal
  ¾ c whole-grain cooked cereal
  1 T wheat germ
0.5 mg in
  1 oz cheese
  1 slice whole-grain bread
  ½ c cooked rice or peas

Vitamin A
15,000 IU in
  1 oz liver (cooked) (beef, lamb, or pork)
8,000 IU in
  ½ c carrots, sweet potato, spinach, pumpkin (cooked)
5,000 IU in
  ½ c dark leafy greens—spinach, turnip, mustard, etc. (cooked)
  ½ c winter squash

  ½ c cantaloupe
  10 dried apricot halves
  ¹⁄₁₆ watermelon
  1½ strained liver (infant)
  9 T strained dark leafy or orange vegetable (infant)
2,000 IU in
  ½ c broccoli (cooked)
  ½ c canned apricots
1,000 IU in
  ½ c tomatoes or tomato juice or 1 small tomato
  ½ c peaches (raw)
  ½ c leaf lettuce, watercress
  ½ c apricot nectar
500 IU in
  ½ c head lettuce
  ½ c light green vegetables (green beans, peas, asparagus, limas, etc.)
  1½ c milk (12 oz)
  1½ oz Cheddar cheese
  1 T butter or margarine
  2 waffles
  1 slice pizza
  1 c ice cream
  9 T strained other vegetables (infant)
  4½ T strained vegetable with meat "dinners" (infant)
200 IU in
  9 T strained fruit (infant)

Thiamine
1.25 mg in
  1 T Brewer's yeast
0.3 mg in
  1 oz pork
  2 oz other meat
0.1 mg in
  ½ c whole-grain or fortified cereal
  2 eggs
  ¼ c dried beans (cooked)
  ¼ c enriched rice (cooked)
  1 slice whole-grain or enriched bread
  ½ c enriched macaroni, spaghetti, noodles (cooked)
0.07 mg in
  ½ c vegetables
  1 c milk
0.06 mg in
  ½ c fruit

Ascorbic Acid
50 mg in
  ½ c orange or juice
  ½ c grapefruit or juice
  1 c tomato (raw or canned)
  1 c cabbage or cauliflower (raw or cooked)
  1 c dark leafy greens—spinach, mustard, etc. (cooked)
  ½ c broccoli or Brussels sprouts (cooked)
  ½ med. sweet pepper (raw)
  1 c cantaloupe or other melon
  1 c strawberries

(continued)

TABLE B-1 "Rough" Food Value Table for Crude Assessment of Vitamin and Mineral Content of Diets *(continued)*

20–40 mg in
  1 potato, baked or boiled
  ½ c rutabaga, cooked
  1 sweet potato, cooked in skin
10 mg in
  ½ c other vegetables (cooked or raw)
  4½ T strained fruit (infant)
  9 T strained vegetable (infant)
5 mg in
  ½ c other fruit (cooked or raw)

Riboflavin
1 mg in
  1 oz liver
  3½ T strained liver (infant)
0.4 mg in
  1 c milk (8 oz)
  1 c yogurt (8 oz)
  1 c oysters (raw) (13–19)
0.3 mg in
  ½ c cottage cheese
  1 T Brewer's yeast
0.1 mg in
  1 c dried beans (cooked)
  1 oz Cheddar cheese
  1 egg
  ½ c dark greens (spinach, turnip, mustard, etc.)
  ½ waffle
  1 slice pizza
  3½ T strained meat, except liver (infant)
  9 T strained dinner, "high meat" (infant)
0.05 mg in
  1 oz meat, fish, poultry
  1 slice whole-grain or enriched bread
  ½ c cereal, whole-grain or enriched
  ½ c cooked or raw vegetable
  ½ c pineapple, pineapple juice
  9 T strained vegetables (infant)
0.03 mg in
  ½ c cooked, raw, or frozen fruit

Niacin (Note that tryptophan, contained in any complete protein, may
  also be a source of niacin)
14 mg or more in
  3 oz liver
10 mg or more in
  3 oz tuna, chicken, turkey
  ½ c peanuts
6 mg or more in
  3 oz salmon
3.0–5.5 mg in
  3 oz beef, lamb, pork
  1 c niacin-enriched cereals
  1 T Brewer's yeast
  2 T peanut butter
1.5 mg in
  1 c enriched pasta products
  2 slices enriched or whole-grain bread

  1 medium potato
  ½ c green peas
Vitamin B6
0.5 mg in
  3 oz beef liver
  1 small banana
0.2–0.3 mg in
  3 oz meat, poultry, fish
  ¾ c legumes, cooked
  1 T wheat germ
  1 medium potato
  ½ c tomato juice
  ½ c cooked corn
0.1 mg in
  1 c milk
  ½ c broccoli, cauliflower, Brussels sprouts, spinach
  ½ c whole pineapple or juice

Vitamin E
2.0 IU or more in
  1 oz nuts
  1 T vegetable oil
  ¾ c leafy greens, cooked
  1 c leafy greens, raw
  1 T wheat germ

Folic Acid (Values are for total folacin)
300 μg in
  1 T Brewer's yeast
50–70 μg in
  ½ c orange juice
  1 orange
  ½ c spinach, beets, or broccoli, cooked
  ¼ cantaloupe
  1 c diced beans, cooked
  ½ c peanuts, roasted
25 μg in
  1 egg
  ½ c peas
  ½ c grapefruit or tomato juice

Vitamin B12
50 μg in
  2 oz fried beef liver
2 μg in
  3 oz beef or lamb
  1 oz fish or shellfish
1 μg in
  3 oz chicken
  1 egg
  ½ c cottage cheese
  1 c milk
0.5 μg in
  3 oz pork
  2 oz Cheddar cheese

TABLE B-2   Fiber Content of Foods

Foods	Serving size	Weight (g)	Dietary Fiber (g/serving)		
			Insoluble	Soluble	Total
Vegetables					
Asparagus, whole spears, canned	1 cup	244	3.0	0.9	3.9
Avocado	1/2 avocado	120	3.1	1.6	4.7
Bean sprouts, canned	1/2 cup	62	0.6	0.1	0.7
Beans, green, whole cut, canned	1 cup	135	1.8	0.6	2.4
Beets, cut, canned	1 cup	170	2.2	0.7	2.9
Broccoli, fresh, cooked, 1/2 in. pieces	1 cup	155	4.8	0.6	5.4
Brussels sprouts, frozen, cooked	1 cup	155	5.5	0.8	6.3
Cabbage, raw, shredded	1 cup	80	1.3	0.1	1.4
Carrots, raw, peeled	1 carrot	81	1.9	0.2	2.1
Cauliflower, fresh, cooked, drained	1 cup	125	2.3	0.4	2.7
Celery, raw, chopped	1 cup	120	2.0	0.1	2.1
Corn, whole kernel, frozen, cooked	1 cup	165	3.3	0.1	3.4
Cucumber, raw, unpeeled	9 slices	28	0.2	tr	0.3
Cucumber, raw, peeled	9 slices	28	0.2	tr	0.2
Mushrooms, canned	1/2 cup	78	1.8	0.2	2.0
Onion, yellow, raw, chopped	1 tbsp	10	0.2	tr	0.2
Peas, green, canned	1 cup	170	5.0	0.6	5.6
Green pepper, raw, chopped	1 cup	150	2.3	0.3	2.6
Potato, baked, with skin	1	202	3.7	1.2	4.9
Potato, boiled, cubed, without skin	1 cup	155	1.5	0.4	1.9
Potato french fries, 2 to 3 1/2 in.	10 strips	50	0.9	0.2	1.1
Pumpkin, canned	1 cup	245	5.8	1.3	7.1
Radish, red, raw	10 radishes	50	0.7	tr	0.7
Squash, zucchini, raw	1 cup	130	1.1	0.1	1.2
Sweet potato, cut, canned	1 cup	200	2.6	0.7	3.3
Tomatoes, canned	1 cup	241	1.4	0.4	1.8
Turnip greens, frozen, cooked	1 cup	165	3.9	0.3	4.2
Vegetarian vegetable soup, canned	1 cup	245	1.6	0.6	2.2
Fruits					
Apple, unpeeled, large (2 1/2 per pound)	1	180	3.3	0.3	3.6
Apple, peeled, large (2 1/2 per pound)	1	180	2.3	0.3	2.6
Apricots, canned in syrup	1 cup	258	3.4	1.3	4.7
Banana	1	175	2.1	0.8	2.9
Blueberries, fresh	1 cup	145	3.6	0.4	4.0
Cantaloupe, raw, cubed	1 cup	160	1.0	0.2	1.2
Cherries, tart, canned	1 cup	244	1.8	0.4	2.2
Grapefruit, with membrane	1/2	184	2.0	0.5	2.5
Grapefruit, sections	1 cup	200	0.7	0.2	0.9

(continued)

TABLE B-2   *(continued)*

Foods	Serving size	Weight (g)	Dietary Fiber (g/serving)		
			Insoluble	Soluble	Total
Grapes, Thompson green, seedless	10 grapes	50	0.4	0.1	0.5
Nectarine, unpeeled	1	150	1.2	0.6	1.8
Orange, large	1	200	2.7	1.1	3.8
Pear, canned	1 cup	244	3.5	0.8	4.3
Pear, Barlett, fresh unpeeled	1	180	4.2	0.8	5.0
Pineapple, canned	1 cup	246	1.5	0.2	1.7
Plum, Friar, fresh, unpeeled	1	66	0.6	0.2	0.8
Strawberries, fresh	1 cup	149	2.1	0.6	2.7
Tangerine	1	135	1.9	0.5	2.4
Watermelon, raw, cubed	1 cup	160	0.5	0.1	0.6
Beans and Nuts					
Almonds, with skin	15 nuts	15	5.0	0.6	5.6
Kidney beans, canned	1 cup	255	10.2	2.9	13.1
Lima beans, green, canned	1 cup	170	6.4	0.7	7.1
Peanuts, roasted in shell	10 nuts	27	1.8	0.1	1.9
Peanut butter	1 tbsp	16	1.0	0.1	1.1
Pork and beans, canned in tomato sauce	1 cup	255	7.7	3.4	11.1
Walnuts, English, chopped	1 cup	120	4.5	0.1	4.6
Bread, cereal, rice, and pasta					
Biscuits, baking powder	1	28	0.5	0.2	0.7
Bread, French	1 slice	35	0.7	0.3	1.0
Bread, white wheat, regular slice	1 slice	28	0.5	0.2	0.7
Bun, hamburger	1 bun	40	0.7	0.3	1.0
Cake, yellow, 1/16 of round cake	1 piece	75	0.8	0.2	1.0
Cereal, All Bran	1/3 cup	28	7.8	0.6	8.4
Cereal, 40% bran flakes	1 cup	39	6.8	0.8	7.6
Cereal, cornflakes	1 cup	25	1.0	0.1	1.1
Cereal, Cream of Wheat, quick, cooked	1 cup	245	1.5	0.4	1.9
Cereal, Frosted Miniwheats	1 cup	55	4.1	0.4	4.5
Cereal, Honey Smacks	3/4 cup	28	0.5	0.1	0.6
Cereal, oat bran, uncooked	1/3 cup	28	3.0	1.8	4.8
Cereal, oatmeal, old fashion, cooked	1 cup	240	2.7	1.7	4.4
Cereal, Product 19	3/4 cup	28	1.4	0.1	1.5
Cereal, rice krispies	1 cup	28	0.4	0.1	0.5
Cereal, shredded wheat	1 biscuit	25	2.5	0.3	2.8
Cereal, Special K	1 1/3 cup	28	0.7	0.1	0.8
Cereal, Total	1 cup	33	1.0	tr	1.0
Cereal, Wheaties	1 cup	28	2.7	0.5	3.2

(continued)

TABLE B-2 Fiber Content of Foods *(continued)*

Foods	Serving size	Weight (g)	Insoluble	Soluble	Total
Cookies, plain sugar, medium size	2 cookies	16	0.1	0.1	0.2
Corn bread	1 piece	55	1.5	0.1	1.6
Cracker, graham, plain	2 squares	14	0.3	0.1	0.4
Cracker, saltine	4 crackers	11	0.2	0.1	0.3
Flour, all-purpose white wheat	1 cup	115	2.2	1.1	3.3
Macaroni, cooked	1 cup	130	2.2	0.3	2.5
English muffin	1	57	1.3	0.4	1.7
Muffin, plain	1	40	0.5	0.1	0.6
Noodles, egg, cooked	1 cup	160	2.2	0.5	2.7
Rice, medium grain, regular, cooked	1 cup	175	1.1	0.1	1.2
Spaghetti, cooked, tender stage	1 cup	140	1.5	0.6	2.1
Sweet roll, cinnamon	1 rectangle	75	1.2	0.5	1.7
Taco shell	1	11	0.7	0.1	0.8
Tortilla, flour	1	28	0.3	0.1	0.4
Wheat germ	1 tbsp	6	0.7	0.1	0.8
Fats, oils, and sweets					
Catsup	1 tbsp	15	0.1	0.1	0.2
Olives, green, with pimento	4 olives	26	0.5	0.1	0.6
Olives, black	10 olives	40	0.9	tr	0.9
Pickle, dill	1 pickle	65	0.7	tr	0.8

Adapted from J.L. Christian, and J.L. Greger, *Nutrition for Living*, 4th ed. Redwood City, CA: Benjamin/Cummings 1992 and J.A. Marlett, Content and Composition of 117 frequently consumed foods. *J. Am. Dietet. Assoc.* 92:(1992)175.

TABLE B-3   Fat Portion Exchange List [*]

Food	Amount
Fats and Oils	
Polyunsaturated Fats	
Margarine, soft, tub-packed diet	1 t
diet	1 T
Mayonnaise, regular	1 1/2 t
diet	1 T
Salad dressing (regular, with vegetable oil)	2 t
(low-cal, with vegetable oil)	2 t
Sunflower seeds, sesame seeds, pumpkin kernels	1 T
Vegetable oil (corn, sunflower, safflower, soybean, sesame	1 t
Walnuts, almonds, pecans	1T or 5 nuts
Other Fats	
Avocado	2 T
Bacon fat, lard	1 t
Butter	1 t
Whipped butter	2 t
Coconut	1/2 oz
Cream cheese	1 T
Oil (olive, palm, coconut, peanut)	1 t
Olives	4
Peanut butter	2 t
Sour cream	2 T
Eggs	
Yolk or whole	1
Dairy Products	
Milk	
Whole milk (regular, homogenized)	1/2 cup
2 % milk, low-fat chocolate milk	1 cup
1 % milk, buttermilk (99 % fat-free)	2 cup
Evaporated whole milk	1/4 cup
Yogurt	
Regular	1/2 cup
Low-fat (4g fat/c)	1 cup
Skim (2 g fat/c)	2 cup
Cream	
Half and half	3 T
Whipping cream, fluid	1 T
whipped	2 T
Light cream	1 1/2 T
Nondairy creamer	3 T
Desserts	
Ice cream	1/3 cup
Ice milk	1 cup
Milk shake	1/2 cup
Tofutti	1/2 cup
Cheese	
American, blue, brick, Cheddar, Cheshire, Colby, Fontina, Gjetost, Gruyere, Monterey, Muenster, Roquefort	1/2 oz
Brie, Edam, Gouda, Jarlsberg, Limberger, provolone, Romano, Swiss	2.3 oz

TABLE B-3   *(continued)*

Food	Amount
Camembert, mozzarella (low moisture), Neufchatel	3/4 oz
Cottage cheese, 1 % milk fat	2 cup
2 % milk fat	1 cup
4 % milk fat	1/2 cup
Meat and Poultry [†]	
Bacon	1 oz
Beef, corned	1/2oz
creamed, chipped lean (choice grade, trimmed of all separable fat)	1 1/2 oz
Round steak	3 oz
Chuck roast or steak	2 1/2 oz
Stew; sirloin, tenderloin or T-bone steak	2 oz
Ground beef (10% fat)	1 1/2oz
Rib roast or steak	1 oz
Bologna: beef	1/2 oz slice
pork or turkey	1 oz slice
Canadian bacon	2 oz
Chicken (broilers or fryers), roasted	
without skin; breast	1 breast
drumstick	2
thigh	1 (2oz)
wing	3
with skin: breast	1/4 to 1/3
drumstick	1
thigh	1/2
Duck, without skin	2 oz
Ham, cured regular (11 % fat)	1 1/2 oz
fresh, lean	3 oz
Lamb: loin chops, lean	2 oz
roast leg, lean	3 oz
Liver	3 oz
Pepperoni	1/2 oz
Pork: loin chop, lean	3/4 chop
roasted blade butt or picnic, lean	2 oz
roasted, lean and marbled	1 oz
Sausage: pork links	1/2 oz
Turkey breast (without skin)	2 oz
Veal (except breast)	3 oz
Fish and Other Seafood [†]	
Cod, flounder, haddock, lobster (spiny), scallops, sea bass (white), sole, and tuna (canned in water)	Unlimited
Halibut [‡], perch [‡], (Atlantic redfish or yellow), pike, pollack, red and gray snapper, shrimp (canned)	16 oz
Catfish	6 oz
Crabs	10 oz
Halibut (Greenland) [‡]	2 oz
Herring, Atlantic	2 oz
Pacific or lake	7 oz
Smoked or kippered	1 1/2 oz
King mackerel	6 oz
Mackerel, Atlantic	1 1/2 oz
canned	2 oz
Perch, Pacific [‡]	12 oz

(continued)

TABLE B-3   Fat Portion Exchange List   *(continued)*

Food	Amount
White (Southern)	4 1/2 oz
Salmon, Atlantic or Chinook	1 oz
chum or pink	2 oz
silver, red or smoked	2 oz
Sardines	2 oz
Tuna, canned in oil	2 oz

Protein Alternatives

Legumes, cooked	
Lima beans, split peas	6 c
Black beans, brown beans, lentils, mung beans, pinto beans	5 c
Black-eyed peas, cowpeas, kidney beans, navy beans, common white beans	4 c
Chick peas	1 c
Soybeans	1/2 c
Tofu	2 to 3 oz
Tempeh	2 to 3 oz

Bread and Starch Group (high-fat snacks and desserts)

Baking powder biscuit	1
Brownies	3/4 oz
Cake	1 oz
Corn chips, potato chips	1/2 oz
Crackers	5
Croissants, Danish, eclairs	1/3 of one
Doughnuts	3/4
French fries, onion rings	7
Pancakes, waffles, French toast, muffins	1

* This exchange list is not suited for use in planning diets for patients with diabetes mellitus. One exchange equals 5 g of fat
† Weight after cooking with no added fat
‡ Different fish with the same name sometimes have different amounts of fat

TABLE B-4   Food Sources of Potassium

Food	Description	Measure	Food	Description	Measure
	5 to 10 mEq/serving		Orange, tangerine, mandarin orange	Fresh	1 medium
Vegetables					
Artichoke	Fresh, cooked	One	Peach	Raw	1 medium
Asparagus	Fresh or frozen	½ c	Pear	Raw	1 medium
Beans, lima	Fresh or frozen, cooked	½ c	Pineapple	Fresh	1 c
Beets	Fresh, cooked	½ c	Pineapple juice	Unsweetened, canned or frozen	1 c
Broccoli	Fresh or frozen, cooked	½ c			
Brussels sprouts	Fresh or frozen	½ c	Plums	Fresh	4
Cabbage	Raw	1 c	Prune juice	Unsweetened, canned	½ c
Carrots	Fresh, raw, or cooked	½ c	Prunes	Dried	8
Cauliflower		1 c	Raspberries	Fresh or frozen	1 c
Celery	Raw	1 c	Strawberries	Fresh or frozen Raw	1 c
Chard, Swiss	Fresh, cooked	½ c	Watermelon	Raw	2 c
Corn	Fresh (5")	1 ear			
Cress	Cooked	½ c	*Meats*		
Dandelion greens	Cooked	½ c	Meat, poultry	Cooked	3 oz
Eggplant	Baked	½ c	Salmon, pink	Canned	3 oz
Kale	Fresh, cooked	½ c	Shrimp	Fresh or cooked	3½ oz
Leeks	Raw	¾ c	Tuna	Fresh or canned	½ c
Lettuce	Raw	½ c			
Mushrooms	Fresh, cooked	½ c	*Milk*		
Parsnips	Cooked	½ c	Skim, 2%, whole, buttermilk		1 c
Peas	Dried, cooked	½ c			
Potato	Cooked	½ c	*Miscellaneous*		
Pumpkin	Fresh	½ c	Brazil nuts		20
Rutabagas	Raw	¾ c	Coffee	instant	1 t
Spinach	Cooked	½ c	Molasses	Brer Rabbit	5 t
Squash, winter	Frozen, cooked	½ c			
Sweet potato	Canned	½ c		**10 to 15 mEq/serving**	
Tomato	Cooked, canned	½ c	*Vegetables*		
Tomato	Fresh	1 medium	Artichokes	Cooked	½ c
Tomato juice	Canned	½ c	Beans	Dried cooked	½ c
Tomato juice	Low-sodium or fresh, unsalted	½ c	Beet greens	Cooked	½ c
			Chard, Swiss	Chopped	2 c
Turnip	Raw	¾ c	Chard, Swiss	Whole leaves	3 c
			Cress, garden	Raw	3 c
Fruits			Dandelion greens	Raw	1 c
Apple juice	Unsweetened, canned or fresh	1 c	Kale	Fresh, whole leaves	3 c
			Kale	Chopped	2 c
Apricots	Fresh	2 medium	Mushrooms	Fresh	10 small, 4 large
Apricots	Canned, unsweetened	½ c			
Apricots	Dried	4 halves	Mushrooms	Sliced	½ c
Banana		1 small	Potatoes	Baked or raw	½ c
Blackberries	Fresh or frozen	1 c	Soybeans	Cooked	½ c
Cherries		15 large	Spinach	Raw, chopped	2 c
Fruit cocktail		½ c			
Grape juice	Unsweetened, canned or fresh	1 c	*Fruits*		
			Avocado		½
Grapefruit	Fresh	½	Cantaloupe	6" in diameter	¼
Grapefruit juice	Unsweetened, canned or fresh	1 c	Honeydew	7" in diameter	⅛
Grapes, white		1 c			
Nectarines	Fresh	2			
Orange juice	Unsweetened, fresh or frozen	½ c			

(continued)

TABLE B-4   *(continued)*

Food	Description	Measure
Meats		
Cod	Cooked	3½ oz
Flounder	Cooked	3½ oz
Halibut	Cooked	3½ oz
Salmon	Fresh or cooked	3½ oz
Scallops	Cooked	3½ oz
Miscellaneous		
Peanuts	Roasted with skins	45
Walnuts		¾ c
	15 to 20 mEq/serving	
Vegetables		
Potato	Baked	1 medium
Turnip greens		1 c
Mustard greens		¾ c
Fruits		
Dates	Dried	15
Figs	Fresh	1 large
Nectarine	Dried	10 large
Peach	Dried	3
Rhubarb	Fresh	1 c
Raisins		1 c
Meats		
Chicken breast		6 oz

TABLE B-5 Fat, Saturated Fat, Cholesterol, and Iron content of Meat, Fish, and Poultry in 3-Ounce Portions Cooked Without Added Fat

Source	Total fat g/3 oz	Saturated fat g/3 oz	Cholesterol mg/3 oz	Iron mg/3 oz
Lean Red Meats				
Beef (rump roast, shank, bottom round, sirloin)	4.2	1.4	71	2.5
Lamb (shank roast, sirloin roast, shoulder roast, loin chops, sirloin chops, center leg chop)	7.8	2.8	78	1.9
Pork (Sirloin cutlet, loin roast, sirloin roast, center roast, butterfly chops, loin chops)	11.8	4.1	77	1.0
Veal (blade roast, sirloin chops, shoulder roast, loin chips, rump roast, shank)	4.9	2.0	93	1.0
Organ Meats				
Liver				
beef	4.2	1.6	331	5.8
calf	5.9	2.2	477	2.2
chicken	4.6	1.6	537	7.2
Sweetbread	21.3	7.3	250	1.3
Kidney	2.9	0.9	329	6.2
Brains	10.7	2.5	1,747	1.9
Heart	4.8	1.4	164	6.4
Poultry				
Chicken (without skin)				
light (roasted)	3.8	1.1	72	0.9
dark (roasted)	8.3	2.3	79	1.1
Turkey (without skin)				
light (roasted)	2.7	0.9	59	1.1
dark (roasted)	6.1	2.0	72	2.0
Fish				
Haddock	0.8	0.1	63	1.1
Flounder	1.3	0.3	58	0.3
Salmon	7.0	1.7	54	0.3
Tuna, light, canned in water	0.7	0.2	25	1.3
Shellfish				
Crustaceans				
Lobster	0.5	0.1	61	0.3
Crab meat				
Alaskan King Crab	1.3	0.1	45	0.6
Blue Crab	1.5	0.2	85	0.8
Shrimp	0.9	0.2	166	2.6
Mollusks				
Abalone	1.3	0.3	144	5.4
Clams	1.7	0.2	57	23.8
Mussels	3.8	0.7	48	5.7
Oysters	4.2	1.3	93	10.2
Scallops	1.2	0.1	27	2.6
Squid	2.4	0.6	400	1.2

Reprinted from: NIH Publication No. 93-3095, Sept. 1993

APPENDIX C

Diabetic Exchange Lists (Part I), 1986 Version

TABLE C-1 Composition of One Serving in Each Diabetic Exchange

		Composition				
Exchange	Approximate measures	Weight (g)	Protein (g)	Fat (g)	Carbohydrates (g)	Kilo-calories
Milk, nonfat	1 c	240	8	Trace	12	90
1 %	1 c	240	8	2	12	100
2 %	1 c	240	8	5	12	120
Whole	1 c	240	8	8	12	150
Vegetable	1/2 c	100	2	—	5	25
Fruit	Varies	Varies	—	—	15	60
Bread / starch	1 slice (other items vary)	25	3	Trace	15	80
Meat or substitute						
Lean	1 oz	30	7	3	—	55
Medium fat	1 oz	30	7	5	—	75
High fat	1 oz	30	7	8	—	100
Fat	1 tsp (other items vary)	5		5	—	45

Tables C-1 through C-10 are adapted from *Exchange Lists for Meal Planning* (1986) prepared by Committees of the American Dietetic Association and the American Diabetes Association, Inc., in cooperation with the Public Health Service: U.S. Department of Health, Education, and Welfare, *Diet Manual Utilizing a Vegetarian Diet Plan,* rev. ed. Loma Linda, Calif.: Seventh-Day Adventist Dietetic Association, 1975; *Modern Nutrition in Health and Disease,* 6th ed., Ed. M.E. Shils and V. Young, Philadelphia: Lea & Febiger, 1988; *Manual of Clinical Dietetics.* University of California, Los Angeles, 1977: *Mayo Clinic Diet Manual* (6th ed.) C.M. Pemberton. ed., Toronto: Decker, 1988; M.J. Franz,. *Exchanges for All Occasions.* Wayzata, MN: International Diabetes Center, 1987; *Ethnic and Regional Practices*: A Series. Chicago: American Dietetic Association, 1989; and L.P. Keall, and R.S.. Beaser, *Joslin Diabetes Manual,* 12th ed.., Philadelphia: Lea & Febiger, 1989.

TABLE C-2 Milk Exchanges*, †, ‡

Type	Amount
Nonfat or very low-fat fortified milk †	
Alba 66 or Alba 77	1 envelop
Skim (1/2 %) or nonfat milk	1 c
Powdered (nonfat dry, before adding liquid)	1/3 c
Evaporated skim milk, canned	1/2 c
Buttermilk (made from skim milk)	1 c
Yogurt (made from skim milk: plain, unflavored)	1 c
1 % fat fortified milk	1 c
Low-fat fortified milk	
Low-fat buttermilk	1 c
2 % fat fortified milk	1 c
Yogurt (made from 2 % fortified milk: plain, unflavored)	8 oz
Acidophilus 2 % milk	1 c
Canned evaporated 2 % milk	1 c
Whole milk	
Whole milk	1 c
Evaporated whole milk, canned	1/2 c
Buttermilk (made from whole milk)	1 c
Yogurt, plain, unflavored, made from whole milk	1 c
Soy milk, unsweetened (add 1/2 bread exchange)	1 c

* Composition: One exchange of each of the three types of milk includes:

	Carbohydrate (g)	Protein (g)	Fat (g)	Calories
Nonfat	12	8	trace	90
Low fat (1%)	12	8	2	100
Low fat (2%)	12	8	5	120
Whole	12	8	8	150

† Italic type indicates nonfat
‡ Contains no dietary fiber

TABLE C-3 Vegetable Exchanges *, †, ‡

Artichoke (1/2 medium)	*Kohlrabi (2/3 c)*
Asparagus (5-7 spears)	*Leeks (2 medium)*
Bamboo shoots (3/4 c)	*Mushrooms, cooked*
Bean sprouts	*Okra*
Beets	*Onions*
Broccoli	*Pea pods, snow peas*
Brussels sprouts	*Rutabaga (1/2 c)*
Cabbage	*Sauerkraut*
Carrots or juice	*Sprouts, raw (1 c)*
Cauliflower	*(alfalfa, mung, soy)*
Chayote	*String beans, green, yellow*
Eggplant	*Summer squash*
Green pepper (1 large)	*Tomato, (1 medium)*
Greens:	*6 cherry*
Beet	*2 tbsp paste*
Chard	*1/4 c puree*
Collards	*1/3 c sauce*
Dandelion	*1/2 c stewed*
Kale	*Turnips*
Mustard	*Vegetable / tomato juice*
Spinach	*Water chestnuts (5)*
Turnip	*Zucchini, cooked*
Jicama, raw	

Ethnic foods ‡

Borscht		
(no sugar, no sour cream)	1/2 c	(J)
Sorrell	1/2 c	(J)
Bitter melon, cooked,	1/2 c	(H)
raw	1 c	(H)
Seaweed, dried, cooked	1/2 c	(A)
Fiddlehead fern, raw	1 c	(A)
Willow greens, cooked	1/2 c	(A)
Sour dock, cooked	1/2 c	(A)

Note: Starchy vegetables are found in the bread / starch exchanges. Raw vegetables are found in the free food list (Table C-8).
* One exchange is 1/2 c of cooked vegetables or vegetable juice unless otherwise noted. Composition: One exchange = 2 g protein, 5 g carbohydrate, 25 kcal, and 2–3 g dietary fiber
† Italic type indicates nonfat

TABLE C-4 Fruit Exchanges *, †, ‡

Fruit	Amount
Apple, 2 in.diam.	1
Applesauce (unsweetened)	1/2 c
Apricots, fresh	4 medium
Apricots canned, unsweetened	4 halves
Apricots, dried	8 halves
Banana, 9 in.	1/2
Berries (raw)	
Blackberries	3/4 c
Blueberries	3/4 c
Gooseberries	1c
Loganberries	3/4 c
Raspberries	1 c
Strawberries	1 1/4 c
Cherries, raw	12 large
Cherries, canned, unsweetened	1/2 c
Dates	3 medium
Figs, fresh, 2 in.	2
Figs, dried	1 1/2
Fruit cocktail, canned, unsweetened	1/2 c
Grapefruit	1/2 or 3/4 c sections
Grapes	17 small
Kiwi, large	1
Kumquat	5 medium
Mango	1/2 small, 1/2 c sliced
Melon	
Cantaloupe, 5 in.	1/3 melon, 1 c cubes
Honeydew, Casaba,	1/8 medium, 1 c cubes
Watermelon	1 1/4 c
Nectarine, 2 1/2 in. diam.	1
Orange, 2 1/2 in. diam.	1
Papaya	1 c., cubed
Peach, 2 3/4 in. diam.	1
Peaches, canned, unsweetened	2 halves
Pear, fresh	1 small or 1/2 large
Persimmon, native	2 medium
Pineapple, canned, unsweetened	2 halves
Pineapple, raw	3/4 cup
Plums	2 medium
Pomegranate, 3 1/2 diam	1/2 medium
Prunes, uncooked	3 medium
Raisins, uncooked	2 tbsp.
Tangelo	1 medium
Tangerine, 2 1/2 in. diam	2

Fruit Juices and Drinks	Amount
Apple juice, unsweetened	1/2 c
Apricot nectar	1/3 c
Cider	1/2 c
Cranberry juice, low calorie	1 1/4 c
Cranberry juice, regular	1/3 c
Del Monte fruit drinks	1/2 c
Gatorade	1 c
Grapefruit or Grape instant breakfast drinks (powder)	3 tsp
Grapefruit juice, unsweetened	1/3c
Hawaiian Punch, low calorie	1 c
Hi-C fruit drinks	1/2 c
Orange juice, unsweetened	1/2 c
Peach nectar	1/3 c
Pineapple juice, unsweetened	1/2 c
Prune juice, unsweetened	1/3 c
Tang (powder)	3 tbsp.

Ethnic foods ‡

Apple, Asian pear, 2 1/2 in. diam	1	(H)
Guava	1 1/2	(H)
Jackfruit	1/2 c	(H)
Highbush cranberries	1 1/2 c	(A)
Huckleberries	1 cup	(A)
Salmonberries	1 1/4 c	(A)

* Composition: One exchange = 15 g carbohydrate, 60 kcal, and 2 g of dietary fiber for fresh, frozen, or dried fruits.
† Italic type indicates low fat
‡ H = Hmong-American: A = Alaska native

TABLE C-5 Bread Exchanges *, †, ‡ (plus Cereals and Starchy Vegetables)

Food	Amount
Bread	
White (including French, Italian)	1 slice
Whole wheat	1 slice
Rye or pumpernickel	1 slice
Cocktail rye	3 slices
Raisin	1 slice
Bagel, small 1 oz.	1/2
Bread sticks, 4 in. × 1/2 in.	2
English muffin, small	1/2
Plain roll, bread	1
Holland Rusk	2
Frankfurter roll	1/2
Hamburger bun	1/2
Syrian or Pita bread, 6 in.	1/2
Dried bread crumbs	3 tbsp
Tortilla, 6 in., not fried	1
Boston Brown Bread, 3 in. × 1/2 in.	1 slice
Cereal	
Bran cereals, concentrated	1/3 c
Flaked bran cereals	1/2 c
Unsweetened flaked cereals	1/2 c
Puffed cereal (unfrosted)	1 1/2 c
Shredded wheat	1/2 c or 1 biscuit
Cereal cooked	1/2 c
Grape Nuts	3 tbsp
Bulgar wheat, cooked	1/2 c
Dried legumes	
Baked beans, no pork (canned)	1/4 c
Beans, peas, lentils, dried	1/3 c
Starchy vegetables	
Corn	1/2 c
Corn on cob, 6 in.	1 small
Lima beans	1/2 c
Parsnips	2/3 c
Peas, green (canned or frozen)	1/2 c
Plantain, cooked	1/2 c
Potato, white, baked, 3 oz	1
Potato (mashed)	1/2 c
Pumpkin	3/4 c
Winter squash, acorn, or butternut	3/4 c
Yam or sweet potato	1/3 c
Prepared foods	
Biscuit, 2 in. diameter (omit 1 fat exchange)	1
Corn bread, 2 in. × 2 in. × 1 in. (omit 1 fat exchange)	1
Corn muffin, 2 in. diameter	1
Crackers, round, butter type (omit 1 fat exchange)	6
Muffin, plain small (omit 1 fat exchange)	1
Pancake, 5 in. × 1/2 in. (omit 1 fat exchange)	1
Popover, 2–3 inches (omit 1 fat exchange)	1
Potatoes, french fried, length 2-3 1/2 in. (omit 1 fat exchange)	10
Potato, corn or other chips (omit 2 fat exchanges)	1 oz
Taco shell (omit 1 fat exchange)	2
Tortilla, fried, 7 1/2 in. (omit 1 fat exchange)	1
Waffle, 5 in. × 1/2 in. (omit 1 fat exchange)	1

TABLE C-5 *(continued)*

Food	Amount	
Flour, wheat	2 1/2 tbsp	
Buckwheat flour, dark	3 tbsp	
Rye flour	3 tbsp	
Tapioca, dry	2 tbsp	
Barley, millet	1/2 c	
Grits, hominy (cooked)	1/2 c	
Miso	3 tbsp	
Pasta, cooked (spaghetti, noodles, macaroni, etc.)	1/2 c	
Popcorn (popped, no fat added, large kernel)	3 c	
Rice, white or brown (cooked)	1/3 c	
Rice, wild	1/2 c	
Wheat germ	3 tbsp	
Crackers		
Arrowroot	3	
Graham, 2 1/2 in. square	3	
Matzo, 4 in. × 6 in.	3/4 oz	
Oyster	24	
Pretzels, 3 1/8 in. long, 1/2 in. diameter	3/4 oz	
Rye wafers, 2 in. × 3 1/2 in.	4	
Saltines	6	
Other (for occasional use only)		
Cookies, 1 3/4 in. diam. (omit 1 fat exchange)	2	
Frozen fruit yogurt	1/3 c	
Ginger snaps	3	
Granola (omit 1 fat exchange)	1/4 c	
Ice cream, any flavor (omit 2 fat exchanges)	1/2 c	
Sherbet, any flavor	1/4 c	
Vanilla wafers, small (omit 1 fat exchange)	6	
Ethnic foods		
Blue corn mush	3/4 c	(N)
Steamed corn hominy	1/2 c	(N)
Cellophane noodles	3/4 c	(H)
Mung bean noodles	3/4 c	(H)
Rice noodles	1/2 c	(H)
Yard long beans	1/2 c	(H)
Pilot bread	1	(A)
Hallak	1 slice, 1 oz	(J)
Kasha, cooked	1/2 c	(J)
raw	2 tbsp.	(J)
Matzoth	3/4 oz.	(J)
Matzoth meal	2 1/2 tbsp	(J)

* Composition: One exchange = 3 g protein, 15 g carbohydrate, a trace of fat, and 80 kcal. Whole grain products average about 2 g of dietary fiber per serving.
† Italic type indicates low fat
‡ N = Navajo; H = Hmong-American; A = Alaska native; J = Jewish

(continued)

TABLE C-6   Meat Exchanges (Lean, Medium-Fat, and High Fat)*,†

Type	Description	Amount
Lean Meat (one exchange = 7 g protein, 3 g fat)		
Beef	*Baby beef (very lean), chipped beef, chuck, flank, steak, London broil, sandwich steaks, tenderloin, plate ribs, plate skirt steak, bottom round, all cuts rump, spare ribs, tripe*	1 oz
Pork	*Leg (whole rump, center shank), ham, smoked (center slices), Canadian bacon*	1 oz
Veal	*Leg, loin, rib, shank, shoulder*	1 oz
Game	*Opossum, rabbit, squirrel, venison*	1 oz
Poultry	*Meat (without skin) of chicken, turkey, Cornish hen, guinea hen, pheasant*	1 oz
Fish	*Any fresh or frozen.*	1 oz
	Drained canned salmon, tuna, mackerel, crab, and lobster.	1 oz
	Clams, oysters, scallops, shrimp	5 or 1 oz
	Sardines (drained)	2 medium
Legumes	*Black-eyed peas, broad beans, garbanzo kidney, lima, mung, navy, or pinto (omit 2 bread exchanges)*	1 c, cooked
Cheeses containing less than 5% butterfat		1 oz
Cottage cheese, dry or 2% butterfat		1 c
Egg whites		3
95% fat-free cold cuts		1 oz
Egg substitute with less than 55 kcal per ¼ c		½ c
Ethnic foods ‡		
Menudo	½ c (M)	
Herring eggs	½ c (A)	
Caribou, moose, venison, walrus, whale	1 oz (A)	
Pike	1 oz (A)	
Gefilte fish	3 oz (J)	
Herring, smoked	1 oz (J)	
Smelts	1 oz (J)	
Medium-Fat Meat (1 exchange = 7 g protein, 5 g fat)		
Beef	Ground (15% fat), roasts and steaks, corned beef (canned), rib eye, round	1 oz
Pork	Loin (all cuts tenderloin), chops, roasts, shoulder arm (picnic), shoulder blade, Boston butt	1 oz
Lamb	Most products	1 oz
Veal	Cutlet	1 oz
Poultry	Chicken with skin, duck, goose, and ground turkey	1 oz
Fish	Tuna, drained, or salmon, drained	¼ c
	Lox, smoked sablefish	1 oz
Cheese	Mozzarella, ricotta, farmer's cheese, Neufchatel, Camembert, Edam, Liederkranz	1 oz
Legumes	Soybeans	⅓ c
	Soybean curd	½ block
	Tofu	4 oz

(continued)

TABLE C-6 Meat Exchanges (Lean, Medium-Fat, and High Fat)[*],[†]

Type	Description	Amount
Liver, heart, kidney, and sweetbreads (high in cholesterol)		1 oz
Cottage cheese, creamed		¼ c
Egg (high in cholesterol); limit to 3 per week		1
Soy beans		½ c
Tofu		4 oz
High-Fat Meat (2 exchange = 7 g protein, 8 g fat); limit choices to 3 times per week		
Beef	Brisket, corned beef (brisket), ground beef (more than 20% fat), hamburger (commercial), chuck (ground, commercial), roasts (rib), steaks (club, rib, Porterhouse, New York strip, T-bone), most prime beef	1 oz
Lamb	Ground	1 oz
Pork	Spare ribs, loin (back ribs), pork (ground), country style ham, deviled ham, hocks, feet, sausage, pastrami	1 oz
Cheeses	Cheddar types, American, blue, roquefort, brick, gorgonzola, gouda, gruyere, limberger, muenster, parmesan, swiss	1 oz
	Cheese spreads	2 tbsp
Peanut butter		1 tbsp
Legumes	Peanuts (omit ½ bread, 2 fat exchanges)	1 tbsp
	Pumpkin seeds (omit 1½ fat exchanges)	8 tsp
	Sesame seeds and sunflower seeds (omit 2½ fat exchanges)	4 tbsp
	Hummus (omit 1 bread exchange)	4 tbsp
	Pignolia nuts (omit ½ vegetable and 1 fat exchange)	6 tbsp
Cold cuts, 4½ in. × ⅛-in. slices		1 slice
Frankfurter (omit additional fat exchange)		1 small

Ethnic foods[‡]

Pastrami	1 oz	(J)
Smoked hooligan	1 oz	(A)
Chorizo	1 oz + 1 fat	(M)

[*] Trim off all visible fat.
[†] Italic type indicates lean (low-fat) meats.
[‡] M = Mexican-American; A = Alaska native; J = Jewish.

TABLE C-7 Fat Exchanges[*]

Fat source	Amount	Fat source	Amount
Margarine, soft in tub or sticks[†, ‡]	1 tsp	Cream	
Margarine, reduced calorie [‡]	1 tbsp	Light‖	2 tbsp
Avocado (4-in. diam)	⅛ (medium)	Sour‖	2 tbsp
		Heavy‖	1 tbsp
Oil: corn, cottonseed, safflower, soy, sunflower [‡]	1 tsp	Cream cheese‖	1 tbsp
Oil, peanut§	1 tsp	French dressing	1 tbsp
Olives [§]	10 small or 5 large	Italian dressing	1 tbsp
Nondairy cream substitute, liquid, powder	2 tbsp / 4 tsp	Lard§	1 tsp
		Mayonnaise	1 tsp
Almonds§	6 whole	Salad dressing, reduced calorie	1 tbsp
Pecans§	5 halves	Salad dressing, mayonnaise type	2 tsp
Peanuts§	20 small or 10 large	Salt pork	¼ oz
Walnuts	4 halves	Tahini	1 tsp
Butter‖	1 tsp	Gravy	2 tbsp
Bacon fat‖	1 tsp	Wine, sweet kosher	¼ c
Bacon, crisp	1 strip	*Ethnic foods#*	
Brazil nuts	2 medium	Pinon nuts 1 tbsp	(N)
Hazel nuts	5	Pig's feet 2½ oz = 2 exchange	(H)
Pistachios	20	Seal oil 1 tsp	(A)
Cashews	4 large	Schmaltz 1 tsp	(J)
Macadamias	4 medium		

[*] Composition: One exchange = 5 g fat and 45 kcal.
[†] Italic type indicates polyunsaturated fat.
[‡] High content of polyunsaturated fat if made with corn, cottonseed, safflower, soy, or sunflower oil.
[§] Fat content is primarily monounsaturated.
[‖] Fat content is predominantly saturated.
[#] N = Navajo; H = Hmong-American; A = Alaska native; J = Jewish.

TABLE C-8   Free Foods*

Condiments

Catsup (1 tbsp)

Horseradish

Mustard

Pickles, dill, unsweetened

Salad dressing

Taco or barbecue sauce (1 tbsp)

Vinegar

Soy sauce, regular

Soy sauce, Low sodium ("lite")

Wine, cooking (¼c)

Worcestershire sauce

Drinks

Bouillon or broth without fat, low sodium

Carbonated drinks, sugar-free

Club soda

Cocoa powder, unsweetened (1 tbsp)

Drink mixes, sugar-free

Tea/coffee (regular, decaffeinated)

Tonic water, sugar-free

Water (carbonated, mineral, regular)

Fruit

Cranberries, unsweetened (½c)

Rhubarb, unsweetened (1c)

Salad Greens

Endive

Escarole

Lettuce

Romaine

Spinach

Seasonings

Basil (fresh)

Celery seeds

Chili powder

Chives

Cinnamon

Curry

Dill

Flavoring extracts (almond, butter, lemon,

peppermint, vanilla, etc.)

Garlic, fresh

Powder

Herbs

Hot pepper sauce

Lemon

Lemon juice

Lime

Mint

Onion powder

Oregano

Paprika

Pepper

Pimento

Spices

Sweet Substitutes

Candy, hard, sugar-free (2–3 pieces)

Gelatin, sugar-free

Gum, sugar-free (2–3 sticks)

Jam/jelly, sugar-free (2 tsp)

Pancake syrup, sugar-free (1–2 tbsp)

Sugar substitutes

(saccharine, aspartame, acesulfame-K)

Whipped topping, low kcal (2 tbsp)

Vegetables (raw, 1c)

Cabbage

Celery

Chicory

Chinese cabbage (bok choy)

Cucumber

Green onion

Hot peppers

Mushrooms

Radishes

Sprouts, beans

Zucchini

Ethnic foods[†]

Jalapeño chiles	(M)
Salsa de chile	(M)
Verdolagas (purslane)	(M)
Beach asparagus	(A)

* Composition: Contains less than 20 calories per serving. Foods without a specified serving size may be eaten as desired. Foods with a specific serving size should be limited to 2 to 3 servings per day.
  † M = Mexican-American; A = Alaska native

TABLE C-9 Combination Foods[*]

Food	Amount	Exchanges
Casserole, homemade	1 cup (8 oz)	2 starch, 2 medium-fat meat, 1 fat
Cheese pizza, thin crust	¼ of 15 oz or ¼ of 10"	2 starch, 1 medium-fat meat, 1 fat
Chili with beans (commercial)	1 cup (8 oz)	2 starch, 2 medium-fat meat, 2 fat
Chow mein (without noodles or rice)	2 cups (16 oz)	1 starch, 2 vegetable, 2 lean meat
Macaroni and cheese	1 cup (8 oz)	2 starch, 1 medium-fat meat, 2 fat
Soup		
Bean	1 cup (8 oz)	1 starch, 1 vegetable, 1 lean meat
Chunky, all varieties	10¾ oz can	1 starch, 1 vegetable, 1 medium-fat meat
Cream (made with water)	1 cup (8 oz)	1 starch, 1 fat
Vegetable or broth	1 cup (8 oz)	1 starch
Spaghetti and meatballs (canned)	1 cup (8 oz)	2 starch, 1 medium-fat meat, 1 fat
Sugar-free pudding (made with skim milk)	½ cup	1 starch
Beans if used as a meat substitute		
Dried beans, peas, lentils	1 cup (cooked)	2 starch, 1 lean meat

[*] This list gives average exchange values for some typical mixed or combination foods.

TABLE C-10   Diabetic Exchange Equivalents of Selected Alcoholic Beverages

Beverages	Serving Size	Comments	Exchange Value
*Beer**	12 oz		
Regular			1 bread. 2 fat
Light			2 fat
Extra light			1½ fat
Near beer			1 bread
Cider, fermented	6 oz		1½ fat
Wine			
Table red, rosé, or dry white	4 oz	Red—Burgundy, Cabernet Sauvignon, Claret, Gamay Beaujolais, Merlot White—Chablis, Chardonnay, dry Chenin blanc, French Colombard, dry Riesling, dry Sauterne, dry Sauvignon, blanc, white burgundy, also dry rosé	2 fat
Sweet*	4 oz		2 fat, ⅓ bread
Light	4 oz		1 fat
Sparkling			
Champagne	4 oz	Dry	2 fat
Sweet kosher	4 oz		2 fat, 1 bread
Dessert Wines			
Sherry	2 oz		1½ fat
Sweet*	2 oz	Sweet sherry, port, muscatel	1½ fat, ½ bread
Vermouth			
Dry	3 oz		2 fat
Sweet *	3 oz		2 fat, 1 bread
Liquors			
Distilled spirits, 80 proof	1.5 oz	Whiskey, scotch, gin, vodka, rum	2 fat
Daiquiri	3.5 oz		½ bread, 2 fat
Manhattan	3.5 oz		½ bread, 3 fat
Martini	3.5 oz		3 fat
Old-Fashioned	4 oz		½ bread, 3½ fat
Tom Collins	10 oz		½ bread, 3½ fat
Brandy, Cognac	1 oz	Dry	1½ fat
Liqueurs, cordials* (anisette, benedictine, creme de menthe, curacao)	—	Sugar content up to 50%. Alcohol content 20%–50% by volume.	½ bread, 1 fat

* Beer, sweet wines, liqueurs, and cordials are best avoided because of their high carbohydrate content.

APPENDIX C

Diabetic Exchange Lists (Part II), 1995 Version

TABLE C-11 Composition of One Serving in Each Diabetic Exchange (1995 Version)

Groups/Lists	Carbohydrate (grams)	Protein (grams)	Fat (grams)	Calories
Carbohydrate Group				
Starch	15	3	1 or less	80
Fruit	15	—	—	60
Milk				
Skim	12	8	0–3	90
Low-fat	12	8	5	120
Whole	12	8	8	150
Other carbohydrates	15	varies	varies	varies
Vegetables	5	2	—	25
Meat and Meat Substitute Group				
Very lean	—	7	0–1	35
Lean	—	7	3	55
Medium-fat	—	7	5	75
High-fat	—	7	8	100
Fat Group	—	—	5	45

Tables C-11 through C-21, from *Exchange Lists for Meal Planning*, revised 1995, are published with permission of the American Dietetic Association.

TABLE C-12   Starch List*

Bread		Potato, baked or boiled	1 small (3 oz)
Bagel	1/2 (1oz)	Potato, mashed	1/2 cup
Bread, reduced-calorie	2 slices (1½ oz)	Squash, winter (acorn, butternut)	1 cup
Bread, white, whole-wheat, pumpernickel, rye	1 slice (1oz)	Yam, sweet potato, plain	1/2 cup
Bread sticks, crisp, 4 in. long x 1/2 in.	2 (⅔ oz)	*Crackers and Snacks*	
English muffin	1/2	Animal crackers	8
Hot dog or hamburger bun	1/2 (1 oz)	Graham crackers, 2 1/2 in. square	3
Pita, 6 in. across	1/2	Matzoth	3/4 oz
Roll, plain, small	1 (1 oz)	Melba toast	4 slices
Raisin bread, unfrosted	1 slice (1 oz)	Oyster crackers	24
Tortilla, corn, 6 in. across	1	Popcorn (popped, no fat added or low-fat microwave)	3 cups
Tortilla, flour, 7–8in. across	1	Pretzels	3/4 oz
Waffle, 4 1/2 in. square, reduced-fat	1	Rice cakes, 4 in. across	2
Cereals and Grains		Saltine-type crackers	6
Bran cereals	1/2 cup	Snack chips, fat-free (tortilla, potato)	15–20 (¾ oz)
Bulgur	1/2 cup	Whole-wheat crackers, no fat added	2–5 (¾ oz)
Cereals	1/2 cup	*Dried Beans, Peas, and Lentils*	
Cereals, unsweetened, ready-to-eat	3/4 cup	(Count as 1 starch exchange, plus 1 very lean meat exchange.)	
Cornmeal (dry)	3 Tbsp	Beans and peas (garbanzo, pinto, kidney, white,	
Couscous	1/3 cup	split, black- eyed)	1/2 cup
Flour (dry)	3 Tbsp	Lima beans	2/3 cup
Granola, low-fat	1/4 cup	Lentils	1/2 cup
Grape-Nuts	1/4 cup	Miso 🔖	3 Tbsp.
Grits	1/2 cup	*Starchy Foods Prepared with Fat*	
Kasha	1/2 cup	(Count as 1 starch exchange, plus 1 fat exchange.)	
Millet	1/4 cup	Biscuit, 2 1/2 in. across	1
Muesli	1/4 cup	Chow mein noodles	1/2 cup
Oats	1/2 cup	Corn bread, 2 in. cube	1 (2 oz)
Pasta	1/2 cup	Crackers, round butter type	6
Puffed cereal	1 1/2 cups	Croutons	1 cup
Rice milk	1/2 cup	French-fried potatoes	16–25 (3 oz)
Rice, white or brown	1/3 cup	Granola	1/4 cup
Shredded Wheat	1/2 cup	Muffin, small	1 (1 1/2 oz)
Sugar-frosted cereal	1/2 cup	Pancake, 4 in. across	2
Wheat germ	3 Tbsp	Popcorn, microwave	3 cups
Starchy Vegetables		Sandwich crackers, cheese or peanut butter filling	3
Baked beans	1/3 cup	Stuffing, bread (prepared)	1/3 cup
Corn	1/2 cup	Taco shell, 6 in. across	2
Corn on cob, medium	1 (5 oz)	Waffle, 4 1/2 in. square	1
Mixed vegetables with corn, peas, or pasta	1 cup	Whole-wheat crackers, fat added	4–6 (1 oz)
Peas, green	1/2 cup	🔖 = 400 mg or more of sodium per serving.	
Plantain	1/2 cup		

*One starch exchange equals 15 g carbohydrate, 3 g protein, 0–1 g fat and 80 calories.

TABLE C-13 Fruit Lists

Fruit			
Apple, unpeeled, small	1 (4oz)	Papaya	1/2 fruit (8 oz) or 1 cup cubes
Applesauce, unsweetened	1/2 cup	Peach, medium, fresh	1 (6 oz)
Apples, dried	4 rings	Peaches, canned	1/2 cup
Apricots, fresh	4 whole (5½ oz)	Pear, large, fresh	1/2 (4 oz)
Apricots, dried	8 halves	Pears, canned	1/2 cup
Apricots canned	1/2 cup	Pineapple, fresh	3/4 cup
Banana, small	1 (4oz)	Pineapple, canned	1/2 cup
Blackberries	3/4 cup	Plums, small	2 (5 oz)
Blueberries	3/4 cup	Plums, canned	1/2 cup
Cantaloupe, small	1/3 melon (11 oz) or 1 cup cubes	Prunes, dried	3
Cherries, sweet, fresh	12 (3 oz)	Raisins	2 Tbsp
Cherries, sweet, canned	1/2 cup	Raspberries	1 cup
Dates	3	Strawberries	1 1/4 cup whole berries
Figs, fresh	1 1/2 large or 2 medium (3½ oz)	Tangerines, small	2 (8 oz)
Figs, dried	1 1/2	Watermelon	1 slice (13½ oz) or 1 1/4 cup cubes
Fruit cocktail	1/2 cup	*Fruit Juice*	
Grapefruit, large	1/2 (11 oz)	Apple juice/cider	1/2 cup
Grapefruit sections, canned	3/4 cup	Cranberry juice cocktail	1/3 cup
Grapes, small	17 (3 oz)	Cranberry juice cocktail, reduced-calorie	1 cup
Honeydew melon	1 slice (10 oz) or 1 cup cubes	Fruit juice blends, 100% juice	1/3 cup
Kiwi	1 (3 ½ oz)	Grape juice	1/3 cup
Mandarin oranges, canned	3/4 cup	Grapefruit juice	1/2 cup
Mango, small	1/2 fruit (5½ oz) or 1/2 cup	Orange juice	1/2 cup
Nectarine, small	1 (5 oz)	Pineapple juice	1/2 cup
Orange, small	1 (6½ oz)	Prune juice	1/3 cup

One fruit equals 15 g carbohydrate and 60 calories. The weight includes skin, core, seeds and rind.

TABLE C-14 Vegetable List[*]

Artichoke

Artichoke hearts

Asparagus

Beans (green, wax, Italian)

Bean sprouts

Beets

Broccoli

Brussels sprouts

Cabbage

Carrots

Cauliflower

Celery

Cucumber

Eggplant

Green onions or scallions

Greens (collard, kale, mustard, turnip)

Kohlrabi

Leeks

Mixed vegetables (without corn, peas, or pasta)

Mushrooms

Okra

Onions

Pea pods

Peppers (all varieties)

Radishes

Salad greens (endive, escarole, lettuce, romaine, spinach)

Sauerkraut   ⚕

Spinach

Summer squash

Tomato

Tomatoes, canned

Tomato sauce   ⚕

Tomato/vegetable juice   ⚕

Turnips

Water chestnuts

Watercress

Zucchini

[*] One vegetable exchange equals 5 g carbohydrate, 2 g protein, 0 g fat, and 25 calories.

⚕   = 400 mg or more sodium per exchange.

TABLE C-15 Milk List

Skim and Very Low-fat Milk (0–3 g fat per serving)

Skim milk	1 cup
1/2% milk	1 cup
1% milk	1 cup
Nonfat or low-fat buttermilk	1 cup
Evaporated skim milk	1/2 cup
Nonfat dry milk	1/3 cup dry
Plain nonfat yogurt	3/4 cup
Nonfat or low-fat fruit-flavored yogurt sweetened with aspartame or with a nonnutritive sweetener	1 cup

Low-fat (5 g fat per serving)

2% milk	1 cup
Plain low-fat yogurt	3/4 cup
Sweet acidophilus milk	1 cup

Whole milk (8 g fat per serving)

Whole milk	1 cup
Evaporated whole milk	1/2 cup
Goat's milk	1 cup
Kefir	1 cup

[*]One milk exchange equals 12 g carbohydrate, and 8 g protein

TABLE C-16   Other Carbohydrates List*

Food	Serving size	Exchanges Per Serving
Angel food cake, unfrosted	1/12th cake	2 carbohydrates
Brownie, small, unfrosted	2 in. square	1 carbohydrate, 1 fat
Cake, unfrosted	2 in. square	1 carbohydrate, 1 fat
Cake, frosted	2 in. square	2 carbohydrates, 1 fat
Cookie, fat-free	2 small	1 carbohydrate
Cookie or sandwich cookie with creme filling	2 small	1 carbohydrate, 1 fat
Cupcake, frosted	1 small	2 carbohydrates, 1 fat
Cranberry sauce, jellied	1/4 cup	2 carbohydrates
Doughnut, plain cake	1 medium (1 1/2 oz)	1 1/2 carbohydrates, 2 fats
Doughnut, glazed	3 3/4 in. across (2 oz)	2 carbohydrates, 2 fats
Fruit juice bars, frozen, 100% juice	1 bar (3 oz)	1 carbohydrate
Fruit snacks, chewy (pureed fruit concentrate)	1 roll (3/4 oz)	1 carbohydrate
Fruit spreads, 100% fruit	1 Tbsp	1 carbohydrate
Gelatin, regular	1/2 cup	1 carbohydrate
Gingersnaps	3	1 carbohydrate
Granola bar	1 bar	1 carbohydrate, 1 fat
Granola bar, fat-free	1 bar	2 carbohydrates
Hummus	1/3 cup	1 carbohydrate, 1 fat
Ice cream	1/2 cup	1 carbohydrate, 2 fats
Ice cream, light	1/2 cup	1 carbohydrate, 1 fat
Ice cream, fat-free, no sugar added	1/2 cup	1 carbohydrate
Jam or jelly, regular	1 Tbsp	1 carbohydrate
Milk, chocolate, whole	1 cup	2 carbohydrates, 1 fat
Pie, fruit, 2 crusts	1/6 pie	3 carbohydrates, 2 fats
Pie, pumpkin or custard	1/8 pie	1 carbohydrate, 2 fats
Potato chips	12–18 (1 oz)	1 carbohydrate, 2 fats
Pudding, regular (made with low-fat milk)	1/2 cup	2 carbohydrates
Pudding, sugar-free (made with low-fat milk)	1/2 cup	1 carbohydrate
Salad dressing, fat-free	1/4 cup	1 carbohydrate
Sherbet, sorbet	1/2 cup	2 carbohydrates
Spaghetti or pasta sauce, canned	1/2 cup	1 carbohydrate, 1 fat
Sweet roll or Danish	1 (2 1/2 oz)	2 1/2 carbohydrates, 2 fats
Syrup, light	2 Tbsp	1 carbohydrate
Syrup, regular	1 Tbsp	1 carbohydrate
Syrup, regular	1/4 cup	4 carbohydrates
Tortilla chips	6–12 (1 oz)	1 carbohydrates, 2 fats
Yogurt, frozen, low-fat, fat-free	1/3 cup	1 carbohydrate, 0–1 fat
Yogurt, frozen, fat-free, no sugar added	1/2 cup	1 carbohydrate
Yogurt, low-fat with fruit	1 cup	3 carbohydrates, 0–1 fat
Vanilla wafers	5	1 carbohydrate, 1 fat

*One exchange equals 15 g carbohydrate, or 1 starch, or 1 fruit, or 1 milk

TABLE C-17   Meats and Meat Substitute List

Very Lean Meat and Substitutes

Poultry: Chicken or turkey (white meat, no skin), Cornish hen (no skin)	1 oz
Fish: Fresh or frozen cod, flounder, haddock, halibut, trout; tuna fresh or canned in water	1 oz
Shellfish: Clams, crab, lobster, scallops, shrimp, imitation shellfish	1 oz
Game: Duck or pheasant (no skin), venison, buffalo, ostrich	1 oz

Cheese with 1 gram or less fat per ounce:

Nonfat or low-fat cottage cheese	1/4 cup
Fat-free cheese	1 oz

Other: Processed sandwich meats with 1 gram or less fat per ounce, such as deli thin, shaved meats, chipped beef 🖉 , turkey ham	1 oz
Egg whites	2
Egg substitutes, plain	1/4 cup
Hot dogs with 1 gram or less fat per ounce	1 oz
Kidney (high in cholesterol)	1 oz
Sausage with 1 gram or less fat per ounce	1 oz

Count as one very lean meat and one starch exchange:

Dried beans, peas, lentils (cooked)	1/2 cup

Lean Meat and Substitutes

Beef: USDA Select or Choice grades of lean beef trimmed of fat, such as round, sirloin, and flank steak; tenderloin; roast (rib, chuck, rump); steak (T-bone, porterhouse, cubed), ground round.	1 oz
Pork: Lean pork, such as fresh ham; canned, cured, or boiled ham; Canadian bacon 🖉 ; tenderloin, center loin chop	1 oz
Lamb: Roast, chop, leg	1 oz
Poultry: Chicken, turkey (dark meat, no skin), chicken white meat (with skin), domestic duck or goose (well-drained of fat, no skin)	1 oz

Fish:

Herring (uncreamed or smoked)	1 oz
Oysters	6 medium
Salmon (fresh or canned), catfish	1 oz
Sardines (canned)	2 medium
Tuna (canned in oil, drained)	1 oz

Game: Goose (no skin), rabbit	1 oz

Cheese:

4.5%-fat cottage cheese	1/4 cup
Grated Parmesan	2 Tbsp
Cheeses with 3 grams or less fat per ounce	1 oz

Other:

Hot dogs with 3 grams or less fat per ounce 🖉	1 1/2 oz
Processed sandwich meat with 3 grams or less fat per ounce, such as turkey pastrami or kielbasa	1 oz
Liver, heart (high in cholesterol)	1 oz

TABLE C-17   *(continued)*

Medium-Fat Meat and Substitutes

Beef: Most beef products fall into this category (ground beef, meatloaf, corned beef, short ribs, Prime grades of meat trimmed of fat, such as prime rib)	1 oz
Pork: Top loin, chop, Boston butt, cutlet	1 oz
Lamb: Rib roast, ground	1 oz
Veal: Cutlet (ground or cubed, unbreaded)	1 oz
Poultry: Chicken dark meat (with skin), ground turkey or ground chicken, fried chicken (with skin)	1 oz
Fish: Any fried fish product	1 oz

Cheese: With 5 grams or less fat per ounce	
Feta	1 oz
Mozzarella	1 oz
Ricotta	1/4 cup (2oz)

Other:

Egg (high in cholesterol, limit of 3 per week)	1
Sausage with 5 grams or less fat per ounce	1 oz
Soy milk	1 cup
Tempeh	1/4 cup
Tofu	4 oz or 1/2 cup

High-Fat Meat and Substitutes

Pork: Spareribs, ground pork, pork sausage	1 oz
Cheese: All regular cheeses, such as American 🖉 , Cheddar, Monterey Jack, Swiss	1 oz
Other: Processed sandwich meats with 8 g or less fat per oz, such as bologna, pimento loaf, salami	1 oz
Sausage, such as bratwurst, Italian, knockwurst, Polish, smoked	1 oz
Hot dog (turkey or chicken) 🖉	1 (10/lb)
Bacon	3 slices (20 slices/lb)

Count as one high-fat meat plus one fat exchange.

Hot dog (beef, pork, or combination) 🖉	1 (10/lb)
Peanut butter (contains unsaturated fat)	2 Tbsp

🖉 -= 400 mg or more sodium per exchange.
* One exchange equals 0 g carbohydrate and 7 g protein
In addition:
Very lean = 0–1 g fat, 35 Calories,
Lean = 3 g fat, 55 Calories
Medium-fat = 5 g fat, 75 Calories, and
High-fat = 8g fat, 100 Calories
** Remember high fat items are high in saturated fat, cholesterol, and calories and may raise blood cholesterol levels if eaten on a regular basis.

(continued)

TABLE C-18 Fat List*

Monounsaturated Fats		Salad dressing: regular 🔗	1 Tbsp
Avocado, medium	1/8 (1 oz)	reduced-fat	2 Tbsp
Oil (canola, olive, peanut)	1 tsp	Miracle Whip Salad Dressing ® : regular	2 tsp
Olives: ripe (black)	8 large	reduced-fat	1 Tbsp
green, stuffed 🔗	10 large	Seeds: pumpkin, sunflower	1 Tbsp
Nuts		**Saturated Fats**	
almonds, cashews	6 nuts	Bacon, cooked	1 slice (20 slices/lb)
mixed (50% peanuts)	6 nuts	Bacon, grease	1 tsp
peanuts	10 nuts	Butter, stick	1 tsp
pecans	4 halves	whipped	2 tsp
Peanut butter, smooth or crunchy	2 tsp	reduced-fat	1 Tbsp
Sesame seeds	1 Tbsp	Chitterlings, boiled	2 Tbsp (1/2 oz)
Tahini paste	2 tsp	Coconut, sweetened, shredded	2 Tbsp
Polyunsaturated Fats		Cream, half and half	2 Tbsp
Margarine: stick, tub, or squeeze	1 tsp	Cream cheese: regular	1 Tbsp (1/2 oz)
lower-fat (30% to 50% vegetable oil)	1 Tbsp	reduced-fat	2 Tbsp (1 oz)
Mayonnaise: regular	1 tsp	Fatback or salt pork†, see below	
reduced-fat	1 Tbsp	Shortening or lard	1 tsp
Nuts, walnuts, English	4 halves	Sour cream: regular	2 Tbsp
Oil (corn, safflower, soybean)	1 tsp	reduced-fat	3 Tbsp

† Use a piece 1 in. × 1 in. × 1/4 in. if you plan to eat the fatback cooked with vegetables. Use a piece 2 in. × 1 in. × 1/2 in. when eating only the vegetables with the fatback removed.

*One fat exchange equals 5 g fat and 45 Calories.

🔗 = 400 mg or more sodium per exchange.

TABLE C-19   Free Foods List

Fat-free or Reduced -fat Foods

Cream cheese, fat-free	1 Tbsp
Creamers, nondairy, liquid	1 Tbsp
Creamers, nondairy, powdered	2 tsp
Mayonnaise, fat-free	1 Tbsp
Mayonnaise, reduced-fat	1 tsp
Margarine, fat-free	4 Tbsp
Margarine, reduced-fat	1 tsp
Miracle Whip ®, nonfat	1 Tbsp
Miracle Whip ®, reduced-fat	1 tsp
Nonstick cooking spray	
Salad dressing, fat-free	1 Tbsp
Salad dressing, fat-free, Italian	2 Tbsp
Salsa	1/4 cup
Sour cream, fat-free, reduced-fat	1 Tbsp
Whipped topping, regular or light	2 Tbsp

Sugar-free or Low-sugar Foods

Candy, hard, sugar-free	1 candy
Gelatin dessert, sugar-free	
Gelatin, unflavored	
Gum, sugar-free	
Jam or jelly, low-sugar or light	2 tsp
Sugar substitutes †	
Syrup, sugar-free	2 Tbsp

Drinks

Bouillon, broth, consomme 🖐	
Bouillon or broth, low-sodium	
Carbonated or mineral water	
Cocoa powder, unsweetened	1 Tbsp
Coffee	
Club soda	
Diet soft drinks, sugar-free	
Drink mixes, sugar-free	
Tea	
Tonic water, sugar-free	

Condiments

Catsup	1 Tbsp
Horseradish	
Lemon juice	

TABLE C-19   *(continued)*

Lime juice	
Mustard	
Pickles, dill 🖐	1 1/2 large
Soy sauce, regular or light 🖐	
Taco sauce	1 Tbsp
Vinegar	

Seasonings

Be careful with seasonings that contain sodium or are salts, such as garlic or celery salt, and lemon pepper.

Flavoring extracts
Garlic
Herbs, fresh or dried
Pimento
Spices
Tabasco ® or hot pepper sauce
Wine, used in cooking
Worcestershire sauce

† Sugar substitutes, alternatives, or replacements that are approved by the Food and Drug Administration (FDA) are safe to use. Common brand names include:
Equal ® (aspartame)
Sprinkle Sweet ® (saccharin)
SweetOne® (acesulfame K)
Sweet-10 ® (saccharin),
Sweet 'n Low ® (saccharin).
🖐 = 400 mg or more of sodium per choice.

(continued)

TABLE C-20   Combination Foods List

Food Entrees	Serving Size	Exchanges per Serving
Tuna noodle casserole, lasagna, spaghetti with meatballs, chili with beans, macaroni and cheese	1 cup (8 oz)	2 carbohydrates, 2 medium-fat meats
Chow mein (without noodles or rice)	2 cups (16 oz)	1 carbohydrate, 2 lean meats
Pizza, cheese, thin crust	1/4 of 10 in. (5 oz)	2 carbohydrates, 2 medium-fat meats, 1 fat
Pizza, meat topping, thin crust	1/4 of 10 in. (5 oz)	2 carbohydrates, 2 medium-fat meats, 2 fats
Pot pie	1 (7 oz)	2 carbohydrates, 1 medium-fat meat, 4 fats
Frozen entrees		
Salisbury steak with gravy, mashed potato	1 (11 oz)	2 carbohydrates, 3 medium-fat meats, 3–4 fats
Turkey with gravy, mashed potato, dressing	1 (11 oz)	2 carbohydrates, 2 medium-fat meats, 2 fats
Entree with less than 300 calories	1 (8 oz)	2 carbohydrates, 3 lean meats
Soups		
Bean	1 cup	1 carbohydrate, 1 very lean meat
Cream (made with water)	1 cup (8 oz)	1 carbohydrate, 1 fat
Split pea (made with water)	1/2 cup (4 oz)	1 carbohydrate
Tomato (made with water)	1 cup (8 oz)	1 carbohydrate
Vegetable beef, chicken noodle or other broth-type	1 cup (8 oz)	1 carbohydrate

⌐ = 400 mg or more sodium per exchange.

TABLE C-21   Fast Foods

Food	Serving Size	Exchanges Per Serving
Burritos with beef	2	4 carbohydrates, 2 medium-fat meats, 2 fats
Chicken nuggets	6	1 carbohydrate, 2 medium-fat meats, 1 fat
Chicken breast and wing, breaded and fried	1 each	1 carbohydrate, 4 medium-fat meats, 2 fats
Fish sandwich/tartar sauce	1	3 carbohydrates, 1 medium-fat meat, 3 fats
French fries, thin	20–25	2 carbohydrates, 2 fats
Hamburger, regular	1	2 carbohydrates, 2 medium-fat meats
Hamburger, large	1	2 carbohydrates, 3 medium-fat meats, 1 fat
Hot dog with bun	1	1 carbohydrate, 1 high-fat meat, 1 fat
Individual pan pizza	1	5 carbohydrates, 3 medium-fat meats, 3 fats
Soft-serve cone	1 medium	2 carbohydrates, 1 fat
Submarine sandwich	1 sub (6 in.)	3 carbohydrates, 1 vegetable, 2 medium-fat meats, 1 fat
Taco, hard shell	1 (6 oz)	2 carbohydrates, 2 medium-fat meats, 2 fats
Taco, soft shell	1 (3 oz)	1 carbohydrate, 1 medium-fat meat, 1 fat

= 400 mg or more of sodium per serving.

APPENDIX D | Medical Terminology

TABLE D-1 Vocabulary

Root Words	Meaning	Root Words	Meaning	Root Words	Meaning
Arterio-	Artery	Forn-	Arch, vault	-osis	Disease
Adeno-	Gland	Gastr-	Stomach	Ot-	Ear
Andro-	Men	Ger-	Old age, aged	Ovar-	Ovary
Ano-	Anus	Glosso-	Tongue	Pancreato-	Pancreas
Antr-	Cavity, cave	Gynec-	Women (especially	Parieto-	Wall
Arthro-	Joint		women's reproduc-	Path-	Disease
-blast	Immature form,		tive organs)	Ped-	Child, feet
	sprout, germ	Hem-, hemat-	Blood	Pneum-, pneumon-	Lung
Broncho-	Bronchus	Hepat-	Liver	Poly-	Many, much
Canc-, carc-	Malignant tumor	Hetero-	Different; other;	Proct-	Anus, rectum
Cardi-	Heart		abnormal	Pseud-	False
Cephal-	Head	Hist-	Tissue	Psych-	Mind
Cero-	Neck	Hydr-	Water	Pulm-	Lung
Cheil-	Lip	Hyster-	Uterus	Pyel-	Pelvis
Chol-	Bile	Idio-	Unknown, strange,	Py-	Pus
Cholecysto-	Gallbladder		peculiar	Pyr-	Fever, fire
Choledocho-	Bile duct	Ileo-	Ileum	Recto-	Rectum
Chondro-	Cartilage	Jejuno-	Jejunum	Ren-	Kidney
Col-	Colon	Laryngo-	Larynx	Retic-, reticulo-	Netlike
Corp-	Body, mass	Leuc-, leuk-	White	Rhino-	Nose
Cost-	Rib	Lip-	Fat	Salping-	Tube
Crani-	Skull	Lith-	Stone	Sang-	Blood
Cyano-	Blue	Lymph-	Waterlike	Sclero-	Hard
Cyst-	Bladder; any fluid-	Mea-	Passage	Seb-	Hard fat
	filled sac	Mening-	Membrane	Sept-	Thin wall
Cyt-	Cell	Morph-	Form, shape	Septic-	Poison
Derm-, dermato-	Skin	My-	Muscle	Sinu-	Curved, hollow
Duoden-	Duodenum	Myel-	Marrow	Spondyl-	Vertebra
Em-	Blood	Naso-	Nose	Sta-	Stand
Encephalo-	Brain, skull	Necro-	Dead	Stomato-	Mouth
Enter-	Intestine	Nephr-	Kidney	Tox-, toxic-	Poison
Erythro-	Red	Neuro-	Nerve	Tracheo-	Trachea
Esophag-	Esophagus	Oligo-	Few, scant	Uretero-	Ureter
Esthe-	Feeling, sensation	Onc-	Tumor; swelling; mass	Urethro-	Urethra
Fibr-	Fiber	Oophor-	Ovary	Utero-	Uterus
Fis-	Cleavage, split	Ophthalm-	Eye	Vari-	Bent, stretched
For-	Opening, aperture	Os-, oss-, ost-	Bone	Veni-, veno-	Vein

(continued)

TABLE D-1 *(continued)*

Modifiers	Meaning	Modifiers	Meaning	Modifiers	Meaning
A-, an-	Without, from	-emia	In blood	-phobia	Fear of
Ab-, abs-	From	En-	In	-plasty	Surgical repair
Ad-	To, toward, at, near, adherence	Endo-, ento-	Within	-pnea	Breathing air
		Epi-	On, at, in addition to	-poiesis	To produce
-algia	Pain in	-esthesia	Feeling, sensation	Poly-	Many
Am-, ambi-, amphi-	Around	Eu-	Well, abundant, easy	Post-	After, behind
-asls	Affected with, disease	Ex-	From, out of, without, away from, over	Pre-, pro-	Before, in front of, forward
Ante-	Before, forward				
Anti-	Against, opposite	Exo-	Outside, beyond	Privia-	Without, lack of
Bi-	Two, both, double	Extra-	Outside, beyond	-ptosis	Falling of, downward, displacement
Brachy-	Short	-genesis, -genic	Producing, forming		
Brady-	Slow	Hemi-	Half	Quad-, quar-	Four
-centesis	Puncture	Hyper-	Over, above, beyond, excessive	Re-	Again
-cele	Hernia of, tumor of, protrusion of			Retro-	Backward, back of, behind
		Hypo-	Under, below, deficiency of		
Circum-	Around			-rrhagia	Bursting from
-cleisis	Closure of	-iasis	Presence of	-rrhaphy	Sewing of, suture
Con-	With, together	Im-, in-	In, Into, not	-rrhea	Flowing
Contra-	Against opposite	Infra-	Below, beneath	-rrhexis	Rupture of
-cyte	Cell	Inter-	Between	-scopy	Viewing of, inspection, examination
De-	Down, from, away	Intra-	Within, during		
Demi-	Half	Iso-	Equal, alike, same	Semi-	Half
-desis	Binding, fixation	-itis	Inflammation of	-spasm	Spasm of
Dextro-	Right	Lev-, levo-	Left	-stenosis	Narrowing of
Dia-	Through	-lith	Stone	-stomy	Making an artificial opening
Dis-	Apart	-lysis, -lytic	Destructive		
-duct	Lead, guide	Mal-	Bad	Sub-	Under, below, beneath
-dynia	Pain in	-malacia	Softening of		
Dys-	Difficult, painful	-megaly	Enlargement of	Supra-, super-	Over, above, beyond, superior
E-	From, out of, without	Meso-	Middle, between		
Ec-	Out, outside	-oid	Formed like	Sym-, Syn-	With, along, together, beside
-ectasis	Dilation of, expansion of	-oma	Tumor		
		-osis	Disease	Tachy-	Swift, fast
Ecto-	Without, outside, external	Pan-	All, every	-tomy	Cutting of, incision, into
		Para-	Beside, around, near, abnormal		
-ectomy	Excision of			Trans-	Above, beyond, through, across, over
-ectopy	Displacement of	-pathy	Disease		
Ek-	From, out of, without	-penia	Without, lack of	-trismus	Spasm of
Em-	In	Peri-	Around, about	-tripsy	Crushing
-emesis	Vomiting	-phagia	To eat	-trophy	Growth or mutation

From Frances J. Zeman, *Clinical Nutrition and Dietetics*, New York Macmillan, 1983, 619–621.

TABLE D-2 Abbreviations Used in Medical Records

a	Before	BM	Bone marrow; bowel movement
A	Artery	BMI	Body mass index
A, Asmt	Assessment	BMR	Basal metabolic rate
AAA	Abdominal aortic aneurysm	BOM	Bilateral otitis media
A&B	Apnea and bradycardia	BP	Blood pressure
Ab	Antibody; abortion; antibiotic	BPD	Biparietal diameter
Abd	Abdomen, abdominal	BPM	Beats per minute
ABG	Arterial blood gases	BRP	Bathroom privileges
a.c.	Before meals, *ante cibum*	BS	Bowel sounds; breath sounds
ACTH	Adrenocorticotropic hormone	BT	Bedtime
ad lib	As needed or desired	BUN	Blood urea nitrogen
AD	Adenovirus	Bx	Biopsy
A.D.C. VAN DISSEL	Mnemonic for Admit, Diagnosis, Condition, Vitals, Activity, Nursing procedures, Diet, Ins and outs, Specific drugs, Symptomatic drugs, Extras, Labs	c	Cup
		$\bar{c}$	With
		ca	Approximately
ADH	Antidiuretic hormone	Ca, Ca++	Calcium
ADL	Activities of daily living	CA	Cancer
AE	Above elbow	CAA	Crystalline amino acids
AEIOU TIPS	Mnemonic for Alcohol, Encephalopathy, Insulin, Opiates, Uremia, Trauma, Infection, Psychiatric, Syncope	CAD	Coronary artery disease
		CAT, CT	Computerized (axial) tomography
		CBC	Complete blood count
AF	Afebrile, aortofemoral, or atrial fibrillation	CC	Chief complaint
AFB	Acid-fast bacilli	CCU	Coronary care-unit; clean catch urine
AFP	Alpha-fetoprotein	CDC	Calculated day of confinement
Ag	Antigen	CF	Cystic fibrosis
AGA	Appropriate for gestational age	CHD	Coronary heart disease
AI	Aortic insufficiency	CHF	Congestive heart failure
A/G	Albumin/globulin ratio	CHI	Creatinine-height index
AIDS	Acquired immune deficiency syndrome	chol	Cholesterol
AKA	Above knee amputation	CHO	Complex carbohydrate
Alb	Albumin	CI	Cardiac index
ALG	Antilymphocyte globulin	CIS	Carcinoma in situ
ALL	Acute lymphocytic leukemia	cm	Centimeter
AML	Acute myelogenous leukemia	CM1	Cell-mediated immunity
Amts	Amounts	CML	Chronic myelogenous leukemia
Amb	Ambulate	CNS	Central nervous system
AOB	Alcohol on breath	C/O	Complains of
AP	Angina pectoris; anteriorposterior; abdominal-perineal	CO	Cardiac output
		COAD	Chronic obstructive airway disease
A&P	Auscultation and percussion	COLD	Chronic obstructive lung disease
ARC	AIDS-related complex	COPD	Chronic obstructive pulmonary disease
ARF	Acute renal failure	CP	Cerebral palsy
AS	Aortic stenosis	CPK	Creatine phosphokinase
ASCVD	Atherosclerotic cardiovascular disease	CPN	Central parenteral nutrition
ASD	Atrial septal defect	CRF	Chronic renal failure
ASAP	As soon as possible	Cr_{Cl}	Creatinine clearance
ASHD	Arteriosclerotic heart; disease	CSF	Cerebrospinal fluid
ASO	Antistreptolysin O	cv	Cardiovascular
AV	Atrioventricular	CVA	Cerebrovascular accident
A-V	Arteriovenous	CVP	Central venous pressure
a&w	Alive and well	CVR	Cardiovascular-renal
B I&II	Billroth I and II	CVS	Cardiovascular system
BBB	Bundle branch block	CXR	Chest X ray
BCAA	Branched-chain amino acids	DAT	Diet as tolerated
BE	Barium enema	DBW	Desirable body weight
BEE	Basal energy expenditure	D/C	Discontinue; discharge; direct current
BF	Breast feeding	DCH	Delayed cutaneous hypersensitivity
b.i.d., b.d.	Twice daily	decaf	Decaffeinated
BJ	Bone and joint	def.	Deficiency
BK	Below knee	dex	Dexter (right)
BKA	Below-knee amputation		

(continued)

TABLE D-2 *(continued)*

DIC	Disseminated intravascular coagulation		HIV	Human immuno deficiency virus
dil	Dilate		H&N	Head and neck
DKA	Diabetic ketoacidosis		HOB	Head of bed
dL	Deciliter		H/O	History of
DM	Diabetes mellitus		H&P	History and physical
DOB	Date of birth		Hp	Hemiplegia
DOE	Dyspnea on exertion		HLP	Hyperlipidemia
DTR	Deep tendon reflexes		HPI	History of present illness
Dx	Diagnosis		HR	Heart rate
D₅LR	5% dextrose in lactated Ringer's solution		HS	At bedtime, *hora somni*
D₅W	5% dextrose in water		HTN, HPN	Hypertension
EAA	Essential amino acids		ht	Height
ECG, EKG	Electrocardiogram		I	Infant
EEG	Electroencephalogram		IBW	Ideal body weight
ENT	Ear, nose, and throat		ICU	Intensive care unit
EENT	Eye, ear, nose, and throat		ID	Identification
EFA (D)	Essential fatty acid (deficiency)		IDDM	Insulin-dependent diabetes mellitus
e.g.	For example		i.e.	That is
elec., lytes	Electrolytes		IHD	Ischemic heart disease
elim.	Eliminate, elimination		IM	Intramuscular
esp.	Especially		IMP	Impression
EtOH	Ethanol, ethyl alcohol		I&O	Intake and output
ESRD	End-stage renal disease		I.P.	Intraperitoneal
FBS	Fasting blood sugar		IRDM	Insulin-resistant diabetes mellitus
FFA	Free fatty acids		IV	Intravenous
FH	Family history		IVC	Intravenous cholangiogram
fl	Fluid		IVP	Intravenous pyelogram
FMH	Family medical history		Jc	Juice
FTT	Failure to thrive		kg	Kilogram
F/U	Follow-up		KOR	Keep-open rate
FUO	Fever of unknown origin		KUB	Kidney, ureter, bladder
Fx	Fracture		KVO	Keep vein open
g	Gram		L	Liter, left
G	Gravida		LA	Left atrium
GA	General appearance		LBV	Low biological value
GB	Gallbladder		LBW	Low birth weight
GC	Gonococcus; gonorrhea		LDH	Lactic acid dehydrogenase
GE	Gastroenteritis		LE	Lupus erythematosus
gest	Gestation		LGA	Large for gestational age
GFR	Glomerular filtration rate		LLE	Left lower extremity
GI	Gastrointestinal		LLL	Left lower lobe (lung)
gluc	Glucose		LLQ	Left lower quadrant
Gt	A drop		LLSB	Left lower sternal border
gr	Grain		LMD	Local medical doctor
gtts	Drops		LML	Left middle lobe (lung)
GTT	Glucose tolerance test		LMP	Last menstrual period
GU	Genitourinary		LOC	Loss of consciousness
GVHD	Graft-versus host disease		LOM	Limitation of motion
GYN	Gynecology		LP	Lumbar puncture
H&H	Hemoglobin & hematocrit		LPN	Licensed practical nurse
Hgb, Hb	Hemoglobin		LS	Lumbosacral; low salt
HbA	Adult hemoglobin		LSB	Left sternal border
HbF	Fetal hemoglobin		LUE	Left upper extremity
HBP	High blood pressure		LV	Left ventricle
HBV	High biological value		l&w	Living and well
HC	High calorie		lytes	Electrolytes
HCG	Human chorionic gonadotropin		MAC	Midarm circumference
Hct, Ht	Hematocrit (*See* PCV)		MAFA	Midarm fat area
HCVD	Hypertensive cardiovascular disease		MAMA	Midarm muscle area
HEENT	Head, eyes, ears, nose, and throat		MAMC	Midarm muscle circumference

(continued)

TABLE D-2 Abbreviations Used in Medical Records *(continued)*

MBF	Meat-base formula	PG	Pregnant, pregnancy
MCH	Mean cell hemoglobin	PH	Past history
mEq	Milliequivalent	PI	Present illness; pulmonary insufficiency
MH	Menstrual history, marital history	PID	Pelvic inflammatory disease
MI	Mitral insufficiency, myocardial infarction	PKU	Phenylketonuria
mL	Milliliter	PMD	Private medical doctor
mm	Millimeter	PMH	Past medical history
mmol	Millimole	PMN	Polymorphonuclear leukocyte (neutrophil)
mos.	Months	po	By mouth, given orally
mOsm	Milliosmole	P.O.	Postoperative
MCH	Mean cell hemoglobin	POD	Postoperative day
MCHC	Mean cell hemoglobin concentration	PP	Patient profile, postprandial
MCL	Midclavicular line	PPN	Peripheral parenteral nutrition
MCT	Medium-chain triglyercide	pr	By rectum, given rectally
MCV	Mean cell volume	PR	Pulse rate
meds	Medications	prn	Whenever necessary
MP	Metatarsal-phalangeal	Pro	Protein
mg	Milligram	Pt	Patient
MS	Mitral stenosis; multiple sclerosis; morphine sulfate	PT	Physical therapy; prothrombin time
MVI	Multivitamin injection	PTA	Prior to admission
N. NML, NL	nal	PTH	Parathormone
NAD	No acute distress; no active disease	PTT	Partial thromboplastin time or prothrombin time
NCAT	Normocephalic atraumatic	PUFAs	Polyunsaturated fatty acids
NCD	Normal childhood disease	PUD	Peptic ulcer disease
NED	No evidence of disease	PVD	Peripheral vascular disease
NERD	No evidence of return disease	PZI	Protamine zinc insulin
ng	Nanogram	q	Every
NG	Nasogastric	q.d.	Every day
NIDDM	Non-insulin-dependent diabetes mellitus	qh	Every hour
NKA	No known allergies	q.i.d.	Four times daily
NKDA	No known drug allergies	q.o.d.	Every other day
NPH	Neutral protein Hagedorn (insulin)	q2h, q3h	Every 2 hours, every 3 hours
NPN	Nonprotein nitrogen	quad	Quadriplegic
NPO	Nothing by mouth, *non per os*	RA	Right atrium
NR	Not remarkable	r.b.c.	Red blood cells
NS	Normal saline; neurosurgery	RBC	Red blood cell count
NSR	Normal sinus rhythm	RCM	Right costal margin
N&V	Nausea and vomiting	RDAs	Recommended dietary allowances
OB	Obstetrics	RLE	Right lower extremity
OBW	Optimal body weight	RLL	Right lower lobe
OC	Oral contraceptives	RLQ	Right lower quadrant
OCG	Oral cystogram	RO, R/O	Rule out
OD	Overdose; right eye	ROM	Range of motion
OK	Okay, suitable	ROS	Review of systems
OOB	Out of bed	RTA	Renal tubular acidosis
O&P	Ova and parasites	RTC	Return to clinic
OR	Operating room	RUE	Right upper extremity
OS	Left eye	RUL	Right upper lobe (lung)
OU	Both eyes	RUQ	Right upper quadrant
oz	Ounce	RV	Right ventricle
PA	Pernicious anemia	rx	Take
Para	Pregnancies; paraplegic	Rx	Prescription, treatment
pc	After eating, *post cibum*	$\bar{s}$	Without
PC	Present complaint	SAA	Synthetic amino acids
PCM	Protein-calorie malnutrition	S&A	Sugar and acetone
PCV	Packed cell volume (hematocrit)	SBS	Short bowl syndrome
PDA	Patent ductus arteriosus	SCr	Serum creatinine
PDR	*Physician's Desk Reference*	SG	Swan-Ganz (catheter)
PE	Pulmonary embolus	SGA	Small for gestational age
pg	picogram	SGOT	Serum glutamic oxaloacetic transaminase

(continued)

TABLE D-2   Abbreviations Used in Medical Records *(continued)*

SGPT	Serum glutamic pyruvic transaminase	TUR	Transurethral resection
SH	Social history	TV	Tidal volume
sig	Label	Tx	Treatment
SL	Sublingual	UA, U.A.	Urine analysis; uric acid
SLE	Systemic lupus erythematosus, St. Louis encephalitis	UBW	Usual body weight
SOAP	Mnemonic for Subjective, Objective, Assessment, Plan	UCD	Usual childhood diseases
		UGI	Upper gastrointestinal
SOB	Short of breath	UNA	Urea nitrogen appearance
SOBOE	Short of breath on exertion	URI	Upper respiratory (tract) infection
sos	If necessary	US	Ultrasound
S/P	Status postoperatively	UTI	Urinary tract infection
SQ	Subcutaneous, given subcutaneously	UUN	Urinary urea nitrogen
S&S	Signs and symptoms	Vag	Vaginal
stat	At once, immediately	VC	Vital capacity
sub	Substitute	V&P	Vagotomy and pyloroplasty
SUN	Serum urea nitrogen	Vit.	Vitamin(s)
Sx	Symptoms	VMA	Vanillylmandelic acid
T	Tablespoon	vs	Versus
t	Teaspoon	VS	Vital Signs
T&A	Tonsillectomy and adenoidectomy	VSS	Vital signs stable
TB, Tbc	Tuberculosis	w.b.c.	White blood cells
TBLC	Term birth, living child	WBC	White blood cell count
TDE	Total daily energy expenditure	WDWN	Well developed, well nourished
temp	Temperature	WNL	Within normal limits
TF	Tube feeding; transferrin	w/o	Without
TG, Trig.	Triglycerides	W/U	Workup
TIA	Transient ischemic attack	w/v	Weight per volume
TIBC	Total iron-binding capacity	yrs	Years
t.i.d.	Three times daily	y.o.	Years old
TKO	To keep open	#	Pounds
TLC	Total lymphocyte count; tender loving care; total lung capacity	2°	Secondary to
		24°	24 hours
TPN	Total parenteral nutrition	37°	37 degrees
TPR	Temperature, pulse, and respiration	↑	High, increased, elevated
TSF	Triceps skinfold	↓	Low, decreased, depressed
TSH	Thyroid stimulating hormone		

APPENDIX E   Clinical Laboratory Values

The preferred method for reporting clinical laboratory data is in terms of SI units, replacing the various "conventional" units previously used. "SI Units" is an abbreviation for, in French, le Systéme international d'Unités, or, in English, International System. The system is in use in many nations and thus promotes understanding of papers written in other countries.

SI units are recommended for use in medicine because they permit reporting in terms of moles per liter or its metric multiples or submultiples. Some of the base units of the SI system and accepted abbreviations are given in Table E-1. Prefixes and symbols for decimal multiples and submultiples are given in Table E-2.

Because the "conventional units" and SI units are both still in use, the tables in this appendix provide both values together with the conversion factors. Conversion factors are used as follows:

Conventional Unit × conversion factor = SI unit   (E-1)
SI unit ÷ conversion factor = conventional unit   (E-2)

TABLE E-1   Base Units of SI

Physical quantity	Base unit	SI Symbol
length	meter	m
mass	kilogram	kg
amount of substance	mole	mol
time, SI	seconds	sec
non-SI	minute	min
	hour	h
	day	d
	week	wk
	month	mo
	year	y

TABLE E-2 Prefixes and Symbols for Decimal Multiples
and Submultiples

Factor	Prefix	Symbol
10^{18}	exa	E
10^{15}	peta	P
10^{12}	tera	T
10^{9}	giga	G
10^{6}	mega	M
10^{3}	kilo	k
10^{-3}	milli	m
10^{-6}	micro	μ
10^{-9}	nano	n
10^{-12}	pico	p
10^{-15}	femto	f
10^{-18}	atto	a

TABLE E-3 SI Units and Conversion Table for Values in Clinical Hematology*

Component	Conventional normal values	Conventional units	Conversion factor	SI normal values	SI units
Erythrocyte count (B)					
female	3.5–5.0	$10^6/mm^3$	1	3.5–5.0	$10^{12}/L$
male	4.3–5.9	$10^6/mm^3$	1	4.3–5.9	$10^{12}/L$
Erythrocyte count (Sf)	0	mm^{-3}	1	0	$10^6/L$
Erythrocyte sedimentation rate [ESR] (BErc)					
female	0–30	mm/h	1	0–30	mm/h
male	0–20	mm/h	1	0–20	mm/h
Hematocrit (BErcs) vol. fraction					
female	33–43	%	0.01	0.33–0.43	1
male	39–49	%	0.01	0.39–0.49	1
Hemoglobin (B) mass concentration					
female	12.0–15.0	g/dL	10	120–150	g/L
male	13.6–17.2	g/dL	10	136–172	g/L
Leukocyte count (B)	3200–9800	mm^{-3}	0.001	3.2–9.8	$10^9/L$
number fraction ["differential"]		%	0.01		1
Leukocyte count (Sf)	0–5	mm^{-3}	1	0–5	$10^6/L$
Mean corpuscular hemoglobin [MCH] (BErc)					
mass	27–33	pg	1	27–33	pg
amount of substance Hb [Fe]	27–33	pg	0.06206	1.70–2.05	fmol
Mean corpuscular hemoglobin concentration [MCHC] (BErc)					
mass concentration	33–37	g/dL	10	330–370	g/L
Mean corpuscular volume [MCV] (BErc)					
erythrocyte volume	76–100	μm^3	1	76–100	fL
Platelet count (B)	130–400	$10^3/mm^3$	1	130–400	$10^9/L$
Reticulocyte count (B)					
adults	10,000–75,000	mm^{-3}	0.001	10–75	$10^9/L$
number fraction	1–24	0/00 (number per 1,000 erythrocytes)	0.001	0.001–0.024	1
	0.1–2.4	%	0.001	0.001–0.024	1

B= blood.   Erc(s) = erythrocytes.   Sf = spinal fluid.   Lkc(s) = leukocytes.   P = plasma.   S = serum.
*Adapted from Young, D.S. Implementation of SI units for clinical laboratory data. *Ann. Int. Med.* 10: (1987) 114–129.

TABLE E-4 SI Units Conversion Factors for Values in Clinical Chemistry*

Component	Conventional normal values	Conventional Units	Conversion factor	SI normal values	SI unit
Acetoacetate (S)	0.3–3.0	mg/dL	97.95	30–300	μmol/L
Acetone (B,S)	0	mg/dL	172.2	0	μmol/L
Acid phosphatase (S)	0–5.5	U/L	16.67	0–90	nkat/L
Adrenocorticotropin [ACTH] (P)	20–100	pg/ml	0.2202	4–22	pmol/L
Alanine Aminotransferase [ALT] (S)	0–35	U/L	0.01667	0–0.58	μkat/L
Albumin (S)	4.0–6.0	g/dL	10.0	40–60	g/L
Aldolase (S)	0–6	U/L	16.67	0–100	nkat/L
Aldosterone (S)					
normal salt diet	8.1–15.5	ng/dL	27.74	220–430	pmol/L
restricted salt diet	20.8–44.4	ng/dL	27.74	580–1240	pmol/L
Aldosterone (U)-sodium excretion					
= 25 mmol/d	18.85	μg/24 h	2.774	50.235	nmol/d
= 17–125 mmol/d	5–26	μg/24 h	2.774	15–70	nmol/d
= 200 mmol/d	1.5–12.5	μg/24 h	2.774	5–35	nmol/d
Alkaline phosphatase (S)	30–120	U/L	0.01667	0.5–2.0	μkat/L
Alpha$_1$-antitrypsin (S)	150–350	mg/dL	0.01	1.5–3.5	g/L
Alpha$_2$-macroglobulin (S)	145–410	mg/dl	0.01	1.5–4.1	g/L
Aluminum (S)	0–15	μg/L	37.06	0–560	nmol/L
Amino acid fractionation (P)					
alanine	2.2–4.5	mg/dL	112.2	245–500	μmol/L
alpha-aminobutyric acid	0.1–0.2	mg/dL	96.97	10–20	μmol/L
arginine	0.5–2.5	mg/dL	57.40	30–145	μmol/L
asparagine	0.5–0.6	mg/dL	75.69	35–45	μmol/L
aspartic acid	0.0–0.3	mg/dL	75.13	0–20	μmol/L
citrulline	0.2–1.0	mg/dL	57.08	15–55	μmol/L
cystine	0.2–2.2	mg/dL	41.61	10–90	μmol/L
glutamic acid	0.2–2.8	mg/dL	67.97	15–190	μmol/L
glutamine	6.1–10.2	mg/dL	68.42	420–700	μmol/L
glycine	0.9–4.2	mg/dL	133.2	120–560	μmol/L
histidine	0.5–1.7	mg/dL	64.45	30–110	μmol/L
hydroxyproline	0–trace	mg/dL	76.26	0–trace	μmol/L
isoleucine	0.5–1.3	mg/dL	76.24	40–100	μmol/L
leucine	1.0–2.3	mg/dL	76.24	75–175	μmol/L
lysine	1.2–3.5	mg/dL	68.40	80–240	μmol/L
methionine	0.1–0.6	mg/dL	67.02	5–40	μmol/L
ornithine	0.4–1.4	mg/dL	75.67	30–400	μmol/L
phenylalanine	0.6–1.5	mg/dL	60.54	35–90	μmol/L
proline	1.2–3.9	mg/dL	86.86	105–340	μmol/L
serine	0.8–1.8	mg/dL	95.16	75–170	μmol/L
taurine	0.3–2.1	mg/dL	79.91	25–170	μmol/L
threonine	0.9–2.5	mg/dL	83.95	75–210	μmol/L
tryptophan	0.5–2.5	mg/dL	48.97	25–125	μmol/L
tyrosine	0.4–1.6	mg/dL	55.19	20–90	μmol/L
valine	1.7–3.7	mg/dL	85.36	145–315	μmol/L
Amino acid nitrogen (P)	4.0–6.0	mg/dL	0.7139	2.9–4.3	mmol/L
Amino acid nitrogen (U)	50–200	mg/24 h	0.07139	3.6–14.3	mmol/d
Delta-aminolevulinate [as levulinic acid] (U)	1.0–7.0	mg/24 h	7.626	8–53	μmol/d
Amitriptyline (P,S) therapeutic	50–200	ng/mL	3.605	180–720	nmol/L

S = serum. B = blood. P = plasma. U = urine. Df = duodenal fluid. aB = arterial blood. kat = katal = mol × s^{-1} × L^{-1} or mol/s × L.   *(continued)*
*Adapted from Young, D.S. Implementation of SI units for clinical laboratory data. *Ann. Int. Med.* 10: (1987) 114–129.

TABLE E-4 *(continued)*

Component	Conventional normal values	Conventional Units	Conversion factor	SI normal values	SI unit
Ammonia (vP)					
as ammonia [NH$_3$]	10–80	µg/dL	0.5872	5–50	µmol/L
as ammonium ion [NH$_4^+$]	10–85	µg/dL	0.5543	5–50	µmol/L
as nitrogen [N]	10–65	µg/dL	0.7139	5–50	µmol/L
Amylase (S)	0–130	U/L	0.01667	0–2.17	µkat/L
Angiotensin converting enzyme (S)	< 40	nmol/mL/min	16.67	< 670	nkat/L
[as AS$_2$O$_3$]	< 25	µg/dL	0.05055	< 1.3	µmol/L
Ascorbate (P) [as ascorbic acid]	0.6–2.0	mg/dL	56.78	30–110	µmol/L
Aspartate aminotransferase [AST] (S)	0–35	U/L	0.01667	0–0.58	µkat/L
Bile acids, total (S) [as chenodeoxycholic acid]	Trace–3.3	µg/mL	2.547	Trace–8.4	µmol/L
cholic acid	Trace–1.0	µg/mL	2.448	Trace–2.4	µmol/L
chendeoxycholic acid	Trace–1.3	µg/mL	2.547	Trace–3.4	µmol/L
deoxycholic acid	Trace–1.0	µg/mL	2.547	Trace–2.6	µmol/L
lithocholic acid	Trace	µg/mL	2.656	Trace	µmol/L
Bile acids, (Df) [after cholecystokinin stimulation]					
total as chenodeoxycholic acid	14.0–58.0	mg/mL	2.547	35.0–148.0	mmol/L
cholic acid	2.4–33.0	mg/mL	2.448	6.8–81.0	mmol/L
chenodeoxycholic acid	4.0–24.0	mg/mL	2.547	10.0–61.4	mmol/L
deoxycholic acid	0.8–6.9	mg/mL	2.547	2.0–18.0	mmol/L
lithocholic acid	0.3–0.8	mg/mL	2.656	0.8–2.0	mmol/L
Bilirubin, total (S)	0.1–1.0	mg/dL	17.10	2–18	µmol/L
Bilirubin, conjugated (S)	0–0.2	mg/dL	17.10	0–4	µmol/L
Calcitonin (S)	< 100	pg/mL	1.00	< 100	ng/L
Calcium (S)					
male	8.8–10.3	mg/dL	0.2495	2.20–2.58	mmol/L
female <50 y	8.8–10.0	mg/dL	0.2495	2.20–2.50	mmol/L
female >50 y	8.8–10.2	mg/dL	0.2495	2.20–2.56	mmol/L
	4.4–5.1	mEq/L	0.500	2.20–2.56	mmol/L
Calcium ion (S)	2.00–2.30	mEq/L	0.500	1.00–1.15	mmol/L
	4.00–4.60	mg/dL	0.2495	1.00–1.15	mmol/L
Calcium (U), normal diet	< 250	mg/24 h	0.02495	< 6.2	mmol/d
Carbamazepine (P) therapeutic	4.0–10.0	mg/L	4.233	17–42	µmol/L
Carbon dioxide content (B,P,S)					
[bicarbonate + CO$_2$]	22–28	mEq/L	1.00	22–28	mmol/L
Beta-carotenes (S)	50–250	µg/dL	0.01863	0.9–4.6	µmol/L
Catecholamines, total (U) [as norepinephrine]	< 120	µg/24 h	5.911	< 675	nmol/d
Ceruloplasmin (S)	20–35	mg/dL	10.0	200–350	mg/L
Chloride (S)	95–105	mEq/L	1.00	95–105	mmol/L
Cholestanol (P) [as a fraction of total cholesterol]	1–3	%	0.01	0.01–0.03	1
Cholesterol (P)					
<29 years	< 200	mg/dL	0.02586	< 5.20	mmol/L
30–39 years	< 225	mg/dL	0.02586	< 5.85	mmol/L
40–49 years	< 245	mg/dL	0.02586	< 6.35	mmol/L
>50 years	< 265	mg/dL	0.02586	< 6.85	mmol/L
Cholesterol esters (P) [as a fraction of total cholesterol]	60–75	%	0.01	0.60–0.75	1
Cholinesterase (S)	620–1370	U/L	0.01667	10.3–22.8	µkat/L
Chorionic gonadotrophin (P) [Beta-HCG]	0 if not pregnant	mIU/mL	1.00	0 if not pregnant	IU/L

S = serum.   B = blood.   P = plasma.   U = urine.   Df = duodenal fluid.   aB = arterial blood.   kat = katal = mol × s^{-1} × L^{-1} or mol/s × L.

(continued)

TABLE E-4   SI Units Conversion Factors for Values in Clinical Chemistry *(continued)*

Component	Conventional normal values	Conventional Units	Conversion factor	SI normal values	SI unit
Citrate (B) [as citric acid}	1.2–3.0	mg/dL	52.05	60–160	µmol/L
Complement, C3 (S)	70–160	mg/dL	0.01	0.7–1.6	g/L
Complement, C4 (S)	20–40	mg/dL	0.01	0.2–O.4	g/L
Copper (S)	70–140	µg/dL	0.1574	11.0–22.0	µmol/L
Copper (U)	< 40	µg/24 h	0.01574	< 0.6	µmol/d
Cortisol (S)					
0800 h	4–19	µg/dL	27.59	110–520	nmol/L
1600 h	2–15	µg/dL	27.59	50–410	nmol/L
2400 h	5	µg/dL	27.59	140	nmol/L
Cortisol, free (U)	10–110	µg/24 h	2.759	30–300	nmol/d
Creatine (S)					
male	0.17–0.50	mg/dL	76.25	10–40	µmol/L
female	0.35–0.93	mg/dL	76.25	30–70	µmol/L
Creatine (U)					
male	0.40	mg/24 h	7.625	0–300	µmol/d
female	0.80	mg/24 h	7.625	0–600	µmol/d
Creatine kinase [CK] (S)					
Creatine kinase isoenzymes (S)	0–130	U/L	0.01667	0–2.16	µkat/L
MB fraction	> 5 in myocardial infarction	%	0.01	> 0.05	1
Creatinine (S)	0.6–1.2	mg/dL	88.40	50–110	µmol/L
Creatinine (U)	Variable	g/24 h	8.840	Variable	mmol/d
Creatinine clearance (S,U)	75–125	mL/min	0.01667	1.24–2.08	mL/s
	creatinine clearance corrected for body surface area		$= \dfrac{\mu mol/L \ (urine\ creatinine)}{\mu mol/L \ (serum\ creatinine)} \times mL/s \times \dfrac{1.73}{A}$		
Cyanocobalamin (S) [Vitamin B$_{12}$]	200–1000	pg/mL	0.7378	150–750	pmol/L
Cyclic AMP (S)	2.6–6.6	µg/L	3.038	8–20	nmol/L
Cyclic AMP (U)					
total urinary	2.9–5.6	µmol/g creatinine	113.1	330–630	nmol/mmol creatinine
renal tubular	< 2.5	µmol/g creatinine	113.1	< 280	nmol/mmol creatinine
Cyclic GMP (S)	0.6–3.5	µg/L	2.897	1.7–10.1	nmol/L
Cyclic GMP (U)	0.3–1.8	µmol/g creatinine	113.1	30–200	nmol/mmol creatinine
Cystine (U)	10–100	mg/24 h	4.161	40–420	µmol/d
Dicoumarol (P) therapeutic	8–30	mg/L	2.974	25–90	µmol/L
Digoxin (P)					
therapeutic	0.5–2.2	ng/mL	1.281	0.6–2.8	nmol/L
	0.5–2.2	µg/mL	1.281	0.6–2.8	nmol/L
toxic	> 2.5	ng/mL	1.281	> 3.2	nmol/L
Electrophoresis, protein (S)					
albumin	60–65	%	0.01	0.60–0.65	1
alpha$_1$-globulin	1.7–5.0	%	0.01	0.02–0.05	1
alpha$_2$-globulin	6.7–12.5	%	0.01	0.07–0.13	1
beta-globulin	8.3–16.3	%	0.01	0.08–0.16	1
gamma-globulin	10.7–20.0	%	0.01	0.11–0.20	1
albumin	3.6–5.2	g/dL	10.0	36–52	g/L
alpha$_1$-globulin	0.1–0.4	g/dL	10.0	1–4	g/L
alpha$_2$-globulin	0.4–1.0	g/dL	10.0	4–10	g/L
beta-globulin	0.5–1.2	g/dL	10.0	5–12	g/L
gamma-globulin	0.6–1.6	g/dL	10.0	6–16	g/L

S = serum.   B = blood.   P = plasma.   U = urine.   Df = duodenal fluid.   aB = arterial blood.   kat = katal = mol × s^{-1} × L^{-1} or mol/s × L.

(continued)

TABLE E-4 SI Units Conversion Factors for Values in Clinical Chemistry *(continued)*

Component	Conventional normal values	Conventional Units	Conversion factor	SI normal values	SI unit
Epinephrine (P)	31–95 (at rest for 15 min)	pg/mL	5.458	170–520	pmol/L
Epinephrine (U)	< 10	µg/24 h	5.458	< 55	nmol/d
Ethanol (P)					
legal limit [driving]	< 80	mg/dL	0.2171	< 17	mmol/L
toxic	>100	mg/dL	0.2171	>22	mmol/L
Ethosuximide (P)					
therapeutic	40–110	mg/L	7.084	280–780	µmol/L
Fat (F) [as stearic acid]	2.0–6.0	g/24 h	3.515	7–21	mmol/d
Fatty acids, non-esterified (P)	8–20	mg/dL	10.00	80–200	mg/L
Ferritin (S)	18–300	ng/mL	1.00	18–300	µg/L
Fibrinogen (P)	200–400	mg/dL	0.01	2.0–4.0	g/L
Folate (S) [as pteroylglutamic acid]	2–10	ng/mL	2.266	4–22	nmol/L
		µg/dL	22.66		nmol/L
Folate (Erc)	140–960	ng/mL	2.266	550–2200	nmol/LF
Fructose (P)	< 10	mg/dL	0.05551	< 0.6	mmol/L
Galactose (P) [children]	< 20	mg/dL	0.05551	< 1.1	mmol/L
Gases (aB)					
pO_2	75–105	mm Hg (=Torr)	0.1333	10.0–14.0	kPa
pCO_2	33–44	mm Hg (=Torr)	0.1333	4.4–5.9	kPa
Gamma-glutamyltransferase [GGT] (S)	0–30	U/L	0.01667	0–0.50	µkat/L
Gastrin (S)	0–180	pg/mL	1	0–180	ng/L
Globulins (S) [see immunoglobulins]	...	...	...	...	...
Glucagon (S)	50–100	pg/mL	1	50–100	ng/L
Glucose (P) fasting	70–110	mg/dL	0.05551	3.9–6.1	mmol/L
Gycerol, free (S)	< 1.5	mg/dL	0.1086	< 0.16	mmol/L
Gold (S) therapeutic	300–800	µg/dL	0.05077	15.0–40.0	µmol/L
Gold (U)	< 500	µg/24 h	0.005077	< 2.5	µmol/d
Haptoglobin (S)	50–220	mg/dL	0.01	0.50–2.20	g/L
Hemoglobin (B)					
male	14.0–18.0	g/dL	10.0	140–180	g/L
female	11.5–15.5	g/dL	10.0	115–155	g/L
Homogentisate (U) [as homogentisic acid]	0	mg/24 h	5.947	0	µmol/d
Homovanillate (U) [as homovanillic acid]	< 8	mg/24 h	5.489	< 45	µmol/d
beta-hydroxybutyrate (S)					
[as beta-hydroxybutyric acid]	< 1.0	mg/dL	96.05	< 100	µmol/L
5-hydroxyindoleacetate (U)					
[as 5-hydroxyindole acetic acid; 5 HIAA]	2.8	mg/24 h	5.230	10–40	µmol/d
Hydroxyproline (U)					
1 wk–1y	55–220	mg/24 h/m²	7.626	420–1680	µmol/(d.m²)
1–13 y	25–80	mg/24 h/m²	7.626	190–610	µmol/(d.m²)
22–65 y	6–22	mg/24 h/m²	7.626	40–170	µmol/(d.m²)
> 65 y	5–17	mg/24 h/m²	7.626	40–130	µmol/(d.m²)
Immunoglobulins (S)					
IgG	500–1200	mg/dL	0.01	5.00–12.00	g/L
IgA	50–350	mg/dL	0.01	0.50–3.50	g/L
IgM	30–230	mg/dL	0.01	0.30–2.30	g/L
IgD	< 6	mg/dL	10	< 60	mg/L
IgE — 0–3 years	0.5–10	IU/mL	2.4	1–24	µg/L
3–80 years	5–100	IU/mL	2.4	12–240	µg/L
Imipramine (P) therapeutic	50–200	ng/mL	3.566	180–710	nmol/L

S = serum.   B = blood.   P = plasma.   U = urine.   Df = duodenal fluid.   aB = arterial blood.   kat = katal = mol $\times$ s^{-1} $\times$ L^{-1} or mol/s $\times$ L.

(continued)

TABLE E-4 SI Units Conversion Factors for Values in Clinical Chemistry *(continued)*

Component	Conventional normal values	Conventional Units	Conversion factor	SI normal values	SI unit
Insulin (P,S)	5–20	μU/mL	7.175	35–145	pmol/L
	5–20	mU/L	7.175	35–145	pmol/L
	0.20–0.84	μg/mL	172.2	35–145	pmol/L
Iron (S)					
male	80–180	μg/dL	0.1791	14–32	μmol/L
female	60–160	μg/dL	0.1791	11–29	μmol/L
Iron binding capacity (S)	250–460	μg/dL	0.1791	45–82	μmol/L
Isoniazid (P)					
therapeutic	< 2.0	mg/L	7.291	< 15	μmol/L
toxic	>3.0	mg/L	7.291	>22	μmol/L
Isopropanol (P)	0	mg/dL	0.1664	0	mmol/L
Lactate (P) [as lactic acid]	0.5–2.0	mEq/L	1.00	0.5–2.0	mmol/L
	5–20	mg/dL	0.1110	0.5–2.0	mmol/L
Lactate dehydrogenase (S)	50–150	U/L	0.01667	0.82–2.66	μkat/L
Lactate dehydrogenase isoenzymes (S)					
LD1	15–40	%	0.01	0.15–0.40	1
LD2	20–45	%	0.01	0.20–0.45	1
LD3	15–30	%	0.01	0.15–0.30	1
LD4	5–20	%	0.01	0.05–0.20	1
LD5	5–20	%	0.01	0.05–0.20	1
LD1	10–60	U/L	0.01667	0.16–1.00	μkat/L
LD2	20–70	U/L	0.01667	0.32–1.16	μkat/L
LD3	10–45	U/L	0.01667	0.22–0.76	μkat/L
LD4	5–30	U/L	0.01667	0.08–0.50	μkat/L
Lipase (S)	5–30	U/L	0.01667	0.02–0.50	μkat/L
Lipids, total (P)	400–850	mg/dL	0.01	4.0–8.5	g/L
Lipoproteins (P)					
low density [LDL] as cholesterol	50–190	mg/dL	0.02586	1.30–4.90	mmol/L
high density[HDL] as cholesterol					
male	30–70	mg/dL	0.02586	0.80–1.80	mmol/L
female	30–90	mg/dL	0.02586	0.80–2.35	mmol/L
Magnesium (S)	1.8–3.0	mg/dL	0.4114	0.80–1.20	mmol/L
	1.6–2.4	mEq/L	0.500	0.80–1.20	mmol/L
Meprobamate (P)					
therapeutic	< 20	mg/L	4.582	< 90	μmol/L
toxic	>40	mg/L	4.582	>180	μmol/L
Beta$_2$-microglobulin (S) <50 y	0.80–2.40	mg/L	84.75	68–204	nmol/L
Beta$_2$-microglobulin (U) <50 y	< 140	μg/24 h	0.08475	< 12	nmol/d
Nitrogen, total (U)	Diet dependent	g/24 h	71.38	Diet Dependent	mmol/d
Norepinephrine (P)	15–475 (at rest for 15 min)	pg/mL	0.005911	1.27–2.81	nmol/L
Norepinephrine (U)	< 100	μg/24 h	5.911	< 590	nmol/d
Osmolality (P)	280–300	mOsm/kg	1.00	280–300	mmol/kg
Osmolality (U)	50–1200	mOsm/kg	1.00	50–1200	mmol/kg
Oxalate (U) [as anhydrous oxalic acid]	10–40	mg/24 h	11.11	110–440	μmol/d
Phenytoin (P)					
therapeutic	10–20	mg/L	3.964	40–80	μmol/L
toxic	>30	mg/L	3.964	>120	μmol/L
Phosphate (S) [as phosphorus, inorganic]	2.5–5.0	mg/dL	0.3229	0.80–1.60	mmol/L
Phosphate (U) [as phosphorus, inorganic]	Diet dependent	g/ 24 h	32.29	Diet dependent	mmol/d
Phospholipid phosphorus, total (P)	5–12	mg/dL	0.3229	1.60–3.90	mmol/L

S = serum.   B = blood.   P = plasma.   U = urine.   Df = duodenal fluid.   aB = arterial blood.   kat = katal = mol $\times$ s^{-1} $\times$ L^{-1} or mol/s $\times$ L.

(continued)

TABLE E-4 SI Units Conversion Factors for Values in Clinical Chemistry *(continued)*

Component	Conventional normal values	Conventional Units	Conversion factor	SI normal values	SI unit
Phospholipid phosphorus, total (Erc)	1.2–12	mg/dL	0.3229	0.40–3.90	mmol/L
Phospholipids (P)					
Substance fraction of total					
phospholipid phosphatidyl choline	65–70	% of total	0.01	0.65–0.70	1
phosphatidyl ethanolamine	4–5	% of total	0.01	0.04–0.05	1
sphingomyelin	15–20	% of total	0.01	0.15–0.20	1
lysophosphatidyl choline	3–5	% of total	0.01	0.03–0.05	1
Phospholipids (Erc)					
Substance fraction of total					
phospholipid phosphatidyl choline	28–33	% of total	0.01	0.28–0.33	1
phosphatidyl ethanolamine	24.31	% of total	0.01	0.24–0.31	1
sphingomyelin	22.29	% of total	0.01	0.22–0.29	1
phosphatidyl serine + phosphatidyl inositol	12.20	% of total	0.01	0.12–0.20	1
lysophosphatidyl choline	1–2	% of total	0.01	0.01–0.02	1
Phytanic acid (P)	Trace–0.3	mg/dL	32.00	<10	µmol/L
Potassium ion (S)	3.5–5.0	mEq/L	1.00	3.5–5.0	mmol/L
		mg/dL	0.2558		mmol/L
Potassium Ion (U) [diet dependent]	25–100	mEq/24 h	1.00	25–100	mmol/d
Protein, total (S)	6.0–8.0	g/dL	10.0	60–80	g/L
Protein, total (U)	>150	mg/24 h	0.001	> 0.15	g/d
Pyruvate (B) [as pyruvic acid]	0.30–0.90	mg/dL	113.6	35–100	µmol/L
Renin (P)					
normal sodium diet	1.1–4.1	ng/mL/h	0.2778	0.30–1.14	ng/ (L's)
restricted sodium diet	6.2–12.4	ng/mL/h	0.2778	1.72–3.44	ng/ (L's)
Salicylate (S) [salicylic acid] toxic	>20	mg/dL	0.07240	>1.45	mmol/L
Serotonin (B) [5-hydroxy-tryptamine]	8–21	µg/dL	0.05675	0.45–1.20	µmol/L
Sodium ion (S)	135–147	mEq/L	1.00	135–147	mmol/L
Sodium ion (U)	Diet dependent	mEq/24 h	1.00	Diet dependent	mmol/d
Steroids					
17-hydroxy-corticosteroids (U) [as cortisol]					
female	2.0–8.0	mg/24 h	2.759	5–25	µmol/d
male	3.0–10.0	mg/24 h	2.759	10–30	µmol/d
17-ketogenic steroids (U) [as dehydroepiandrosterone]					
female	7.0–12.0	mg/24 h	3.467	25–40	µmol/d
male	9.0–17.0	mg/24 h	3.467	30–60	µmol/d
17-ketosteroids (U) [as dehydroepiandrosterone]					
female	6.0–17.0	mg/24 h	3.467	20–60	µmol/d
male	6.0–20.0	mg/24 h	3.467	20–70	µmol/d
ketosteroid fractions (U) androsterone					
female	0.5–3.0	mg/24 h	3.443	1–10	µmol/d
male	2.0–5.0	mg/24 h	3.443	7–17	µmol/d
dehydroepiandrosterone					
female	0.2–1.8	mg/24 h	3.467	1–6	µmol/d
Theophylline (P) therapeutic	10.0–20.0	mg/L	5.550	55–110	µmol/L
Thyroid tests:					
thyroid stimulating hormone [TSH] (S)	2–11	µU/mL	1.00	2.11	mU/L
thyroxine [T4] (S)	4.0–11.0	µg/dL	12.87	51–142	nmol/L
thyroxine binding globulin [TBG] (S)					
[as thyroxine]	12.0–28.0	µg/dL	12.87	150–360	nmol/L
thyroxine, free (S)	0.8–2.8	ng/dL	12.87	10–36	pmol/L
tri iodothyronine [T3] (S)	75–220	ng/dL	0.01536	1.2–3.4	nmol/L
T_3 uptake (S)	25–35	%	0.01	0.25–0.35	1

S = serum.   B = blood.   P = plasma.   U = urine.   Df = duodenal fluid.   aB = arterial blood.   kat = katal = mol × s⁻¹ × L⁻¹ or mol/s × L.   *(continued)*

TABLE E-4   SI Units Conversion Factors for Values in Clinical Chemistry *(continued)*

Component	Conventional normal values	Conventional Units	Conversion factor	SI normal values	SI unit
Tolbutamide (P) therapeutic	50–120	mg/L	3.699	180–450	µmol/L
Transferrin (S)	170–370	mg/dL	0.01	1.70–3.70	g/L
Triglycerides (P) [as triolein]	< 160	mg/dL	0.01129	< 1.80	mmol/L
Urate (S) [as uric acid]	2.0–7.0	mg/dL	59.48	120–420	µmol/L
Urate (U) [as uric acid]	Diet dependent	g/ 24 h	5.948	Diet dependent	mmol/d
Urea nitrogen (S)	8–18	mg/dL	0.3570	3.0–6.5	mmol/L UREA
Urea nitrogen (U)	2.0–20.0 diet dependent	g/24 h	35.700	450–700	mmol/d UREA
Urobilinogen (U)	0.0–4.0	mg/24 h	1.693	0.0–6.8	µmol/d
Valproic acid (P) therapeutic	50–100	mg/L	6.934	350–700	µmol/L
Vanillylmandelic acid [VMA] (U)*	< 6.8	mg/24 h	5.046	< 35	µmol/d
Vitamin A [retinol] (P,S)	10–50	µg/dL	0.03491	0.35–1.75	µmol/L
Vitamin B_1 [thiamine hydrochloride] (U)	60–500	µg/24 h	0.002965	0.18–1.48	µmol/d
Vitamin B_2 [riboflavin] (S)	2.6–3.7	µg/dL	26.57	70–100	nmol/L
Vitamin B_6 [pyridoxal] (B)	20–90	ng/mL	5.982	120–540	nmol/L
Vitamin B_{12} [cyanocobalamin] (P,S)	200–1000	pg/mL	0.7378	150–750	pmol/L
		ng/dL	7.378		pmol/L
Vitamin C [see ascorbate] (B,P,S)	…	…	…	…	…
Vitamin D_3					
[cholecalciferol] (P)	24–40	µg/mL	2.599	60–105	nmol/L
25 OH-cholecalciferol	18–36	ng/mL	2.496	45–90	nmol/L
Vitamin E [alpha-tocopherol] (P,S)	0.78–1.25	mg/dL	23.22	18–29	µmol/L
Warfarin (P) therapeutic	1.0–3.0	mg/L	3.243	3.3–9.8	µmol/L
Xanthine (U)	5–30	mg/24 h	6.574	30–200	µmol.d
hypoxanthine		mg/24 h	7.347		µmol/d
D-xylose (B) [25 g dose]	30–40 (30–60 min)	mg/dL	0.06661	.0–2.7 (30–60 min)	mmol/L
D-xylose excretion (U) [25 g dose]	21–31 (excreted in 5 h)	%	0.01	0.21–0.31 (excreted in 5 h)	1
Zinc (S)	75–120	µg/dL	0.1530	11.5–18.5	µmol/L
Zinc (U)	150–1200	µg/24 h	0.01530	2.3–18.3	µmol/d

S = serum.   B = blood.   P = plasma.   U = urine.   Df = duodenal fluid.   aB = arterial blood.   kat = katal = mol × s^{-1} × L^{-1} or mol/s × L.

TABLE E-5 Typical Test Panels*

Preliminary Screening (SMA 6)
Bicarbonate (CO₂)
Sodium
Potassium
Chloride
Blood urea nitrogen (BUN)
Blood glucose
(Reported in patient's chart as follows:

Na	Cl	BUN
K	HCO₃	Glucose

e.g.,

142	102	10
4.0	28	102)

Health Survey Screening
Albumin
Alkaline phosphatase
SGOT
Bilirubin (total)
Blood urea nitrogen (BUN)
Calcium
Cholesterol
Glucose
Lactic dehydrogenase (LDH)
Phosphorus
Protein total
Uric acid

Routine Urinalysis
Color
Appearance
Specific gravity
pH
Albumin, qualitative
Glucose, qualitative
Ketone bodies, qualitative
Bilirubin, qualitative
Occult blood
Casts
Organisms
Mucus
Epithelial cells
Crystal
White blood cells
Red blood cells

Hemogram
Hemoglobin
Hematocrit
Red cells
White cells

Differential
Neutrophils, segmented
Neutrophils, nonsegmented
Lymphocytes
Monocytes
Eosinophils
Basophils
Atypical lymphocytes
Other
RBC morphology
Platelets:
morphology
count
Mean corpuscular volume (calc)
Mean corpuscular hemoglobin (calc)
Mean corpuscular hemoglobin concentration (calc)
(Some of the above values are reported in the patient's chart as follows:
Hgb Segs/Bands/Lymphs/Monos/Basos/Eos
WBC—MCV-MCH-MCHC Hct Platelet count
e.g., 10.2 40S, 20B, 30L, 6M, 1B, 3E
11,000 ---- 80/27/32 30.4 286,000
A complete blood count (CBC) usually includes Hgb, Hct, RBC, WBC, MCV, MCH, MCHC)

Broad Spectrum Screening (SMA 20)
Albumin
Alkaline phosphatase
Bicarbonate (CO₂)
Bilirubin, total
direct
indirect
Blood urea nitrogen (BUN)
BUN/creatinine ratio
Calcium
Ionized calcium (est)
Chloride
Cholesterol
Creatinine
Globulin
Glucose
Lactic dehydrogenase (LDH)
Inorganic phosphorus
Potassium
Serum glutamic oxaloacetic transaminase (SGOT)
Serum glutamic pyruvic transaminase (SGPT)
Sodium
Total protein
Triglycerides
Uric acid
Anion gap (calc)

*Test panels are the result of the development of automated analytical instruments. It is common for the physician to order an automated panel of tests, rather than ordering individual tests. The contents of some typical test panels are shown in this table.

(continued)

TABLE E-5 *(continued)*

Lipid panel
Cholesterol, total
Cholesterol, LDL
Cholesterol, HDL
Cholesterol, VLDL
LDL:HDL ratio
Triglycerides
VLDL:triglycerides ratio
Lipoprotein electrophoresis
Phospholipids
Total lipids
Glucose

CHD Risk Profile
HDL
Cholesterol, total
Triglycerides
Glucose

Hypertension Panel
Renal panel
Blood gases:
 pH
 pCO₂
 Bicarbonate
Cholesterol
Glucose
LDH
Triglycerides

Liver Panel
Alkaline phosphatase
Bilirubin, total
  direct
LDH
LDH isozymes
SGOT (AST)
SGPT (ALT)
Protein, total
Protein electrophoresis
Urine bile pigment
Albumin
Globulin

Pancreatic Panel
Serum amylase
Serum lipase
Urine amylase

Acute heart panel
Creatinine phosphokinase (CPK)
Hydroxybutyric dehydrogenase (HBD)
Lactate dehydrogenase (LDH)
LDH isozymes
Potassium
SGOT

Renal Panel
BUN
Creatinine
Creatinine clearance
Calcium
Chloride
Phosphorus
Potassium
Protein, total
Protein electrophoresis
Sodium
Urine specific gravity
Urine culture

Diabetes Mellitus Panel
Glucose
Glucose tolerance (if not contraindicated)
Serum ketones
Triglycerides
Urine glucose/24 hours
Urine ketones

Diabetes Management Profile
Glucose
Hemoglobin A$_{lc}$

TABLE E-6   Clinical Laboratory Values in Serum, Whole Blood and Plasma in Pregnancy

Measurement	Typical Reference Intervals	
	Common units	SI Units
Acetone (serum)		
Qualitative	Negative	Negative
Quantitiative	0.3–0.2 mg/dL	51.6–344 µmol/L
Amylase (serum)	60–160 Somogyi units/dL	111–296 U/L
Base excess		
(male whole blood)	–2.4 ± 2.3 mEq/L	–2.4–2.3 mmol/L
Base total (serum)	145–160 mEq/L	145–160 mmol/L
Bicarbonate (plasma)	21–28 mM	21–28 mmol/L
Bilirubin (serum)		
Direct (conjugated)	up to 0.3 mg/dL	up to 5.1 µmol/L
Indirect (unconjugated)	0.1–1.0 mg/dL	1.7–17.1 µmol/L
Total	0.1–1.2 mg/dL	1.7–20.5 µmol/L
Newborns total	1–12 mg/dL	17.1–205 µmol/L
Blood gases (whole blood)		
pH	7.38–7.44 (arterial)	7.38–7.44
	7.36–7.41 (venous)	7.36–7.41
pCO_2	35–40 mm Hg (arterial)	4.6–5.32 kPa
	40–45 mm Hg (venous)	5.32–5.99 kPa
pO_2	95–100 mm Hg (arterial)	12.64–13.30 kPa
Calcium (serum)		
Ionized	4.4–4.9 mg/dL	1.0–1.2 mmol/L
	or 2.0–2.4 mEq/L	
	30–58% of total	0.3–0.58 of total
Total (serum)	9.2–11.0 mg/dL	2.3–2.8 mmol/L
Carbon dioxide (CO_2 content)		
Whole blood (arterial)	19–24 mM	19–24 mmol/L
Plasma or serum (arterial)	21–28 mM	21–28 mmol/L
Plasma or serum (venous)	24–30 mM	24–30 mmol/L
Chloride (serum)	95–103 mEq/L	95–103 mmol/L
Complete blood count		
Hematocrit (female)		
Nonpregnant	37–48%	
Pregnant	↓ **to 32.5–41% in 2d and early 3d trimester with rise to prepregnant value at term**	
Hemoglobin (whole blood)	13–15 g/dL (female)	1.86–2.48 mmol/L
Pregnant nadir 30–34 weeks	↓ **to 10–13 g/dL in 2d to early 3d trimester with rise to prepregnant value at term**	
Leukocyte count		
Nonpregnant	4,300–10,800 mm³	4.3–10.8 × 10⁹/L
Pregnant	**6,000–16,000 mm³**	**6.0–16.0 × 10⁹/L**
(2d and 3d trimesters)	**(mean 10,5000)**	
Erythrocyte count	4.2–5.9 million/mm³	4.2–5.9 × 10¹²/L
Mean corpuscular hemoglobin (MCH)	27–32 pg/RBC	1.7–2.0 pg/cell
Mean corpuscular hemoglobin concentration (MCHC)	32–36%	0.32–0.36
Mean corpuscular volume (MCV)	86–98 µm³/cell	86–98 fL
Creatinine (serum or plasma)		
Non-pregnant	0.6–1.2	53–106
Pregnant	**0.5–0.6**	**44.2–53**
Children < 2 yr	**0.3–0.6**	**27–54**
Creatinine clearance (serum or plasma and urine)		
Non-pregnant	87–107 mL/min	1.45–1.79 mL/s
Pregnant	**increases about 50%**	
Ferritin (serum)	12–150 ng/mL	12–150 µg/L
Folate (serum)	>2.3 ng/mL (RIA)	>5.2 nmol/L

(continued)

TABLE E-6   *(continued)*

Measurement	Typical Reference Intervals				
	Common units			SI Units	
Glucose tolerance test (serum or plasma)	*mg/dL*			*mmol/L*	
	Time	*Normal*	*Diabetic*	*Normal*	*Diabetic*
Nonpregnant	0	70–105	> 140	3.9–5.8	≥ 7.8
(GTT) oral	1-h	120–170	≥ 200	6.7–9.4	≥ 11
	1.5-h	100–140	≥ 200	5.6–7.8	≥ 11
	2-h	70–120	≥ 140	3.9–6.7	≥ 7.8
Pregnant	**0**	**≥ 105**		**5.8**	
(100-g loading test)	**1-h**	**190**		**10.5**	
For diagnosis of GDM	**2-h**	**165**	**2 Abnormal values**	**9.1**	**2 Abnormal values**
	3-h	**145**		**8.0**	
α-Hydroxybutyrate dehydrogenase (serum)	140–350 U/ml			140–350 kU/L	
Insulin (plasma) fasting					
Nonpregnant (RIA)	4–24 µIU/mL			0.17–1.0 µg/L	
Pregnant (RIA)	**23 ± 9 µIU/mL**			**0.96 ± 0.38**	
Iron, total (serum)	60–150 µg/dL			11–27 µmol/L	
Iron binding capacity (serum)	200–400 µg/dL			56–64 µmol/L	
Iron saturation (serum)	20–50%			Fraction of total iron binding	
Ketone bodies (serum)	Negative			Negative	
Lactate (whole blood, heparin, as lactic acid)	Venous 4.5–19.8 mg/dL			0.5–2.2 mmol/L	
	Arterial 4.5–14.4 mg/dL			0.5–1.6 mmol/L	
Lactic acid dehydrogenase (LDH) (serum)	25–175 IU/L			25–175 IU/L	
Lipids (serum)					
Nonpregnant					
Cholesterol	150–250 mg/dL			3.9–6.5 mmol/L	
Triglycerides	10–190 mg/dL			1.09–20.71 mmol/L	
Phospholipids	130–380 mg/dL			1.50–380 g/L	
Fatty acids (free)	9.0–15 mM/L			9.0–15.0 mmol/L	
Pregnant					
Cholesterol					
2d trimester	**251 ± 8**			**6.5 ± 0.2**	
3d trimester	**259 ± 13**			**6.7 ± 0.3**	
3 months postpartum	**204 ± 10**			**5.3 ± 0.3**	
Triglyceride					
2d trimester	**185 ± 22**			**20.2 ± 2.4**	
3d trimester	**224 ± 24**			**24.4 ± 2.6**	
3 months postpartum	**82 ± 5**			**8.9 ± 0.5**	
Osmolality (serum)	280–295 mOsm/kg			280–295 mmol/L	
Pregnant	**270–280 mOsm/kg**			**270–280 mmol/L**	
Proteins (serum)	g/dL			g/L	
Total	6.0–7.8			60–78	
Albumin	3.2–4.5			32–45	
Globulin	2.3–3.5			23–35	
SGOT (AST, aspartate amino transaminase) (serum)	10–45 IU/L			10–45 IU/L	
SGPT (ALT, alanine amino transaminase) (serum)	10–45 IU/L			10–45 IU/L	
Sodium (plasma)	136–142 mEq/L			136–142 mmol/L	
Thyroid hormones (serum)					
Nonpregnant					
T_4 (RIA)	5.5–12.5 µg/dL			76–163 nmol/L	
T_3 (RIA)	70–190 ng/dL			1.85–3.0 nmol/L	
Free T_4 (total)	0.9–2.3 ng/dL			12–30 pmol/L	
T_3 resin uptake (%)	25–38 relative % uptake			Relative uptake fraction 0.25–0.38	

(continued)

TABLE E-6 Clinical Laboratory Values in Serum, Whole Blood and Plasma in Pregnancy *(continued)*

Measurement	Typical Reference Intervals	
	Common units	SI Units
Thyroxin binding globulin (TBG)	10–26 µg/dL	100–260 µg/L
Pregnant (serum)		
T₄ (RIA)	**8.0–14.5 µg/dL**	**104–188 nmol/L**
T₃ (RIA)	**150–220 ng/dL**	**2.3–3.4 nmol/L**
Free T₄	**0.9–2.3 ng/dL**	**12–30 pmol/L**
T₃ resin uptake (%)	**15–25**	**0.15–0.02**
Thyroxin binding globulin (TBG)	**↑ to twice normal**	
TSH (serum) "sensitive" method		
Nonpregnant	0.5–3.5 µU/mL	0.5–3.5 µU/mL
Pregnant	**Not increased**	
Urea nitrogen (serum)	mg/dL	mmol/L
Nonpregnant	8–23	2.9–8.2
Pregnant	**8–9**	**2.9–3.2**
Uric acid (serum)		0.16–0.43
Nonpregnant	2.7–7.3	
Pregnant (to 24 weeks)	**2.0–3.0**	**0.12–0.18**
Zinc (serum)	50–150 µg/dL	7.65–22.95 µmol/L

TABLE E-7   Urine Values in Pregnancy

Measurement	Typical Reference Intervals	
	Common units	SI Units
Albumin		
Qualitative (random)	Negative	Negative
Quantitative (24 h)	15–150 mg/24 h	0.015–0.150 g/24 h
Chloride (24 h)	140–250 mEq/24 h	140–250 mmol/24 h
Creatinine (24 h)	14–22 mg/kg/24 h	0.12–0.19 mmol/kg/24 h
	0.8–1.8 g/24 h	7.0–15.8 mmol/24 h
Osmolality (random)	500–800 mOsm/kg water	500–800 mmol/kg
Potassium (24 h)	40–80 mEq/24 h	40–80 mmol/24 h
Protein (24 h)	40–150 mg/24 h	40–150 mg/24 h
Sodium (24 h)	75–200 mEq/24 h	75–200 mmol/24 h

TABLE E-8 Conversion Factors

1. *Metric system weights*
   1 kilogram   = 1,000 grams (g)
   1 milligram = 0.001 g
   1 microgram = 10^{-6} g or μ
   1 nanogram   = 10^{-9} g or mμ
   1 picogram   = 10^{-12} g or $\mu\mu$
   1 femtogram = 10^{-15} g or m$\mu\mu$

2. *Metric and avoirdupois systems of volume (fluid)*
   1 liter (L) = 1,000 milliliters (mL) or 1.06 quarts (qt)
   1 milliliter = 1,000 microliters (μL)

3. *Conversion factors*
   1 kg = 2.2046 pounds (usually rounded to 2.2)
   1 fl oz = 29.573 mL (usually rounded to 30)
   Degrees Celsius = (°F − 32) $\times$ 5/9
   Degrees Fahrenheit = (°C $\times$ 9/5) + 32
   Parts per million (ppm) to percent:

1 ppm	= 0.0001%
10 ppm	= 0.001%
100 ppm	= 0.01%
1,000 ppm	= 0.1%
10,000 ppm	= 1%

   Milliequivalents (mEq) to milligrams:
   mEq $\times$ *atomic weight* / *valence* = mg
   e.g.: (30 mEq Na $\times$ 23) / 1 = 690 mg Na
   Milligrams to milliequivalents:
   (mg / *atomic weight*) $\times$ *valence* = mEq
   e.g.: (1,482 mgK / 39) $\times$ 1 = 38 mEqK
   Milliequivalents (mEq) to millimoles (mmol)
   mEq / *molecular weight* = mmol
   e.g.: (5.0 mEq Ca^{++}) / 2 = 2.5 mmol
   Milligrams to millimoles:
   (mg / *molecular weight*) = mmol
   e.g.: (10 mg Ca^{++}) / 40 = 0.25 mmol

For other values, use these atomic weights:

		Atomic weight
Calcium	Ca	40
Chlorine	Cl	35.4
Magnesium	Mg	24.3
Phosphorus	P	31
Potassium	K	39
Sodium	Na	23
Sulfur	S	32
Zinc	Zn	65.37

APPENDIX F

Nutritional Assessment Data

Table F-1   Means, Standard Deviations and Percentiles of Weight (kg) by Height (cm) for Males of 2 to 74 Years

Height (cm)	N	Mean	SD	Percentiles								
				5	10	15	25	50	75	85	90	95
Boys: 2 to 11 years												
84–86	75	12.1	1.1	10.7	10.9	11.1	11.3	11.9	12.8	13.1	13.5	14.3
87–87	170	12.8	1.1	11.2	11.4	11.7	12.0	12.7	13.4	13.8	14.2	14.6
90–92	207	13.5	1.0	11.9	12.1	12.5	12.8	13.6	14.2	14.6	14.9	15.2
93–95	278	14.4	1.2	12.7	13.0	13.4	13.6	14.3	15.1	15.5	15.8	16.3
96–98	310	15.0	1.3	13.3	13.6	13.8	14.2	15.0	15.6	16.1	16.4	17.0
99–101	300	16.0	1.3	13.9	14.4	14.7	15.1	15.9	16.7	17.2	17.6	18.3
102–104	290	16.9	1.4	15.1	15.4	15.6	15.9	16.8	17.7	18.0	18.5	19.3
105–107	291	17.6	1.6	15.4	15.9	16.2	16.6	17.5	18.4	19.0	19.4	19.8
108–110	298	18.7	1.7	16.7	17.0	17.1	17.6	18.5	19.6	20.1	20.5	21.3
111–113	274	20.0	2.2	17.0	17.8	18.1	18.7	19.6	21.0	21.7	22.4	23.4
114–116	223	20.9	2.2	18.6	19.0	19.2	19.6	20.5	21.7	22.3	22.7	23.6
117–119	199	21.9	2.3	19.0	19.6	20.2	20.5	21.5	23.0	23.8	24.3	26.0
120–122	177	23.3	2.4	19.8	20.8	21.2	21.9	23.1	24.5	25.4	26.0	27.3
123–125	174	25.0	2.8	21.5	22.0	22.7	23.4	24.5	26.2	27.0	28.2	30.0
126–128	185	26.5	3.8	22.6	23.1	23.8	24.3	25.9	27.8	29.4	30.6	32.0
129–131	174	27.6	3.1	23.5	24.4	24.7	25.6	27.3	28.9	30.0	31.0	32.9
132–134	180	29.3	3.5	25.1	25.7	25.8	26.8	28.5	31.0	33.0	34.4	35.4
135–137	175	31.4	4.6	26.2	27.1	27.6	28.5	30.4	33.0	34.9	37.4	41.5
138–140	150	33.5	4.7	28.2	28.9	29.4	30.5	32.3	35.1	37.8	39.9	42.0
141–143	153	36.1	5.0	30.4	31.3	31.8	33.0	34.9	38.2	40.5	43.3	45.4
144–146	114	38.9	6.6	31.6	32.7	33.1	35.1	37.6	41.2	43.9	46.3	50.7
147–149	87	40.9	6.8	33.6	34.3	35.3	35.9	39.2	43.8	47.3	51.5	56.7
Boys: 12 to 17 years												
144–146	59	38.1	5.5	31.1	32.4	33.6	34.6	36.5	40.3	42.1	46.1	53.0
147–149	77	40.9	7.1	33.6	34.0	34.7	36.5	38.3	43.8	47.4	49.4	59.8
150–152	103	43.4	6.6	36.3	37.2	38.0	38.7	41.4	46.5	51.5	54.7	56.7
153–155	106	45.9	7.9	36.5	38.1	39.1	40.6	43.7	49.7	51.9	55.2	60.9
156–158	113	48.5	9.2	39.9	40.7	41.3	42.5	45.8	50.0	57.9	62.0	67.3
159–161	146	51.1	9.2	40.8	42.9	43.9	45.6	48.6	53.6	60.9	65.4	68.4
162–164	177	54.8	8.9	44.7	45.9	46.9	49.1	53.2	58.4	61.8	64.3	69.1
165–167	197	57.3	9.2	47.1	48.8	49.9	51.3	55.3	61.0	64.8	68.6	73.3
168–170	235	61.4	10.4	49.2	51.4	52.4	55.0	59.9	65.5	69.6	72.5	79.1
171–173	233	62.8	8.8	51.4	53.4	54.8	56.9	61.3	66.1	71.2	73.7	78.2
174–176	202	66.7	10.9	52.3	55.7	57.4	60.0	64.8	71.2	75.5	81.4	89.9
177–179	166	68.8	12.0	55.8	58.7	59.6	61.6	66.3	72.3	75.5	79.6	88.0
180–182	103	71.8	9.7	60.2	60.9	62.1	64.0	70.1	79.5	82.2	85.2	88.7
183–185	64	73.5	9.1	62.4	63.6	65.4	67.8	72.1	77.3	79.4	89.9	91.1
Males: 18 to 74 years												
153–155	56	64.6	13.0	48.6	51.3	54.5	57.1	62.0	66.8	76.8	80.6	83.5
156–158	140	65.5	11.2	48.3	51.4	54.0	57.4	64.9	72.0	77.3	79.3	86.0
159–161	292	66.2	10.8	49.1	53.8	56.4	59.2	66.0	71.2	76.9	80.2	84.3
162–164	643	68.0	10.5	52.2	55.2	57.0	60.4	67.3	74.5	79.1	81.6	86.9
165–167	1147	70.8	11.6	53.0	56.6	59.6	62.7	70.3	77.6	82.3	85.2	90.1
168–170	1582	73.5	12.0	55.9	58.6	61.3	65.9	72.7	80.2	84.5	87.9	93.4
171–173	2047	76.1	12.5	58.2	61.3	63.6	67.6	75.1	83.2	88.1	92.0	97.8
174–176	2053	78.3	12.7	60.0	63.8	66.1	69.5	77.3	84.9	90.1	93.8	99.7
177–179	1750	80.3	12.8	61.9	65.1	67.5	71.4	79.4	87.3	92.6	96.5	102.6
180–182	1252	82.6	13.6	63.4	67.3	69.6	72.9	81.4	90.1	95.0	99.4	105.7
183–185	833	85.2	13.9	65.1	69.2	71.5	75.3	83.3	93.4	99.1	103.2	110.4
186–188	398	88.0	13.3	68.9	72.3	74.8	79.4	86.6	95.1	100.4	103.5	109.8
189–191	161	92.0	16.0	71.3	75.3	77.8	80.7	89.9	99.4	105.0	110.8	123.7
192–194	66	95.9	15.8	71.8	78.6	80.2	84.8	94.2	105.2	109.1	111.8	123.8

Reproduced from A.R. Frisancho. *Anthropometric Standards for Assessment of Growth and Nutritional Status*, Ann Arbor, MI: University of Michigan Press, 1990

TABLE F-2 Means, Standard Deviations and Percentiles of Weight (kg) by Height (cm) for Females of 2 to 74 Years

Height (cm)	N	Mean	SD	Percentiles 5	10	15	25	50	75	85	90	95
Girls: 2 to 10 years												
81–83	36	11.2	.8	10.1	10.2	10.3	10.4	11.0	11.7	12.1	12.6	12.6
84–86	118	11.9	.9	10.5	10.8	11.0	11.3	12.0	12.5	12.7	13.0	13.6
87–89	156	12.5	1.2	11.0	11.3	11.6	11.8	12.4	13.0	13.6	13.8	14.6
90–92	229	13.2	1.2	11.6	11.8	12.0	12.3	13.0	13.8	14.3	14.6	15.2
93–95	259	13.9	1.2	12.0	12.6	12.8	13.1	13.8	14.6.	15.1	15.5	16.1
96–98	275	15.0	1.3	13.1	13.5	13.7	14.1	14.9	15.6	16.3	16.7	17.2
99–101	272	15.8	1.6	13.8	14.1	14.3	14.6	15.5	16.6	17.2	17.6	18.4
102–104	278	16.6	2.0	14.2	14.6	15.0	15.5	16.4	17.3	18.0	18.5	19.4
105–107	290	17.6	1.6	15.3	15.8	16.1	16.6	17.3	18.4	19.2	19.4	20.1
108–110	275	18.3	1.6	15.9	16.6	16.8	17.2	18.1	19.2	20.0	20.4	21.1
111–113	251	19.4	1.9	16.6	17.1	17.3	17.9	19.4	20.4	21.2	21.8	22.8
114–116	215	20.7	2.5	17.5	18.3	18.6	19.0	20.2	21.8	22.9	23.9	25.7
117–119	191	21.9	2.6	19.0	19.4	19.5	20.2	21.4	23.6	24.0	24.8	26.6
120–122	181	23.1	2.5	20.1	20.4	20.9	21.5	22.6	24.0	25.3	26.2	27.7
123–125	162	24.5	2.5	21.2	21.8	22.3	22.8	24.0	25.9	26.5	27.2	29.0
126–128	172	26.2	3.1	22.6	23.0	23.4	23.9	25.6	27.7	29.4	30.0	31.5
129–131	157	28.0	3.8	23.6	24.3	24.8	25.6	27.3	29.4	31.1	33.4	36.6
132–134	148	30.3	4.4	25.1	25.8	26.2	27.0	29.4	32.3	34.5	37.2	39.9
135–137	135	32.1	5.4	25.6	27.2	27.7	28.3	30.8	33.9	35.8	41.6	44.1
138–140	124	34.6	7.3	27.6	28.8	29.1	30.6	32.5	35.5	40.9	43.5	47.5
141–143	97	36.0	6.3	28.8	29.8	30.7	32.2	34.8	37.9	41.3	45.6	49.9
144–146	65	39.2	7.0	31.0	31.9	32.9	34.5	37.6	42.9	45.3	48.4	51.8
147–149	45	40.0	7.3	30.7	32.3	34.0	35.0	38.3	44.2	48.0	50.8	54.8
Girls: 11 to 17 years												
141–143	54	37.1	7.8	28.9	29.8	31.1	32.2	34.9	38.6	42.4	45.7	59.5
144–146	67	38.5	6.8	30.4	30.8	31.6	32.9	38.4	41.4	44.1	46.5	52.4
147–149	127	43.4	10.0	32.7	34.3	35.4	37.0	40.7	46.7	51.3	56.4	61.2
150–152	180	45.8	9.1	34.7	36.3	37.4	39.5	44.1	49.9	54.3	56.1	61.9
153–155	235	48.8	8.9	38.0	39.5	40.6	43.1	46.7	53.6	56.5	60.0	66.3
156–158	352	52.3	10.4	39.7	41.7	43.1	45.1	49.9	57.5	62.5	66.0	72.3
159–161	372	55.1	11.0	42.2	44.3	46.0	48.3	52.8	59.2	62.9	68.4	77.6
162–164	344	56.6	9.9	44.9	46.6	47.5	50.2	54.4	60.6	65.4	68.6	73.8
165–167	243	60.0	12.5	46.3	48.8	50.1	52.8	57.6	62.7	69.4	74.7	84.7
168–170	124	61.2	10.8	48.9	49.2	51.1	53.5	59.0	65.7	73.4	75.1	82.4
171–173	74	67.5	15.0	53.0	54.3	54.9	57.7	62.1	72.3	80.1	89.1	104.2
Females: 18 to 74 years												
141–143	64	55.9	10.2	39.2	41.3	43.9	49.0	56.5	63.3	64.9	67.7	76.6
144–146	178	57.1	14.2	38.7	42.0	44.3	48.1	54.3	64.4	71.3	74.6	82.0
147–149	430	59.4	13.2	41.5	44.6	46.8	50.1	56.9	66.9	71.9	76.1	84.8
150–152	928	61.1	13.2	43.1	46.5	48.1	51.5	59.0	68.3	74.3	78.4	86.2
153–155	1685	63.0	13.7	45.3	47.5	49.8	53.2	60.7	70.2	77.3	81.6	88.6
156–158	2670	63.8	14.6	46.6	49.1	50.8	53.5	60.7	70.9	77.1	82.3	90.0
159–161	3041	65.3	14.5	47.7	50.2	52.0	55.2	62.3	72.6	79.4	84.6	92.9
162–164	2849	66.9	14.6	49.4	51.5	53.4	56.6	63.5	74.2	81.4	86.0	94.9
165–167	2327	68.2	15.3	50.3	52.8	54.9	57.8	64.5	74.7	82.4	88.6	98.2
168–170	1327	69.5	15.1	52.5	54.7	56.5	59.2	65.4	76.1	83.5	90.1	99.4
171–173	685	71.8	15.8	54.1	55.9	57.9	60.5	67.6	78.9	86.1	93.9	105.0
174–176	334	72.9	17.3	56.1	57.9	59.6	62.3	68.4	77.6	85.7	93.1	106.9
177–179	97	75.3	16.5	57.6	59.9	60.7	64.4	71.2	81.8	89.6	102.1	112.8

Reproduced from A.R. Frisancho. *Anthropometric Standards for Assessment of Growth and Nutritional Status*, Ann Arbor, MI: University of Michigan Press, 1990

TABLE F-3 An Approximation of Frame Size

Height, men	Elbow breadth for medium frame	Height, women	Elbow breadth for medium frame
5'1"–5'2"	2½"–2⅞"	4'9"–4'10"	2¼"–2½"
5'3"–5'6"	2⅝"–2⅞"	4'11"–5'2"	2¼"–2½"
5'7"–5'10"	2¾"–3"	5'3"–5'6"	2⅜"–2⅝"
5'11"–6'0"	2¾"–3⅛"	5'7"–5'10"	2⅜"–2⅝"
6'1"–6'3"	2⅞"–3¼"	5'11"	2½"–2¾"

Adapted from Metropolitan Life Insurance Company

TABLE F-4 Means, Standard Deviations and Percentiles of Weight (kg) by Age for Adult Males of Small, Medium, and Large Frames

Age (yrs)	N	Mean	SD	5	10	15	25	Percentiles 50	75	85	90	95
Males with small frames												
18.0–24.9	444	69.9	11.5	54.5	57.4	59.0	62.3	68.3	76.1	80.5	83.8	89.8
25.0–29.9	318	73.4	12.0	56.7	60.3	61.9	65.1	71.8	79.4	84.7	87.5	97.9
30.0–34.9	239	75.7	12.5	57.9	61.6	63.2	67.0	74.6	83.1	87.8	92.9	98.0
35.0–39.9	212	75.5	12.0	56.0	59.9	62.1	66.6	75.9	83.5	87.8	91.4	96.0
40.0–44.9	210	78.3	12.4	58.8	62.8	65.4	70.3	76.1	86.3	92.3	94.8	101.0
45.0–49.9	220	76.3	11.7	57.7	60.9	63.2	67.6	76.2	83.6	89.0	92.1	95.8
50.0–54.9	225	75.4	11.9	57.3	60.2	64.5	67.1	74.7	82.8	88.2	90.5	99.3
55.0–59.9	204	74.5	12.0	54.7	58.2	61.5	66.7	74.8	81.9	87.2	90.6	94.7
60.0–64.9	318	74.0	12.3	54.2	59.2	62.5	65.9	73.4	80.7	85.7	88.4	93.8
65.0–69.9	446	70.7	12.1	50.8	55.4	57.8	61.9	70.3	79.0	83.3	86.8	92.4
70.0–74.9	315	70.5	12.5	49.9	54.4	57.3	61.9	70.1	78.4	83.0	85.5	92.8
Males with medium frames												
18.0–24.9	87.7	74.0	12.7	57.5	60.6	62.3	65.3	71.5	80.3	86.0	91.6	99.6
25.0–29.9	627	77.0	13.2	58.5	61.8	64.5	68.4	75.9	84.1	88.3	92.4	100.4
30.0–34.9	473	78.5	12.9	59.8	63.0	65.9	69.5	77.8	85.8	91.1	93.8	98.8
35.0–39.9	419	80.5	12.8	58.7	64.8	68.4	72.9	80.4	87.4	91.5	95.9	102.5
40.0–44.9	414	80.1	12.4	60.8	64.2	67.9	71.9	79.3	88.1	92.4	96.8	102.6
45.0–49.9	436	80.7	13.0	60.3	65.1	67.1	71.9	79.8	88.7	93.3	96.7	101.3
50.0–54.9	441	79.0	13.7	58.4	62.5	65.8	70.0	78.3	86.3	91.7	96.6	103.1
55.0–59.9	404	78.8	12.7	59.9	64.5	66.7	70.5	77.9	85.3	91.1	95.4	102.2
60.0–64.9	629	76.7	11.9	58.3	61.5	64.5	68.7	76.3	84.4	88.4	91.6	97.8
65.0–69.9	886	75.0	12.2	56.1	59.5	62.5	66.9	74.5	82.9	86.9	90.8	97.2
70.0–74.9	627	73.6	12.2	54.3	58.3	61.1	65.5	72.6	81.0	86.1	89.8	93.9
Males with large frames												
18.0–24.9	433	77.5	15.4	58.2	61.3	62.6	67.4	74.7	85.0	91.2	95.0	104.9
25.0–29.9	310	84.3	17.4	61.2	66.0	68.4	72.6	82.2	91.6	99.8	102.8	115.2
30.0–34.9	233	86.5	16.6	65.5	68.4	70.2	75.2	85.4	92.0	101.6	106.7	116.7
35.0–39.9	206	85.0	15.0	59.6	67.4	71.8	75.4	84.1	93.1	98.9	104.1	113.3
40.0–44.9	205	85.8	16.4	63.7	67.7	68.8	74.3	84.9	94.5	100.3	107.4	113.3
45.0–49.9	215	85.5	16.5	62.7	67.0	69.4	74.0	84.0	94.0	101.3	105.9	119.2
50.0–54.9	216	84.7	14.7	64.4	66.9	68.8	73.3	83.1	94.3	101.7	103.6	108.4
55.0–59.9	199	85.7	15.7	64.5	67.1	70.3	74.8	84.5	93.5	100.5	103.5	121.1
60.0–64.9	313	82.1	14.6	61.5	66.6	69.3	73.1	80.7	89.4	94.5	98.9	107.7
65.0–69.9	440	79.5	13.8	57.0	61.5	64.9	70.4	78.9	87.8	93.0	96.3	104.0
70.0–74.9	310	77.1	13.8	55.3	59.9	63.6	67.9	76.7	84.1	90.5	95.8	101.4

Reproduced from A.R. Frisancho. *Anthropometric Standards for Assessment of Growth and Nutritional Status*, Ann Arbor, MI: University of Michigan Press, 1990

TABLE F-5 Means, Standard Deviations and Percentiles of Weight (kg) by Age for Adult Females of Small, Medium, and Large Frames

Age (yrs)	N	Mean	SD	5	10	15	25	Percentiles 50	75	85	90	95
Females with small frames												
18.0–24.9	652	56.2	8.75	44.0	46.1	48.0	50.3	55.1	60.9	64.4	66.9	71.5
25.0–29.9	487	56.9	9.50	44.1	47.3	48.6	50.9	55.6	61.1	64.5	67.6	72.6
30.0–34.9	413	59.1	10.0	45.7	48.2	50.0	52.7	57.6	63.4	68.1	71.8	77.7
35.0–39.9	369	61.1	11.4	45.8	48.2	50.8	53.4	59.5	66.7	71.9	76.0	79.5
40.0–44.9	353	60.6	9.4	48.1	50.3	51.8	54.5	59.1	66.1	70.0	73.6	80.3
45.0–49.9	244	61.4	11.1	46.3	47.8	50.8	53.6	60.3	67.3	71.4	75.1	80.8
50.0–54.9	257	61.3	10.8	46.3	49.1	51.7	54.5	60.3	66.9	71.0	73.1	78.4
55.0–59.9	224	61.3	11.1	47.3	49.5	52.2	54.7	59.9	65.3	70.2	73.6	81.5
60.0–64.9	351	61.9	11.0	46.4	48.9	50.6	54.2	60.9	68.5	71.7	74.0	82.2
65.0–69.9	491	61.1	10.7	44.9	48.4	50.7	53.6	60.2	67.4	71.7	74.0	79.3
70.0–74.9	369	60.6	12.1	42.6	45.9	48.5	51.6	60.2	67.0	72.3	75.4	81.0
Females with medium frames												
18.0–24.9	1297	59.5	10.4	46.0	48.4	50.0	52.5	58.1	64.4	69.5	72.8	78.4
25.0–29.9	967	60.9	11.5	46.9	49.1	50.6	53.0	58.6	66.3	72.2	76.9	83.0
30.0–34.9	815	63.5	13.4	47.2	50.0	51.7	54.3	60.7	69.3	76.7	80.6	87.2
35.0–39.9	730	64.1	12.1	49.2	51.7	53.0	56.1	61.8	69.8	74.7	79.4	87.9
40.0–44.9	700	65.6	13.3	48.8	51.3	53.6	57.0	62.8	71.8	77.3	82.4	92.1
45.0–49.9	484	65.8	13.4	48.3	51.4	53.3	56.4	63.4	72.2	77.8	83.1	91.6
50.0–54.9	504	66.4	12.2	48.9	52.0	54.4	57.7	64.4	73.1	79.3	82.8	89.7
55.0–59.9	444	68.0	15.3	48.2	51.1	54.3	58.1	66.3	74.8	81.0	86.2	92.1
60.0–64.9	695	66.2	12.4	49.1	52.3	54.0	57.5	64.5	73.5	78.1	82.2	89.0
65.0–69.9	973	66.2	12.7	48.1	51.4	53.6	57.1	64.9	73.1	78.7	82.4	88.8
70.0–74.9	731	64.3	11.9	46.8	50.5	52.5	56.8	62.9	70.8	76.9	80.2	84.7
Females with large frames												
18.0–24.9	642	68.0	17.2	48.9	51.3	53.1	56.3	62.9	76.2	83.8	89.0	102.7
25.0–29.9	480	72.6	17.7	49.9	53.4	55.6	59.3	68.7	82.9	90.9	98.8	105.0
30.0–34.9	402	76.4	19.7	51.1	54.9	57.7	61.1	72.7	88.4	97.3	102.8	111.9
35.0–39.9	361	79.1	19.5	52.8	56.1	59.1	64.5	76.7	90.4	98.1	106.0	117.9
40.0–44.9	346	79.7	19.8	53.4	57.3	60.7	65.7	77.1	91.3	99.2	104.9	114.2
45.0–49.9	240	80.1	19.6	54.5	60.1	63.2	66.7	76.8	86.6	97.6	105.0	116.9
50.0–54.9	250	79.4	16.9	55.6	60.0	63.0	67.8	77.7	88.8	97.1	103.3	112.1
55.0–59.9	218	79.8	17.5	56.4	60.2	62.5	67.6	77.6	89.9	97.0	101.6	111.3
60.0–64.9	346	77.8	15.6	56.0	59.4	62.8	66.8	76.8	85.7	92.8	100.0	104.8
65.0–69.9	484	76.6	15.4	55.3	59.4	62.0	65.8	74.5	84.6	91.7	97.8	105.0
70.0–74.9	363	74.9	14.0	53.5	57.9	60.9	65.8	74.5	82.7	87.9	91.3	99.1

Reproduced from A.R. Frisancho. *Anthropometric Standards for Assessment of Growth and Nutritional Status*, Ann Arbor, MI: University of Michigan Press, 1990

TABLE F-6 Age Correction Factors for Weight Percentiles for Ages 25 to 74

	Men		Women	
	Median age	Correction Factor	Median age	Correction factor
Age 25–54				
Frame: small	39	0.074	37	0.165
medium	39	0.080	37	0.234
large	40	0.080	37	0.284
Age 55–74				
Frame: small	66	−0.329	67	−0.027
medium	67	−0.435	66	−0.196
large	67	−0.562	67	−0.466

Adapted from R. Frisancho. New standards of weight and body composition by frame size and height for assessment of nutritional status of adults and the elderly. Am. J. Clin. Nutr. 40:808, 1984

TABLE F-7   Means, Standard Deviations and Percentiles of Body Mass Index (w/s²) by Age for Males and Females of 1 to 74 Years

Age (yrs)	N	Mean	SD	Percentiles 5	10	15	25	50	75	85	90	95
Males												
1.0–1.9	366	17.3	2.4	15.2	15.6	15.9	16.4	17.1	18.0	18.6	19.0	19.6
2.0–2.9	664	16.2	1.3	14.3	14.6	15.0	15.4	16.2	17.1	17.5	17.8	18.4
3.0–3.9	716	16.0	1.4	14.2	14.6	14.8	15.1	15.8	16.6	17.1	17.5	18.2
4.0–4.9	709	15.7	1.3	13.9	14.2	14.5	14.9	15.6	16.4	16.8	17.2	17.8
5.0–5.9	675	15.6	1.5	13.8	14.1	14.3	14.7	15.5	16.3	16.8	17.2	18.1
6.0–6.9	298	15.8	1.9	13.7	14.1	14.3	14.8	15.3	16.4	17.2	18.0	19.3
7.0–7.9	312	16.0	1.8	13.7	14.1	14.3	14.9	15.6	16.7	17.5	18.2	19.5
8.0–8.9	296	16.3	2.2	13.8	14.3	14.6	15.0	15.9	17.1	18.0	19.1	20.1
9.0–9.9	322	16.9	2.4	14.1	14.6	14.8	15.3	16.3	17.7	19.0	19.9	21.8
10.0–10.9	334	17.7	2.8	14.6	15.0	15.3	15.8	17.1	18.7	19.8	21.2	23.4
11.0–11.9	324	18.4	3.6	14.7	15.1	15.7	16.2	17.4	19.8	21.5	22.5	25.3
12.0–12.9	349	18.9	3.5	15.2	15.7	16.1	16.7	17.9	20.2	21.7	23.7	25.8
13.0–13.9	348	19.5	3.5	15.6	16.4	16.6	17.2	18.7	20.7	22.2	24.0	25.9
14.0–14.9	359	20.3	3.3	16.5	17.0	17.5	18.1	19.5	21.6	23.1	24.2	26.4
15.0–15.9	359	20.8	3.1	16.8	17.5	18.0	19.0	20.4	22.0	23.4	24.1	26.6
16.0–16.9	349	21.9	3.3	18.0	18.5	19.0	19.6	21.3	23.0	24.8	25.9	27.3
17.0–17.9	338	21.8	3.5	17.8	18.4	18.9	19.5	21.1	23.4	24.9	26.1	28.3
18.0–24.9	1755	23.6	3.8	18.8	19.6	20.1	21.0	23.0	25.5	27.2	28.5	31.0
25.0–29.9	1255	24.9	4.3	19.5	20.4	21.1	21.9	24.3	27.0	28.5	30.0	32.8
30.0–34.9	947	25.7	4.2	19.9	21.0	21.9	23.0	25.1	27.8	29.3	30.5	32.9
35.0–39.9	839	25.9	4.0	19.7	21.0	21.9	23.3	25.6	28.0	29.5	30.6	32.8
40.0–44.9	829	26.2	4.0	20.4	21.5	22.2	23.4	26.0	28.5	29.9	31.0	32.5
45.0–49.9	871	26.3	4.2	20.1	21.5	22.4	23.5	26.0	28.6	30.1	31.2	33.4
50.0–54.9	882	26.1	4.2	19.9	21.1	22.0	23.3	25.9	28.2	30.1	31.3	33.3
55.0–59.9	807	26.2	4.3	19.8	21.3	22.1	23.5	26.1	28.5	30.2	31.6	33.6
60.0–64.9	1261	25.8	3.8	20.1	21.3	22.0	23.4	25.6	28.0	29.4	30.4	32.4
65.0–69.9	1773	25.5	4.0	19.1	20.5	21.4	22.7	25.5	27.8	29.6	30.7	32.3
70.0–74.9	1257	25.3	4.0	19.0	20.3	21.4	22.6	25.1	27.7	29.3	30.5	32.3
Females												
1.0–1.9	333	16.7	1.5	14.4	14.9	15.2	15.7	16.7	17.6	18.2	18.6	19.3
2.0–2.9	610	16.0	1.5	14.1	14.4	14.7	15.1	15.9	16.8	17.3	17.8	18.4
3.0–3.9	651	15.7	1.4	13.6	14.1	14.4	14.7	15.5	16.4	17.0	17.5	18.0
4.0–4.9	678	15.5	1.4	13.6	13.9	14.2	14.6	15.3	16.2	16.7	17.2	18.0
5.0–5.9	673	15.5	1.7	13.3	13.7	14.0	14.5	15.2	16.3	16.9	17.5	18.6
6.0–6.9	296	15.5	1.7	13.5	13.7	13.9	14.3	15.2	16.2	17.0	17.5	18.7
7.0–7.9	331	15.9	1.9	13.7	14.1	14.2	14.7	15.4	16.8	17.5	18.3	19.6
8.0–8.9	276	16.5	2.7	13.8	14.1	14.4	14.9	15.8	17.4	18.7	19.8	21.7
9.0–9.9	322	17.3	3.1	14.0	14.6	14.8	15.3	16.5	18.1	19.8	21.5	23.3
10.0–10.9	330	17.7	3.1	14.0	14.5	15.0	15.6	16.9	18.9	20.7	22.0	24.1
11.0–11.9	303	18.9	3.8	14.8	15.3	15.6	16.3	18.1	20.3	21.8	23.4	26.2
12.0–12.9	324	19.6	3.7	15.0	15.6	16.2	17.0	18.9	21.2	23.1	24.6	27.0
13.0–13.9	361	20.4	4.1	15.4	16.3	16.7	17.7	19.4	22.2	23.8	25.2	28.6
14.0–14.9	370	21.1	3.9	16.5	17.1	17.7	18.4	20.3	22.8	24.7	26.2	28.9
15.0–15.9	309	21.1	3.8	17.0	17.5	18.0	18.8	20.3	22.4	24.1	25.6	28.7
16.0–16.9	343	22.1	4.0	17.7	18.3	18.7	19.3	21.1	23.5	25.7	26.8	30.1
17.0–17.9	293	22.5	4.7	17.1	17.9	18.7	19.6	21.4	24.0	26.2	27.5	32.1
18.0–24.9	2592	22.9	4.6	17.7	18.4	19.0	19.9	21.8	24.5	26.5	28.6	32.1
25.0–29.9	1935	23.7	5.2	18.0	18.8	19.2	20.1	22.3	25.6	28.4	30.8	34.3
30.0–34.9	1633	24.8	5.9	18.5	19.4	19.9	20.8	23.1	27.2	30.4	33.0	36.6
35.0–39.9	1461	25.3	5.8	18.7	19.5	20.2	21.3	23.8	28.0	31.0	33.1	36.9
40.0–44.9	1399	25.7	5.9	18.8	19.8	20.5	21.5	24.2	28.3	31.6	33.7	36.6
45.0–49.9	969	26.0	6.2	19.0	20.1	20.8	21.9	24.5	28.6	31.4	33.4	37.1
50.0–54.9	1012	26.3	5.5	19.2	20.3	21.0	22.4	25.2	29.2	32.1	33.8	36.5
55.0–59.9	887	26.9	6.1	19.2	20.5	21.3	22.8	25.7	30.1	32.7	34.7	38.2
60.0–64.9	1392	26.7	5.5	19.3	20.7	21.4	22.9	25.8	29.7	32.1	33.8	36.6
65.0–69.9	1952	26.8	5.5	19.5	20.7	21.7	23.0	26.0	29.6	32.0	33.8	36.6
70.0–74.9	1467	26.6	5.3	19.3	20.5	21.5	23.0	26.0	29.5	31.7	33.1	35.8

Reproduced from A.R. Frisancho. *Anthropometric Standards for Assessment of Growth and Nutritional Status*, Ann Arbor, MI: University of Michigan Press, 1990

TABLE F-8   Evaluation of Weight Loss

Time	Significant weight loss (% of change)	Severe weight loss (% of change)
1 week	1–2	> 2
1 mo	5	> 5
3 mo	7.5	> 7.5
6 mo	10	> 10

Reprinted with permission from G.L. Blackburn, B.R. Bristrian, B.S. Maini et al., Nutritional metabolic assessment of the hospitalized patient. JPEN 1:(1977) 15.

TABLE F-9 Means, Standard Deviations and Percentiles of Triceps Skinfold Thickness (mm) by Age for Males and Females of 1 to 74 Years

Age (yrs)	N	Mean	SD	5	10	15	25	Percentiles 50	75	85	90	95
Males												
1.0–1.9	681	10.4	2.9	6.5	7.0	7.5	8.0	10.0	12.0	13.0	14.0	15.5
2.0–2.9	677	10.0	2.9	6.0	6.5	7.0	8.0	10.0	12.0	13.0	14.0	15.0
3.0–3.9	717	9.9	2.7	6.0	7.0	7.0	8.0	9.5	11.5	12.5	13.5	15.0
4.0–4.9	708	9.2	2.7	5.5	6.5	7.0	7.5	9.0	11.0	12.0	12.5	14.0
5.0–5.9	677	8.9	3.1	5.0	6.0	6.0	7.0	8.0	10.0	11.5	13.0	14.5
6.0–6.9	298	8.9	3.8	5.0	5.5	6.0	6.5	8.0	10.0	12.0	13.0	16.0
7.0–7.9	312	9.0	4.0	4.5	5.0	6.0	6.0	8.0	10.5	12.5	14.0	16.0
8.0–8.9	296	9.6	4.4	5.0	5.5	6.0	7.0	8.5	11.0	13.0	16.0	19.0
9.0–9.9	322	10.2	5.1	5.0	5.5	6.0	6.5	9.0	12.5	15.5	17.0	20.0
10.0–10.9	334	11.5	5.7	5.0	6.0	6.0	7.5	10.0	14.0	17.0	20.0	24.0
11.0–11.9	324	12.5	7.0	5.0	6.0	6.5	7.5	10.0	16.0	19.5	23.0	27.0
12.0–12.9	348	12.2	6.8	4.5	6.0	6.0	7.5	10.5	14.5	18.0	22.5	27.5
13.0–13.9	350	11.0	6.7	4.5	5.0	5.5	7.0	9.0	13.0	17.0	20.5	25.0
14.0–14.9	358	10.4	6.5	4.0	5.0	5.0	6.0	8.5	12.5	15.0	18.0	23.5
15.0–15.9	356	9.8	6.5	5.0	5.0	5.0	6.0	7.5	11.0	15.0	18.0	23.5
16.0–16.9	350	10.0	5.9	4.0	5.0	5.1	6.0	8.0	12.0	14.0	17.0	23.0
17.0–17.9	337	9.1	5.3	4.0	5.0	5.0	6.0	7.0	11.0	13.5	16.0	19.5
18.0–24.9	1752	11.3	6.4	4.0	5.0	5.5	6.5	10.0	14.5	17.5	20.0	23.5
25.0–29.9	1251	12.2	6.7	4.0	5.0	6.0	7.0	11.0	15.5	19.0	21.5	25.0
30.0–34.9	941	13.1	6.7	4.5	6.0	6.5	8.0	12.0	16.5	20.0	22.0	25.0
35.0–39.9	832	12.9	6.2	4.5	6.0	7.0	8.5	12.0	16.0	18.5	20.5	24.5
40.0–44.9	828	13.0	6.6	5.0	6.0	6.9	8.0	12.0	16.0	19.0	21.5	26.0
45.0–49.9	867	12.9	6.4	5.0	6.0	7.0	8.0	12.0	16.0	19.0	21.0	25.0
50.0–54.9	879	12.6	6.1	5.0	6.0	7.0	8.0	11.5	15.0	18.5	20.8	25.0
55.0–59.9	807	12.4	6.0	5.0	6.0	6.5	8.0	11.5	15.0	18.0	20.5	25.0
60.0–64.9	1259	12.5	6.0	5.0	6.0	7.0	8.0	11.5	15.5	18.5	20.5	24.0
65.0–69.9	1774	12.1	5.9	4.5	5.0	6.5	8.0	11.0	15.0	18.0	20.0	23.5
70.0–74.9	1251	12.0	5.8	4.5	6.0	6.5	8.0	11.0	15.0	17.0	19.0	23.0
Females												
1.0–1.9	622	10.4	3.1	6.0	7.0	7.0	8.0	10.0	12.0	13.0	14.0	16.0
2.0–2.9	614	10.5	2.9	6.0	7.0	7.5	8.5	10.0	12.0	13.5	14.5	16.0
3.0–3.9	652	10.4	2.9	6.0	7.0	7.5	8.5	10.0	12.0	13.0	14.0	16.0
4.0–4.9	681	10.3	3.0	6.0	7.0	7.5	8.0	10.0	12.0	13.0	14.0	15.5
5.0–5.9	673	10.4	3.5	5.5	7.0	7.0	8.0	10.0	12.0	13.5	15.0	17.0
6.0–6.9	296	10.4	3.7	6.0	6.5	7.0	8.0	10.0	12.0	13.0	15.0	17.0
7.0–7.9	330	11.1	4.2	6.0	7.0	7.0	8.0	10.5	12.5	15.0	16.0	19.0
8.0–8.9	276	12.1	5.4	6.0	7.0	7.5	8.5	11.0	14.5	17.0	18.0	22.5
9.0–9.9	322	13.4	5.9	6.5	7.0	8.0	9.0	12.0	16.0	19.0	21.0	25.0
10.0–10.9	329	13.9	6.1	7.0	8.0	8.0	9.0	12.5	17.5	20.0	22.5	27.0
11.0–11.9	302	15.0	6.8	7.0	8.0	8.5	10.0	13.0	18.0	21.5	24.0	29.0
12.0–12.9	323	15.1	6.3	7.0	8.0	9.0	11.0	14.0	18.5	21.5	24.0	27.5
13.0–13.9	360	16.4	7.4	7.0	8.0	9.0	11.0	15.0	20.0	24.0	25.0	30.0
14.0–14.9	370	17.1	7.3	8.0	9.0	10.0	11.5	16.0	21.0	23.5	26.5	32.0
15.0–15.9	309	17.3	7.4	8.0	9.5	10.5	12.0	16.5	20.5	23.0	26.0	32.5
16.0–16.9	343	19.2	7.0	10.5	11.5	12.0	14.0	18.0	23.0	26.0	29.0	32.5
17.0–17.9	291	19.1	8.0	9.0	10.0	12.0	13.0	18.0	24.0	26.5	29.0	34.5
18.0–24.9	2588	20.0	8.2	9.0	11.0	12.0	14.0	18.5	24.5	28.5	31.0	36.0
25.0–29.9	1921	21.7	8.8	10.0	12.0	13.0	15.0	20.0	26.5	31.0	34.0	38.0
30.0–34.9	1619	23.7	9.2	10.5	13.0	15.0	17.0	22.5	29.5	33.0	35.5	41.5
35.0–39.9	1453	24.7	9.3	11.0	13.0	15.5	18.0	23.5	30.0	35.0	37.0	41.0
40.0–44.9	1391	25.1	9.0	12.0	14.0	16.0	19.0	24.5	30.5	35.0	37.0	41.0
45.0–49.9	962	26.1	9.3	12.0	14.5	16.5	19.5	25.5	32.0	35.5	38.0	42.5
50.0–54.9	1006	26.5	9.0	12.0	15.0	17.5	20.5	25.5	32.0	36.0	38.5	42.0
55.0–59.9	880	26.6	9.4	12.0	15.0	17.0	20.5	26.0	32.0	36.0	39.0	42.5
60.0–64.9	1389	26.6	8.8	12.5	16.0	17.5	20.5	26.0	32.0	35.5	38.0	42.5
65.0–69.9	1946	25.1	8.5	12.0	14.5	16.0	19.0	25.0	30.0	33.5	36.0	40.0
70.0–74.9	1463	24.0	8.5	11.0	13.5	15.5	18.0	24.0	29.5	32.0	35.0	38.5

Reproduced from A.R. Frisancho. *Anthropometric Standards for Assessment of Growth and Nutritional Status*, Ann Arbor, MI: University of Michigan Press, 1990

TABLE F-10 Means, Standard Deviations and Percentiles of Subscapular Skinfold Thickness (mm) by Age for Males and Females of 1 to 74 Years

Age (yrs)	N	Mean	SD	5	10	15	25	Percentiles 50	75	85	90	95
Males												
1.0–1.9	681	6.3	1.9	4.0	4.0	4.5	5.0	6.0	7.0	8.0	8.5	10.0
2.0–2.9	677	5.9	2.0	3.5	4.0	4.0	4.5	5.5	7.0	7.5	8.5	10.0
3.0–3.9	716	5.5	1.8	3.5	4.0	4.0	4.5	5.0	6.0	7.0	7.0	9.0
4.0–4.9	708	5.3	1.8	3.0	3.5	4.0	4.0	5.0	6.0	6.5	7.0	8.0
5.0–5.9	677	5.2	2.4	3.0	3.5	4.0	4.0	5.0	5.5	6.5	7.0	8.0
6.0–6.9	298	5.5	3.3	3.0	3.5	3.5	4.0	4.5	5.5	6.5	8.0	13.0
7.0–7.9	312	5.7	3.3	3.0	3.5	4.0	4.0	5.0	6.0	7.0	8.0	12.0
8.0–8.9	296	6.0	3.8	3.0	3.5	4.0	4.0	5.0	6.0	7.5	9.0	12.5
9.0–9.9	322	6.8	4.8	3.0	3.5	4.0	4.0	5.0	7.0	9.5	12.0	14.5
10.0–10.9	334	7.6	5.5	3.5	4.0	4.0	4.5	6.0	8.0	11.0	14.0	19.5
11.0–11.9	324	9.0	7.6	4.0	4.0	4.0	5.0	6.0	9.0	15.0	18.5	26.0
12.0–12.9	349	8.9	7.1	4.0	4.0	4.5	5.0	6.0	9.5	15.0	19.0	24.0
13.0–13.9	350	8.8	7.0	4.0	4.0	5.0	5.0	6.5	9.0	13.0	17.0	25.0
14.0–14.9	358	9.0	6.5	4.0	5.0	5.0	5.5	7.0	9.0	12.0	15.5	22.5
15.0–15.9	357	9.4	6.8	5.0	5.0	5.5	6.0	7.0	10.0	13.0	16.0	22.0
16.0–16.9	349	10.1	6.2	5.0	6.0	6.0	7.0	8.0	11.0	14.0	16.0	22.0
17.0–17.9	339	10.1	6.0	5.0	6.0	6.0	7.0	8.0	11.0	14.0	17.0	21.5
18.0–24.9	1750	13.4	7.6	6.0	7.0	7.0	8.0	11.0	16.0	20.0	24.0	30.0
25.0–29.9	1247	15.5	8.2	7.0	7.0	8.0	9.0	13.0	20.0	24.5	26.5	31.0
30.0–34.9	938	17.3	8.5	7.0	8.0	9.0	11.0	15.5	22.0	25.5	29.0	33.0
35.0–39.9	835	17.6	8.3	7.0	8.0	9.5	11.0	16.0	22.5	25.5	28.0	33.0
40.0–44.9	818	17.4	8.2	7.0	8.0	9.0	11.5	16.0	22.0	25.5	29.5	33.0
45.0–49.9	860	18.2	8.6	7.0	8.0	9.5	11.5	17.0	23.5	27.0	30.0	34.5
50.0–54.9	872	17.7	8.4	7.0	8.0	9.0	11.5	16.0	22.5	26.5	29.5	34.0
55.0–59.9	802	17.6	8.1	6.5	8.0	9.5	11.5	16.5	23.0	26.0	28.5	32.0
60.0–64.9	1251	18.1	8.4	7.0	8.0	10.0	12.0	17.0	23.0	26.0	29.0	34.0
65.0–69.9	1770	16.8	8.2	6.0	7.5	8.5	10.5	15.0	21.5	25.0	28.0	32.5
70.0–74.9	1247	16.3	7.8	6.5	7.0	8.0	10.3	15.0	21.0	25.0	27.5	31.0
Females												
1.0–1.9	622	6.5	2.0	4.0	4.0	4.5	5.0	6.0	7.5	8.5	9.0	10.0
2.0–2.9	615	6.4	2.3	4.0	4.0	4.5	5.0	6.0	7.0	8.0	9.0	10.5
3.0–3.9	652	6.1	2.2	3.5	4.0	4.0	5.0	5.5	7.0	7.5	8.5	10.0
4.0–4.9	681	6.0	2.3	3.5	4.0	4.0	4.5	5.5	7.0	8.0	9.0	10.5
5.0–5.9	672	6.2	3.0	3.5	4.0	4.0	4.5	5.0	7.0	8.0	9.0	12.0
6.0–6.9	296	6.3	3.4	3.5	4.0	4.0	4.5	5.5	7.0	8.0	10.0	11.5
7.0–7.9	330	6.7	3.5	3.5	4.0	4.0	4.5	6.0	7.5	9.5	11.0	13.0
8.0–8.9	276	7.8	5.8	3.5	4.0	4.0	5.0	6.0	8.0	11.5	14.5	21.0
9.0–9.9	322	9.0	6.5	4.0	4.5	5.0	5.0	6.5	9.5	13.0	18.0	24.0
10.0–10.9	329	9.7	6.5	4.0	4.5	5.0	5.5	7.0	11.5	16.0	19.5	24.0
11.0–11.9	300	10.7	7.6	4.5	5.0	5.0	6.0	8.0	12.0	16.0	20.0	28.5
12.0–12.9	323	11.5	7.7	5.0	5.5	6.0	6.5	9.0	13.0	17.0	22.0	30.0
13.0–13.9	360	12.3	7.8	5.0	6.0	6.0	7.0	10.0	15.5	19.0	23.0	26.5
14.0–14.9	370	13.0	7.7	6.0	6.0	7.0	7.5	10.0	16.0	20.5	25.0	30.0
15.0–15.9	308	13.0	7.5	6.0	7.0	7.5	8.0	10.0	15.0	20.0	23.0	28.0
16.0–16.9	343	14.7	8.7	7.0	7.5	8.0	9.0	11.5	16.5	24.0	26.0	34.0
17.0–17.9	291	15.4	8.9	6.0	7.0	7.5	9.0	12.5	19.0	24.5	28.0	34.0
18.0–24.9	2587	16.1	9.4	6.5	7.0	8.0	9.5	13.0	20.0	25.5	29.0	36.0
25.0–29.9	1913	17.5	10.4	6.5	7.0	8.0	10.0	14.0	23.0	29.0	33.0	38.5
30.0–34.9	1615	19.7	11.7	6.5	7.5	8.5	10.5	16.0	26.5	32.5	37.0	43.0
35.0–39.9	1446	20.6	11.6	7.0	8.0	9.0	11.0	18.0	28.5	34.0	36.5	43.0
40.0–44.9	1382	20.9	11.4	6.5	8.0	9.0	11.5	19.0	28.5	34.0	37.0	42.0
45.0–49.9	956	21.8	11.4	7.0	8.5	10.0	12.5	20.0	29.5	34.0	37.5	43.5
50.0–54.9	995	23.0	11.4	7.0	9.0	11.0	14.0	21.9	30.0	35.0	39.0	43.5
55.0–59.9	870	23.2	11.7	7.0	9.0	11.0	13.5	22.0	31.0	35.0	38.0	45.0
60.0–64.9	1376	22.8	11.3	7.5	9.0	11.0	14.0	21.5	30.5	35.0	38.0	43.0
65.0–69.9	1933	21.4	10.6	7.0	8.0	10.0	13.0	20.0	28.0	33.0	36.0	41.0
70.0–74.9	1460	20.5	10.1	6.5	8.5	10.0	12.0	19.5	27.0	32.0	35.0	38.5

Reproduced from A.R. Frisancho. *Anthropometric Standards for Assessment of Growth and Nutritional Status*, Ann Arbor, MI: University of Michigan Press, 1990

TABLE F-11   Means, Standard Deviations and Percentiles of Upper Arm Fat Area (cm²) by Age for Males and Females of 1 to 74 Years

Age (yrs)	N	Mean	SD	5	10	15	25	Percentiles 50	75	85	90	95
Males												
1.0–1.9	681	7.5	2.2	4.5	4.9	5.3	5.9	7.4	8.9	9.6	10.3	11.1
2.0–2.9	672	7.4	2.3	4.2	4.8	5.1	5.8	7.3	8.6	9.7	10.6	11.6
3.0–3.9	715	7.6	2.4	4.5	5.0	5.4	5.9	7.2	8.8	9.8	10.6	11.8
4.0–4.9	707	7.3	2.5	4.1	4.7	5.2	5.7	6.9	8.5	9.3	10.0	11.4
5.0–5.9	676	7.4	3.1	4.0	4.5	4.9	5..5	6.7	8.3	9.8	10.9	12.7
6.0–6.9	298	7.7	4.1	3.7	4.3	4.6	5.2	6.7	8.6	10.3	11.2	15.2
7.0–7.9	312	8.1	4.2	3.8	4.3	4.7	5.4	7.1	9.6	11.6	12.8	15.5
8.0–8.9	296	8.9	5.0	4.1	4.8	5.1	5.8	7.6	10.4	12.4	15.6	18.6
9.0–9.9	322	10.1	6.2	4.2	4.8	5.4	6.1	8.3	11.8	15.8	18.2	21.7
10.0–10.9	333	12.0	7.3	4.7	5.3	5.7	6.9	9.8	14.7	18.3	21.5	27.0
11.0–11.9	324	13.6	9.4	4.9	5.5	6.2	7.3	10.4	16.9	22.3	26.0	32.5
12.0–12.9	348	13.9	9.6	4.7	5.6	6.3	7.6	11.3	15.8	21.1	27.3	35.0
13.0–13.9	350	13.0	9.2	4.7	5.7	6.3	7.6	10.1	14.9	21.2	25.4	32.1
14.0–14.9	358	13.3	10.2	4.6	5.6	6.3	7.4	10.1	15.9	19.5	25.5	31.8
15.0–15.9	356	12.8	9.0	5.6	6.1	6.5	7.3	9.6	14.6	20.2	24.5	31.3
16.0–16.9	350	13.9	9.5	5.6	6.1	6.9	8.3	10.5	16.6	20.6	24.8	33.5
17.0–17.9	337	12.9	8.9	5.4	6.1	6.7	7.4	9.9	15.6	19.7	23.7	28.9
18.0–24.9	1752	16.9	10.8	5.5	6.9	7.7	9.2	13.9	21.5	26.8	30.7	37.2
25.0–29.9	1250	18.8	11.6	6.0	7.3	8.4	10.2	16.3	23.9	29.7	33.3	40.4
30.0–34.9	940	20.4	11.4	6.2	8.4	9.7	11.9	18.4	25.6	31.6	34.8	41.9
35.0–39.9	832	20.1	10.5	6.5	8.1	9.6	12.8	18.8	25.2	29.6	33.4	39.4
40.0–44.9	828	20.4	11.2	7.1	8.7	9.9	12.4	18.0	25.3	30.1	35.3	42.1
45.0–49.9	867	20.1	11.0	7.4	9.0	10.2	12.3	18.1	24.9	29.7	33.7	40.4
50.0–54.9	879	19.4	10.3	7.0	8.6	10.1	12.3	17.3	23.9	29.0	32.4	40.0
55.0–59.9	807	19.2	10.2	6.4	8.2	9.7	12.3	17.4	23.8	28.4	33.3	39.1
60.0–64.9	1259	19.1	10.2	6.9	8.7	9.9	12.1	17.0	23.5	28.3	31.8	38.7
65.0–69.9	1773	18.0	9.8	5.8	7.4	8.5	10.9	16.5	22.8	27.2	30.7	36.3
70.0–74.9	1250	17.5	9.4	6.0	7.5	8.9	11.0	15.9	22.0	25.7	29.1	34.9
Females												
1.0–1.9	622	7.3	2.3	4.1	4.6	5.0	5.6	7.1	8.6	9.5	10.4	11.7
2.0–2.9	614	7.7	2.3	4.4	5.0	5.4	6.1	7.5	9.0	10.0	10.8	12.0
3.0–3.9	651	7.8	2.5	4.3	5.0	5.4	6.1	7.6	9.2	10.2	10.8	12.2
4.0–4.9	680	8.0	2.6	4.3	4.9	5.4	6.2	7.7	9.3	10.4	11.3	12.8
5.0–5.9	672	8.5	3.4	4.4	5.0	5.4	6.3	7.8	9.8	11.3	12.5	14.5
6.0–6.9	296	8.7	3.9	4.5	5.0	5.6	6.2	8.1	10.0	11.2	13.3	16.5
7.0–7.9	329	9.8	4.5	4.8	5.5	6.0	7.0	8.8	11.0	13.2	14.7	19.0
8.0–8.9	275	11.3	6.5	5.2	5.7	6.4	7.2	9.8	13.3	15.8	18.0	23.7
9.0–9.9	321	13.1	7.3	5.4	6.2	6.8	8.1	11.5	15.6	18.8	22.0	27.5
10.0–10.9	329	14.1	7.7	6.1	6.9	7.2	8.4	11.9	18.0	21.5	25.3	29.9
11.0–11.9	302	16.3	9.7	6.6	7.5	8.2	9.8	13.1	19.9	24.4	28.2	36.8
12.0–12.9	323	16.9	8.9	6.7	8.0	8.8	10.8	14.8	20.8	24.8	29.4	34.0
13.0–13.9	360	19.1	11.0	6.7	7.7	9.4	11.6	16.5	23.7	28.7	32.7	40.8
14.0–14.9	370	20.4	11.0	8.3	9.6	10.9	12.4	17.7	25.1	29.5	34.6	41.2
15.0–15.9	309	20.7	11.4	8.6	10.0	11.4	12.8	18.2	24.4	29.2	32.9	44.3
16.0–16.9	343	23.5	10.9	11.3	12.8	13.7	15.9	20.5	28.0	32.7	37.0	46.0
17.0–17.9	291	23.9	13.0	9.5	11.7	13.0	14.6	21.0	29.5	33.5	38.0	51.6
18.0–24.9	2588	25.2	13.4	10.0	12.0	13.5	16.1	21.9	30.6	37.2	42.0	51.6
25.0–29.9	1921	28.1	14.7	11.0	13.3	15.1	17.7	24.5	34.8	42.1	47.1	57.5
30.0–34.9	1619	31.6	16.1	12.2	14.8	17.2	20.4	28.2	39.0	46.8	52.3	64.5
35.0–39.9	1453	33.6	16.8	13.0	15.8	18.0	21.8	29.7	41.7	49.2	55.5	64.9
40.0–44.9	1390	34.3	16.2	13.8	16.7	19.2	23.0	31.3	42.6	51.0	56.3	64.5
45.0–49.9	961	36.0	17.2	13.6	17.1	19.8	24.3	33.0	44.4	52.3	58.4	68.8
50.0–54.9	1004	36.7	15.9	14.3	18.3	21.4	25.7	34.1	45.6	53.9	57.7	65.7
55.0–59.9	879	37.6	17.7	13.7	18.2	20.7	26.0	34.5	46.4	53.9	59.1	69.7
60.0–64.9	1389	37.1	16.0	15.3	19.1	21.9	26.0	34.8	45.7	51.7	58.3	68.3
65.0–69.9	1946	34.7	15.1	13.9	17.6	20.0	24.1	32.7	42.7	49.2	53.6	62.4
70.0–74.9	1463	32.9	14.6	13.0	16.2	18.8	22.7	31.2	41.0	46.4	51.4	57.7

Reproduced from A.R. Frisancho. *Anthropometric Standards for Assessment of Growth and Nutritional Status*, Ann Arbor, MI: University of Michigan Press, 1990

TABLE F-12 Means, Standard Deviations and Percentiles of Upper Arm Muscle Area (cm²) by Age for Males and Females of 1 to 74 Years

Age (yrs)	N	Mean	SD	5	10	15	25	50	75	85	90	95
Males												
1.0–1.9	681	13.2	2.3	9.7	10.4	10.8	11.6	13.0	14.6	15.4	16.3	
2.0–2.9	672	14.1	3.2	10.1	10.9	11.3	12.4	13.9	15.6	16.4	16.9	
3.0–3.9	715	15.2	3.1	11.2	12.0	12.6	13.5	15.0	16.4	17.4	18.3	
4.0–4.9	707	16.3	2.7	12.0	12.9	13.5	14.5	16.2	17.9	18.8	19.8	
5.0–5.9	676	17.8	3.7	13.2	14.2	14.7	15.7	17.6	19.5	20.7	21.7	
6.0–6.9	298	19.3	4.0	14.4	15.3	15.8	16.8	18.7	21.3	22.9	23.8	
7.0–7.9	312	21.0	4.5	15.1	16.2	17.0	18.5	20.6	22.6	24.5	25.2	
8.0–8.9	296	22.1	4.2	16.3	17.8	18.5	19.5	21.6	24.0	25.5	26.6	
9.0–9.9	322	24.5	5.1	18.2	19.3	20.3	21.7	23.5	26.7	28.7	30.4	
10.0–10.9	333	26.7	5.9	19.6	20.7	21.6	23.0	25.7	29.0	32.2	34.0	
11.0–11.9	324	28.8	6.7	21.0	22.0	23.0	24.8	27.7	31.6	33.6	36.1	
12.0–12.9	348	31.9	7.4	22.6	24.1	25.3	26.9	30.4	35.9	39.3	40.9	
13.0–13.9	350	36.8	9.0	24.5	26.7	28.1	30.4	35.7	41.3	45.3	48.1	
14.0–14.9	358	42.4	9.1	28.3	31.3	33.1	36.1	41.9	47.4	51.3	54.0	
15.0–15.9	356	46.8	9.6	31.9	34.9	36.9	40.3	46.3	53.1	56.3	57.7	
16.0–16.9	350	52.6	10.0	37.0	40.9	42.4	45.9	51.9	57.8	63.6	66.2	
17.0–17.9	337	54.7	10.5	39.6	42.6	44.8	48.0	53.4	60.4	64.3	67.9	
18.0–24.9	1752	50.5	11.6	34.2	37.3	39.6	42.7	49.4	57.1	61.8	65.0	
25.0–29.9	1250	54.1	11.9	36.6	39.9	42.4	46.0	53.0	61.4	66.1	68.9	
30.0–34.9	940	55.6	12.1	37.9	40.9	43.4	47.3	54.4	63.2	67.6	70.8	
35.0–39.9	832	56.5	12.4	38.5	42.6	44.6	47.9	55.3	64.0	69.1	72.7	
40.0–44.9	828	56.6	11.7	38.4	42.1	45.1	48.7	56.0	64.0	68.5	71.6	
45.0–49.9	867	55.9	12.3	37.7	41.3	43.7	47.9	55.2	63.3	68.4	72.2	
50.0–54.9	879	55.0	12.5	36.0	40.0	42.7	46.6	54.0	62.7	67.0	70.4	
55.0–59.9	807	54.7	11.8	36.5	40.8	42.7	46.7	54.3	61.9	66.4	69.6	
60.0–64.9	1259	52.8	11.7	34.5	38.7	41.2	44.9	52.1	60.0	64.8	67.5	
65.0–69.9	1773	49.8	11.6	31.4	35.8	38.4	42.3	49.1	57.3	61.2	64.3	
70.0–74.9	1250	47.8	11.5	29.7	33.8	36.1	40.2	47.0	54.6	59.1	62.1	
Females												
1.0–1.9	622	12.3	2.3	8.9	9.7	10.1	10.8	12.3	13.8	14.6	15.3	
2.0–2.9	614	13.3	2.3	10.1	10.6	10.9	11.8	13.2	14.7	15.6	16.4	
3.0–3.9	651	14.3	2.4	10.8	11.4	11.8	12.6	14.3	15.8	16.7	17.4	
4.0–4.9	680	15.4	2.8	11.2	12.2	12.7	13.6	15.3	17.0	18.0	18.6	
5.0–5.9	672	16.7	3.1	12.4	13.2	13.9	14.8	16.4	18.3	19.4	20.6	
6.0–6.9	296	18.0	3.9	13.5	14.1	14.6	15.6	17.4	19.5	21.0	22.0	
7.0–7.9	329	19.3	4.0	14.4	15.2	15.8	16.7	18.9	21.2	22.6	23.9	
8.0–8.9	275	21.1	4.7	15.2	16.0	16.8	18.2	20.8	23.2	24.6	26.5	
9.0–9.9	321	22.9	4.6	17.0	17.9	18.7	19.8	21.9	25.4	27.2	28.3	
10.0–10.9	329	24.3	5.5	17.6	18.5	19.3	20.9	23.8	27.0	29.1	31.0	
11.0–11.9	302	27.6	6.7	19.5	21.0	21.7	23.2	26.4	30.7	33.5	35.7	
12.0–12.9	323	29.7	6.5	20.4	21.8	23.1	25.5	29.0	33.2	36.3	37.8	
13.0–13.9	360	31.9	7.4	22.8	24.5	25.4	27.1	30.8	35.3	38.1	39.6	
14.0–14.9	370	33.9	7.7	24.0	26.2	27.1	29.0	32.8	36.9	39.8	42.3	
15.0–15.9	309	33.8	7.0	24.4	25.8	27.5	29.2	33.0	37.3	40.2	41.7	
16.0–16.9	343	34.8	8.0	25.2	26.8	28.2	30.0	33.6	38.0	40.2	43.7	
17.0–17.9	291	36.1	8.8	25.9	27.5	28.9	30.7	34.3	39.6	43.4	46.2	
18.0–24.9	2588	29.8	8.4	19.5	21.5	22.8	24.5	28.3	33.1	36.4	39.0	
25.0–29.9	1921	31.1	9.1	20.5	21.9	23.1	25.2	29.4	34.9	38.5	41.9	
30.0–34.9	1619	32.8	10.4	21.1	23.0	24.2	26.3	30.9	36.8	41.2	44.7	
35.0–39.9	1453	34.2	11.5	21.1	23.4	24.7	27.3	31.8	38.7	43.1	46.1	
40.0–44.9	1390	35.2	13.3	21.3	23.4	25.5	27.5	32.3	39.8	45.8	49.5	
45.0–49.9	961	34.9	11.8	21.6	23.1	24.8	27.4	32.5	39.5	44.7	48.4	
50.0–54.9	1004	35.6	11.0	22.2	24.6	25.7	28.3	33.4	40.4	46.1	49.6	
55.0–59.9	879	37.1	13.3	22.8	24.8	26.5	28.7	34.7	42.3	47.3	52.1	
60.0–64.9	1389	36.3	11.3	22.4	24.5	26.3	29.2	34.5	41.1	45.6	49.1	
65.0–69.9	1946	36.3	11.3	21.9	24.5	26.2	28.9	34.6	41.6	46.3	49.6	
70.0–74.9	1463	36.0	10.8	22.2	24.4	26.0	28.8	34.3	41.8	46.4	49.2	

Note: Values for males and females aged 18 Years and older have been adjusted for bone area by subtracting 10.0 cm² and 6.5 cm², respectively, from the calculated mid upper muscle area.

Reproduced from A.R. Frisancho. *Anthropometric Standards for Assessment of Growth and Nutritional Status*, Ann Arbor, MI: University of Michigan Press, 1990

TABLE F-13a   Means, Standard Deviations and Percentiles of Muscle Area (cm²) by Age for Adult Males of Small, Medium and Large Frames

Age (yrs)	N	Mean	SD	5	10	15	25	Percentiles 50	75	85	90	95
Males with small frames												
18.0–24.9	443	45.6	10.6	30.8	33.8	35.8	38.7	44.6	51.3	55.2	58.1	63.2
25.0–29.9	318	48.2	9.8	33.5	36.8	39.2	41.8	47.6	53.5	57.7	61.2	63.7
30.0–34.9	237	49.6	10.2	35.0	37.5	38.9	42.0	48.8	56.4	60.0	62.7	66.9
35.0–39.9	212	51.2	10.4	34.7	38.7	40.9	44.1	50.7	57.5	61.7	63.8	70.0
40.0–44.9	210	51.5	10.1	34.9	38.1	40.6	44.2	51.6	58.2	61.6	64.5	66.9
45.0–49.9	220	49.7	10.8	32.8	36.5	38.9	42.9	49.1	55.7	59.5	63.5	68.8
50.0–54.9	225	49.1	11.2	33.8	36.0	38.2	41.5	47.6	55.5	60.7	63.8	69.3
55.0–59.9	204	47.9	10.1	31.2	35.4	37.8	41.7	47.8	54.3	58.8	61.4	64.2
60.0–64.9	318	48.7	11.2	32.5	36.3	38.7	41.4	48.0	54.6	59.6	62.2	68.0
65.0–69.9	446	45.1	10.7	26.7	31.5	34.7	37.6	44.7	52.5	56.1	58.5	62.7
70.0–74.9	314	43.5	10.3	27.7	30.8	32.9	36.1	43.4	49.6	53.4	56.6	59.9
Males with medium frames												
18.0–24.9	875	50.5	10.5	35.5	38.2	40.8	43.6	49.5	56.5	60.8	63.2	69.3
25.0–29.9	626	54.0	11.3	37.0	40.1	42.9	46.8	53.2	60.9	65.6	67.7	73.0
30.0–34.9	472	55.0	10.4	38.5	42.2	44.8	48.0	54.3	61.8	65.7	68.6	72.7
35.0–39.9	416	56.7	11.7	39.9	43.1	45.2	48.8	55.9	64.0	69.0	71.6	75.0
40.0–44.9	413	56.7	11.0	39.2	42.6	45.8	49.2	56.3	64.0	68.0	71.1	74.4
45.0–49.9	433	56.6	11.2	39.0	42.6	45.6	49.4	55.9	63.7	69.6	72.8	76.2
50.0–54.9	440	55.3	11.7	37.6	41.8	44.5	47.7	54.2	62.5	65.9	69.6	74.1
55.0–59.9	403	55.4	10.8	39.2	42.5	44.4	48.5	54.8	62.2	66.7	69.5	75.0
60.0–64.9	627	52.3	10.8	34.5	38.3	41.6	45.0	52.1	59.2	63.3	66.3	70.4
65.0–69.9	886	49.8	10.5	33.4	37.2	39.6	43.0	49.2	56.7	60.1	62.4	68.1
70.0–74.9	626	47.8	10.8	30.8	34.6	36.9	40.6	47.5	54.4	59.1	62.0	66.8
Males with large frames												
18.0–24.9	431	55.7	12.2	37.6	40.8	43.0	47.3	54.6	63.5	67.0	71.6	76.7
25.0–29.9	305	60.3	12.0	42.6	45.7	48.4	52.6	60.4	67.3	72.8	75.8	81.2
30.0–34.9	230	62.8	13.4	44.2	46.9	49.2	53.3	62.6	70.6	75.3	78.8	84.0
35.0–39.9	203	61.6	13.3	43.2	46.0	48.9	51.8	59.9	70.3	76.6	79.4	82.8
40.0–44.9	204	61.8	12.3	44.9	47.4	49.6	53.2	60.0	69.8	74.4	79.4	83.7
45.0–49.9	214	61.1	13.0	42.9	46.3	48.1	52.4	59.6	67.5	71.1	74.9	86.4
50.0–54.9	214	60.5	12.8	41.8	46.0	47.8	51.6	59.4	67.6	72.5	77.6	85.4
55.0–59.9	198	60.2	12.0	42.3	45.0	47.9	52.9	59.8	66.9	71.8	75.3	83.8
60.0–64.9	311	57.9	12.1	38.9	43.9	46.8	50.1	57.5	65.8	69.0	71.8	77.4
65.0–69.9	439	54.5	12.7	35.6	39.4	41.7	46.0	53.7	62.7	66.9	70.7	75.6
70.0–74.9	310	52.0	12.4	33.2	38.3	40.3	43.6	51.6	59.0	63.8	67.2	72.2

Values for males aged 18 years and older have been adjusted for bone area for subtracting 10.0 cm² from the calculated upper arm muscle area (see text).
Reproduced from A.R. Frisancho. *Anthropometric Standards for Assessment of Growth and Nutritional Status*, Ann Arbor, MI: University of Michigan Press, 1990

TABLE F-13b Means, Standard Deviations and Percentiles of Muscle Area (cm²) by Age for Adult Females of Small, Medium and Large Frames

Age (yrs)	N	Mean	SD	5	10	15	25	50	75	85	90	95
								Percentiles				
Females with small frames												
18.0–24.9	651	26.2	6.0	18.2	19.6	20.7	22.5	25.5	29.2	31.2	32.8	36.2
25.0–29.9	486	27.8	7.4	19.5	20.6	21.6	23.2	26.9	30.8	33.3	35.2	38.1
30.0–34.9	413	28.6	7.8	19.1	21.6	22.4	24.5	27.8	31.4	33.7	36.2	38.8
35.0–39.9	368	29.8	10.1	19.7	21.4	22.9	24.4	28.8	32.5	35.4	37.5	42.2
40.0–44.9	350	29.8	6.6	20.9	22.1	23.4	25.7	28.9	33.2	36.0	37.9	41.8
45.0–49.9	241	29.2	7.4	19.1	21.5	22.6	24.3	28.3	33.3	36.1	38.7	41.2
50.0–54.9	256	30.3	7.3	20.8	22.1	23.9	25.5	29.1	33.4	36.7	38.5	41.3
55.0–59.9	223	30.9	7.6	20.4	22.3	23.6	25.8	30.2	34.8	37.6	41.3	45.1
60.0–64.9	351	31.9	8.7	20.9	22.4	23.6	25.8	31.2	36.4	39.1	41.1	46.2
65.0–69.9	491	31.3	8.1	19.4	22.1	23.7	25.7	30.6	35.4	39.8	41.8	45.7
70.0–74.9	367	32.0	9.9	20.3	22.5	24.1	25.9	30.3	36.1	39.8	42.6	47.3
Females with medium frames												
18.0–24.9	1296	29.3	7.0	19.8	21.9	23.2	24.9	28.4	32.8	35.2	37.2	40.7
25.0–29.9	964	30.0	7.2	20.7	22.1	23.3	25.0	29.0	33.9	36.8	39.0	43.3
30.0–34.9	814	32.0	9.1	21.4	23.1	24.2	26.3	30.8	36.1	39.4	41.8	46.6
35.0–39.9	728	32.7	8.4	21.4	23.6	24.9	27.3	31.4	37.3	40.8	43.0	47.0
40.0–44.9	696	33.7	12.1	21.2	23.2	25.1	27.2	31.6	37.7	43.1	47.1	52.3
45.0–49.9	484	33.8	8.8	22.2	23.6	25.5	27.9	32.2	37.9	42.5	45.4	49.6
50.0–54.9	502	35.0	9.7	22.8	25.2	26.2	28.5	33.7	40.0	43.5	46.7	51.4
55.0–59.9	442	36.3	11.5	23.7	25.3	26.6	28.7	34.5	41.5	44.9	49.2	53.4
60.0–64.9	695	35.1	9.1	23.0	25.3	26.5	29.2	33.9	39.9	43.7	46.1	49.4
65.0–69.9	971	35.7	10.0	22.4	24.8	26.4	29.1	34.6	40.7	44.5	48.1	51.9
70.0–74.9	731	35.3	9.7	22.2	24.3	26.1	28.9	34.0	40.0	44.4	46.7	51.3
Females with large frames												
18.0–24.9	641	34.4	10.7	21.9	23.8	25.3	27.3	31.9	38.7	43.9	47.5	55.8
25.0–29.9	471	36.7	11.5	22.2	25.4	26.8	29.3	34.5	42.0	46.8	50.3	60.1
30.0–34.9	392	36.8	12.3	24.0	25.8	27.3	30.1	36.3	45.1	50.7	55.1	61.2
35.0–39.9	357	41.6	14.4	23.9	27.4	29.1	32.2	39.1	47.2	53.7	61.0	72.1
40.0–44.9	344	43.5	16.6	26.2	28.8	30.5	32.9	40.3	49.5	54.4	58.7	71.6
45.0–49.9	236	43.0	15.8	25.0	28.0	29.4	32.5	39.7	49.0	58.3	62.8	69.9
50.0–54.9	246	42.4	13.1	25.1	28.4	30.1	33.4	39.6	49.5	54.8	59.7	68.4
55.0–59.9	213	45.2	16.9	27.0	30.0	32.4	35.8	42.0	51.0	58.5	62.2	65.7
60.0–64.9	341	43.1	14.2	26.6	29.1	31.2	33.9	40.7	49.8	54.8	57.5	67.6
65.0–69.9	482	42.5	13.4	26.4	28.4	30.6	33.5	40.0	48.7	55.3	58.7	66.5
70.0–74.9	363	41.5	11.6	25.7	28.8	30.2	32.8	40.1	48.7	51.4	54.8	60.3

Values for females aged 18 years and older have been adjusted for bone area by subtracting 6.5cm² from the calcualted mid-upper arm area (see text).

Reproduced from A.R. Frisancho. *Anthropometric Standards for Assessment of Growth and Nutritional Status*, Ann Arbor, MI: University of Michigan Press, 1990

TABLE F-14 Normal 24-hour Creatinine Excretion (mg/24 hours)

Height (cm)	Children aged 0–9 years	Males	Females
50.0	36		
53.5	45		
56.9	55		
60.4	66		
64.4	79		
66.4	85		
69.6	96		
73.8	113		
76.3	124		
80.7	143		
84.7	165		
88.5	189		
94.1	231		
98.0	264		
102.2	290		
105.6	308		
108.7	337		
113.2	385		
117.2	408		
121.5	478		
124.5	528		
126.0	557		
129.0	617		
130.0		448	525
135.0		480	589
140.0		556	653
145.0		684	717
150.0		812	781
155.0		940	845
160.0		1,068	909
165.0		1,196	
170.0		1,324	
175.0		1,452	

The usual creatine excretion rates is 20–26 mg/kg/day in men, and 14–22 mg/kg/day in women.

Adapted from F.E. Viteri and J. Alvardo. The creatinine-height index: its use in the estimation of the degree of protein depletion and repletion in protein-calorie malnourished children. *Pediatrics* 46:(1970) 696–706; J.E. Graystone, Creatinine excretion during growth. In D.B. Cheek, *Human Growth, Body Composition, Cell Growth, Energy, and Intelligence*, 18–97, Philadelphia: Lea & Febiger, 1968.

TABLE F-15 Clinical Evaluation of Nutritional Status

	Clinical findings	Deficiency	Differential diagnosis
Skull	In infants; bossing of the skulls over ossification centers, delayed closure of anterior fontanelle	Vitamin D, calcium	Syphilis, sickle-cell disease, positional deformity, hydrocephalus
	Decreased head circumference	Protein-calorie	
Hair	Dry, wirelike, easily pluckable, brittle, depigmented, sparse	Protein-calorie	
	Impaired keratinization (hair is "steely")	Copper	
	Hair loss	Zinc, biotin, protein, essential fatty acids	
Skin	Malar pigmentation (darkened pigment over malar eminences)	Calories, B complex, especially niacin	Melasma in pregnancy or from oral contraceptives, Addison's disease
	Nasolabial seborrhea	Niacin, riboflavin, B_6	
	Ecchymosis	Vitamin C	Hematologic disorders (thrombocytopenia), trauma, liver disease, anticoagulant overdose, orthostatic purpura, Fabry's disease, emboli, stasis, clotting factor deficiency
	Perifollicular petechiae	Vitamin K	
	Follicular hyperkeratosis (skin is rough, surrounding skin is dry)	Vitamin A	Fungus infection, perifolliculitis or scurvy, keratosis pilaris, Darier's disease
	Xerosis (skin is dry, with fine flaking)	Vitamin A, essential fatty acids	Aging, environmental drying, hypothyroidism, uremia, poor hygiene, ichthyosis
	Hyperpigmentation (seen more frequently on hands and face)	Niacin, folic acid, B_{12}	Addison's disease, environmental factors, trauma
	Scrotal dermatitis	Riboflavin, zinc	Fungus infection
	Pellagrous dermatitis (lesions are symmetric and in areas exposed to the sun)	Niacin	Chemical injury, sunburn, thermal burn
	Thickened skin at pressure points (predominantly in belt area)		
	Delayed wound healing	Zinc, vitamin C, protein	
Eyes	Circumcorneal injection (bilateral)	Riboflavin	
	Xerophthalmia (conjunctiva is dull, lusterless, exhibits a striated or rough surface)	Vitamin A	
	Bitot's spots (small circumscribed, dull, dry lesions usually seen on the lateral aspect of the bulbar conjunctiva)	Vitamin A	Pterygium
	Keratomalacia	Vitamin A	
	Night blindness	Vitamin A	
	Xanthomatosis, hyperlipidemia, and hyper-cholesterolemia leading to localized deposits of lipids	Excess intake of fat with elevated serum lipoproteins	
Lips	Cheilosis (lips may be swollen)	Niacin, riboflavin	Herpes simplex, arid or arctic environmental exposure
	Angular fissures (corners of mouth broken or macerated)	Niacin, riboflavin, iron B_6	Herpes, syphilis
Gums	Bleeding gums (spongy)	Vitamin C	Dilantin toxicity, periodontal disease
Teeth	Dental caries	Fluoride	Poor oral hygiene
	Mottled enamel	Excess fluoride	Staining from tetracyclines

(continued)

TABLE F-15 *(continued)*

	Clinical findings	Deficiency	Differential diagnosis
Tongue	Glossitis (red, painful tongue-may be fissured)	Folic acid, niacin, riboflavin, B_{12}, B_6, iron	Uremia, antibiotics, malignancy, aphthous stomatitis, monilial infection
	Atrophy of filiform papillae (low or absent)	Niacin, folic acid, B_{12}, iron	Non-nutritional anemias
	Hypertrophy of fungiform papillae	General malnutrition	Dietary irritants
	Pale, atrophic tongue	Iron, folic acid, B_{12}, niacin, riboflavin, B_6	Nonnutritional anemias
Exocrine	Parotid enlargement	Protein (?)	Mumps
Endocrine	Goiter	Iodine	Thyroglossal duct cyst, bronchial cleft, cysts and tumors, hyperthyroidism, thyroiditis, thyroid carcinoma
Oral	Dysgeusia (disordered taste)	Zinc	Cancer therapy
	Hypogeusia (loss of taste acuity)		
Nails	Koilonychia (spoon nails; nails are thin, concave)	Iron	Cardiac or pulmonary disease
Cardiac	Cardiac enlargement, tachycardia	Thiamine, iron	
Abdominal	Heptomegaly	Chronic malnutrition	Liver disease
Skeletal	Rickets (bowed legs, deformities may also be seen in pelvic bones)	Calcium, phosphates, vitamin D	Renal rickets, malabsorption, congenital deformity
	Costochondral beading (?)	Calcium, vitamin D	
	Scorbutic rosary (costochondral junctions may have sharp edges caused by epiphyseal separation)	Vitamin C	
	Epiphyseal swelling secondary to epiphyseal hyperplasia (in rickets, secondary to tenderness and swelling caused by hemorrhage)	Vitamin D, calcium, vitamin C	Renal disease, malabsorption, congenital deformity
Neurologic	Absence of tendon reflexes (bilateral)	Thiamine, B_{12}	Peripheral neuropathy from other causes
	Absence of vibratory sense (bilateral)		
	Calf tenderness	Thiamine	
	Pseudoparalysis (movement restricted because of pain)	Vitamin C	Hypokalemia
Extremities	Calf tenderness	Thiamine	Muscle strain, trauma, other causes of peripheral neuropathy, deep venous thrombosis
	Bilateral edema of lower extremities	Protein (occurs late in deficiency)	Congestive heart failure, renal failure, protein-losing enteropathy
Growth	Nutritional dwarfism, subcutaneous fat loss	Calories, protein	
	Dwarfism, hypogonadism	Zinc	

Reproduced with permission from W.W. Walker and K.M. Hendricks, *Manual of Pediatric Nutrition*, Philadelphia: Saunders, 1985

TABLE F-16 Clinical Examination in Nutritional Deficiencies and Excesses

	Major physiologic functions	Deficiency signs	Excess signs	Important food sources
Nutrient				
Protein	Constitutes part of the structure of every cell; regulates body processes as part of enzymes, some hormones, body fluids, and antibodies that increase resistance to infection; provides nitrogen and has caloric density of 4 kcal/g	Dry, depigmented, easily pluckable hair; bilateral, dependent edema, cirrhosis, fatty liver, decreased visceral proteins; skin is dry with pellagroid dermatoses in severe cases	Azotemia, acidosis, hyperammonemia	Meat, poultry, fish, legumes, eggs, cheese, milk and other dairy products, nuts, breast milk, infant formula
Carbohydrate	Supplies energy at an average of 4 kcal/g of glucose (sparing protein) and is the major energy source for CNS function; unrefined, complex carbohydrates supply fiber that aids in normal bowel function	Seizures	May cause diarrhea	Breads, cereals, crackers, potatoes, corn, simple sugars (sugar, honey), fruits and vegetables, milk, breast milk, infant formula
Fat	Concentrated calorie source at an average 9 kcal/g; constitutes part of the structure of every cell; supplies essential fatty acids and provides and carries fat-soluble vitamins (A, D, E, K)	Essential fatty acid deficiency; dry, scaly skin, poor weight gain, hair loss	Atherosclerosis may be affected by excessive intakes of certain dietary fats; altered blood lipid level	Shortening, oil, butter, margarine, protein-rich foods (meat, dairy, nuts) breast milk, infant formula
Fat-Soluble Vitamins				
Vitamin A (serum carotene)	Formation and maintenance of skin and mucous membranes; necessary for the formation of rhodopsin (the photo-sensitive pigment of the rods governing vision in dim light), and regulation of membrane structure and function	Night blindness, degeneration of the retina, xerophthalmia, follicular hyperkeratosis, poor growth, keratomalacia, Bitot's spots	Fatigue, malaise, lethargy, abdominal pain, hepatomegaly, alopecia, headache with increased intracranial pressure, vomiting	Carrots, liver, green vegetables, sweet potatoes, butter, margarine, apricots, melons, peaches, broccoli, cod liver oil, breast milk, infant formula
Vitamin D	Promotes intestinal absorption of calcium and phosphate, renal conservation of calcium and phosphorus	Rickets, osteomalacia, costochondral beading, epiphyseal enlargement, cranial bossing, bowed legs, persistently open anterior fontanelle	Hypercalcemia, vomiting, anorexia, irritability, azotemia, diarrhea, convulsions	Cod liver oil, fish, eggs, liver, butter, fortified milk, sunlight (activation of 7-dehydrocholesterol in the skin), infant formula
Vitamin E	Acts as an antioxidant and free radical scavenger to prevent peroxidation of polyunsaturated fatty acids in the body; enhances absorption and utilization of vitamin A	Hemolytic anemia in the premature and new-born, enhanced fragility of red blood cells, increased peroxidative hemolysis	None known	Oils high in polyunsaturated fatty acids, milk, eggs, breast milk, infant formula
Vitamin K	Necessary for prothrombin and the three blood-clotting factors VII, IX and X; half of the vitamin K in humans is of intestinal origin, synthesized by gut flora; necessary for bone mineralization	Hemorrhagic manifestations (especially in newborns), cirrhosis	Hemolytic anemia, nerve palsy	Green leafy vegetables, fruits, cereals, dairy products, soybeans, breast milk, infant formula

(continued)

TABLE F-16 *(continued)*

Water-Soluble Vitamins

	Major physiologic functions	Deficiency signs	Excess signs	Important food sources
Vitamin C	Forms collagen cross-linkages of proline hydroxylase, thus strengthening tissue and improving wound healing and resistance to infection; aids utilization of iron; is a water-soluble antioxidant and thus protects other lipid-soluble vitamins	Joint tenderness, scurvy (capillary hemorrhaging), impaired wound healing, acute periodontal gingivitis, petechiae, purpura	Increased incidence of renal oxalate stones	Heat-labile; broccoli, papaya, orange, mango, grapefruit, strawberries, tomatoes, potatoes, leafy vegetables, breast milk, infant formula
Thiamine (B$_1$)	Aids in energy utilization as part of a coenzyme component to promote the utilization of carbohydrate; promotes normal functions of the nervous system; co-enzyme for oxidative carboxylation of 2-keto acids	Beriberi, neuritis, edema, cardiac failure, anorexia, restlessness, confusion, loss of vibration sense and deep tendon reflexes, calf tenderness	None known	Pork (lean), and nuts, whole grain and fortified cereal products, breast milk, infant formula
Riboflavin (B$_2$)	Functions primarily as the reactive portion of flavoproteins concerned with biologic oxidations (cellular metabolism)	Cheilosis, glossitis, photophobia, angular stomatitis, corneal vascularization, scrotal skin changes, seborrhea, magenta tongue	None known	Dairy products, liver, almonds, lamb, pork, breast milk, infant formula
Niacin	Aids in energy utilization as part of a coenzyme (NAD$^+$ and NADP$^+$) in fat synthesis, tissue respiration, and carbohydrate utilization; aids digestion and fosters normal appetite; synthesized from the amino acid tryptophan	Pellagra (dermatitis, diarrhea, dementia, death), cheilosis, angular stomatitis, inflammation of mucous membranes, weakness	Dilation of the capillaries, vasomotor instability, "flushing" (utilization of muscle glycogen, serum lipids, mobilization of fatty acids during exercise)	Liver, meat, fish, poultry, peanuts, fortified cereal products, yeast, breast milk, infant formula
Pyridoxine (B$_6$)	Coenzyme component for many of the enzymes of amino acid metabolism	Convulsions, loss of weight, abdominal distress, vomiting, hyper-irritability, depression, confusion, hypochromic and macrocytic anemia	None known	Fish, poultry, meat, wheat, breast milk, infant formula
Folacin	Utilized in carbon transfer and thus nucleotide synthesis	Megaloblastic anemia, stomatitis, glossitis	None known	Liver, leafy vegetables, fruit, breast milk, infant formula
Cobalamin (B$_{12}$; intrinsic factor required)	Cobalamin-containing coenzymes function in the degradation of certain odd-chain fatty acids and in the recycling of tetrahydrofolate	Megaloblastic anemia, neurologic deterioration	None known	Animal products, breast milk, infant formula
Biotin	Component of several carboxylating enzymes; plays an important role in the metabolism of fat and carbohydrate	Anorexia, nausea; vomiting, glossitis; depression; dry, scaly dermatitis; thin hair; loss of eyebrows	None known	Liver, kidney, egg yolk, breast milk, infant formula
Pantothenic Acid	Component of coenzyme A; plays a role in release of energy from carbohydrates and in synthesis and degradation of fatty acids	Infertility, abortion, slowed growth, depression	None known	Meat, fish, poultry, whole grains, legumes, breast milk, infant formula

(continued)

TABLE F-16 Clinical Examination in Nutritional Deficiences and Excesses (*continued*)

	Major physiologic functions	Deficiency signs	Excess signs	Important food sources
Minerals				
Calcium	Essential for calcification of bone (matrix formation); assists in blood clotting; functions in normal muscle contraction and relaxation and in normal nerve transmission	Osteomalacia, osteoporosis	Hypercalcemia (vomiting, anorexia)	Dairy products (i.e., milk, cheese), sardines, oysters, salmon, herring, greens, breast milk, infant formula
Phosphorus	Important intracellular anion; involved in many chemical reactions within the body; necessary for energy turnover (ATP)	Weakness, anorexia, malaise, bone pain, growth arrest	Hypocalcemia (when parathyroid gland not fully functioning)	Dairy products, fish, legumes, pork, breast milk, infant formula
Magnesium	Essential part of many enzyme systems; important for maintaining electrical potential in nerves and muscle membranes and for energy turnover.	Tremor, convulsions, hyperexcitability (hypocalcemic tetany)	Sedation	Widely distributed, especially in food of vegetable origin; breast milk, infant formula
Trace Elements				
Iron	Part of hemoglobin molecule; prevents nutritional anemia and fatigue; increases resistance to infection; functions as a part of enzymes involved in tissue respiration	Anemia, malabsorption, irritability, anorexia, pallor, lethargy	Hemosiderosis, hemochromatosis	Red meats, liver, dried beans and peas, enriched farina, breast milk, iron-fortified infant formula, infant cereal
Zinc	Constituent of enzymes involved in most major metabolic pathways (specifically nucleic acid synthesis for cellular growth and repair)	Growth failure, skin changes, delayed wound healing, hypogeusia, sexual immaturity, hair loss, diarrhea	Acute gastrointestinal upset, vomiting	Whole grains, legumes, beef, lamb, pork, poultry, nuts, seeds, shellfish, eggs, some cheeses, breast milk, infant formula
Iodine	Component of thyroid hormones triiodothyronine and thyroxine, important in regulation of cellular oxidation and growth	Goiter, depressed thyroid function, cretinism	Thyroid suppression (thyrotoxicosis)	Iodized table salt, salt water, fish, shellfish (content of most other goods geographically dependent) breast milk, infant formula
Copper	Constituent of proteins and enzymes, some of which are essential for the proper utilization of iron	Anemia (hemolytic), neutropenia, bone disease	Excess accumulation in the liver, brain, kidney, cornea	Oysters, nuts, liver, kidney, corn-oil margarine, dried legumes
Manganese	Essential part of several enzyme systems involved in protein and energy metabolism and in the formation of mucopolysaccharides	Impaired growth, skeletal abnormalities, lowered reproductive function, neonatal ataxia	In extremely high exposure of contamination: severe psychiatric and neurologic disorders	Nuts, whole grains, dried fruits, fruits, vegetables (nonleafy)

(*continued*)

TABLE F-16 Clinical Examination in Nutritional Deficiences and Excesses (*continued*)

	Major physiologic functions	Deficiency signs	Excess signs	Important food sources
Fluoride	The main target organs of fluoride in humans are the enamel of teeth and bones, where fluoride is incorporated into the crystalline structure of hydroxyapatite and produces increased caries resistance	Poor dentition, caries, osteoporosis	Mottling, brown staining of teeth (in excess of 4 ppm); fluorosis occurs after prolonged (10–20 yrs) ingestion of 20–80 mg/day	Fluoridated water; depends on the geochemical environment and therefore amount in foods varies widely
Chromium	Maintenance of normal glucose metabolism, cofactor for insulin	Disturbed glucose metabolism (lower glucose tolerance caused by insulin resistance)		Brewer's yeast, meat products, cheeses
Selenium	Functions as a part of the enzyme glutathione peroxidase, which protects cellular components from oxidative damage	Cardiomyopathy, probably secondary to oxidative damage	In animals, blindness, abdominal pain, lack of vitality	Seafoods, kidney, liver, meat, grains (depending on growing area)
Molybdenum	Essential for the function of flavin-dependent enzymes involved in the production of uric acid and in the oxidation of aldehydes and sulfites	Not described in humans	Acts as an antagonist to the essential element copper; goutlike syndrome associated with elevated blood levels of molybdenum, uric acid, and xanthine oxidase	Varies considerably, depending on growing environment; main contributions come from meat, grains and legumes

Reproduced with permission from W.A. Walker and K.M. Hendricks, *Manual of Pediatric Nutrition*, Philadelphia: Saunders, 1985.

TABLE F-17   Current Guidelines for Laboratory Evaluation of Nutritional Status

Nutrient and units	Age of subject (yrs)	Deficient	Marginal	Acceptable
		Criteria of Status		
Visceral Protein				
Serum albumin (g/L)*	<1		<25	25+
	1–5		<30	30+
	6–16		<35	35+
	16+	<28	<28–34	35+
	Pregant	<30	<30–34	40–60
Hematological Indices				
Hemoglobin (g/L)	1 wk			130–200
	1 mo			>140
	6–23 mo	<90	90–99	100+
	2–5	<100	100–109	110+
	6–12	<100	100–114	115+
	13–16 M	<120	120–129	130+
	13–16 F	<100	100–114	115+
	16+ M	<120	120–139	140+
	16+ F	<100	100–119	120+
	Pregnant			
	2nd trimester	<95	95–109	110+
	3rd trimester	<90	90–105	—
Hematocrit*	1 wk			0.43–0.66
(volume fraction)	1 mo			>0.50
	3 mo			>0.35
	6 mo–5 yr			>0.38
	6–12	<0.30	0.30–0.35	0.36+
	13–16 M	<0.37	0.37–0.39	0.40+
	13–16 F	<0.31	0.31–0.35	0.36+
	16+ M	<0.37	0.37–0.43	0.44+
	16+ F	<0.31	0.31–0.37	0.33+
	Pregant	<0.30	0.30–0.32	0.33+
Mean corpuscular hemoglobin, pg	All ages			27–35
Mean corpuscular hemoglobin concentration, g/L	All ages			320–360
Mean corpuscular volume (μm3) /L	All ages			80–94

M= male subjects; F= female subjects
*Adapted from the Ten-State Nutritional Survey
†Criteria may vary with methodology
Compiled from *Critical Resources in Clinical Laboratory Sciences*, 119, J. W. King and W.R. Faukner, eds. Cleveland: CRC Press, 1973; D. Ney, Nutritional assessment. In D. G. Kelts and E.G. Jones, eds., *Manual of Pediatric Nutrition*, Boston: Little, Brown, 1984.

TABLE F-18 Laboratory Tests in the Differential Diagnosis of Anemias

Type of anemia	Hgb	Hct	MCV	Serum iron	TIBC	Transferrin saturation	Ferritin	Marrow hemosiderin	Sidero-blasts	RBC	Retic	Other
Iron deficiency	D*	D	D	D	I	D	D	D	D	N	D	Hypochromic, microcytic, or normocytic
Vitamin B$_{12}$	D	D	I	I	D or N	I, D or N	N	I	I	D	D or N	Macrocytic, megaloblastic, hypersegmented neutrophils, low-serum B$_{12}$, thrombocytopenia, leukopenia
Folic acid	D	D	I	I	D or N	I,D, or N	D	I	I	D	D or N	Macrocytic, megaloblastic, normal or slightly low B$_{12}$, decreased red cell folate
Vitamin E	D	D	I or N	I	D	N	N	I	I	D	I	Hemolytic anemia, low serum vitamin E, increased RBC hemolysis, normochromic, normocytic
Anemia of chronic disease	D	D	N	D	D	D	N	N or I	D	D	D	Usually normocytic, normochromic, may be hypochromic, microcytic
Anemia of chronic infection	D	D	N or D	D	D	D or N	I or N	I, N or D	D	D	D	Normochromic and normocytic, may be hypochromic and microcytic

*D: decreased; N: normal; I: increased.
Reproduced with permission from W.A. Walker and K.M. Hendricks, *Manual of Pediatric Nutrition*, Philadelphia: Saunders, 1985.

Nutritional Assessment Tools for Pregnancy

TABLE G-1

NUTRITIONAL ASSESSMENT
FOR
PREGNANT WOMEN

Source	Date

NUTRITIONAL RISK FACTORS

Very overweight	☐	Hypovolemia	☐	Medical/obstet. complications	☐
Underweight	☐	Prev. obstet. complications	☐	Low income	☐
Inadequate gain	☐	Adolescence	☐	Substance abuse	☐
Excessive gain	☐	High parity	☐	Pica	☐
Anemia	☐	Short inter-preg. interval	☐	Psychological problems	☐

VISIT 1

Week gest. _____ Weight _____

BP _____ Alb _____ Ket _____

Comment _____ Glu _____ Edema _____

COMMENTS:

LABORATORY OBSERVATIONS

TEST	Values			
	Date	Date	Date	Date
Hemoglobin (g/dL)				
Hematocrit (%)				
MCV (μ3 or fL)				
Cervical cytology				
1-hour oral glucose load				

DIETARY ASSESSMENT   Daily average from _____ days:

Food Group	Minimum Amt./Serv.	Amt./Serv. Eaten	Sugg. Change
Animal protein	6 oz.		
Vegetable protein	1		
Milk products	3		
Breads/cereals/grains	7		
Vitamin C-rich frt./veg.	1		
Vitamin A-rich frt./veg.	1		
Other fruit/veg.	3		
Unsaturated fats	3		

Excessive: ☐ Fat   ☐ Sugar   ☐ Salt   ☐ Caffeine

California Department of Health Services. MCH/WIC. Nutrition During Pregnancy and the postpartum Period, 6/90.

TABLE G-1 *(continued)*

NUTRITIONAL RISK FACTORS

VISIT 2	Dietary Assessment	Daily avg. from ___ days:

Food Group	Min. Amt./ Serv.	Amt./ Serv. Eaten	Sugg. Change
Animal protein	6 oz.		
Vegetable protein	1		
Milk products	3		
Breads/cereals/grains	7		
Vit. C-rich frt./veg.	1		
Vit. A-rich frt./veg.	1		
Other fruit/veg	3		
Unsaturated fats	3		

VISIT 2

Date_____
Week gest._____
Weight_____
BP_____
Comment_____
Alb_____
Glu_____
Ket_____
Edema_____

Excessive: ☐ Fat ☐ Sugar ☐ Salt ☐ Caffeine

COMMENTS:

VISIT 3

Date_____
Week gest._____
Weight_____
BP_____
Comment_____
Alb_____
Glu_____
Ket_____
Edema_____

Food Group	Min. Amt./ Serv.	Amt./ Serv. Eaten	Sugg. Change
Animal protein	6 oz.		
Vegetable protein	1		
Milk products	3		
Breads/cereals/grains	7		
Vit. C-rich frt./veg.	1		
Vit. A-rich frt./veg.	1		
Other fruit/veg	3		
Unsaturated fats	3		

Excessive: ☐ Fat ☐ Sugar ☐ Salt ☐ Caffeine

COMMENTS:

California Department of Health Services. MCH/WIC. Nutrition During Pregnancy and the postpartum Period, 6/90.

NUTRITIONAL QUESTIONNAIRE FOR PREGNANT WOMEN

Name: _____ I.D.#: _____ Date: _____

Please answer the following questions by checking the appropriate box "yes" or "no" or by filling in the blank. Answer only the questions that apply to you. All information is confidential.

1. a. How many times have you been pregnant?_____

    b. If you have children, list their birth dates and birthweights below.

    Birth date and birthweight   Birth date and birthweight

    _____   _____

    _____   _____

    _____   _____

2. Do you now or have you ever had any of the following?

Yes No		Yes No		Yes No	
☐ ☐	Abnormal pap smear	☐ ☐	Liver disease/hepatitis	☐ ☐	Premature infant
☐ ☐	Allergy/asthma	☐ ☐	Tuberculosis	☐ ☐	Infant weighing less than
☐ ☐	Anemia	☐ ☐	Venereal disease		5.5 lbs. (2,500 g)
☐ ☐	Cancer	☐ ☐	Miiscarriage	☐ ☐	Infant weighing more than
☐ ☐	Diabetes	☐ ☐	Twins/triplets		8 lbs., 13 oz. (4,000 g)
☐ ☐	Heart disease	☐ ☐	Cesarean delivery	☐ ☐	Infant with medical
☐ ☐	High blood pressure	☐ ☐	Excessive bleeding		problems
☐ ☐	Intestinal problems		during/after delivery	☐ ☐	Infant death
☐ ☐	Kidney disease				
☐ ☐	Other_____				

3. Have you had any of the following during this pregnancy?

Yes No		Yes No		Yes No	
☐ ☐	Nausea	☐ ☐	Diarrhea	☐ ☐	Stress
☐ ☐	Vomiting	☐ ☐	Heartburn	☐ ☐	Cold/flu
☐ ☐	Constipation/ hemorrhoids	☐ ☐	Leg cramps	☐ ☐	Other illness _____

4. a. Before this pregnancy, what was your usual weight? _____ Pounds/kilos   ☐ Don't know

    b. If you have been pregnant before, how much weight did you gain during your last pregnancy?

    _____ Pounds/kilos   _____ Don't know

    c. How much weight do you expect to gain during this pregnancy?

    _____ Pounds/kilos   _____ Don't know

5. a. How often do you exercise (besides housework, child care?)_____

    b. What types of exercise do you do?_____

6. During your pregnancy, have you wanted to eat any of the following?

Yes No		Yes No		Yes No	
☐ ☐	Ice/freezer frost	☐ ☐	Laundry starch	☐ ☐	Plaster
☐ ☐	Cornstarch	☐ ☐	Dirt or clay	☐ ☐	Other: _____

7. Are there any foods that you avoid eating?   ☐ Yes ☐ No   If yes, what:_____

    _____ Why? _____

8. Are you now on any of these special diets?

Yes No		Yes No		Yes No	
☐ ☐	Diabetic	☐ ☐	Low salt	☐ ☐	High protein
☐ ☐	Low fat	☐ ☐	Weight loss	☐ ☐	Other: _____

    If yes, who suggested the diet?_____

For office use only

NUTRITIONAL QUESTIONNAIRE FOR PREGNANT WOMEN (continued)

9. a. Are you a vegetarian? ☐ Yes ☐ No
    b. If yes, do you consume milk products (milk, cheese, yogurt) and/or eggs? ☐ Yes ☐ No

10. During this pregnancy, are taking the following?

Yes No		Yes No		Yes No	
☐ ☐	Prenatal vitamin-mineral formula	☐ ☐	Antihistamines/cold remedies	☐ ☐	Birth control pills
☐ ☐	Iron	☐ ☐	Laxatives/antacids	☐ ☐	Other prescription drugs
☐ ☐	Other vitamins	☐ ☐	Other nonprescription drugs	☐ ☐	Marijuana/cocaine
☐ ☐	Other minerals			☐ ☐	Other drugs
☐ ☐	Aspirin				

11. How many cups of the following liquids do you usually drink per day?

    _____ Water   _____ Sodas with sugar   _____ Coffee

    _____ Juice   _____ Diet soda, diet punch   _____ Tea

    _____ Milk   _____ Punch, Kool-Aid, Tang   _____ Other: _____

12. a. How often do you drink beer, wine, hard liquor, or mixed drinks? ☐ Daily ☐ Weekly ☐ Monthly
    b. When you drink, how many drinks do you have? ☐ One ☐ Two ☐ Three ☐ More
    c. During this pregnancy, how many times have you had more than four drinks on any single occasion? _____

13. How many cigarettes do you smoke each day?
    ☐ Do not smoke ☐ Fewer than 10 cigarettes ☐ 11-20 cigarettes ☐ More than 20 cigarettes

14. What is the highest grade or year of regular school you have completed?
    ☐ Less than 6 years   ☐ Two-year college (14 years)
    ☐ Elementary school (6 years)   ☐ Four-year college (16 years)
    ☐ Junior high school (9 years)   ☐ Graduate school (17+ years)
    ☐ High school (12 years)

15. Do you live: ☐ Alone ☐ With own family ☐ With other people

16. Check if you have the following: ☐ Stove ☐ Oven ☐ Refrigerator

17. a. Do you plan your own meals? ☐ Yes ☐ No
    b. Do you buy your own food? ☐ Yes ☐ No
    c. Do you prepare your own food? ☐ Yes ☐ No

18. How would describe the type and amount of food in your household?
    ☐ Enough of the kind you want   ☐ Sometimes not enough
    ☐ Enough, but not always the kind you want ☐ Often not enough

19. Are you receiving any of the following?
    ☐ Food stamps   ☐ Medi-Cal   ☐ Donated food/meals
    ☐ WIC   ☐ AFDC/welfare ☐ Other: _____

20. a. How do you plan to feed your baby?
    ☐ Breast-feed   ☐ Both breast and formula
    ☐ Formula-feed   ☐ Other: _____
    b. Have you ever breast-fed or tried to breast-feed before? ☐ Yes ☐ No
    c. If yes, how long did you breast-feed? _____
    d. Why did you stop breast-feeding? _____

For office use only

Reviewed by:

California Department of Health Services, MCH/WIC, Nutrition During Pregnancy and the Postpartum Period, 4/89.

TABLE G-3

DIETARY INTAKE
RECORD DE COMIDA

<table>
<tr><td colspan="2"></td><td colspan="5" align="center">DO NOT WRITE IN THIS SPACE
NO ESCRIBA EN ESTE EPACIO</td></tr>
<tr><td colspan="2"></td><td colspan="5" align="center">INTAKE SUMMARY</td></tr>
</table>

Name/Nombre				Age/Edad	Height/Altura	Weight/PESO	Animal protein	Veg. protein	Milk products	Breads/cereals/ grains	Vit. C-frt./veg.	Vit. A-frt./veg.	Other fruits/veg.	Unsaturated fats
TIME HORA	PLACE LUGAR	AMOUNT CANTIDAD	FOODS EATEN ALIMENTOS CONSUMIDOS											

INFLUENCES ON DIET, COMMENTS, AND FOLLOW-UP	SUMMARY	Servings eaten								
		Servings needed								
		Difference								

Condition/diagnosis	Visit no.	Weeks gestation	Date	Interviewer

California Department of Health Services. MCH/WIC. Nutrition During Pregnancy and the postpartum Period, 6/90.

TABLE G-4   Guidelines for Laboratory Evaluation of Anemia

Determination	Not acceptable	Determination	Not acceptable
Hemoglobin, g/dL		Serum ferritin (ng/mL)	
12–14-yr female, nonpregnant	<11.8	Female, nonpregnant	<10
15 + yr female, nonpregnant	<12.0	Female, pregnant	<10
Pregnant, first trimester	<11.0	Transferrin saturation (%)	
Pregnant, second trimester	<10.5	Female, nonpregnant	<15
Pregnant, third trimester	<11.0	Female, pregnant	<15
Hematocrit, %		Free erythrocyte protoporphyrin	
12–14-yr female, nonpregnant	<35.5	(mcg/dL RBC)	
15 + yr female, nonpregnant	<36.0	Female, nonpregnant	>70
Pregnant, first trimester	<33.0	Female, pregnant	>70
Pregnant, second trimester	<32.0	Red cell folate, ng/mL	
Pregnant, third trimester	<33.0	All ages	<160
Mean corpuscular volume, cu. microns		Serum folate, ng/mL	
		All ages	<6
Female, nonpregnant	<80 or >101*	Serum vitamin B-12,** pg/mL	
Female, pregnant	<83 or >94*	All ages	<200

* These values indicate risk of folate deficiency.
** Criteria may vary with different methodology.

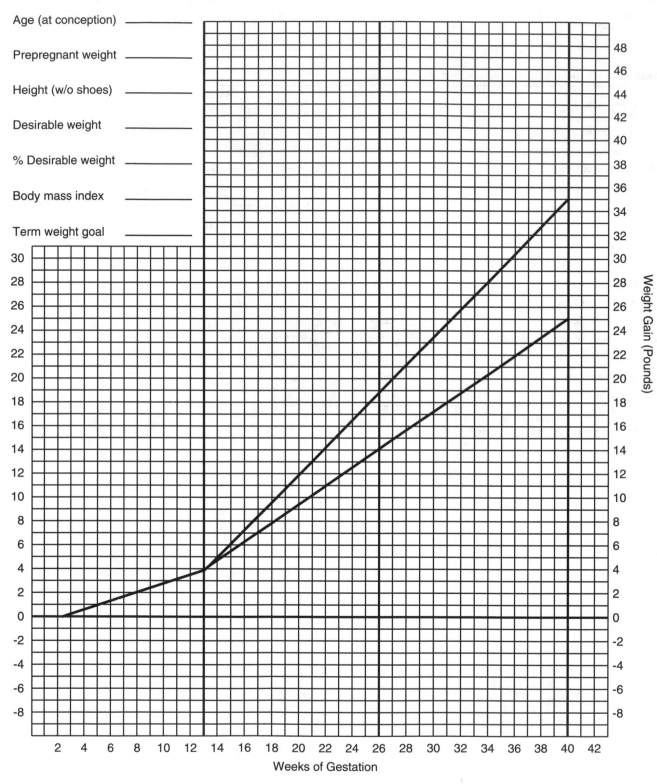

Age (at conception) _____

Prepregnant weight _____

Height (w/o shoes) _____

Desirable weight _____

% Desirable weight _____

Body mass index _____

Term weight goal _____

Weeks of Gestation

Weight Gain (Pounds)

Note: Young adolescents, African American women, and smokers should strive for gains at the upper end of the recommended ranges. Short women (<62 inches) should strive for gains at the lower end of the range.

California Department of Health Services, MCH/WIC. Nutrition During Pregnancy and the Postpartum Period, 6/90.

FIGURE G-1 Prenatal Weight Gain Grid for Normal Weight Women

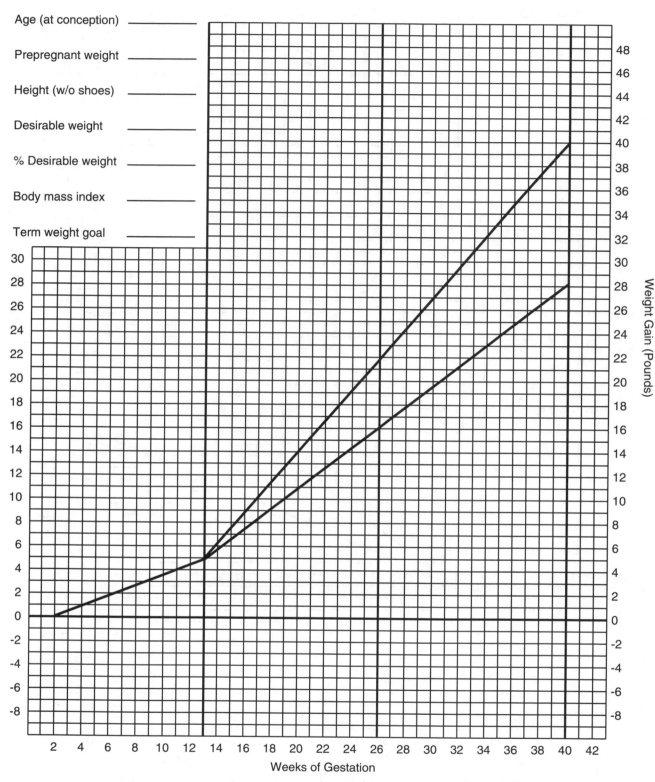

Age (at conception) _____

Prepregnant weight _____

Height (w/o shoes) _____

Desirable weight _____

% Desirable weight _____

Body mass index _____

Term weight goal _____

Weeks of Gestation

Weight Gain (Pounds)

Note: Young adolescents, African American women, and smokers should strive for gains at the upper end of the recommended ranges. Short women (<62 inches) should strive for gains at the lower end of the range.

California Department of Health Services, MCH/WIC. Nutrition During Pregnancy and the Postpartum Period, 6/90.

FIGURE G-2 Prenatal Weight Gain Grid for Underweight Women

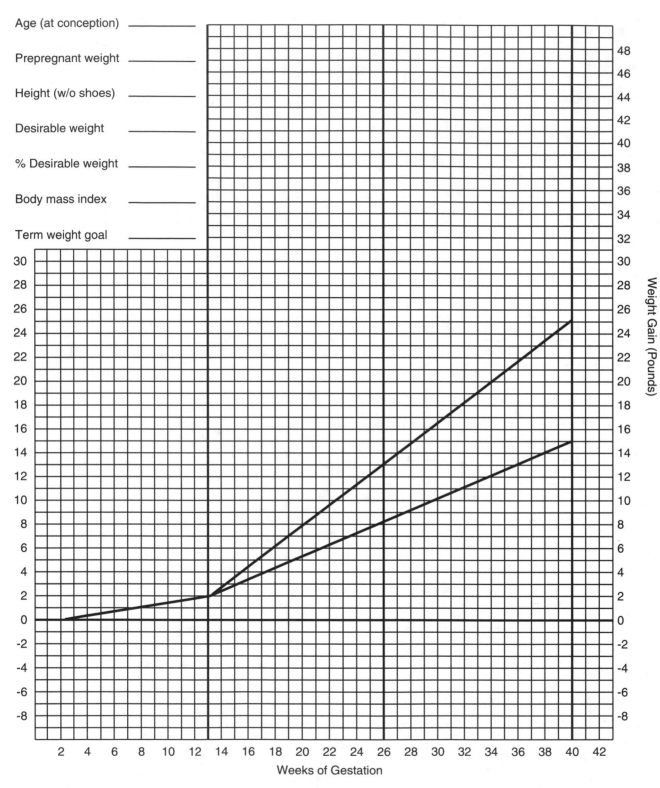

Age (at conception) _____

Prepregnant weight _____

Height (w/o shoes) _____

Desirable weight _____

% Desirable weight _____

Body mass index _____

Term weight goal _____

Weeks of Gestation

Weight Gain (Pounds)

Note: Young adolescents, African American women, and smokers should strive for gains at the upper end of the recommended ranges. Short women (<62 inches) should strive for gains at the lower end of the range. Very overweight women should gain at least 15 pounds.

California Department of Health Services, MCH/WIC. Nutrition During Pregnancy and the Postpartum Period, 6/90.

FIGURE G-3 Prenatal Weight Gain Grid for Overweight Women

Infant Formulas

TABLE H-1 Infant Formula Composition—Infant Formulas for Full-Term Infants

Formula	Manufacturer	Caloric density at normal dilution	Osmolality (mOsm/kg H$_2$O)	Iron (mg/quart)	Protein source	Fat source	Carbohydrate source	Caloric distribution (% kcal; g/100 mL)
Cow's Milk Based								
Carnation Good Start w/Iron	Carnation	20 kcal/fl oz 67 kcal/100 ml	265	9.6	whey hydrolysate	palm olein, high oleic safflower oil coconut oil	lactose, maltodextrim	pro-9.8%; 1.6 g fat-46.0%; 3.4 g cho-44.2%; 7.4 g
Carnation Follow-up Formula w/Iron	Carnation	20 kcal/fl oz 67 kcal/100 ml	345	12.0	nonfat milk	palm oil, high oleic safflower oil, corn oil	glucose high maltose corn syrup, lactose	pro-12%; 2.0 g fat-35%; 2.6 g cho-53%; 8.9 g
Gerber Baby Formula w/Iron; Gerber Baby Formula	Gerber Products Company	20 kcal/fl oz 67 kcal/100 ml	320	11.5 1.0	nonfat milk	soy or corn and coconut oils	lactose	pro-9%; 1.5 g fat-48%; 3.6 g cho-43%; 7.2 g
Enfamil w/Iron; Enfamil	Mead Johnson Nutritionals	20 kcal/fl oz 67 kcal/100 ml	300	12.0 1.0	reduced minerals whey, nonfat milk*	coconut and soy or corn oils	lactose	pro-9%; 1.5 g fat-50%; 3.7 g cho-41%; 6.9 g
Similac w/Iron; Similac	Ross Laboratories	20 kcal/fl oz 67 kcal/100 ml	300	11.5 1.4	nonfat milk	coconut and soy or corn oils	lactose	pro-8.9%; 1.5 g fat48.3%; 3.6 g cho-42.8%; 7.2 g
SMA; SMA Low-Iron	Wyeth-Ayerst Laboratories	20 kcal/fl oz 67 kcal/100 ml	300	11.4 1.4	nonfat milk, reduced minerals, whey*	oleo, coconut, oleic and soy oils	lactose	pro-8.9%; 1.5 g fat-48.6%; 3.6 g cho-42.9%; 7.2 g
Soy Based								
Soyalac	Loma Linda Foods	20 kcal/fl oz 67 kcal/100 ml	240	12.2	soybean solids, L-methionine	soy oil	corn syrup, sucrose, soybean carbohydrate	pro-12.2%; 2.0 g fat-48.2%; 3.6 g cho-39.2%; 6.6 g
I-Soyalac	Loma Linda Foods	20 kcal/fl oz 67 kcal/100 ml	270	12.2	soy protein isolate, L-methionine	soy oil	sucrose, tapioca dextran	pro-12.2%; 2.0 g fat-48.6%; 3.6 g cho-39.2%; 6.6 g
ProSobee	Mead Johnson Nutritionals	20 kcal/fl oz 67 kcal/100 ml	200	12.0	soy protein isolate, L-methionine	coconut and corn or soy oils	corn syrup solids	pro-12%;; 2.0 g fat-48%; 3.6 g cho-40%; 6.7 g
Isomil	Ross laboratories	20 kcal/fl oz 67 kcal/100 ml	240	11.5	soy protein isolate	coconut and soy or corn oils	corn syrup, sucrose	pro-10.6%; 1.8 g fat-49.1%; 3.7 g cho-40.4%; 6.8 g

*Whey: casein ratio is 60:40.

(continued)

426

TABLE H-1 (continued)

Formula	Manufacturer	Caloric density at normal dilution	Osmolality (mOsm/kg H₂0)	Iron (mg/quart)	Protein source	Fat source	Carbohydrate source	Caloric distribution (% kcal; g/100 mL)
Isomil SF	Ross Laboratories	20 kcal/fl oz 67 kcal/100 ml	150	11.5	soy protein isolate	soy and coconut oils, mono- and diglycerides	glucose ploymers	pro-10.6%; 1.8 g fat-49.1%; 3.7 g cho-40.4%; 6.8 g
Nursoy	Wyeth-Ayerst Laboratories	20 kcal/fl oz 67 kcal/100 ml	296	10.9	soy protein isolate	oleo, coconut, oleic and soy oils	sucrose or corn syrup solids	pro-12.3%; 2.1 g fat-47.4%; 3.5 g cho-40.3%; 6.8 g
Cow's Milk + Soy Based								
Advance	Ross Laboratories	16 kcal/fl oz 53 kcal/100 ml	200	9.5	nonfat milk, soy protein isolate	soy and corn oils	corn syrup, lactose	pro-15%; 2.0 g fat-45%; 2.7 g cho-40%; 5.3 g

*Whey: casein ratio is 60:40.

TABLE H-2 Infant Formula Composition—Specialized Infant Formulas Exempt from the Infant Formula Act of 1980 and 1986 Amendments

Manufacturer formula	Caloric density at normal dilution	Osmolality (mOsm/kg H₂0)	Iron (mg/quart)	Protein source	Fat source	Carbohydrate source	Caloric distribution (% kcal)
Preterm & Low-Birthweight Infants							
MEAD JOHNSON NUTRITIONALS:							
Enfamil Premature Formula w/Iron; Enfamil Premature Formula	20 kcal/fl oz 67 kcal/100 mL	240	12.0 1.6	whey protein concentrate, nonfat milk	soy oil, MCT, coconut oil	corn syrup solids, lactose	pro–12% fat–44% cho–44%
Enfamil Premature Formula w/Iron; Enfamil Premature Formula	24 kcal/fl oz 80 kcal/100 mL	300	14.4 1.9	whey protein concentrate, nonfat milk	soy oil, MCT, coconut oil	corn syrup solids, lactose	pro–12% fat–44% cho–44%
Enfamil Human Milk Fortifier	not available	+120 420 (when added to breastmilk)	0	whey protein concentrate, casein	negligible	corn syrup solids, lactose	pro–20% fat–3% cho–77%
ROSS LABORATORIES:							
Similac Special Care 20	20kcal/fl oz 67 kcal/100 mL	250	2.4	nonfat milk, whey protein concentrate	MCT, soy and coconut oils	hydrolyzed cornstarch, lactose	pro–11% fat–47% cho–42%
Similac Special Care 24 w/Iron; Similac Special Care 24	24 kcal/fl oz 80 kcal/100 mL	300	14.2 2.8	nonfat milk, whey protein concentrate	MCT, soy and coconut oils	hydrolyzed cornstarch, lactose	pro–11% fat–47% cho–42%
Similac Natural Care	24 kcal/fl oz 80 kcal/100 mL	300	2.8	nonfat milk, whey protein concentrate	MCT, soy and coconut oils	hydrolyzed cornstarch, lactose	pro–11% fat–47% cho–42%
Similac PM 60/40	20kcal/fl oz 67 kcal/100 mL	280	1.4	whey protein concentrate, sodium caseinate	corn and coconut oils	lactose	pro–9% fat–50% cho–41%
WYETH-AYERST LABORATORIES:							
"Preemie" SMA 20	20 kcal/fl oz 67 kcal/100 mL	268	2.8	nonfat milk, whey protein concentrate	coconut, oleic, oleo, and soy oils, MCT	maltodextrins, lactose	pro–11.9% fat 46.7% cho–41.5%
"Preemie" SMA 24	24 kcal/fl oz 80 kcal/100 mL	280	2.8	nonfat milk, whey protein concentrate	coconut, oleic, oleo, and soy oils, MCT	maltodextrins, lactose	pro–9.6% fat–48.5% cho–41.9%

(continued)

TABLE H-2 *(continued)*

Manufacturer formula	Caloric density at normal dilution	Osmolality (mOsm/kg H$_2$0)	Iron (mg/quart)	Protein source	Fat source	Carbohydrate source	Caloric distribution (% kcal)
Special Indication Formulas							
MEAD JOHNSON NUTRITIONALS:							
Nutramigen	20 kcal/fl oz 67 kcal/100 mL	320	12	casein hydrolysate, amino acids	corn oil	corn syrup solids, modified cornstarch	pro-11% fat-35% cho-54%
Pregestimil	20 kcal/fl oz 67 kcal/100 mL	320	12	casein hydrolysate, amino acids	corn oil, MCT, high oleic safflower oil	corn syrup solids, modified cornstarch, dextrose	pro-11% fat-48% cho-41%
Portagen	20 kcal/fl oz 67 kcal/100 mL	230	12	sodium caseinate	MCT, corn oil	cornsyrup solids, sucrose	pro-14% fat 40% cho-46%
ROSS LABORATORIES							
Alimentum Protein Hydrolysate	20 kcal/fl oz 67 kcal/100 mL	370	11.4	amino acids, peptides	MCT, safflower and corn oils	sucrose, tapioca starch	pro-11% fat-48% cho-41%
Calcilo XD	20 kcal/fl oz 67 kcal/100 mL	280	1.4	whey protein concentrate, sodium caseinate	corn and coconut oils	lactose	pro-9% fat-50% cho-41%
RCF-Ross Carbohydrate Free	20 kcal/fl oz 67 kcal/100 mL	74	1.4	soy protein isolate	soy and coconut oils	none	pro-11% fat-48% cho-41%
WYETH-AYERST LABORATORIES:							
S-14	20 kcal/fl oz 67 kcal/100 mL	280	11.8	nonfat milk	oleo, coconut, oleic, and soybean oils	lactose	pro-5.6% fat-50.4% cho-43.0%
S-29 and S-44	20 kcal/fl oz 67 kcal/100 mL	360	11.8	reduced minerals, whey, whey protein concentrate	oleo, coconut, oleic, and soybean oils	lactose	pro-10.3% fat-30.1% cho-59.6%

APPENDIX
I

Growth Charts

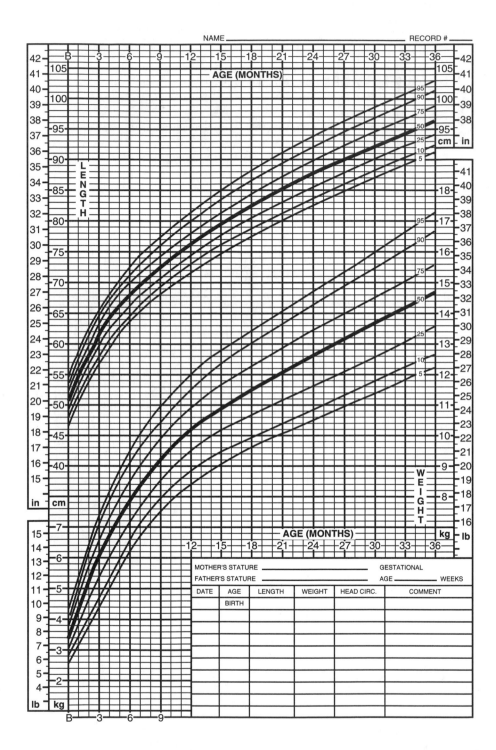

FIGURE I-1   Boys: Birth to 36 months physical growth, NCHS percentiles. (Adapted with permission from P.V.V. Hamill, T.A. Drizd, C.L. Johnson, R.B. Reed, A.F. Roche, and W.M. Moore. Physical growth: National Center for Health Statistics percentiles. *Am. J. Clin. Nutr.* 32:(1979)607–629. Data from the Fels Research Institute, Wright State University School of Medicine, Yellow Springs, OH. Used with permissions of Ross Products Division, Abbott Laboratories, Columbus, OH 43216, from NCHS Growth Charts, © 1982. *Ross Products Division, Abbott Laboratories.*

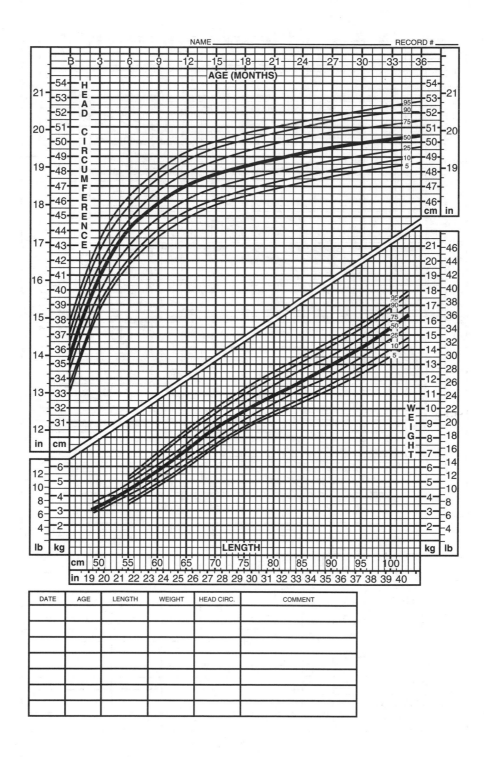

FIGURE I-2 Boys: Birth to 36 months physical growth, NCHS percentiles. (Adapted with permission from P.V.V. Hamill, T.A. Drizd, C.L. Johnson, R.B. Reed, A.F. Roche, and W.M. Moore. Physical growth: National Center for Health Statistics percentiles. *Am. J. Clin. Nutr.* 32:(1979)607–629. Data from the Fels Research Institute, Wright State University School of Medicine, Yellow Springs, OH. Used with permissions of Ross Products Division, Abbott Laboratories, Columbus, OH 43216, from NCHS Growth Charts, © 1982. *Ross Products Division, Abbott Laboratories.*

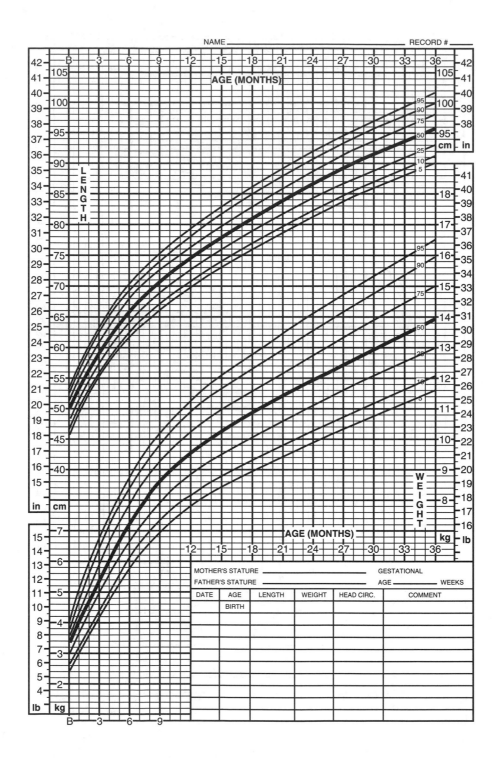

FIGURE I-3 Girls: Birth to 36 months physical growth, NCHS percentiles. (Adapted with permission from P.V.V. Hamill, T.A. Drizd, C.L. Johnson, R.B. Reed, A.F. Roche, and W.M. Moore. Physical growth: National Center for Health Statistics percentiles. *Am. J. Clin. Nutr.* 32:(1979)607–629. Data from the Fels Research Institute, Wright State University School of Medicine, Yellow Springs, OH. Used with permissions of Ross Products Division, Abbott Laboratories, Columbus, OH 43216, from NCHS Growth Charts, © 1982. *Ross Products Division, Abbott Laboratories.*

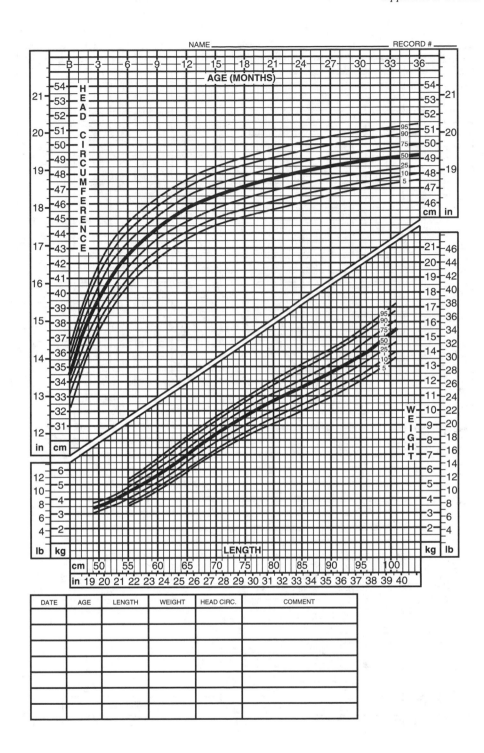

DATE	AGE	LENGTH	WEIGHT	HEAD CIRC.	COMMENT

FIGURE I-4 Girls: Birth to 36 months physical growth, NCHS percentiles. (Adapted with permission from P.V.V. Hamill, T.A. Drizd, C.L. Johnson, R.B. Reed, A.F. Roche, and W.M. Moore. Physical growth: National Center for Health Statistics percentiles. *Am. J. Clin. Nutr.* 32:(1979)607–629. Data from the Fels Research Institute, Wright State University School of Medicine, Yellow Springs, OH. Used with permissions of Ross Products Division, Abbott Laboratories, Columbus, OH 43216, from NCHS Growth Charts, © 1982. *Ross Products Division, Abbott Laboratories.*

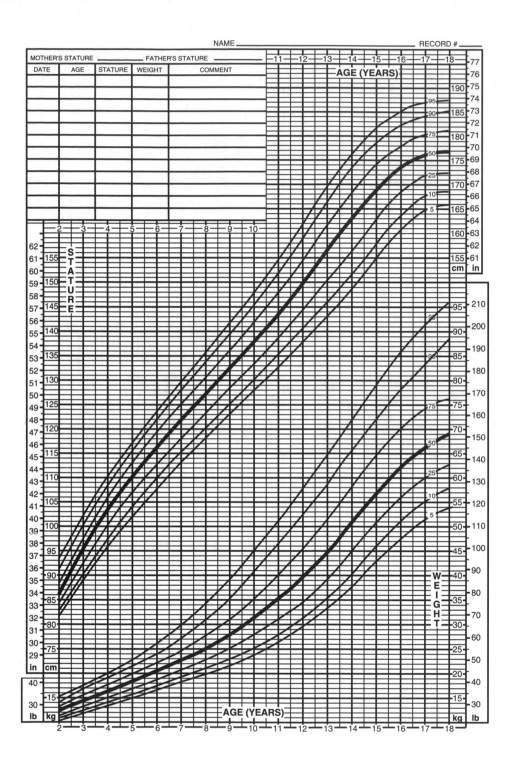

FIGURE I-5 Boys: 2 to 18 years physical growth, NCHS percentiles. (Adapted with permission from P.V.V. Hamill, T.A. Drizd, C.L. Johnson, R.B. Reed, A.F. Roche, and W.M. Moore. Physical growth: National Center for Health Statistics percentiles. *Am. J. Clin. Nutr.* 32:(1979)607–629. Data from the Fels Research Institute, Wright State University School of Medicine, Yellow Springs, OH. Used with permissions of Ross Products Division, Abbott Laboratories, Columbus, OH 43216, from NCHS Growth Charts, © 1982. *Ross Products Division, Abbott Laboratories.*

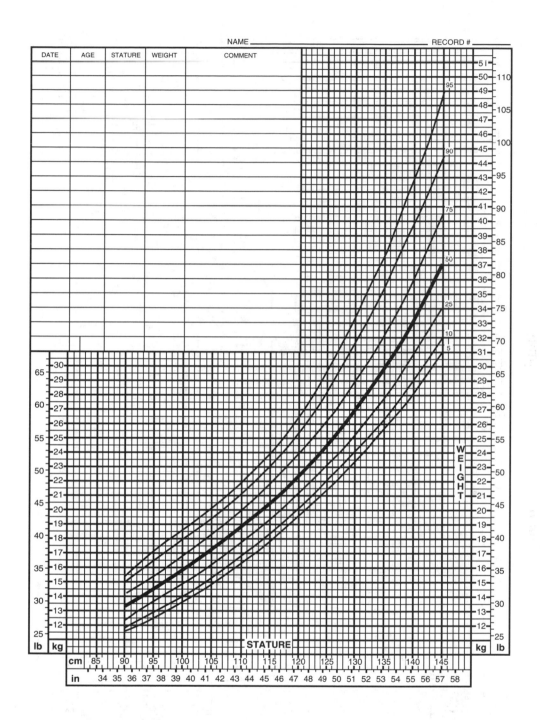

FIGURE I-6 Boys: Prepubescent physical growth, NCHS percentiles. (Adapted with permission from P.V.V. Hamill, T.A. Drizd, C.L. Johnson, R.B. Reed, A.F. Roche, and W.M. Moore. Physical growth: National Center for Health Statistics percentiles. *Am. J. Clin. Nutr.* 32:(1979)607–629. Data from the National Center for Health Statistics (NCHS), Hyattsville, MD, Used with permissions of Ross Products Division, Abbott Laboratories, Columbus, OH 43216, from NCHS Growth Charts, © 1982. *Ross Products Division, Abbott Laboratories.*

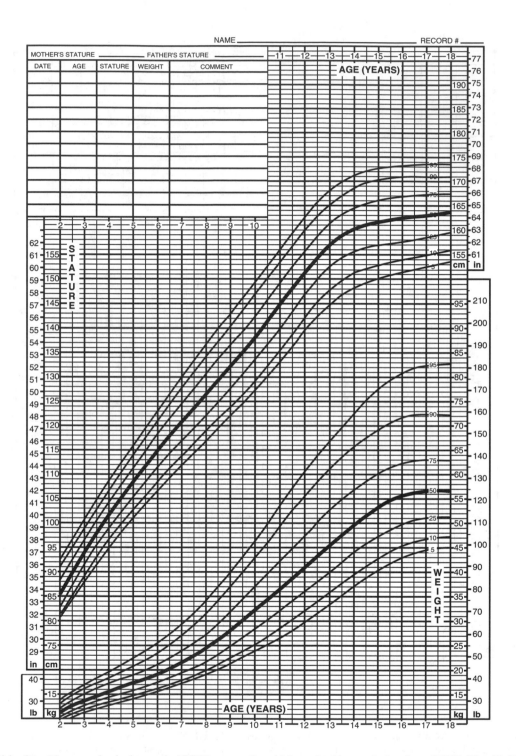

FIGURE I-7   Girls: 2 to 18 years physical growth, NCHS percentiles. (Adapted with permission from P.V.V. Hamill, T.A. Drizd, C.L. Johnson, R.B. Reed, A.F. Roche, and W.M. Moore. Physical growth: National Center for Health Statistics percentiles. *Am. J. Clin. Nutr.* 32:(1979)607–629. Data from the National Center for Health Statistics (NCHS), Hyattsville, MD, Used with permissions of Ross Products Division, Abbott Laboratories, Columbus, OH 43216, from NCHS Growth Charts, © 1982. *Ross Products Division, Abbott Laboratories.*

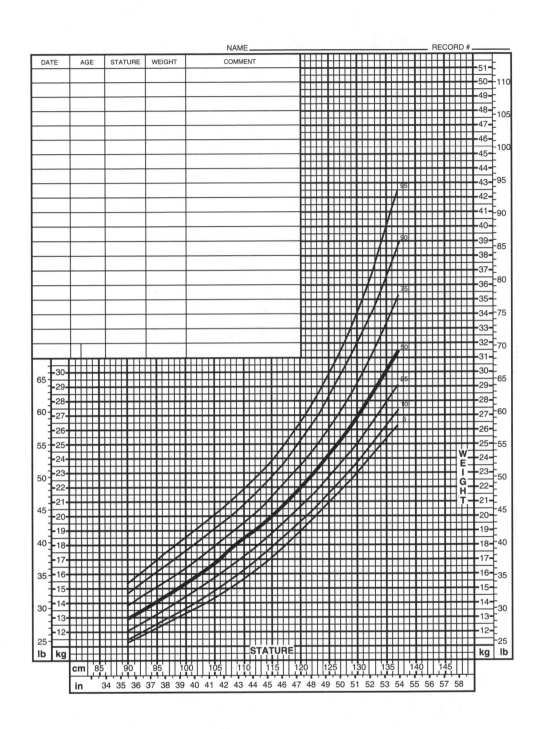

FIGURE I-8 Girls: Prepubescent physical growth, NCHS percentiles. (Adapted with permission from P.V.V. Hamill, T.A. Drizd, C.L. Johnson, R.B. Reed, A.F. Roche, and W.M. Moore. Physical growth: National Center for Health Statistics percentiles. *Am. J. Clin. Nutr.* 32:(1979)607–629. Data from the National Center for Health Statistics (NCHS), Hyattsville, MD, Used with permissions of Ross Products Division, Abbott Laboratories, Columbus, OH 43216, from NCHS Growth Charts, © 1982. *Ross Products Division, Abbott Laboratories.*

APPENDIX J

Characteristic Food Choices of Cultural Groups

TABLE J-1 Characteristic African American Food Choices

Protein foods	Milk products	Breads & cereals	Vegetables	Fruits	Fats & oils	Beverages, condiments, other foods	Preparation methods
Legumes:	Cheese:	Biscuits	Beans, green	Apple	Bacon	Beverages:	Frying, boiling
black-eyed peas	American	Bread:	Broccoli	Banana	Butter	coffee	Overcooked
kidney beans	cheddar	white	Cabbage	Grapefruit	Cream	Kool Aid	vegetables
pinto beans	cottage	Cereals, cooked	Carrots	Grapes	Gravy	fruit drinks	Barbecuing
red beans	Ice Cream	hominy grits	Corn	Lemon	Lard	fruit punch	High-sodium
Meat:	Milk:	Cereals, dry	Greens:	Nectarine	Salt pork	soda	foods
beef	buttermilk	Cornbread	chard	Orange	Shortening	tea	
ham	evaporated	Crackers	collard	Peach	Vegetable oil	pot liquor	
hot dogs	fluid	Macaroni	kale	Pineapple	Chitterlings	Sauces:	
luncheon meats	Milkshakes	Muffins	mustard	Plums		barbecue	
organ meats		Pancakes	pokeweed	Tangerine			
pork sausage		Rice	spinach turnip	Watermelon			
Nuts:		Rolls	Lettuce				
peanuts		Spaghetti	Lima beans				
peanut butter			Okra				
Poultry:			Peas				
chicken			Potato				
eggs			Pumpkin				
turkey			Sweet potato				
Seafood:			Tomato				
catfish			Yam				
perch							
red snapper							
salmon							
sardines							
shrimp							

Compiled from *Nutrition During Pregnancy and the Postpartum Period: A Manual for Health Professionals*. Sacramento, CA: California Department of Health Services, 1990; L.D. McBean, Diet and Nutrition related consensus of blacks and other ethnic minorities. *Dairy Council Digests* 59(6): 1-6, 1988; and P. Kittler and K. Sucher, *Food and Culture in America*. New York: Van Nostrand, 1989.

TABLE J-2 Characteristic Native American Foods

Protein foods	Milk products	Breads and cereals	Vegetables	Fruits	Fats & oils	Beverages, condiments, other foods
Legumes:	Buttermilk	Cornmeal (blue or yellow)	Squash	Berries	Lard	Culinary ash from juniper or green cedar
kidney beans	Yogurt	Flours made from acorn, wheat, or rye	Pumpkin	Lemons	Butter	Coffee
pinto beans	Cottage cheese	Tortillas	Carrots	Oranges	Margarine	Tea
lentils	Monterey jack cheese	Fry bread from white flour	Onions	Melons	Cooking oil	Soft drinks
peanuts	Nonfat dry milk in cooking	Cornbread	Potatoes	Grapefruit	Pinon nuts	Sugar
Meat:	Evaporated milk	Rice	Celery	Dried fruit:		Candy
beef		Bean bread (bean and cornmeal mix)	Cabbage	cherries		Jams
lamb/mutton			Peas	berries		Jellies
pork		Ta fulla (hominy and bean ashes)	Greens:	grapes		
goat			dandelion	Apples		
wild when available:		Rice	mustard	Pears		
rabbit		Sugared cereals	turnip	Bananas		
venison			milkweed	Peaches		
groundhog			Corn	Pineapple		
canned and cured meats			Eggplant			
Nuts:			Green beans			
pinenuts			Cucumbers			
acorn			Wild tullies (tuber)			
Poultry			Beets			
chicken			Cassava			
wild geese						
wild duck						
eggs						
Fish						
fresh fish						
roe						
Eggs						

Compiled from *Nutrition During Pregnancy and the Postpartum Period: A Manual for Health Professionals.* Sacramento, CA: California Department of Health Services, 1990; L.D. McBean, Diet and Nutrition related consensus of blacks and other ethnic minorities. *Dairy Council Digests* 59(6): 1–6, 1988; and P. Kittler and K. Sucher, *Food and Culture in America.* New York: Van Nostrand, 1989.

TABLE J-3 Food Plans for Selected European Ethnic Groups

	Italian	Greek	German/Hungarian	Polish	Czechoslovak
Milk Group	Very little milk used; cheese popular, *casiscavallo; gorgonzola, locatelli, Parmesan, provolone, mozarella, ricotta;* ice cream desserts as gelati, spumoni, and tortoni.	Cow, goat, or sheep milk (boiled for children); many cheeses, *feta* cheese popular, fermented milk (*yaourti*) for dessert	Milk, buttermilk, sour milk, or cream used in cooking, cottage, cream, and brick cheese in cheese cake, strudels, and noodle dishes.	Cow or goat milk; sour cream on vegetables, meats, salads; cream in soup, Brick, cottage and cream cheese. Cottage cheese in kuchens and dumplings.	Cow milk (fresh for children), fermented milk and buttermilk (preferred by adults). Cheese from sheep milk preferred. Use in baking.
Bread-Cereal	Cornmeal (*polenta*), farina, macaroni, spaghetti and similar *pastas;* crusty Italian white bread, whole wheat bread (facaccia); pizza.	Corn, rice, wheat	Barley, farina, rye, *mehl* (Hungarian flour); noodles, dumplings (*spaetzel*), strudel.	Barley, buckwheat, cornmeal, oats, rice, rye, whole wheat, kasha (buckwheat), oats, millet; rice in meats and vegetables; barley and kasha in soup; dark rye bread with every meal.	Corn, rye, wheat. Cornmeal as a mush; white flour in pastry and dumplings; sour rye bread preferred.
Vegetable Group	Artichokes, string beans, broccoli, cauliflower, celery, chicory, Savoy cabbage, dandelion greens, endive, eggplant, fennel, garlic, mushrooms, peas, peppers, radishes, romaine, spinach, Italian squash and tomatoes. Greens are served raw with oil and wine, tomatoes are cooked into sauce, soups, or cooked with meat or fish.	Cabbage, cauliflower, cucumbers, eggplant, greens, okra, onions, peppers, some potatoes, vine leaves, zucchini, tomatoes, salad greens, oranges, and lemons. Boiled or fried in a small amount of olive oil, served hot or cold, cooked with meat and fish. Lemon juice on salads and cold foods.	Cabbage (red and white), carrots, cauliflower, cucumbers, beets, beans, broccoli, kale, kohlrabi, onions, potatoes, sauerkraut, tomatoes, and lettuce. Lettuce with bacon and hot vinegar, red cabbage with bacon sauce, potato salad with herring.	Butter beans, cabbage, carrots, cucumbers, kale, lettuce, mushrooms, onions, parsnips, potatoes, sauerkraut, sorrel, radishes, leeks, turnips, beets, and split peas. Cabbage (sauerkraut) and root vegetables primarily. Potatoes at most of the meals. Vegetables cooked with meat (pig's knuckles) and noodles, cabbage, and split peas, stuffed cabbage, potato pancakes, and borscht (beet soup).	Beets, cabbage, carrots, cauliflower, celeriac, kale, leeks, mushrooms, parsnips, potatoes, spinach, turnips, and tomatoes; potatoes and vegetables boiled and served with cream. Cabbage as sauerkraut.
Fruit Group	Fresh, glazed and dried fruits, grapes, pears, plums, melons, quinces, cherries, peaches, figs, dates, apricots, apples, oranges, persimmon, and raisins. Served for dessert.	Apricots, cherries, dates, figs, grapes, melons, nuts, plums, peaches, pears, quinces, and raisins. Served as dessert. Grapes are pressed into wine or dried as raisins.	Apples, apricots, bananas, cherries, berries, grapes, melons, oranges, quinces, pears, peaches, and prunes for dessert.	Apples, apricots, cherries, grapes, pears, plums, prunes, and strawberries in fruit, soup, dried or raw.	Apples, apricots, berries, cherries, pears, plums, and some imported bananas, pineapple, dried fruits, citrus fruits, raw or preserved; dried fruits in baking.

(continued)

TABLE J-3 (continued)

	Italian	Greek	German/Hungarian	Polish	Czechoslovak
Meat Group	Beef, lamb, veal, pork, fowl, and sausages, bologna and salami. Small quantity of meat slow simmered, served with sauce, such as tomato sauce, prepared with garlic, onion, green peppers, tomato; or fried. Usually cut up and stewed, fried or ground and cooked with pasta such as chicken cacciatora, veal (cutlet) scallopine, meat balls with tomato sauce; all fish, and clams, mussels, octopus, fresh sardines, squid and snails; eggs, dried beans, lentils and peas. Eggs fried plain or with spinach, onions, and peppers; used as thickening agent; and omelet with cheese. Dried beans, lentils and peas cooked in thick soups such as *minestrone* and *pastafasiole.*	Lamb, some beef, goat, mutton, pork products; poultry; cut into small pieces or ground. Poultry is cooked into broth. Lamb is cooked on skewers or cut up and browned in oil or fat with rice or flour and vegetables. Salt water fish (fresh, smoked, or salted), shellfish, smoked roe, squid, and octopus; fried or steamed with vegetables, used frequently. Eggs, white beans and legumes, boiled, mashed, stewed, and eaten either hot or cold. Soup made of dried beans, onions, celery, and carrots is a national dish. Eggs are popular.	Beef (muscle and organs), pork, veal, bacon, sausage, poultry (especially goose), and game; fresh-water fish and shrimp; in stews served with dumplings or noodles as chicken and anchovies, beef and noodle soup, beans with pork, veal and peas, and crawfish and tomatoes. Eggs, used in noodles, as thickening agent, or as garnish.	Beef, pork (ham), veal (lungs, tongue, tripe, brain, liver, kidneys), fowl, geese, and salami; all varieties of fish, fresh in summer, pickled in winter; eggs, in soups and dumplings.	Beef, pork (fresh and smoked), veal, poultry; fresh water fish; eggs, in cooking and baking, lentils, yellow peas, kidney and white beans, boiled, cooked in soups or stews, or served as a relish.
Other	Fats: Olive or cotton seed oil, lard, salt pork. Desserts: Fruit, fancy cakes, chestnuts, gelati (brick ice cream), marzipan (almond cakes), spumone ice cream, and tortoni; served on feast days and special occasions. Seasoning: Aniseed, cloves, garlic, onions, parsley, pepper, salt, thyme, vinegar. Beverages: Coffee with hot milk and sugar, dry wines in cooking and as beverage for adults, and liquors.	Fats: Olive oil, seed oils, salted black olives, and little butter. Seasoning: Caraway and pumpkin seeds, herbs, honey, nuts (hazel, pignolia, and pistachio), and sesame; seeds and nuts as snack or dessert. Beverages: Coffee and wine at meals.	Fats: Butter in cooking and meat fats. Desserts: Fruits, cheese cakes and strudels. Seasonings: Caraway seed, horseradish, garlic, onions, paprika, peppers, pickles, poppy seed, parsley, and vinegar. Beverages: Tea, coffee, beer, Tokay wine, schnapps, and Hungarian whiskey.	Desserts: Fruits, cookies, small cakes and pancakes with preserves. Seasonings: Almonds, chili sauce, dried mushrooms, horseradish, mace, onions, pickles, poppy seeds, peppers, and saffron. Beverages: Tea, coffee, Polish beer.	Fats: Butter for baking, lard in cooking, poultry fat spread on bread. Seasonings: Caraway, poppy, and sesame seeds, garlic, honey, dried mushrooms, nuts, and spices. Beverages: Coffee, cocoa, beer (Czech), and wine (Slovak).

TABLE J-4 Characteristic Mexican-American Food Choices

Protein foods	Milk products	Breads and cereals	Vegetables	Fruits	Fats & oils	Beverages, condiments, other foods
Legumes: black beans garbanzo beans kidney beans lentils pinto beans	Cheese: American Monterey jack queso fresco Ice Cream ("helado" or "nieve")	Bread: sweet ("pan dulce") white Cereals, cooked: oatmeal	Beans, green Cabbage Cactus leaf (nopales) Carrots	Banana Cactus fruit (prickly pear, tunas) Guava	Avocado Bacon Cracklings (chicharrones) Cream	Beverages: beer coffee cornstarch drinks (atole de maizena)
Meat: beef luncheon meats (carnes frias) organ meats pork sausage (chorizo)	Milk: condensed evaporated flavored fluid Licuado Yogurt	Cereals, dry: cornflakes Cornmeal (masa harina) Cornstarch (maizena) Pasta (fideo) Rice; rice pudding	Cauliflower Cilantro Corn Cucumber Lettuce Onion Peas	Lemon Lime Mango Melon Orange Papaya Peach	Lard (manteca) Sour cream Vegetable oil	fruit drinks (aqua de fruta) herb teas yerba buena, mint, camomile Kool-Aid sodas
Nuts: peanuts peanut butter Poultry: chicken eggs, raw or cooked	Custard (flan)	Tortillas: corn wheat Atole (oats, flour, cornstarch and hot milk)	Peppers: chile sweet Potato Spinach Squash: chayote zucchini squash flowers	Persimmon Pineapple Plantain Pomegranate Sapote (zapote) Strawberries Tangerine		Sauces: mole salsa
Seafood: crab fish shrimp			Sweet potato Tomatillo Tomato			

Compiled from *Nutrition During Pregnancy and the Postpartum Period: A Manual for Health Professionals*. Sacramento, CA: California Department of Health Services, 1990; L.D. McBean, Diet and Nutrition related consensus of blacks and other ethnic minorities. *Dairy Council Digests* 59(6): 1-6, 1988; and P. Kittler and K. Sucher, *Food and Culture in America*. New York: Van Nostrand, 1989

TABLE J-5 Typical Diets of Indochinese Refugees in Minnesota

Group	Breakfast	Lunch & dinner	Snacks
Vietnamese	Soup—"pho"—containing rice noodles, thin slices of beef or chicken, bean sprouts, and greens *or* Boiled eggs and crusty bread *or* Rice and leftover meat Tea or coffee	Rice (prefer long-grain) Fish and/or meat and vegetable dish Fish sauce-"nuoc mam" Clear soup with vegetables and/or meat Tea, coffee, soft drinks, or alcoholic beverages	Fruits Clear soup Rice
Laotian	Rice (prefer sweet, glutinous) Boiled egg, roasted meat, or fish with sauce Tea or coffee	Fish—"padek"—and/or meat stew with hot peppers and other vegetables Rice Cucumber salad Tea, coffee, soft drinks, or alcoholic beverages	Bananas Stew
Cambodian	Soup with meat and noodles or rice Tea or coffee	Rice Fermented fish—"prahoc" Fish sauce—"tuk-trey"—with cabbage, cucumbers, and/or turnips Tea, coffee, soft drinks, or alcoholic beverages	Sweets made from palm sugar Bananas Clear soup
Hmong*	(Most adults do not eat breakfast but may eat first meal early in day. Children eat cereal and milk, or egg and American-type bread.)	Chicken, pork, and/or fish, vegetables, and rice or noodles *or* Tofu, rice (short-grain), and vegetables *or* Rice and soup containing meat and vegetables Tea, coffee, juice, or soft drinks	Fruits Commercial baked goods

*Most Hmong eat only two daily meals, the menus for which are listed in the lunch and dinner column. Some families eat meals early and other families eat late. Typical times of early first and second meals are 7:00 AM and 3:30 PM; late first and second meals are eaten at 11:00 AM and 6:00 PM.

Reproduced with permission from P.L. Splett, Indochinese refugees in the WIC program, *WIC Currents* 7(1981)7-20.

Formula Feeding Products

TABLE K-1 Oral Supplementary Feedings

Product	Composition (Source) Carbohydrate (g/100 kcal)	Protein (g/100 kcal)	Fat (g/100 kcal)	Caloric Density (Kcal/mL)	Lactose	Residue	Notes
Citrisource[a] (liquid)	20	5 (whey protein concentrate)	0	0.76	No	Low	Osmolality 700 mOsm/kg C: N ratio 105:1 Low Na and K for renal disease
Citrotein[a] (powder)	18.25 (Maltodextrins, sucrose)	6.25 (Egg albumin)	0.26 (Soy oil, monoglycerides diglycerides)	0.66	No	Low	Protein and vitamin supplement to clear liquid diet 263.4 g dry weight needed to give 1,000 kcal; 3.1 mEq Na/dL; 1.8 mEq K/dL Nonpro C:N ration = 76.1. Gluten free; 496 mOsm/kg
Delmark Eggnog[b]	13 (nonfat dry milk, malodextrins, sugar)	5.25 (nonfat dry milk, egg white, egg yolk solids)	3.0 (Cottonseed oil, soy oil, egg yolk)	1.16	Yes		
Delmark Milkshake[b]	12.5 (Sugar, maltodextrins, ice cream mix)	3.8 (Egg, milk)	3.85 (Vegetable oil)	0.95	Yes		
Dietene[a]	15.75 (Nonfat milk, sucrose)	8.75 (Nonfat milk)	0.2	0.8	Yes		Add powder to milk.
dp High p.e.r. Protein[c]	2.0	20.6	1.0	2.58 kcal/g			Protein supplement; low electrolyte; 258 g dry weight to give 1,000 kcal.
Duocal[d]	15.5 (Maltodextrins)	0	47 (Vegetable: 34% MCT, 23% linoleate)	4.7	No	Low	Energy supplement; low electrolyte; 100 g = 28 mg Na, 3.5 mg K.
Forta Pudding[e]	13.6 (Sucrose, modified starch)	2.72 (Nonfat milk)	3.88 (Soy oil)	1.69	Yes		Vanilla, chocolate, butterschotch, tapioca. 240 mg Na/serving; 330 mg K/serving.
Gevral[f]	6.68 (Lactose, sucrose)	17.1 (Ca Caseinate)	0.57 (Milk fat)	0.653	Yes	Low	Protein-calorie supplement; artificial flavors; 248.8 g dry weight to give 1,000 kcal.
Lolactene[a]	13 (Corn syrup solids, sucrose)	6.6 (Caseinate)	2.3 (Vegetable oil, mono and diglycerides)	0.8	Low	None	1.150 mL gives 1,100 kcal.
Lonalac[g]	30 (Lactose)	21 (Casein)	49 (coconut oil)	0.67	High	Low	Low Na (4 mg/dL); high K, high protein; do not reconstitute with water high in Na.
MCT Duocal[d]	15.7 Malodextrins	0	4.94 (82.5% MCT: 12.5% linoleate; 5% LCT vegetable oil)	4.7	No	Low	Energy supplement; 100 g contains 175 mg Na and 6 mg K.

(continued)

| Product | Compostion (Source) | | | Caloric Density (Kcal/mL) | Lactose | Residue | Notes |
	Carbohydrate (g/100 kcal)	Protein (g/100 kcal)	Fat (g/100 kcal)				
Nutrex broth[h]	87 (Corn syrup solids)	13 (Caseinate)	0	1.39	No	Low	Clear soup: chicken, beef, vegetable. PER=2.5; Nonpro C:N ratio=175:1; mOsm/kg=350.
Nutrex CLD[h]	12.9 (Sucrose)	11.4 (Egg white solids; gelatin)	0	0.95	No	Low	Clear gel; semisolid; mOsm/kg = 680
Nutrex drink[h]	20 (Corn syrup solids; sucrose)	5.3 (Egg white solids)	0	0.71	No	Low	Clear liquid diet; six flavors
Nutrex Protamin[h]	15 (Corn syrup solids; sucrose)	3.1 (Caseinate)	3 (Corn oil)	1.27	No	Low	Full liquid diet; three flavors; mOsm/kg = 450.
Nutricare[i]	11.8 (Maltodextrins; sucrose)	5.7 (Whey protein concentrate)	3.2 (Whey concentrate lecithin)	1.16	Yes		Mix with 8 oz. whole milk per serving
Opti[j]	82.2 (Glucose polymers; fructose)	15.3 (lactalbumen; BCAA)	<2	1.5	No	Low	Non pro C:N 136:1;
Peptamen Oral[k]	51 (Maltodextrim; sucrose; starch)	16 (Hydrolyzed whey protein)	33 (70% MCT; sunflower seed oil)	1.0	No	Low	Nonpro C:N 131:1; 380 mOsm/kg; Contains taurine,carnitine
Restore Plus	5.5 (Corn syrup, sucrose)	15 (Caseinate)	30 (Corn oil)	1.5	No	Low	Oral use only; Low cholesterol
Ross SLD[e] (840)	78 (Hydrolyzed cornstarch; sucrose)	21.4 (Egg white solids)	0.6	0.7	No	Low	Clear liquid; 3.6 mEq N/dL and 2.1 mEq K/dL; Nonpro C:N ratio = 92:1; mOsm/kg = 545.
Sustacal Pudding[f]	53 (Nonfat milk; sucrose)	11 (Milk)	36 (Soy oil)	48/oz.	Yes		Vanilla, chocolate, butterscotch; 120 mg Na per serving; 46.2 mOsm per 5 oz. serving; Nonpro C:N ratio = 200:1.

[a]Sandoz
[b]Delmark
[c]General Mills
[d]Scientific Hospital Supplies
[e]Ross Laboratories
[f]Clintec
[g]Mead Johnson Nutriitionals
[h]Nutrex
[i]Advanced Healthcare
[j]Metagenics
Note: The composition of these products is subject to change. Current product literature should be consulted before use. This table is not intended to be comprehensive.

TABLE K-2 Sources of Single Nutrients

Product (form)	Composition (Source)			Caloric Density	Osmolality (mOsm/kg)	Lactose	Residue	Notes
	Carbohydrate (g/100 kcal)	Protein (g/100 kcal)	Lipid (g/100 kcal)					
Protein sources								
Casec[a] (powder)	0	23.78 (caseinate)	0.54	3.7/g		No	Low	Add to liquid or food; 270 g gives 1,000 kcal; low Na; no vitamins.
Dialume[b] (powder)	17.22	6.9	Trace	3.6/g	918 at 1:5 dilution	No		For oral or tube feeding; contains all essential amino acids, cystine, and histidine; gluten-free; orange flavor tartrazine-free; 168 mg. Na and 9.2 mg K/10 g.
Elementra	0.52	21	1.36	3.8/g		No	Low	
Maxipro HBV[b] (powder)	Trace	22.56	1.02	3.09/g	165 at 1:5 dilution	Trace		For oral or tube feeding: 230 mg Na and 450 mg K/100g; gluten-free
ProMix[d] (powder)	1.39	20.85 (whey protein)	1.1	3.52g		No		Add to liquids; no vitamins.
ProMod[e] (powder)	2.4	18.9 (whey protein)	2	4.3/g		0.4/5 g protein		Add to liquids; unflavored.
Pro-pac[f] (powder)	1.25	19.2 (whey protein)	20	4/g		Yes		Add to liquids; no vitamins.
Carbohydrate sources								
Cal-Power[c] (liquid)	27.2 (deionized corn syrup)	0.06	0	1.8/mL		No		For oral or tube feeding: 550 g gives 1,000 kcal; 30 mg Na and 3 mg K/8 fl. oz.; high osmolality.
Controlyte[g] (powder)	14.3 (cornstarch hydrolysate)	Trace	4.8 (soy oil)	2.0/mL 5.0/g	598	No	Low	For oral or tube feeding; add to liquid or food; high osmolality; 198 g gives 1,000 kcal; 60 mg Na and 16 mg K/14-oz. can.
Hy-Cal[h] (liquid)	24.41	0.01	0.01	2.5/mL	2,781	No	Low	Oral supplement; 16 mg Na and 0.7 mg K/4 oz.; 407 mL gives 1,000 kcal.
L.C. Liquid Carbohydrate Supplement[d]	25 (glucose polymers)	0	0	2.5/mL		No		
Liquid Maxijul[b] (liquid)	26.7 (maltodextrins)	0	0	1.87/mL	400	No	Low	55% Maxijul powder in water; 23 mg Na and 0.42 mg K/dL.
Maxijul[b] (powder)	25.6 (maltodextrins)	0	0	3.75/g	525 in 40% solution	No	Low	Oral use; 46 mg Na and 3.9 mg K/100g.

(continued)

TABLE K-2 (continued)

Product (form)	Composition (Source)			Caloric Density	Osmolality (mOsm/kg)	Lactose	Residue	Notes
	Carbohydrate (g/100 kcal)	Protein (g/100 kcal)	Lipid (g/100 kcal)					
Maxijul LE[b] (powder)	25.6 (maltodextrins)	0	0	3.75/g	525 in 40% solution	No	Low	Oral use; 0.23 mg Na and 0.4 mg K/100g.
Pure Carbohydrate Supplement[d] (powder)	25 (glucose polymers)	0	0	4/g	131 at usual dilution	No	Low	
Moducal[a] (liquid or powder)	25 (maltodextrins)	0	0	2/mL; 3.8/g	725 (liquid 206/60 g in 250 mL water	No	Low	
Pedialyte[ae]	25	0	0	0.2/mL				Calorie and electrolyte source.
Polycose[ae] (liquid or powder)	25 (hydrolyzed cornstarch)	0	0	2.8/mL 3.8 g	570	No	Low	100 g powder contains 380 kcal, 110 mg K; 100 mL liquid contains 200 kcal, 70 mg Na, and 6 mg K.
Sumacal[f] (liquid or powder)	25 (maltodextrins)	0	0	3.8/g	680	No	Low	150 mg Na and 40 mg K/12-oz. bottle.
Sumacal Plus[f] (powder)	32.	0	0	2.5/g	890	No	Low	Low electrolyte.
Lipid sources								
Calogen[h] (liquid)	0	0	11.1 (Arachis oil)	4.5/mL		No	Low	Long-chain triglycerides; 77% linoleate; 20.7 mg Na and 19.6 mg K/100 mL.
High Fat Supplement[i] (powder)	6.5	0.75	7.7(Partly hyrogenated corn oil)	6.12/g				
MCT Oil[a] (liquid)	0	0	12.05 (Coconut oil fraction)	8.3/mL	Negligible	No		Oral supplement; 60% C$_8$ and 24% C$_{10}$ fatty acids; 120.5 g gives 1,000 kcal; low electrolytes
Microlipid[f] (liquid)	0	0	11.11 (Soy, corn, or safflower oil)	4.5/mL	80	No	Low	Oral supplement; P:S = 7.3:1; 73.7% linoleate; low electrolyte.

(continued)

TABLE K-2 Sources of Single Nutrients *(continued)*

| Product (form) | Composition (Source) | | | Caloric Density | Osmolality (mOsm/kg) | Lactose | Residue | Notes |
	Carbohydrate (g/100 kcal)	Protein (g/100 kcal)	Lipid (g/100 kcal)					
Electrolyte sources								
Lytren[a] (powder)	25.3	0	0	0.333/g	290	No	Low	Electrolytes (mEq/L:Na, 30; K, 25: Ca.4; Mg,, 4; citrate, 36; SO$_4$, 4; Cl, 25; PO$_4$,5.
Pedialyte Maintenance Solution	25.0	0	0	0.333/g	250	No	Low	Electrolytes (mEq/L): Na, 45; K,20; Cl 35; citrate, 30.
Pedialyte RS	25.0	0	0	0.333/g	305	No	Low	Electrolytes (mEq/L): Na, 75; K,20; Cl, 65; citrate, 30; rehydration solution.
Resol[j]	25	0	24 g/dL		290	No	Low	Electrolytes (mEq/L): Na, 50; K, 20; Cl, 50; Ca, 4; Mg, 4, citrate, 34.

[a] Sandoz
[b] Delmark
[c] General Mills
[d] Scientific Hospital Supplies
[e] Ross Laboratories
[f] Clintec
[g] Mead Johnson Nutritionals
[h] Nutrex
[i] Advanced Healthcare
[j] Metagenics

Note: The composition of these products is subject to change. Current product literature should be consulted before use. This table is not intended to be comprehensive.

TABLE K-3 Complete Liquid Formula Diets

Product	Source	Form	Concentration (Kcal/mL)	Protein Source	Protein g/1000 Kcal	Protein % Kcal	Carbohydrate Source	Carb g/1000 Kcal	Carb % Kcal	Fat Source	Fat g/1000 Kcal	Fat % Kcal	MC:LCT Ratio	Osmolality (mOsm/kgH₂O)	Volume To Meet 100% US RDA For Vit/Min (mL)*	Nonprotein Calorie: Nitrogen Ratio
Elemental Formulas																
Accupep™ HPF	Sherwood Medical	Powder	1.0	Hydrolyzed Lactabumin	40	16	Maltodextrin	188.8	75.5	MCT Oil, Corn Oil	10	8.5	50:50	490	1600	134:1
AlitraQ™	Ross	Powder	1.0	Soy & Lactalbumin Hydrolysate, Whey Protein Concentrate, Free Amino Acids	52.5	21	Hydrolyzed Cornstarch, Sucrose, Fructose	65	66	MCT, Safflower Oil	15.5	13	53:47	575	1500	120:1
Criticare® HN	Mead Johnson	Liquid	1.06	Enzymatically Hydrolyzed Casein	36	14	Maltodextrin, Modified Cornstarch	208	83	Safflower Oil	4.7	3	No MCT	650	1890	148:1
Peptamen® Diet	Clintec	Liquid	1.0	Enzymatically Hydrolyzed Whey	40	16	Maltodextrin, Starch	127	51	MCT Oil, Sunflower Oil, Lecithin	39	33	70:30	270	1500	131:1
Peptamen®—Oral Diet	Clinitec	Liquid	1.0	Enzymatically Hydrolyzed Whey	40	16	Maltodextrin, Sucrose, Starch	127	51	MCT Oil, Sunflower Oil, Lecithin	39	33	70:30	380	1500	131:1
Reabilan®	Elan Pharma	Liquid	1.0	Enzymatically Hydrolyzed, Whey Casein	31.5	12.5	Maltodextrin, Tapioca Starch	131.5	52.5	MCT Oil, Soy Oil, Oneothera Biennis Oil, Soy Lecithin	38.9	35	40:60	350	3000	175:1
Reabilan® HN	Elan Pharma	Liquid	1.33	Enzymatically Hydrolyzed Whey, Casein	44	17.5	Maltodextrin, Tapioca Starch	119	47.5	MCT Oil, Soy Oil, Oneothera Biennis Oil, Soy Lecithin	39	35	40:60	490	2857	125:1
Tolerex®	Sandoz	Powder	1.0	Free Amino Acids	21	8	Glucose Oligosaccharides	230	91	Safflower Oil	1.5	1	No MCT	550	3160	282:1
Vital® HN	Ross	Powder	1.0	Partially Hydrolyzed Whey, Meat, Soy, Free Essential Amino Acids	41.7	16.7	Hydrolyzed Cornstarch, Sucrose	185	73.9	Safflower Oil, MCT Oil	10.8	9.4	45:55	500	1500	125:1
Vivonex® TEN	Sandoz	Powder	1.0	Free Amino Acids	38	15	Maltodextrin, Modified Starch		82	Safflower Oil	2.8	3	No MCT	630	2000	149:1

*For vitamin and mineral content, see pages 463 to 466.

(continued)

TABLE K-3 (continued)

Product	Source	Form	Concentration (Kcal/mL)	Protein Source	Protein g/1000 Kcal	Protein % Kcal	Carbohydrate Source	Carbohydrate g/1000 Kcal	Carbohydrate % Kcal	Fat Source	Fat g/1000 Kcal	Fat % Kcal	n6:n3	MCT:LCT Ratio	Osmolality (mOsm/kg H₂O)	Volume To Meet 100% US RDA For Vit/Min (mL)*	Nonprotein Calorie: Nitrogen Ratio
Standard Intake Protein Formulas																	
Attain®	Sherwood Medical	Liquid	1.0	Sodium, Calcium Caseinates	40	16	Maltodextrin	135	54	Corn Oil, MCT	35	30	N/A	50:50	300	1250	134:1
Comply®	Sherwood Medical	Liquid	1.0	Sodium, Calcium Caseinates	40	16	Hydrolyzed Cornstarch (Sucrose only in flavored)	120	48	Corn Oil	40	36	N/A	No MCT	410	1000	134:1
Deliver 2.0	Mead Johnson	Liquid	1.06	Casein, Soy	42	17	Maltodextrin	117	47	Soy Oil, MCT	42	36	N/A	40:60	300	1179	125:1
Ensure®	Ross	Liquid	1.06	Sodium, Calcium Caseinates, Soy Protein Isolate	35.2	14	Corn Syrup, Sucrose	137.2	54.5	Corn Oil	35.2	31.5	N/A	No MCT	470	1887	153:1
Ensure® HN	Ross	Liquid	1.06	Sodium, Calcium Caseinates, Soy Protein Isolate	42	16.7	Corn Syrup, Sucrose	113.6	53.2	Corn Oil	33.6	30.1	N/A	No MCT	470	1321	125:1
Ensure® Plus	Ross	Liquid	1.5	Sodium, Calcium Caseinates, Soy Protein Isolate	36.6	14.7	Corn Syrup, Sucrose	133.2	53.3	Corn Oil	35.5	32	N/A	No MCT	690	1420	146:1
Ensure® Plus HN	Ross	Liquid	1.5	Sodium, Calcium Caseinates, Soy Protein Isolate	41.7	16.7	Hydrolyzed Cornstarch, Sucrose	133.2	53.3	Corn Oil	33.2	30	N/A	No MCT	650	947	125:1
Entrition™ 0.5 Diet	Clintec	Liquid	0.5	Casein	35	14	Maltodextrin	136	54.5	Corn Oil	35	31.5	N/A	No MCT	120	4000	153:1
Entrition™ HN Diet	Clintec	Liquid	1.0	Casein, Soy	44	17.6	Maltodextrin	114	45.6	Corn Oil	41	36.8	N/A	No MCT	300	1300	117:1
Isocal®	Mead Johnson	Liquid	1.06	Casein, Soy	32	13	Maltodextrin	125	50	Soy Oil, MCT	42	37	N/A	20:80	300	1890	167:1
Isocal® HCN	Mead Johnson	Liquid	2.0	Casein	38	15	Corn Syrup	100	40	Soy Oil, MCT	51	45	N/A	30:70	690	1000	145:1
Isolan®	Elan Pharma	Liquid	1.06	Caseinates	38	15.1	Maltodextrin	136	54.3	Corn Oil, MCT	34	30.6	N/A	50:50	300	1250	139:1
Isosource®	Sandoz	Liquid	1.2	Sodium, Calcium Caseinates, Soy Protein Isolate	36	14	Hydrolyzed Cornstarch	140	56	Canola Oil, MCT	34	30	N/A	53:47	360	1500	148:1
Isosource® HN	Sandoz	Liquid	1.2	Sodium, Calcium Caseinates, Soy Protein Isolate	44	18	Hydrolyzed Cornstarch	130	52	Canola Oil, MCT	34	30	N/A	53:47	330	1500	116:1

*For vitamin and mineral content, see pages 463 to 466.

(continued)

TABLE K-3 Complete Liquid Formula Diets *(continued)*

Product	Source	Form	Concentration (Kcal/mL)	Protein Source	Protein g/1000 Kcal	Protein % Kcal	Carbohydrate Source	CHO g/1000 Kcal	CHO % Kcal	Fat Source	Fat g/1000 Kcal	Fat % Kcal	n6:n3	MCT:LCT Ratio	Osmolality (mOsm/kgH₂O)	Volume To Meet 100% US RDA For Vit/Min (mL)*	Nonprotein Calorie: Nitrogen Ratio
Lipisorb®	Mead Johnson	Powder	1.0	Sodium Caseinate	35	14	Corn Syrup Solids, Sucrose	117	46	MCT, Corn Oil	48	40	N/A	86:14	320	2000	157:1
Magnacal®	Sherwood Medical	Liquid	2.0	Sodium, Calcium Caseinates	35	14	Maltodextrin, Sucrose	125	50	Soy Oil	40	36	N/A	No MCT	590	1000	157:1
Nutren® 1.0 Diet	Clintec	Liquid	1.0	Casein	40	16	Maltodextrin, Corn Syrup Solids	127	51	MCT, Canola Oil, Corn Oil, Lecithin	38	33	4:1	24:76	300–390	1500	131:1
Nutren® 1.5 Diet	Clintec	Liquid	1.5	Casein	40	16	Maltodextrin	113	45	MCT, Canola Oil, Corn Oil, Lecithin	45	39	4:1	48:52	410–590	1000	131:1
Nutren® 2.0 Diet	Clintec	Liquid	2.0	Casein	40	16	Corn Syrup Solids, Maltodextrin, Sucrose	98	39	MCT Canola Oil, Lecithin	53	45	4:1	73:27	710	750	131:1
Nutrilan®	Elan Pharma	Liquid	1.06	Caseinates	36	14:4	Maltodextrin, Sugar	135	54.1	Corn Oil, MCT	35	31.5	N/A	19:81	450	1585	149:1
Osmolite®	Ross	Liquid	1.06	Sodium, Calcium Caseinates, Soy Protein Isolate	35.2	14	Glucose Polymers	137.2	54.6	MCT, Corn Oil, Soy Oil	36.4	31.4	N/A	50:50	300	1887	153:1
Osmolite® HN	Ross	Liquid	1.06	Sodium, Calcium Caseinates, Soy Protein Isolate	42	16.7	Glucose Polymers	133.6	53.3	MCT, Corn Oil, Soy Oail	34.8	30	N/A	50:50	300	1321	125:1
Resource® Liquid	Sandoz	Liquid	1.06	Sodium, Calcium Caseinates, Soy Protein Isolate	35	14	Hydrolyzed Cornstarch, Sugar	140	54	Corn Oil	35	32	N/A	No MCT	430	1890	154:1
Resource® Plus	Sandoz	Liquid	1.5	Sodium, Calcium Caseinates, Soy Protein Isolate	37	15	Hydrolyzed Cornstarch, Sugar	130	53	Corn Oil	35	32	N/A	No MCT	600	1400	146:1
Sustacal® 8.8	Mead Johnson	Liquid	1.06	Casein, Soy Protein Isolate	35.2	14	Corn Syrup, Sucrose	140	56	Soy Oil	33.2	30	N/A	No MCT	500	1890	153:1
Sustacal® HC	Mead Johnson	Liquid	1.5	Casein	41	16	Corn Syrup Solids, Sucrose	127	50	Corn Oil	39	34	N/A	No MCT	650	1200	134:1
TwoCal® HN	Ross	Liquid	2.0	Sodium, Calcium Caseinates	41.7	16.7	Hydrolyzed Cornstarch, Sucrose	108.2	43.2	Corn Oil, MCT	45.3	40.1	N/A	20:80	690	950	125:1
Ultralan®	Elan Pharma	Liquid	1.5	Caseinates, Soy Isolate	40	16	Maltodextrin	135	54	Corn Oil, MCT	33	30	N/A	50:50	610	1000	131:1

*For vitamin and mineral content, see pages 463 to 466.

(continued)

TABLE K-3 Complete Liquid Formula Diets *(continued)*

Product	Source	Form	Concentration (Kcal/mL)	Protein Source	Protein g/1000 Kcal	Protein % Kcal	Carbohydrate Source	Carbohydrate g/1000 Kcal	Carbohydrate % Kcal	Fat Source	Fat g/1000 Kcal	Fat % Kcal	Fat n6:n3	MC:LCT Ratio	Osmolality (mOsm/kgH₂O)	Volume To Meet 100% US RDA For Vit/Min (mL)*	Nonprotein Caloric: Nitrogen Ratio
High Protein Formulas																	
Citrotein®	Sandoz Nutrition	Powder	0.67	Egg White Solids	62	25	Sugar, Maltodextrin	183	73	Soybean Oil	2.4	2	1.0	No MCT	480	1100	76:1
Isotein® HN	Sandoz Nutrition	Powder	1.19	Delactosed Lactalbumin	57	23	Hydrolyzed Cornstarch, Fructose	130	52	Partially Hydrogenated Soybean Oil, MCT	29	25	N/A	19:81	300	1770	86:1
Nitrolan®	Elan Pharma	Liquid	1.24	Caseinates	48	19.3	Maltodextrin	129	51.6	Corn Oil, MCT	32	29	N/A	50:50	310	1250	104:1
Promote®	Ross	Liquid	1.0	Sodium Calcium Caseinates, Soy Protein Isolate	62.4	25	Hydrolyzed Cornstarch, Sucrose	130	52	Hi-Oleic Safflower Oil, Canola Oil, MCT	26	23	6.8:1	20:80	350	1250	75:1
Replete ®—Oral	Clintec	Liquid	1.0	Casein	62.5	25	Maltodextrin, Sucrose	113	45	Corn Oil, Lecithin	34	30	N/A	No MCT	350	1500	75:1
Sustacal®	Mead Johnson	Liquid	1.0	Casein, Soy	61	24	Corn Syrup, Sucrose	140	55	Partially Hydrogenated Soy Oil	23	21	20.5:1	No MCT	620	1080	79:1

*For vitamin and mineral content, see pages 463 to 466.

(continued)

TABLE K-3 Complete Liquid Formula Diets *(continued)*

Product	Source	Form	Concentration (Kcal/mL)	Protein Source	Protein g/1000 Kcal	Protein % Kcal	Carbohydrate Source	Carbohydrate g/1000 Kcal	Carbohydrate % Kcal	Fat Source	Fat g/1000 Kcal	Fat % Kcal	MC:LCT Ratio	Osmolality (mOsm/kgH₂O)	Volume To Meet 100% US RDA For Vit/Min (mL)*	Nonprotein Calorie: Nitrogen Ratio	Fiber Source	Fiber g/1000 Kcal
Intact Protein Formulas with Fiber																		
Ensure® with Fiber	Ross	Liquid	1.1	Sodium, Calcium Caseinates, Soy Protein Isolate	36	14.5	Hydrolyzed Cornstarch, Sucrose	147	55	Corn Oil	34	30.5	No MCT	480	1530	148:1	Soy Polysaccharide	13.1
Fiberlan®	Elan Pharma	Liquid	1.2	Sodium, Calcium Caseinates	42	16.7	Maltodextrin	133	53.3	Corn Oil, MCT	33	30	50:50	310	1250	122:1	Soy Polysaccharide	12
Fibersource®	Sandoz	Liquid	1.2	Sodium, Calcium Caseinates	36	14	Hydrolyzed Cornstarch	140	56	Canola Oil, MCT	34	30	53:47	390	1800	151:1	Soy Polysaccharide	8
Fibersource HN	Sandoz	Liquid	1.2	Sodium, Calcium Caseinates	44	18	Hydrolyzed Cornstarch	130	52	Canola Oil, MCT	34	30	53:47	390	1800	118:1	Soy Polysaccharide	6
Jevity®	Ross	Liquid	1.06	Sodium, Calcium Caseinates	42	16.7	Hydrolyzed Cornstarch	144	53.3	MCT, Corn Oil, Soy Oil	35	30	50:50	310	1321	125:1	Soy Polysaccharide	13.6
Nutren® 1.0 with Fiber Diet	Clinitec	Liquid	1.0	Casein	40	16	Maltodextrin, Corn Syrup Solids	127	51	Canola Oil, MCT, Lecithin	38	33	24:76	303–412	1500	131:1	Soy Polysaccharide	14
Profiber®	Sherwood Medical	Liquid	1.0	Sodium, Calcium Caseinates	40	16	Hydrolyzed Cornstarch	132	48	Corn Oil	40	36	No MCT	300	1500	134:1	Soy Polysaccharide	12
Sustacal® with Fiber	Mead Johnson	Liquid	1.06	Sodium, Calcium Caseinates, Soy Protein Isolate	43	17	Sodium, Calcium Caseinate, Soy Protein Isolate	132	53	Corn Oil	33	30	No MCT	480	1420	120:1	Soy Polysaccharide	5.6
Ultracal®	Mead Johnson	Liquid	1.06	Sodium, Calcium Caseinates	42	17	Maltodextrin	116	46	Soy Oil, MCT	43	37	40:60	310	1250	128:1	Soy Polysaccharide, Oat Fiber	13.6

*For vitamin and mineral content, see pages 463 to 466.

(continued)

TABLE K-3 Complete Liquid Formula Diets (continued)

Product	Source	Form	Concentration (Kcal/mL)	Protein Source	Protein g/1000 Kcal	Protein % Kcal	Carbohydrate Source	CHO g/1000 Kcal	CHO % Kcal	Fat Source	Fat g/1000 Kcal	Fat % Kcal	n6:n3	MCT:LCT Ratio	Osmolality (mOsm/kg H₂O)	Volume To Meet 100% US RDA For Vit/Min (mL)*	Nonprotein Calorie: Nitrogen Ratio	Fiber Source	Fiber g/1000 Kcal
Disease-Specific Formulas																			
Critical Care																			
Immun-Aid®	Kendall McGaw	Powder	1.0	Lactalbumin, Supplemental Amino Acids	80	32	Maltodextrin	120	48	MCT, Canola Oil	22	20	2.1:1	50:50	460	2000	53:1	N/A	N/A
Impact®	Sandoz	Liquid	1.0	Sodium, Calcium Caseinates L-Arginine	56	22	Hydrolyzed Cornstarch	132	53	Structured Lipid, Menhaden Oil	28	25	1.4:1	27:73	375	1500	71:1	N/A	N/A
Impact® with Fiber	Sandoz	Liquid	1.0	Sodium, Calcium Caseinates, L-Arginine	56	22	Hydrolyzed Cornstarch, Enzymatically Modified Guar	140	53	Structured Lipid, Menhaden Oil	28	25	1.4:1	27:73	375	1500	71:1	Soy Polysaccharide, Enzymatically Modified Guar	10
Perative™	Ross	Liquid	1.3	Partially Hydrolyzed Sodium Caseinate, Lactalbumin Hydrolysate, L-Arginine	51	20.5	Hydrolyzed Cornstarch	136	55	Canola Oil, MCT, Corn Oil	29	25	N/A	40:60	425	1155	97:1	N/A	
Protain XL™	Sherwood Medical	Liquid	1.0	Sodium, Calcium Caseinates	55	22	Maltodextrin	138	51	MCT, Corn Oil	30	27	N/A	50:50	340	1250	93:1	Soy Polysaccharide	8
Replete® Diet	Clintec	Liquid	1.0	Casein	62.5	25	Maltodextrin, Corn Syrup Solids	113	45	Canola Oil, MCT, Lecithin	34	30	3:1	25:75	300	1000	75:1	Soy Polysaccharide	14
Replete with Fiber Diet	Clintec	Liquid	1.0	Casein	62.5	25	Maltodextrin, Corn Syrup Solids	113	45	Canola Oil, MCT, Lecithin	34	30	3:1	25:75	300	1000	75:1	Soy Polysaccharide	14
Stresstein®	Sandoz	Powder	1.21	Free Amino Acids	58	23	Hydrolyzed Cornstarch	142	57	MCT, Soybean Oil	23	21	8:1	53:47	910	2000	97:1	N/A	N/A
TraumaCal®	Mead Johnson	Liquid	1.5	Calcium, Sodium Caseinates	55	22	Corn Syrup, Sugar	95	38	Soy Oil, MCT	45	40	6.3:1	30:70	490	2000	91:1	N/A	N/A

*For vitamin and mineral content, see pages 463 to 466.

(continued)

TABLE K-3 Complete Liquid Formula Diets (*continued*)

Product	Source	Form	Concentration (Kcal/mL)	Protein Source	Protein g/1000 Kcal	Protein % Kcal	Carbohydrate Source	Carb g/1000 Kcal	Carb % Kcal	Fat Source	Fat g/1000 Kcal	Fat % Kcal	n6:n3	MC:LCT Ratio	Osmolality (mOsm/kg H₂O)	Volume To Meet 100% US RDA For Vit/Min (mL)*	Nonprotein Calorie: Nitrogen Ratio	Fiber Source	Fiber g/1000 Kcal
Glucose Intolerance																			
Glucerna®	Ross	Liquid	1.0	Casein	41.8	16.7	Hydrolyzed Cornstarch, Fructose	93.7	33.3	Hi-oleic Safflower Oil, Soy Oil, Soy Lecithin	55.7	50	N/A	N/A	375	1422	140:1	Soy Polysaccharide	14.4
Hepatic																			
Hepatic-Aid® II	Kendall McGaw	Powder	1.2	L-Amino Acids (46% BCAA)	38	15	Maltodextrin, Sucrose	144	57.3	Soybean Oil	31	27.7	N/A	No MCT	560	N/A	148:1	N/A	N/A
NutriHep	Clintec	Liquid	1.5	L-Amino Acids (50% BCAA)	26.7	10.6		19.4	77.3	MCT 66%	13	12.1	N/A	66:34	690	1000	209:1	N/A	N/A
Travasorb® Hepatic Diet	Clintec	Powder	1.1	L-Amino Acids (50% BCAA)	26.7	10.6	Glucose Oligo-saccharides, Sucrose	196	77.4	MCT, Sunflower Oil	13	12	N/A	70:30	600	2060	211:1	N/A	N/A
Fat Malabsorption																			
Lipisorb	Mead Johnson	Liquid	1.35	Calcium, Sodium Caseinates		17	Maltodextrin Sucrose		48	MCT, Soy Oil		35		85:15		1600		N/A	N/A
Pulmonary																			
NutriVent™ Diet	Clintec	Liquid	1.5	Casein	45	18	Maltodextrin, Sucrose	67	27	Canola Oil, MCT, Corn Oil, Lecithin	63	55	4:1	40:60	450	1000	116:1	N/A	N/A
Pulmocare®	Ross	Liquid	1.5	Sodium, Calcium Caseinates	41.7	16.7	Sucrose, Hydrolyzed Cornstarch	70.4	28.1	Corn Oil	61.4	55.2	43.5:1	No MCT	465	947	125:1	N/A	N/A
Respalor	Mead Johnson	Liquid	1.5			20			39			41		70:30	580	2160	102:1	N/A	
Renal																			
Alterna®	Ross	Powder	0.36	Whey, Nonfat Dry Milk, Sodium Caseinate	26.9	11	Corn Syrup Solids, Nonfat Dry Milk, Sucrose	128	51	Soybean Oil	43	39	N/A	No MCT	N/A	N/A	209:1	N/A	N/A
Amin-Aid®	Kendall McGaw	Powder	2.0	Essential L-Amino Acids plus Histidine	10	4	Maltodextrin, Sucrose	187	74.8	Soybean Oil	24	21.2	N/A	No MCT	700	N/A	800:1	N/A	N/A

*For vitamin and mineral content, see pages 463 to 466.

(*continued*)

461

TABLE K-3 Complete Liquid Formula Diets (continued)

Product	Source	Form	Concentration (Kcal/mL)	Protein Source	g/1000 Kcal	% Kcal	Carbohydrate Source	g/1000 Kcal	% Kcal	Fat Source	g/1000 Kcal	% Kcal	n6:n3	MCT:LCT Ratio	Osmolality (mOsm/kgH$_2$O)	Volume To Meet 100% US RDA For Vit/Min (mL)*	Nonprotein Calorie: Nitrogen Ratio	Fiber Source	g/1000 Kcal
Aminess® Essential Amino Acid Tablets	Clintec	Tablet	3 Kcal/Tablet	8 Essential Amino Acids plus Histidine	0.69 g/Tablet	85	Lactose (added as excipient)	0.05 g/Tablet	6	Magnesium stearate (added as excipient)	0.03 g/Tablet	8	N/A	N/A	N/A	N/A	N/A	N/A	N/A
Nepro®	Ross	Liquid	2.0	Calcium, Magnesium, Sodium Caseinates	34.9	14	Hydrolyzed Cornstarch, Sucrose	107.6	43	Hi-oleic Safflower Oil, Soy Oil	47.8	43	N/A	No MCT	635	947	157:1	N/A	N/A
Suplena®	Ross	Liquid	2.0	Sodium, Calcium Caseinates	15	6	Hydrolyzed Cornstarch, Sucrose	128	51	Hi-oleic Safflower Oil, Soy Oil	48	43	N/A	No MCT	600	947	392:1	N/A	N/A
Travasorb® Renal Diet	Clintec	Powder	1.35	Essential L-Amino Acids, Select Nonessential Amino Acids	17	6.9	Glucose Oligosac-carides, Sucrose	200	81.1	MCT, Sunflower Oil	13	12	N/A	70:30	590	N/A	339:1	N/A	N/A
HIV, AIDS		Liquid	1.28	Soy Hydrolysate, Sodium Caseinates		18.7	Hydrolyzed Cornstarch		65.5	Canola Oil, MCT, Sardine Oil	15.8		1.64:1		1184			N/A	N/A

*For vitamin and mineral content, see pages 463 to 466.

TABLE K-3 Complete Liquid Formula Diets *(continued)*

Vitamins per 1000 Kcal

Product	Vitamin A (IU)	Vitamin D (IU)	Vitamin E (IU)	Vitamin K (μg)	Vitamin C (mg)	Thiamine-B₁ (mg)	Riboflavin-B₂ (mg)	Niacin (mg)	Vitamin B₆ (mg)	Folic Acid (μg)	Pantothenic Acid (mg)	Vitamin B₁₂ (μg)	Biotin (μg)	Choline (mg)	Taurine (mg)	L-Carnitine (mg)
Elemental Formulas																
Accupep™ HPF	3125	250	30	35	60	1.13	1.28	15	1.5	300	7.5	4.5	230	200	N/A	N/A
AlitraQ™	3998	267	30	54	200	2	2.3	27	2.7	265	14	8	400	400	200	100
Criticare® HN	2453	200	37.8	125	150	1.9	2.2	24.5	2.5	200	12.5	7.5	150	245	N/A	N/A
Peptamen® Diet	4000	280	28	80	140	2	2.4	28	4	540	14	8	400	448	80	80
Peptamen®—Oral Diet	4000	280	28	80	140	2	2.4	28	4	540	14	8	400	448	80	80
Reabilan®	2660	200	15	50	100	1.5	1.5	20	2	250	5	2	98.4	200	N/A	N/A
Reabilan® HN	2662	105	15	50.2	100	1.5	1.5	20.1	2	250	5	2.3	100.2	200	142.4	N/A
Tolerex®	2800	220	17	37	33	0.8	0.9	11	1.1	220	5.6	3.3	170	41	N/A	N/A
Vital® HN	3332	267	30	54	200	2	2.3	26.7	2.7	533	13.4	8	400	400	N/A	N/A
Vivonex® TEN	2500	200	15	22	60	1.5	1.7	20	2	400	10	6	300	74	N/A	N/A
Standard Intake Protein Formulas																
Attain®	4000	320	48	80	144	1.8	2.04	24	2.4	360	12	6	240	400	N/A	N/A
Comply®	3333	267	40	33.3	120	1.5	1.7	20	2	400	10	6	300	300	N/A	N/A
Ensure®	2500	200	22.5	40	150	1.5	1.7	20	2	400	10	6	300	300	N/A	N/A
Ensure® HN	3572	286	32.2	57	215	1.61	1.83	21.5	2.15	429	10.8	6.43	322	429	N/A	N/A
Ensure® Plus	2349	189	21.1	38	141	1.41	1.61	18.79	1.89	377	9.41	5.63	282	282	N/A	N/A
Ensure® Plus HN	3522	282	31.7	85	212	2.11	2.4	28.2	2.83	564	14.1	8.5	423	423	158*	158*
Entrition™ 0.5 Diet	2500	200	30	100	150	1.5	1.7	20	2	400	10	6	300	400	N/A	N/A
Entrition™ HN Diet	3845	308	23	54	116	1.7	2	23.1	2.31	460	11.5	6.92	346	346	N/A	N/A

Minerals Per 1000 Kcal

Product	Sodium (mg)	Sodium (mEq)	Potassium (mg)	Potassium (mEq)	Chloride (mg)	Chloride (mEq)	Calcium (mg)	Phosphorus (mg)	Magnesium (mg)	Iron (mg)	Iodine (μg)	Copper (mg)	Zinc (MG)	Manganese (mg)	Selenium (μg)	Molybdenum (μg)	Chromium (μg)
Elemental Formulas																	
Accupep™ HPF	680	29.6	1150	29.5	1064	30	625	625	250	11.3	100	1.5	15	2.5	N/A	N/A	N/A
AlitraQ™	1000	43.5	1200	30.7	1300	36.7	733	733	267	15	100	1.3	20	3.4	50	110	75
Criticare® HN	595	25.8	1245	31.9	1000	28.2	500	500	200	9	75	1	10	2.5	N/A	N/A	N/A
Peptamen® Diet	500	21.7	1252	32.1	1000	28.2	800	700	400	12	100	1.4	14	2.7	40	120	40
Peptamen®—Oral Diet	500	21.7	1252	32.1	1000	28.2	800	700	400	12	100	1.4	14	2.7	40	120	40
Reabilan®	699	30.4	1251	32.1	2000	56.3	499	499	251	10	74.7	1.6	10	2	50.7	N/A	82.5
Reabilan® HN	752	32.7	1249	31.9	1880	52.9	339	375	248	10	76.2	0.95	10	2	50.1	N/A	62.2
Tolerex®	470	20	1200	31	950	27	560	560	220	10	83	1.1	8.3	1.6	83	83	28
Vital® HN	566	24.6	1400	35.8	1032	29.1	667	667	267	12	100	1.4	15	3.4	47	100	67
Vivonex® TEN	460	20	780	20	820	23	500	500	200	9	75	1	10	0.9	50	50	17
Standard Intake Protein Formulas																	
Attain®	805	35	1600	41	1346	38	960	800	320	14.4	120	1.6	24	4	100	150	100
Comply®	733	31.9	1233	31.6	1133	31.9	667	667	267	12	100	1.3	20	3	N/A	N/A	N/A
Ensure®	800	34.8	1480	37.9	1240	34.9	500	500	200	9	75	1	11.25	2.5	35	50	75
Ensure® HN	760	33	1480	37.8	1240	34.9	715	715	286	12.86	107.2	1.43	16.08	3.57	50	108	72
Ensure® Plus	704	30.6	1296	33.1	1268	35.7	470	470	189	8.5	70	0.96	10.6	2.34	33	71	47
Ensure® Plus HN	786	34.2	1265	32.4	1066	30.1	705	705	282	12.7	106	1.42	15.9	3.52	50	106	71
Entrition™ 0.5 Diet	700	30.4	1200	30.8	1000	28.2	500	500	200	9	75	1	7.5	2	N/A	N/A	N/A
Entrition™ HN Diet	845	36.7	1579	40.5	1540	43.4	770	770	308	13.9	116	1.54	11.6	1.54	N/A	N/A	N/A

(continued)

463

TABLE K-3 Complete Liquid Formula Diets *(continued)*

Product	Vitamin A (IU)	Vitamin D (IU)	Vitamin E (IU)	Vitamin K (µg)	Vitamin C (mg)	Thiamine-B₁ (mg)	Riboflavin-B₂ (mg)	Niacin (mg)	Vitamin B₆ (mg)	Folic Acid (µg)	Pantothenic Acid (mg)	Vitamin B₁₂ (µg)	Biotin (µg)	Choline (mg)	Taurine (mg)	L-Carnitine (mg)	Sodium (mg)	Sodium (mEq)	Potassium (mg)	Potassium (mEq)	Chloride (mg)	Chloride (mEq)	Calcium (mg)	Phosphorus (mg)	Magnesium (mg)	Iron (µg)	Iodine (µg)	Copper (mg)	Zinc (MG)	Manganese (mg)	Selenium (µg)	Molybdenum (µg)	Chromium (µg)
Isocal®	2455	200	38	125	150	1.9	2.2	25	2.5	200	12.5	7.5	150	245	N/A	N/A	500	21.7	1245	31.9	1000	28.2	595	500	200	9	75	1	10	2.5	N/A	N/A	N/A
Isocal® HN	3962	320	60	100	235	3	3.4	40	4	320	20	12	235	400	N/A	N/A	877	38.1	1500	38.5	1360	38.2	800	800	320	14	120	1.6	12	4.3	80	200	80
Isocal® HCN	2500	200	37.5	125	150	1.9	2.2	25	2.5	200	12.5	7.5	150	250	N/A	N/A	400	17.5	850	21.5	600	17	500	500	200	9	75	1.5	15	1.7	N/A	N/A	N/A
Isolan®	3774	302	22.6	75.5	136	1.1	1.3	15.1	1.5	302	7.5	4.5	226	283	N/A	N/A	651	28.3	1100	28.3	1037	29.2	755	755	13.5	113	1.5	11.3	1.9	113	226	113	
Isosource®	2800	220	25	40	170	1.7	1.9	22	2.2	220	11	6.7	330	280	N/A	N/A	1000	43	1400	36	940	27	560	560	220	10	83	1.1	14	2.8	83	170	83
Isosource® HN	2800	220	25	40	170	1.7	1.9	22	2.2	220	11	6.7	330	280	N/A	N/A	1000	43	1400	36	940	27	560	560	220	10	83	1.1	14	2.8	83	170	83
Lipisorb®	3753	300	22.5	60.1	45	1.2	1.3	15	1.5	300	7.5	4.5	225	342	N/A	N/A	734	31.9	1251	31.1	1168	32.9	701	701	200	9.2	75.1	1	10	1.5	N/A	N/A	N/A
Magnacal®	2500	200	30	150	150	1.5	1.7	20	2	200	5	6	150	250	N/A	N/A	500	21.8	625	16	475	13.4	500	500	200	9	75	1	15	2.5	N/A	N/A	N/A
Nutren® 1.0 Diet	4000	280	28	80	140	2	2.4	28	4	540	14	8	400	452	80	80	500	21.74	1252	32.1	1000	28.2	700	700	340	12	100	1.4	1.4	2.7	40	120	40
Nutren® 1.5 Diet	400	280	28	80	140	2	2.4	28	4	533	13.3	8	400	448	80	80	500	21.74	1253	32.1	1000	28.2	693	333	12	100	1.3	13.3	2.7	40	120	40	
Nutren® 2.0 Diet	4000	280	28	80	140	2	2.4	28	4	540	14	8	400	450	80	80	500	21.74	1250	32.1	1000	28.2	700	700	340	12	100	1.4	14	2.6	40	120	40
Nutrilan®	2985	239	23.6	35.8	142	1.5	1.7	20	2	239	6	6	179	199	N/A	N/A	597	26	1000	25.6	700	19.7	595	595	239	10.8	119	1.2	9	1.9	N/A	N/A	N/A
Osmolite®	2500	200	22.5	40	150	1.5	1.7	20	2	400	10	6	300	300	75	75	600	26.1	960	24.6	800	22.5	500	500	200	9	75	1	11.5	2.5	35	75	50
Osmolite® HN	3572	286	32.2	5	215	1.61	1.83	21.5	2.15	429	10.8	6.43	322	429	108	108	880	38.3	1480	37.8	1360	38.3	715	715	286	12.86	107.2	1.43	16.08	3.57	50	108	72
Resource® Liquid	2500	200	23	36	150	1.5	1.7	20	2	200	5	6	150	520	N/A	N/A	840	36	1500	39	950	27	500	500	9	75	1	15	2	N/A	N/A	N/A	
Resource® Plus	2500	200	22	37	110	1.8	1.8	21	2.1	210	5.6	6.3	160	360	N/A	N/A	850	37	1400	35	1100	30	470	470	210	9.6	70	1.1	16	1.4	N/A	N/A	N/A
Suscatal® 8.8	2520	200	37.6	62.4	92	1.52	1.72	20	2	400	10	6	300	300	N/A	N/A	800	34.8	1520	39	1360	38.9	500	500	1.52	9.2	75.2	1	10	200	50	124	50
Suscatal® HC	2800	227	16.7	140	50.7	1.3	1.4	16.7	1.7	340	8.7	5.1	253	140	N/A	N/A	567	24.6	987	25.2	847	23.8	567	567	227	10	86.7	1.1	8.7	1.7	N/A	N/A	N/A
TwoCal® HN	2632	211	23.68	43	158	1.26	1.43	16.8	1.68	337	8.4	5.1	253	316	N/A	N/A	653	28.4	1221	31.2	821	23.1	526	526	211	9.5	78.9	1.05	11.85	2.63	37	79	53
Ultralan®	333	267	20	83.3	120	1	1.1	13.3	1.3	267	6.7	4	200	250	N/A	N/A	690	30	1170	30	1136	32	667	667	267	12	100	1.3	10	1.7	80	160	80

(continued)

TABLE K-3 Complete Liquid Formula Diets (continued)

(continued)

Product	Vitamin A (IU)	Vitamin D (IU)	Vitamin E (IU)	Vitamin K (µg)	Vitamin C (mg)	Thiamine-B1 (mg)	Riboflavin-B2 (mg)	Niacin (mg)	Vitamin B6 (mg)	Folic Acid (µg)	Pantothenic Acid (mg)	Vitamin B12 (µg)	Biotin (µg)	Choline (mg)	Taurine (mg)	L-Carnitine (mg)	Sodium (mg)	Sodium (mEq)	Potassium (mg)	Potassium (mEq)	Chloride (mg)	Chloride (mEq)	Calcium (mg)	Phosphorus (mg)	Magnesium (mg)	Iron (µg)	Iodine (µg)	Copper (mg)	Zinc (MG)	Manganese (mg)	Selenium (µg)	Molybdenum (µg)	Chromium (µg)
High Protein Formulas																																	
Citrotein®	7824	629	47	N/A	353	4.7	5.4	62.9	6.5	1235	31.2	18.8	941	52	N/A	N/A	1000	43.5	824	21	1176	33	1588	1588	629	56	235	3.1	24	7.6	N/A	N/A	N/A
Isotein® HN	2400	190	14	48	43	1.1	1.2	9.5	1.4	190	4.8	2.9	140	48	N/A	N/A	520	23	900	23	810	23	480	480	190	8.6	71	0.95	7.1	1.9	71	140	71
Nitrolan®	3226	258	19.3	64.5	116	0.97	1.1	12.9	1.3	258	6.5	3.9	194	242	N/A	N/A	557	24.2	945	24.2	887	25	645	645	258	11.6	96.8	1.3	9.7	1.6	96.8	194	96.8
Promote®	4000	320	36	64	240	1.8	2.1	24	2.4	480	12	7.2	360	480	120	120	928	40.4	1980	50.6	1263	35.6	960	960	320	14.4	120	1.6	18	4	56	120	80
Replete®—Oral	5000	280	28	80	140	2	2.4	28	4	540	14	8	400	450	N/A	N/A	500	21.74	1560	40	1000	28.2	800	720	400	12	100	1.4	14	2.7	N/A	N/A	N/A
Sustacal®	4700	370	29	230	56.0	1.4	1.7	20	2	370	9.8	5.6	290	230	N/A	N/A	940	41	2100	54.0	1490	42	930	380	16.9	140	2.	14.1	2.9	N/A	N/A	N/A	
Intact Protein Formulas with Fiber																																	
Ensure® with Fiber	3269	262	29.6	46	196	1.5	1.69	19.6	1.96	392	9.81	6.1	296	392	N/A	N/A	769	33.4	1538	39.4	1231	34.5	654	654	262	11.77	98.1	1.31	14.73	3.27	N/A	N/A	N/A
Fiberlan®	333	267	20	67	120	1	1.1	13.3	1.3	267	6.7	4	200	250	N/A	N/A	767	33.3	1300	33.3	1155	32.5	667	667	267	12	100	1.3	10	1.7	100	200	100
Fibersource®	2800	220	25	40	170	1.7	1.9	22	2.2	220	11	6.7	330	280	N/A	N/A	940	41	1500	38	940	27	560	4560	220	10	83	1.1	14	2.8	83	170	83
Fibersource® HN	2800	220	25	40	170	1.7	1.9	22	2.2	220	11	6.7	330	280	N/A	N/A	940	41	1500	38	940	27	560	560	220	10	83	1.1	14	2.8	83	170	83
Jevity®	3572	288	32.4	58	214	1.64	1.84	21.4	2.16	432	10.7	6.8	324	428	108	108	880	38.3	1480	37.8	1240	34.9	860	716	286	12.9	107	1.44	16.1	3.56	50	108	72
Nutren® 1.0 with Fiber Diet	4000	280	28	80	140	2	2.4	28	4	540	14	8	400	452	80	80	500	21.74	1252	32.1	1000	28.2	7000	7000	340	12	100	1.4	14	2.7	40	120	40
Profiber®	3334	267	40	50	120	1.5	1.7	20	2	400	10	6	300	300	N/A	N/A	730	32	1250	32	1200	34	667	667	267	12	100	1.5	20	3	80	200	80
Sustacal® with Fiber	3300	396	20	91.5	120	1.5	1.7	20	2	396	10	6	300	N/A	N/A	N/A	680	29.5	1310	33.6	1310	36.9	792	660	265	12	100	1.3	13.1	1.7	N/A	N/A	N/A
Ultracal®	4000	320	60.4	100	240	3	3.4	40	4	321	20	12	240	400	120	179	877	38.1	1518	38.9	1340	37.7	800	800	320	14.1	120	1.6	16	2.4	80	200	80

Minerals Per 1000 Kcal · *Vitamins per 1000 Kcal*

TABLE K-3 Complete Liquid Formula Diets *(continued)*

Product	Vitamin A (IU)	B-Carotene (IU)	Vitamin D (IU)	Vitamin E (IU)	Vitamin K (µg)	Vitamin C (mg)	Thiamine-B_1 (mg)	Riboflavin-B_2 (mg)	Niacin (mg)	Vitamin B_6 (mg)	Folic Acid (µg)	Pantothenic Acid (mg)	Vitamin B_{12} (µg)	Biotin (µg)	Choline (mg)	Taurine (mg)	L-Carnitine (mg)	Sodium (mg)	Sodium (mEq)	Potassium (mg)	Potassium (mEq)	Chloride (mg)	Chloride (mEq)	Calcium (mg)	Phosphorus (mg)	Magnesium (mg)	Iron (mg)	Iodine (µg)	Fluoride (mg)	Copper (mg)	Zinc (MG)	Manganese (mg)	Selenium (µg)	Molybdenum (µg)	Chromium (µg)
Disease Specific Formulas																																			
Critical Care																																			
Immun-Aid®	2665	N/A	200	50	40	60	0.75	0.85	10	10	200	5	3	150	210	100	200	575	25	1055	27	888	25.1	500	500	200	9	75	0.76	2	25	2.5	100	75	75
Impact®	3400	3400	270	60	67	80	2	1.7	20	1.5	400	6.7	8	200	270	N/A	N/A	1100	48	1300	33	1300	37	800	800	270	12	100	N/A	1.7	15	2	100	200	100
Impact® with Fiber	3400	3400	270	60	67	80	2	1.7	20	1.5	400	6.7	8	200	270	N/A	N/A	1100	48	1300	33	1300	37	800	800	270	12	100	N/A	1.7	15	2	100	200	100
Perative™	6663	N/A	267	30	54	200	1.5	1.7	20	2	400	10	6	300	400	100	100	800	34.8	1330	34.1	1269	35.8	667	667	267	12	100	N/A	1.34	15	3.34	47	100	67
Protain XL™	8000	N/A	400	48	60	240	2.4	2.72	32	3.2	480	12	9.6	360	500	N/A	N/A	860	37.4	1500	38.4	1350	38.1	800	800	320	21.6	120	N/A	2.4	36	6	10	150	100
Replete® Diet	4000	3332	400	60	80	340	3	2.4	28	4	540	14	8	400	450	100	100	500	21.74	1560	40	1000	28.2	1000	1000	400	18	160	N/A	2	24	4	100	220	140
Replete® with Fiber Diet	4000	3332	400	60	80	340	3	2.4	28	4	540	14	8	400	450	100	100	500	21.74	1560	40	1000	28.2	1000	1000	400	18	160	N/A	2	24	4	100	220	140
Stresstein®	2100	N/A	170	13	29	25	0.63	0.71	8.3	0.92	170	4.2	2.5	130	42	N/A	N/A	540	23	920	24	830	23	420	420	170	7.5	63	N/A	0.8	6.3	1.7	50	130	50
TraumaCal®	1667	N/A	133	25.3	84.7	98.7	1.3	1.5	16.7	1.7	133	8.5	5	98.7	167	N/A	N/A	787	34.2	927	23.8	1067	30	500	500	133	5.9	50	N/A	1	9.9	1.7	N/A	N/A	N/A
Glucose Intolerance																																			
Glucerna®	3520	N/A	282	31.7	57	212	1.6	1.8	21.2	2.2	423	10.6	6.4	317	423	106	141	928	40.3	1561	40	1435	41	704	704	282	12.7	106	N/A	1.5	15.9	3.6	50	106	71
Hepatic																																			
Hepatic-Aid® II	N/A	N/A	N/A	N/A	N/A	N/A	N/A	N/A	N/A	N/A	N/A	N/A	N/A	N/A	N/A	N/A	N/A	<288	<12.5	<196	<5	N/A	N/A	N/A	N/A	N/A	N/A	N/A	N/A	N/A	N/A	N/A	N/A	N/A	N/A
Travasorb® Hepatic Diet	668	N/A	179	9.1	46.8	40.1	0.63	0.71	8	0.97	179	4.5	2.7	134	179	N/A	N/A	213.6	9.3	818	20.6	634	17.8	446	446	179	8	66.8	N/A	0.9	6.7	1.2	N/A	N/A	N/A
Pulmonary																																			
NutriVent™ Diet	4000	N/A	280	28	80	140	2	2.4	28	4	540	14	8	400	450	80	80	500	21.74	1493	38.3	1000	28.2	800	800	400	12	100	N/A	1.4	14	2.7	40	120	40
Pulmocare®	3521	N/A	282	31.8	56.4	211	2.1	2.4	28	2.8	563	14.1	8.4	423	423	N/A	N/A	873	38	1155	29.5	1126	31.8	704	704	282	12.7	106	1.4	1.4	15.9	3.5	50	106	71
Renal																																			
Alterna®	N/A	N/A	N/A	N/A	N/A	N/A	N/A	N/A	N/A	N/A	N/A	N/A	N/A	N/A	N/A	N/A	N/A	1103	48	2988	76.4	2161	61	<977	<1379	138	N/A	N/A	N/A	N/A	N/A	N/A	N/A	N/A	N/A
Amin-Aid®	N/A	N/A	N/A	N/A	N/A	N/A	N/A	N/A	N/A	N/A	N/A	N/A	N/A	N/A	N/A	N/A	N/A	<173	<7.5	<117	<3	N/A	N/A	N/A	N/A	N/A	N/A	N/A	N/A	N/A	N/A	N/A	N/A	N/A	N/A
Aminess® Essential Amino Acid Tablets	N/A	N/A	N/A	N/A	N/A	N/A	N/A	N/A	N/A	N/A	N/A	N/A	N/A	N/A	N/A	N/A	N/A	N/A	N/A	N/A	N/A	N/A	N/A	N/A	N/A	N/A	N/A	N/A	N/A	N/A	N/A	N/A	N/A	N/A	N/A
Nepro®	526	N/A	42	24	42	53	1.26	1.43	16.8	4.29	526	8.4	5.1	253	316	80	131	415	18.1	528	13.5	505	14.2	686	343	105	9.5	78.9	N/A	1.1	11.8	2.63	51.1	N/A	N/A
Suplena®	526	N/A	42	23.8	42	53	1.26	1.43	16.8	4.3	526	8.4	5.1	253	316	80	80	392	17.1	558	14.3	463	13.1	693	364	105	9.5	78.9	N/A	1.05	11.8	2.63	38	N/A	N/A
Travasorb® Renal Diet	N/A	N/A	N/A	N/A	N/A	31.6	0.53	0.59	7.03	3.59	35.3	1.94	N/A	105.6	140.8	N/A	N/A	N/A	N/A	N/A	N/A	N/A	N/A	N/A	N/A	N/A	N/A	N/A	N/A	N/A	N/A	N/A	N/A	N/A	N/A

Vitamins per 1000 Kcal · *Minerals Per 1000 Kcal*

APPENDIX L

Data for Evaluation in Cardiovascular Disease

TABLE L-1 Total Serum Cholesterol Levels in Milligrams per Deciliter for Persons 20 years of Age and Older by Race/Ethnicity, Sex, and Age: United States, 1988–91

Race/ethnicity, sex, and age	Number of examined persons	Mean	Selected Percentile								
			5th	10th	15th	25th	50th	75th	85th	90th	95th
Men											
20 years and older	3,953	205	143	153	162	176	201	231	247	260	276
20–34 years	1,186	189	134	145	151	162	186	211	225	236	260
35–44 years	653	207	144	155	167	182	205	231	245	258	269
45–54 years	508	218	152	170	180	191	215	242	257	268	283
55–64 years	535	221	154	169	180	195	221	245	264	274	285
65–74 years	557	218	157	173	179	190	214	241	256	270	286
75 and older	514	205	145	156	164	175	202	232	248	257	275
Women											
20 years and older	3,885	207	143	154	162	175	202	233	252	269	287
20–34 years	1,177	185	134	143	150	160	182	204	218	229	254
35–44 years	709	195	142	152	159	170	193	215	232	242	254
45–54 years	464	217	158	165	171	187	212	240	264	279	297
55–64 years	503	237	168	184	191	204	228	264	280	291	323
65–74 years	493	234	168	180	186	205	232	261	278	290	308
75 and older	539	230	163	175	184	198	227	263	279	287	316
Mexican Americans											
Men	1,092	202	140	151	159	172	199	225	245	257	277
Women	1,046	200	139	149	158	169	195	224	241	258	279
Non-Hispanic black											
Men	922	199	136	149	156	170	195	224	242	252	276
Women	985	203	137	150	159	172	200	227	248	262	286
Non-Hispanic white											
Men	1,816	206	144	154	163	177	203	232	247	260	276
Women	1,734	208	144	155	163	176	202	234	254	271	288

Reprinted from NIH Publication No. 93-3095, Sep. 1993.

TABLE L-2 Low-density Lipoprotein Cholesterol in Milligrams per Deciliter for Persons 20 years of Age and Older by Race/Ethnicity, Sex, and Age: United States, 1988–91

Race/ethnicity, sex, and age	Number of examined persons	Mean	Selected Percentile								
			5th	10th	15th	25th	50th	75th	85th	90th	95th
Men											
20 years and older	1,669	131	75	87	95	106	129	154	167	179	194
20–34 years	487	120	67	78	86	97	121	139	152	165	186
35–44 years	274	134	85	92	98	111	131	156	166	176	192
45–54 years	224	138	78	91	100	118	136	163	174	187	195
55–64 years	228	142	78	90	104	117	143	165	175	194	205
65–74 years	259	141	93	104	109	119	134	163	177	185	199
75 and older	197	132	83	88	93	106	130	154	170	186	196
Women											
20 years and older	1,673	126	69	81	88	99	122	150	165	175	191
20–34 years	525	110	59	70	75	88	108	129	142	155	173
35–44 years	316	117	67	85	88	97	116	138	146	155	165
45–54 years	214	132	70	87	93	107	130	157	173	182	198
55–64 years	213	145	79	90	101	122	145	170	184	189	209
65–74 years	202	147	92	97	109	119	148	169	185	192	206
75 and older	203	147	90	102	109	121	143	168	189	197	209
Mexican Americans											
Men	448	124	70	77	85	96	120	148	161	172	188
Women	471	122	67	80	86	95	118	144	158	166	189
Non-Hispanic black											
Men	393	126	69	76	82	96	123	146	168	186	206
Women	422	126	67	76	86	100	124	147	162	174	192
Non-Hispanic white											
Men	773	132	76	88	97	108	129	154	168	179	194
Women	729	126	69	82	89	99	122	151	166	176	192

Reprinted from NIH Publication No. 93-3095, Sep. 1993.

TABLE L-3 High-density Lipoprotein Cholesterol in Milligrams per Deciliter for Persons 20 years of Age and Older by Race/Ethnicity, Sex, and Age: United States, 1988–91

Race/ethnicity, sex, and age	Number of examined persons	Mean	Selected Percentile								
			5th	10th	15th	25th	50th	75th	85th	90th	95th
Men											
20 years and older	3,920	46.5	28.0	31.0	34.0	37.0	44.1	53.1	59.1	64.0	73.0
20–34 years	1,178	47.1	30.0	34.0	35.1	38.0	46.0	54.0	60.1	64.0	71.0
35–44 years	642	46.3	28.0	30.0	33.0	37.0	44.0	53.0	58.1	63.0	73.0
45–54 years	502	46.6	28.0	30.0	33.0	36.0	43.1	53.0	61.0	66.1	77.1
55–64 years	533	45.6	29.0	31.0	33.0	36.1	43.0	53.0	59.0	62.0	72.0
65–74 years	553	45.3	28.0	31.0	32.0	36.0	43.0	53.0	58.0	62.1	71.0
75 and older	512	47.2	28.0	32.0	34.0	38.0	45.0	54.0	62.0	67.0	75.1
Women											
20 years and older	3,855	55.7	34.0	38.0	41.0	44.1	54.0	65.0	71.0	76.1	83.0
20–34 years	1,167	55.7	34.0	38.0	41.0	44.1	54.0	64.1	70.1	75.1	83.1
35–44 years	701	54.3	33.0	37.0	40.0	44.0	530	64.1	69.1	72.1	79.0
45–54 years	459	56.7	37.0	38.1	41.0	46.0	56.0	65.0	72.1	77.1	84.1
55–64 years	500	56.1	33.0	37.0	40.0	44.0	53.0	66.0	73.0	79.0	87.1
65–74 years	492	55.7	34.0	37.0	40.0	44.1	54.0	65.1	73.0	78.0	83.1
75 and older	536	57.1	33.0	39.0	41.0	44.1	56.0	66.1	73.1	78.1	87.0
Mexican Americans											
Men	1,077	46.9	30.0	33.0	34.1	38.0	45.0	54.0	59.0	64.0	69.0
Women	1,040	53.3	34.0	37.0	40.0	44.0	52.0	61.0	68.0	72.1	78.0
Non-Hispanic black											
Men	918	53.3	30.0	35.0	38.0	42.0	51.0	62.0	69.1	75.1	86.1
Women	978	57.8	37.0	40.0	43.0	47.0	55.1	67.1	74.0	78.1	86.0
Non-Hispanic white											
Men	1,803	45.5	28.0	30.0	33.1	36.1	44.0	52.1	58.0	62.0	71.1
Women	1,717	55.7	33.1	37.0	40.0	44.0	54.0	65.1	71.1	77.0	83.1

Reprinted from NIH Publication No. 93-3095, Sep. 1993.

Name _____

Date _____

MEDFICTS: Dietary Assessment Questionnaire
(**M**eats, **E**ggs, **D**airy, **F**ried foods, **I**n baked goods, **C**onvenience foods, **T**able fats, **S**nacks)

Directions: For each food category for both Group 1 and Group 2 listings: Please check a box in the "Weekly Consumption" column and in the "Serving Size" column. If patient rarely or never eats the food listed, please check only the "Weekly Consumption" box.

FOOD CATEGORY	WEEKLY CONSUMPTION			SERVING SIZE			SCORE
	Rarely/ Never	3 or less serv/wk	4 or more serv/wk	Small	Average	Large	For office use

M Meats

• Average amount per day: 6 oz (equal in size to 2 decks of playing cards)

Group 1 • Base your estimate on the food you consume the most of

Beef	Processed meats	Pork % Others
Ribs	Ribs	Pork shoulder
Steak	Steak	Pork chops, roast
Chuck blade	Chuck blade	Pork ribs
Brisket	Brisket	Ground pork
Ground Beef	Ground Beef	Regular ham
Meatloaf	Meatloaf	Lamb steaks, ribs, chops
Corned Beef	Corned Beef	Organ meats

Group 1: Weekly Consumption — 3 pts / 7 pts; Serving Size — 1 pts / 2 pts / 3 pts =

Group 2

Poultry with skin

Lean Cuts of Beef	Low-fat Processed Meats	Poultry, Fish, Meat
Sirloin tip	Low-fat lunch meat	Poultry without skin
Flank steak	Low-fat hot dogs	Fish, seafood
Round steak	Canadian bacon	Lamb flank, leg-shank,
Rump roast		sirloin, roast
Chuck arm roast		Lean ham cured and fresh
		Pork loin chops, tenderloin
		Veal chops, cutlets, roast
		Venison

Group 2: Large serving — 6 pts =   +

E Eggs

• Weekly consumption is express as times/week

How many eggs do you eat each time?

Group 1

Whole eggs, Yolks

Weekly Consumption — 3 pts / 7 pts; ≤1 (1 pts) / 2 (2 pts) / ≥3 (3 pts) =

Group 2

Egg whites, Egg substitutes (1/2 cup = 2 eggs)

≤1 / 2 / ≥3

D Dairy

Milk • Average serving: 1 cup

Group 1

Whole milk, 2% milk, 2% buttermilk, Yogurt (whole milk)

Weekly Consumption — 3 pts / 7 pts; Serving Size — 1 pts / 2 pts / 3 pts =

Group 2

Skim milk, 1% milk, Skim milk-buttermilk
Yogurt (nonfat & low-fat)

Cheese • Average serving: 1 oz.

Group 1

Cream cheese, Cheddar, Monterey Jack, Colby, Swiss
American processed, Blue cheese
Regular cottage cheese and Ricotta (1/2 cup)

Weekly Consumption — 3 pts / 7 pts; Serving Size — 1 pts / 2 pts / 3 pts =

Group 2

Low-fat & fat-free cheeses, Skim milk mozzarella
String cheese
Low-fat & fat-free cottage cheese, and Skim milk ricotta (1/2/ C)

Frozen Desserts • Average serving: 1/2 cup

Group 1

Ice cream, Milk shakes

Weekly Consumption — 3 pts / 7 pts; Serving Size — 1 pts / 2 pts / 3 pts =

Group 2

Ice milk, Frozen yogurt

+ Score 6 points if this box is checked.

Comments: _____

Total _____

(Continued)

FIGURE L-1   MEDFICTS: Dietary Assessment Questionnaire

FOOD CATEGORY	WEEKLY CONSUMPTION			SERVING SIZE			SCORE
	Rarely/ Never	3 or less serv/wk	4 or more serv/wk	Small	Average	Large	For office use

F **Fried Foods** • Average serving: see below

Group 1
French fries, Fried vegetables: (1/2 cup)
*Fried chicken, fish, and meat: (3 oz.)
  *Check meat category also

☐ □3 pts□ □7 pts□ | x □1 pts□ 2 pts□ 3 pts□ =

Group 2
Vegetables, - not deep fried
Meat, Poultry, or fish - prepared by baking, broiling,
  grilling, poaching, roasting, stewing

☐ ☐ ☐ | ☐ ☐ ☐

I **In Baked Goods** • Average serving: 1 serving

Group 1
Doughnuts, Biscuits, Butter rolls, Muffins, Croissants,
Sweet rolls, Danish, Cakes, Pies, Coffee cakes, Cookies

☐ 3 pts 7 pts | x 1 pts 2 pts 3 pts =

Group 2
Fruit bars, Low-fat cookies/cakes/pastries, Angel food cake,
Homemade baked goods with vegetable oils

☐ ☐ ☐ | ☐ ☐ ☐

C **Convenience Foods** • Average serving: see below

Group 1
Canned, Packaged, or Frozen dinners: e.g. Pizza (1 slice),
Macaroni & cheese (about 1 cup), Pot pie (1), Cream soups (1 cup)

☐ 3 pts 7 pts | x 1 pts 2 pts 3 pts =

Group 2
Diet/Reduced calorie or reduced fat dinners (1 dinner)

☐ ☐ ☐ | ☐ ☐ ☐

T **Table Fats** • Average serving: see below

Group 1
Butter, Stick margarine: 1 pat
Regular salad dressing or mayonnaise, Sour cream: 1-2 Tbsp

☐ 3 pts 7 pts | x 1 pts 2 pts 3 pts =

Group 2
Diet and tub margarine, Low-fat & fat-free salad dressings
Low-fat & fat-free mayonnaise

☐ ☐ ☐ | ☐ ☐ ☐

S **Snacks** • Average serving: see below

Group 1
Chips (potato, corn, taco), Cheese puffs, Snack mix, Nuts,
Regular crackers, Regular popcorn,
Candy (milk chocolate, caramel, coconut)

☐ 3 pts 7 pts | x 1 pts 2 pts 3 pts =

Group 2
Air-popped or low-fat popcorn, Low-fat crackers, Hard candy,
Licorice, Fruit rolls, Bread sticks, Pretzels, Fat-free chips
Fruit

☐ ☐ ☐ | ☐ ☐ ☐

Directions for scoring:
Multiply Weekly Consumption points (3 or 7) by Serving
Size points (1, 2, 3) for Group 1 foods only except for
a large serving of Group 2 meats

Example: 3 pts ✓ 7 pts 1 pts 2 pts ✓ 3 pts
3 x 7 = 21 points

Add score on page 1 and 2 to get Final Score

Key
40 - 70   - Step I Diet
less than 40   - Step II Diet

▨ = Foods high in fat, saturated fat, and/or cholesterol

Total _____

Score from
page 1   + _____

Final Score _____

Comments: _____
      (Note frequent use of foods high in fat or saturated fat, e.g. coffee creamer, whipped topping)

FIGURE L-1 *(continued)*   Reprinted from NIH Publication No. 93-3095, Sep. 1993.

| APPENDIX M | **Forms** |

FORM A

University Medical Center
24-Hour Recall Form

Patient's name_____   Date _____

Level of activity_____
Person responsible for shopping?_____
Food preparation?_____
Dentition (circle one)   Normal; Dentures, partial or complete; Edentulous

List of food eaten yesterday

Wake-up time? _____   Is this usual? _____

Time	Where eaten	Food	Description	Amount

Was this day typical?
If not, why not?
How much salt do you add to your food at the table?
Do you take vitamins?
What kind and how much?
Are there foods you do not eat because of religious beliefs?

Form B

University Medical Center
Food-Frequency Checklist

Patient's name_____ Date _____

How often do you consume the following foods?

Food	Servings per day	Servings per week	Seldom	Never	Food	Servings per day	Servings per week	Seldom	Never
Beef, hamburger					Potatoes				
Pork, ham					Dried beans, peas				
Bacon									
Liver					Fruit or juice, citrus				
Lamb									
Veal					Other				
Lunch meat					Tomatoes				
Poultry					Dried fruit				
Fish					Margarine				
Shellfish					Butter				
Cheese (type)					Cooking fat/ oil				
Milk (type)									
Yogurt					Salad dressing				
Ice cream					Salt pork				
Ice milk					Cream (type, % fat)				
Bread (type)									
Cereal (type)					Fried foods				
Pasta (type)					Nuts				
Baked goods (type)					Seeds				
					Sprouts				
Dark green vegetables					Snack crackers				
Dark yellow vegetables					Chips				
					Candy				
Other vegetables					Soft drinks				
					Coffee (decaf?)				
					Tea				
					Alcohol				

Are there other foods not listed that you eat regularly?_____

_____

_____

FORM C

University Medical Center Summary of Daily Nutrient Intake				
Food Group	No. of Exchanges	PRO g	FAT g	CHO g
Starch/Bread exchanges				
Milk exchanges (Circle non-fat, low-fat, or whole)				
Fruit exchanges				
Vegetable exchanges				
Meat exchanges (Circle low, medium, or high fat)				
Fat exchanges				
Other				
TOTAL g		_____	_____	_____

Kcal = _____ g protein   × 4 = _____
          _____ g fat   × 9 = _____
          _____ g carbohydrate × 4 = _____
                              _____ TOTAL kcal

FORM D

University Medical Center Nutritional Assessment

Patient's Name _____

Sex(Circle one)   M   F   Date of Admission _____

Age:_____Years   Date of Assessment _____

Height and Weight:

Height: _____ ft.   _____in.   _____cm.

Body weight:				
On admission	_____ #			_____ kg
Current	_____ #			_____ kg
Usual	_____ #			_____ kg
Ideal	_____ #			_____ kg
Recent loss	_____ #	in _____ mos		_____ kg
% weight change	_____ #	_____ gain	or _____ loss	

Interpretation:	Severely underweight	(20% < ideal)	_____
(Mark X where appro-	Severely overweight	(+20 % > ideal)	_____
priate)	Unplanned weight change,	> 10%	_____
	Stable and within normal limits		_____

Somatic Protein

Value Measured	Standard Value	Patient's Value	Mark X for interpretation			
			50th % ile	50th – 15th % ile	15th – 5th % ile	<5th % ile
TSF, mm						
MAFA cm^2						
MAMA cm^2						

Visceral Protein: Value Measured	Normal Value	Patient's Value	Mark X for interpretation Deficit			
			None	Mild	Moderate	Severe
Albumin, g/L						
TIBC umol/L						
Total Lymphocytes mm^3						

Cellular immunity, 48 hrs

                                       Interpretation:

PPD _____   Normal Reactivity _____

Mumps _____   Subnormal Reactivity _____

Candida _____   Anergy _____

Hematological: Value Measured	Normal Value	Patient's Value	Mark x for interpretation		
			Acceptable	Marginal	Deficient
RBC, 10 ^{12}/L					
Hct					
Hgb, g/L					
MCV, L					
MCH, pg					
MCHC, g/L					

(continued)

FORM D *(continued)*

Nutritional Status: (Mark X where appropriate)

_____ Normal

_____ Marasmus

_____ Kwashiorkor-like syndrome

_____ Combined Marasmus-kwashiorkor

Diet Evaluation

Intake _____ kcal/24 hrs

_____ g protein/24 hrs

Nitrogen Balance: Positive _____ g

Negative _____ g

BEE = _____ kcal

Total Daily Energy Expenditure for maintenance assuming patient is ambulatory = _____ × BEE = _____ kcal.

Recommended Intake:

Energy: Oral anabolic requirement

kg actual body weight × _____ to _____ = _____ to _____ g protein

kcal: gN = _____ N required = _____ g:

N × 6.25 = _____ g.

FORM E

Calculating a Meal Pattern

Total kcal _____
Carbohydrate (% kcal) _____ (g) _____
Protein   (% kcal) _____ (g) _____
Fat   (% kcal) _____ (g) _____
Division of carbohydrate: _____

Daily Meal Pattern

Exchange	# of Exchanges	Protein (g)	Fat (g)	Carbohydrate (g)
* Milk—NF, LF, whole				
Fruit				
Vegetable				
Subtotal				
* Bread/Starch				
Subtotal				
* Meat—lean, medium, high fat				
Fat				
TOTAL				

* Circle the one used in calculating the meal pattern

Distribution of Exchanges at Meals and Snacks

Exchanges	Total # of Exchanges	Breakfast	AM Snack	Lunch	PM Snack	Dinner	HS Snack
Milk		( )	( )	( )	( )	( )	( )
Fruit		( )	( )	( )	( )	( )	( )
Vegetable		( )	( )	( )	( )	( )	( )
Bread		( )	( )	( )	( )	( )	( )
Meat		( )	( )	( )	( )	( )	( )
Fat		( )	( )	( )	( )	( )	( )
Total		( )	( )	( )	( )	( )	( )

FORM F: Renal Diet

Diet Prescribed:

Energy, kcal   _____
Protein, g   _____   HBV   _____
Sodium, mg   _____
Potassium, mg   _____
Phosphorus, mg   _____

Choices	Number	kcal	Pro (g)	Na (mg)	K (mg)	P (mg)
Milk						
Non-dairy milk sub						
Meat						
SUBTOTAL						
Starch						
Vegetable Lo K						
Med K						
High K						
Fruit Lo K						
Med K						
High K						
HiCal						
Salt						
Fat						
TOTAL						

FORM G

Phenylalanine-Restricted Meal Plan

Date _____   Age _____   Name _____

Weight _____   Height _____
Phenylalanine _____ mg   Tyrosine _____mg
Protein _____g   Energy _____ kcal

Medical Food Mixture	*Phenylalanine* (mg)	*Tyrosine* (mg)	*Protein* (g)	*Energy* (kcal)
_____ g Phenex ™-2	_____	_____	_____	_____
Add _____ mL _____	_____	_____	_____	_____
Add _____ g _____	_____	_____	_____	_____
Add water to make _____ mL				

Breakfast

_____ mL medical food mixture	_____	_____	_____	_____
_____ Servings breads/cereals	_____	_____	_____	_____
_____ Servings fats	_____	_____	_____	_____
_____ Servings fruits	_____	_____	_____	_____
_____ Servings.free foods A	_____	_____	_____	_____

Midmorning

_____ mL Medical food mixture	_____	_____	_____	_____
_____ Servings _____	_____	_____	_____	_____

Lunch

_____ mL medical food mixture	_____	_____	_____	_____
_____ Servings breads/cereals	_____	_____	_____	_____
_____ Servings fats	_____	_____	_____	_____
_____ Servings fruits	_____	_____	_____	_____
_____ Servings vegetables	_____	_____	_____	_____
_____ Servings free foods A	_____	_____	_____	_____

Mid afternoon

_____ mL medical food mixture	_____	_____	_____	_____
_____ Servings _____	_____	_____	_____	_____

Supper

_____ mL medical food mixture	_____	_____	_____	_____
_____ Servings breads/cereals	_____	_____	_____	_____
_____ Servings fats	_____	_____	_____	_____
_____ Servings fruits	_____	_____	_____	_____
_____ Servings vegetables	_____	_____	_____	_____
_____ Servings free foods A	_____	_____	_____	_____

Bedtime

_____ Servings _____	_____	_____	_____	_____
_____ Servings _____	_____	_____	_____	_____

| *Total* | _____ | _____ | _____ | _____ |

Index